Surgical Management of Cerebrovascular Disease

Surgical Management of Cerebrovascular Disease

Robert G. Ojemann, M.D.
Professor of Surgery
Harvard Medical School
Visiting Neurosurgeon
Massachusetts General Hospital
Boston, Massachusetts

Robert M. Crowell, M.D.
Professor and Head,
Department of Neurosurgery
University of Illinois at Chicago
Chicago, Illinois

Illustrations by
 Edith Tagrin
 Chief, Medical Art Unit
 Massachusetts General Hospital

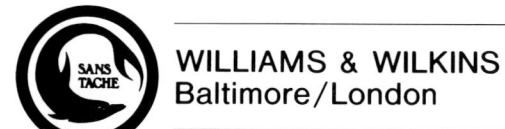

WILLIAMS & WILKINS
Baltimore/London

Copyright ©, 1983
Williams & Wilkins
428 East Preston Street
Baltimore, MD 21202, U.S.A.

All rights reserved. This book is protected by copyright. No part of this book may be reproduced in any form or by any means, including photocopying, or utilized by any information storage and retrieval system without written permission from the copyright owner.

The Publishers have made every effort to trace the copyright holders for borrowed material. If they have inadvertently overlooked any, they will be pleased to make the necessary arrangements at the first opportunity.

Made in the United States of America

Library of Congress Cataloging in Publication Data

Ojemann, Robert G.
   Surgical Management of cerebrovascular disease.

   Includes bibliographical references and index.
   1. Nervous system—Blood-vessels—Surgery. 2. Cerebrovascular disease—Surgery. I. Crowell, Robert M. II. Title. [DNLM: 1. Cerebrovascular disorders—Surgery. 2. Neurosurgery. WL 355 039n]
RD594.2.36 1983   617'.481   82-8551
ISBN 0-683-06639-0   AACR2

Composed and printed at the
Waverly Press, Inc.
Mt. Royal and Guilford Aves.
Baltimore, MD 21202, U.S.A.

DEDICATION

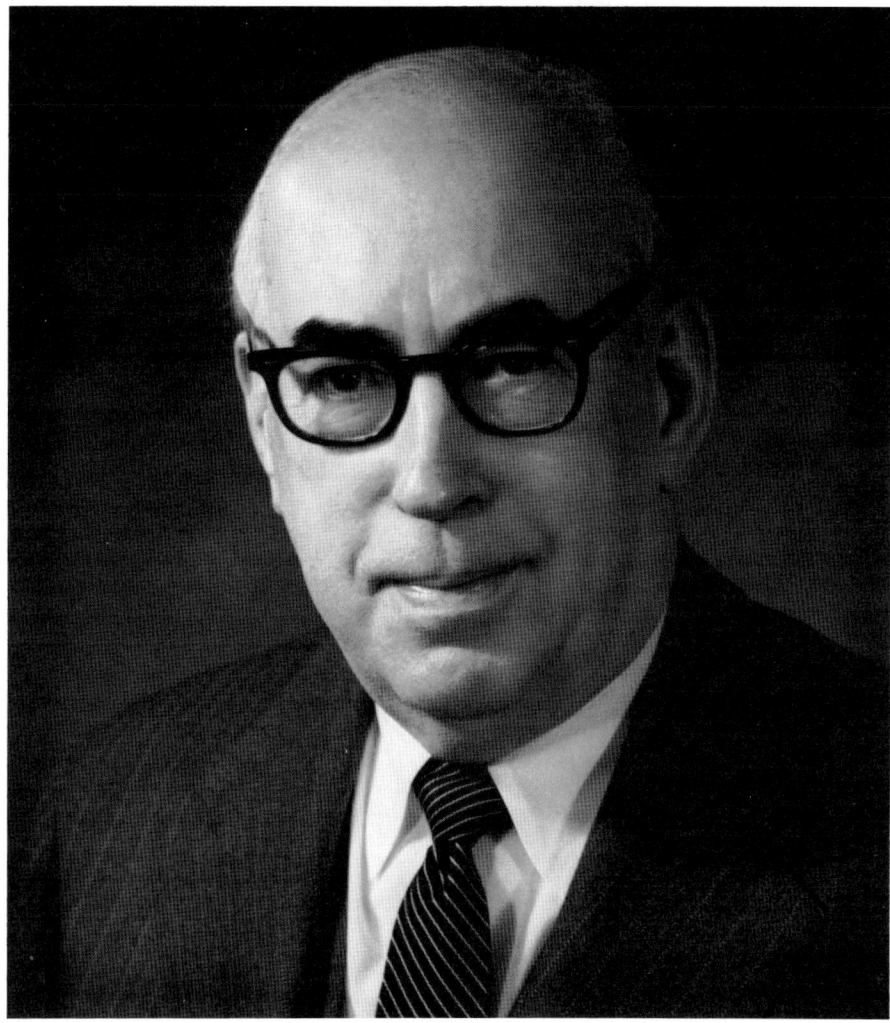

C. Miller Fisher M.D.

For his remarkable accomplishments in the field of cerebrovascular disease, we dedicate this book to Dr. C. Miller Fisher. His ability to observe and describe clinical phenomenon, his insistence on establishing, whenever possible, a definite diagnosis in the stroke patient and to then plan a rational program of treatment, his publications, and his teaching have all done as much to advance the field of cerebrovascular disease as any other single factor.

We are fortunate to be able to continue a most pleasant association which began many years ago with this outstanding dedicated physician. Every discussion of a patient's problem is a learning experience, for each case will be reviewed in relationship to his vast background. His unique ability to organize clinical observations into well-ordered patterns has led to a method and style which have been a constant inspiration.

As one listens to his teachings, a series of basic principles emerge which he has followed in the practice of medicine. Caplan has nicely summarized these into "Fisher's Rules" (1):

1. The bedside can be your laboratory. Study the patient seriously.
2. Settle an issue as it arises at the bedside.
3. Make a hypothesis and then try as hard as you can to disprove it or find the exception before accepting it as valid.
4. Always be working on one or more projects; it will make the daily routine more meaningful.
5. In arriving at a clinical diagnosis, think of the five most common findings (historical, physical, or laboratory) found in a given disorder.
6. Describe quantitatively and precisely.
7. The details of the case are important; their analysis distinguishes the expert from the journeyman.
8. Collect and categorize phenomena; their mechanism and meaning may become clearer later if enough cases are gathered.
9. Fully accept what you have heard or read only when you have verified it yourself.
10. Learn from your own past experience and that of others (literature and experienced colleagues).
11. Didactic talks benefit most the lecturer. We teach others best by listening, questioning, and demonstrating.

12. Write often and carefully. Let others gain from your work and ideas.
13. Pay particular attention to the specifics of the patient with a known diagnosis; it will be helpful later when similar phenomena occur in an unknown case.
14. Be a good listener; even from the mouths of beginners may come wisdom.
15. Resist the temptation to prematurely place a case or disorder into a diagnostic cubbyhole that fits poorly.
16. The patient is always doing the best he can.
17. Maintain a lively interest in patients as people.

A review of C. Miller Fisher's publications from the last three decades reveals the range of his accomplishments in cerebrovascular disease. His clinical and pathological studies beginning in 1951 established the clinical syndrome related to carotid artery atherosclerosis which was the foundation for development of the surgical treatment of carotid artery occlusive disease. He called attention to the frequency and pathology of cerebral embolism, described syndromes associated with lacunar disease and vertebrovascular disease, studied the clinical manifestations of vasospasm and carotid dissection, described the syndromes and pathology of brain hemorrhage, and reported numerous other observations pertaining to cerebrovascular disease. He has also made many other important contributions to the field of neurology, and these have been summarized by Adams and Richardson in a "Salute to C. Miller Fisher." (2)

1. Caplan LR: Fisher's rules. Arch Neurol 39:389–390, 1982.
2. Adams RD, Richardson EP: Salute to C. Miller Fisher. Arch Neurol 38:137–139, 1981.

C. Miller Fisher's Publications on Cerebrovascular Disease (1951–1981)

1. Fisher CM: Occlusion of the internal carotid artery. Arch Neurol Psychiat 65:346–377, 1951.
2. Fisher CM, Adams RD: Observation on brain embolism. J Neuropathol Exp Neurol 10:92, 1951.
3. Fisher CM, Vander Eecken HM, Adams RD: The arterial anastomoses of the human brain and their importance in the delimitation of human brain infarction. J Neuropathol Exp Neurol 11:91, 1952.
4. Fisher CM: Transient monocular blindness associated with hemiplegia. Arch Ophthalmol 47:167–203, 1952.
5. Fisher CM: Concerning strokes. Can Med Assoc J 69:257–268, 1953.
6. Fisher CM, Cameron, DG: Concerning cerebral vasospasm. Neurology 3:468–473, 1953.
7. Fisher CM: Concerning cerebral arteriosclerosis. J Am Geriatr Soc 2:1–18, 1954.
8. Fisher CM: Occlusion of the carotid arteries. Arch Neurol Psychiat 72:187–204, 1954.
9. Fisher CM: Clinical picture of cerebral arteriosclerosis. Minnesota Med 38:839–851, 1955.
10. Fisher CM: Left hemiplegia and motor impersistence. J Nerv Ment Dis 123:201–218, 1956.
11. Fisher CM: Cranial bruit associated with occlusion of the internal carotid artery. Neurology 7:299–306, 1957.
12. Hakim S, Fisher CM: A new technique for the microscopic examination of cerebral vessels in vivo. J Neurosurg 14:405–412, 1957.
13. Fisher CM: Cerebral thromboangitis obliterans. Medicine 36:169–209, 1957.
14. Fisher CM, Adams RD: Transient global amnesia. Trans Amer Neurol Assoc 83:143–146, 1958.
15. Fisher CM: The use of anticoagulants in cerebral thrombosis. Neurology 8:311–332, 1958.
16. Fisher CM: Cerebrovascular diseases: Pathophysiology, diagnosis, and treatment. J Chronic Dis 8:419–447, 1958.
17. Fisher CM: Intermittent cerebral ischemia, in Wright and Millikan (eds): *Cerebral Vascular Disease (Second Conference)*. New York, Grune and Stratton, 1958, pp 81–97.
18. Fisher CM, Karp HR, Adams RD: Cerebrovascular diseases, in Harrison TR, et al (eds): *Principles of Internal Medicine*, 3rd Ed. New York, McGraw-Hill, 1958, pp 1560–1606.
19. Fisher CM: Cerebral embolism, in Conn HF (ed): *Current Therapy*. Philadelphia, WB Saunders, 1958, pp 548–550.
20. Fisher CM: Early-life carotid-artery occlusion associated with late intracranial hemorrhage. Observations on the ischemic pathogenesis of mantle sclerosis. Lab Invest 8:680–700, 1959.
21. Fisher CM: Observations of the fundus oculi in transient monocular blindness. Neurology 9:337–347, 1959.
22. Fisher CM: The pathologic and clinical aspects of thalamic hemorrhage. Trans Am Neurol Assoc 84:56–59, 1959.
23. Fisher CM: Ocular palsy in temporal arteritis. Minnesota Med 42:1258–1268, 1430–1437, 1617–1630, 1959.
24. Fisher CM: Present trends in the treatment of the cerebral vascular diseases. R I Med J 43:27–34, 44, 1960.
25. Fisher CM, Adams RD: Subarachnoid hemorrhage due to ruptured aneurysm, in HF Conn (ed): *Current Therapy*. Philadelphia, WB Saunders, 1960, pp 523–524.
26. Fisher CM: Clinical syndromes in cerebral arterial occlusion, in WS Fields (ed): *Pathogenesis and Treatment of Cerebrovascular Disease*. Springfield, Charles C Thomas, 1961, pp 151–177.
27. Adams RD, Fisher CM: Pathology of cerebral arterial occlusion, in Fields WS (ed): *Pathogenesis and Treatment of Cerebrovascular Disease*. Springfield, Charles C Thomas, 1961, pp 126–142.
28. Fisher CM: Clinical syndromes in cerebral hemorrhage, in Fields WS (ed): *Pathogenesis and Treatment of Cerebrovascular Disease*. Springfield, Charles C Thomas, 1961, pp 318–338.
29. Fisher CM: The pathology and pathogenesis of intracerebral hemorrhage, in Fields WS, (ed): *Pathogenesis and Treatment of Cerebrovascular Disease*. Springfield, Charles C Thomas, 1961, pp 295–311.
30. Fisher CM: Palpation of arteries in temporal arteritis. JAMA 175:325, 1961.
31. Fisher CM: Anticoagulant therapy in cerebral thrombosis and cerebral embolism. Neurology 11:119–131, 1961.
32. Fisher CM, Karnes WE, Kubik CS: Lateral medullary infarction—the pattern of vascular occlusion. J Neuropathol Exp Neurol 20:323–379, 1961.
33. Fisher CM, Dalal PM, Adams RD: Cerebrovascular disease and the stroke syndrome, in Harrison TR, et al (eds): *Principles of Internal Medicine*, 4th Ed. New York, McGraw-Hill, 1962, pp 1746–1795.
34. Fisher CM: Concerning recurrent transient cerebral ischemic attacks. Can Med Assoc 86:1091–1099, 1962.

35. Fisher CM: Cerebral arterial occlusion—remarks on pathology, pathophysiology, and diagnosis. Clin Neurosurg 9:88–105, 1963.
36. Fisher CM, Curry HB: Pure motor hemiplegia. Trans Am Neurol Assoc 89:94–97, 1964.
37. Fisher CM: Pure sensory stroke involving face, arm, and leg. Neurology 15:76–80, 1965.
38. Fisher CM: The circle of Willis: Anatomical variations. Vasc Dis 2:99–105, 1965.
39. Fisher CM, Picard EH, Polak A, Dalal P, Ojemann RG: Acute hypertensive cerebellar hemorrhage: Diagnosis and surgical treatment. J Nerv Ment Dis 140:38–57, 1965.
40. Fisher CM, Cole M: Homolateral ataxia and crural paresis: A vascular syndrome. J Neurol Neurosurg Psychiat 28:48–55, 1965.
41. Fisher CM, Curry HB: Pure motor hemiplegia of vascular origin. Arch Neurol 13:130–140, 1965.
42. Fisher CM, Gore I, Okabe N, White PD: Atherosclerosis of the carotid and vertebral arteries—extracranial and intracranial. J Neuropath Exper Neurol 24:455–476, 1965.
43. Fisher CM: Lacunes: Small, deep cerebral infarcts. Neurology 15:774–784, 1965.
44. Fisher CM, Gore I, White PD, Okabe N: Calcification of the carotid siphon. Circulation 32:538–548, 1965.
45. Fisher CM: Diagnosis and management of cerebrovascular disease. Postgrad Med 38:130–140, 1965.
46. Fisher CM: The vascular lesion in lacunae. Trans Am Neurol Assoc 90:243–245, 1965.
47. Fisher CM: Augmentation bruit of the vertebral artery. J Neurol Neurosurg Psychiat 29:343–345, 1966.
48. Fisher CM: Capsular infarcts—the underlying vascular lesions. Trans Am Neurol Assoc 91:227–229, 1966.
49. Fisher CM: Dilated pupil in carotid occlusion. Trans Am Neurol Assoc 91:230–231, 1966.
50. Fisher CM: Vertigo in cerebrovascular disease. Arch Otolaryngol 85:529–534, 1967.
51. Fisher CM: A lacunar stroke. The dysarthria-clumsy hand syndrome. Neurology 17:614–617, 1967.
52. Fisher CM, Pearlman A: The nonsudden onset of cerebral embolism. Neurology 17:1025–1032, 1967.
53. Fisher CM: Some neuro-ophthalmological observations. J Neurol Neurosurg Psychiat 30:383–392, 1967.
54. Fisher CM: Headache in cerebrovascular disease, in Vinken PJ, Bruyn GW (eds): Handbook of Clinical Neurology. Amsterdam, North-Holland, 1967, pp 124–156.
55. Fisher CM: Dementia in cerebral vascular disease. Cerebral Vascular Diseases (Sixth Princeton Conference). Grune and Stratton, 1968, pp 232–236.
56. Fisher CM: Migraine accompaniments versus arteriosclerotic ischemia. Trans Am Neurol Assoc 93:211–213, 1968.
57. Fisher CM: The arterial lesions underlying lacunes. Acta Neuropath 12:1–15, 1969.
58. Fisher CM: Occlusion of the vertebral arteries. Arch Neurol 22:13–19, 1970.
59. Fisher CM: Facial pulses in internal carotid artery occlusion. Neurology 20:476–478, 1970.
60. Fisher CM, Mohr JP, Adams RD: Cerebrovascular diseases, in Harrison TR, et al (eds): Principles of Internal Medicine, 6th Ed. New York, McGraw-Hill, 1970, pp 1727–1764.
61. Fisher CM, Kaplan LR: Basilar artery branch occlusion—a cause of pontine infarction. Neurology 21:900–905, 1971.
62. Fisher CM: Cerebral ischemia—less familiar types. Clin Neurosurg 18:267–336, 1971.
63. Fisher CM: Pathological observations in hypertensive cerebral hemorrhage. J Neuropathol Exp Neurol 30:536–550, 1971.
64. Fisher CM: Cerebral miliary aneurysms in hypertension. Am J Pathol 66:313–324, 1972.
65. Ojemann RG, Fisher CM, Rich JC: Spontaneous dissecting aneurysm of the internal carotid artery. Stroke 3:434–440, 1972.
66. Fisher CM: Acute headache and tender scalp arteries in the elderly. Trans Am Neurol Assoc 97:280–281, 1972.
67. Hochberg FH, Fisher CM, Roberson GH: Subarachnoid hemorrhage from a small non-aneurysmal artery. Neurology 24:319–321, 1974.
68. Duncan GW, Parker SW, Fisher CM: Acute cerebellar infarction in the PICA territory. Arch Neurol 32:364–368, 1975.
69. Hochberg FH, Bean CS, Fisher CM, Roberson GH: Stroke in a 15 year old girl secondary to terminal carotid dissection. Neurology 25:725–729, 1975.
70. Fisher CM: Clinical syndromes in cerebral thrombosis, hypertensive hemorrhage and ruptured saccular aneurysm. Clin Neurosurg 22:117–147, 1975.
71. Fisher CM: Anatomy and pathology of cerebral vasculature, in Meyer JJ (ed): Modern Concepts of Cerebrovascular Disease. New York, Spectrum, 1975.
72. Ojemann RG, Crowell RM, Roberson GH, Fisher CM: Surgical treatment of extracranial carotid occlusive disease. Clin Neurosurg 22:214–263, 1975.
73. Altemus LR, Roberson GH, Fisher CM, Pessin M: Embolic occlusion of the superior and inferior divisions of the middle cerebral artery with angiographic-clinical correlation. Am J Roentgenol Radium Ther Nucl Med 126:576–581, 1976.
74. Fisher CM: The microembolic theory of transient ischemic attacks. Cerebrovascular Disease, Princeton Conference. 1976, pp 50–53.
75. Fisher CM, Roberson GH, Ojemann RG: Cerebral vasospasm with ruptured saccular aneurysm—the clinical manifestations. Neurosurgery 1:245–248, 1977.
76. Walshe TM, Davis KR, Fisher CM: Thalamic hemorrhage: A computed tomographic-clinical correlation. Neurology 27:217–222, 1977.
77. Groothuis DR, Duncan GW, Fisher CM: The human thalamocortical sensory path in the internal capsule: Evidence from a small capsular hemorrhage causing a pure sensory stroke. Ann Neurol 2:328–331, 1977.
78. Fisher CM: Bilateral occlusion of basilar artery branches. J Neurol Neurosurg Psychiat 40:1182–1189, 1977.
79. Hinton R, Kistler JP, Fallon JT, Friedlich A, Fisher CM: Influence of etiology of atrial fibrillation on incidence of systemic embolism. Am J Cardiol 40: 509–513, 1977.
80. Fisher CM, Ojemann RG, Roberson GH; Spontaneous dissection of cervico-cerebral arteries. Can J Neurol Sci 5:9–19, 1978.
81. Fisher CM, Ojemann RG: Basal rupture of saccular aneurysm. J Neurosurg 48:642–644, 1978.
82. Mohr JP, Kase CS, Meckler MD, Fisher CM: Sensorimotor stroke due to thalamocapsular ischemia. Arch Neurol 34:739–741, 1977.
83. Fisher CM: Thalamic pure sensory stroke: A pathologic study. Neurology 28:1141–1144, 1978.
84. Fisher CM: Bilateral capsular infarcts—the mechanism of recovery from hemiplegia. J Neuropathol Exp Neurol 37:613, 1978.
85. Ropper AH, Fisher CM, Kleinman GM: Pyramidal infarction in the medulla: A cause of pure motor hemiplegia sparing the face. Neurology 29:91–95, 1979.
86. Fisher CM: Reducing risks of cerebral embolism. Geriatrics 34:59–66, 1979.
87. Fisher CM: Capsular infarcts—the underlying vascular lesions. Arch Neurol 36:65–73, 1979.
88. Hinton RC, Mohr JP, Ackerman RH, Adair LB, Fisher CM: Symptomatic middle cerebral artery stenosis. Ann Neurol 5:152–157, 1979.
89. Fisher CM: Late-life migraine accompaniments as a cause of unexplained transient ischemic attacks. Can J Neurol Sci 7:9–17, 1980.
90. Fisher CM, Kistler JP, Davis JM: Relation of cerebral vasospasm to subarachnoid hemorrhage visualized by computerized tomographic scanning. Neurosurgery 6:1–9, 1980.
91. Beal MF, Park TS, Fisher CM: Cerebral atheromatous embolism following carotid sinus pressure. Arch Neurol 38:310–312, 1981.
92. Fisher CM: Visual disturbances associated with quinidine and quinine. Neurology 31:1569–1571, 1981.

PREFACE

During the past several years, medicine has achieved remarkable progress in the diagnosis, prevention, and treatment of cerebrovascular disease, and a more thorough understanding of the pathology and physiology of these problems. New technology allows earlier and more precise diagnosis. Improved medical programs have been developed. Microsurgical techniques have provided improved surgical treatment for more patients. These and other factors have contributed to the reduction in morbidity and mortality from surgical procedures.

The purpose of this book is to give the reader a concise summary of those cerebrovascular diseases that may require consideration for surgical treatment. The guidelines for the surgical management of the diseases presented are based on the clinical experience of the authors while working at the Massachusetts General Hospital.

For each problem, the clinical aspects of the disease are outlined, diagnostic studies that can be used are considered, and the problems encountered are illustrated with appropriate CT scans and angiograms. Indications for the surgical procedures are discussed. We have illustrated the steps in many of the operative procedures, going into some detail for the more common operations, and have supplemented this with a full description in the text. The results of the operative procedures are presented, including a discussion of the complications.

No attempt has been made to present a historical review of the literature. Included are appropriate pertinent references, the majority from the past decade, to which the physician can turn to obtain more detailed information on specific subjects of interest.

ACKNOWLEDGMENTS

It is not possible to acknowledge the contributions from all who helped with this book or to list all those from the clinical services at the Massachusetts General Hospital who participated in the care of the patients with cerebrovascular disease. We would like to thank Dr. Nicholas T. Zervas, Chief of Neurological Surgery at the Massachusetts General Hospital, and Dr. William H. Sweet, former Chief who helped make it possible for us to acquire the clinical series that forms the basis for this book. We also received invaluable help from Dr. Roberto Heros of the Neurosurgical Service, from Dr. Kenneth Davis, Chief of the Neuroradiology Service, and from Dr. Gerard Debrun.

For the beautifully detailed drawings, we are indebted to Edith Tagrin, Chief of the Medical Art Unit at the Massachusetts General Hospital, who spent countless hours attending to every aspect of the illustrations. Thanks also goes to Stanley Bennett, Chief of the Photography Unit at the Massachusetts General Hospital, who did the reproductions of the radiographic studies.

The staff at Williams & Wilkins was a great help to us. We want to especially mention Alice Reid (Editor), Jonathan Pine (Associate Editor), Carol Eckhart (Production Coordinator), and Reginald Stanley (Illustration Planner).

Finally, we thank Jean Ojemann and Suzanne Sampson for their assistance in preparation of the manuscript.

CONTENTS

Dedication v
Preface ix
Acknowledgments xi

SECTION 1: Occlusive Cerebrovascular Disease

1. Atherosclerosis of the Carotid Circulation: Evaluation and Management 1
2. Carotid Endarterectomy 29
3. Asymptomatic Carotid Bruit 66
4. Superficial Temporal Artery to Middle Cerebral Artery Bypass Graft 71
5. Atherosclerosis of the Vertebrobasilar Circulation: Evaluation, Management, and Operative Procedures 93
6. Fibromuscular Dysplasia of the Internal Carotid Artery 107
7. Dissection of Internal Carotid, Vertebral, and Intracranial Arteries 111
8. Embolism 122
9. Cerebral and Cerebellar Infarction 126

SECTION 2: Intracranial Aneurysms, Arteriovenous Malformations, and Brain Hemorrhage

10. Intracranial Aneurysms and Subarachnoid Hemorrhage: Incidence, Pathology, Clinical Features, and Medical Management 128
11. Intracranial Aneurysms: General Aspects of Surgical Treatment 141
12. Internal Carotid Aneurysms 157
13. Carotid-Ophthalmic Aneurysms 171
14. Anterior Communicating Aneurysms 183
15. Distal Anterior Cerebral Aneurysms 196
16. Middle Cerebral Aneurysms 201
17. Basilar Bifurcation Aneurysms 210
18. Basilar Trunk and Vertebral Aneurysms 223
19. Multiple, Unruptured, and Asymptomatic Aneurysms 233
20. Giant Aneurysms 240
21. Infectious Intracranial Aneurysms 255
22. Arteriovenous Malformations of the Brain 264
23. Dural Arteriovenous Malformations 287
24. Carotid-Cavernous Fistula 291
25. Brain Hemorrhage 297

Index 309

Section 1 OCCLUSIVE CEREBROVASCULAR DISEASE

Chapter 1 ATHEROSCLEROSIS OF THE CAROTID CIRCULATION: EVALUATION AND MANAGEMENT

DIAGNOSIS

Clinical Presentation

Transient ischemic attacks (TIAs) with transient monocular blindness (TMB), transient hemispheral attacks (THA), or both are often caused by carotid artery atherosclerosis. When this is the case, the most frequent site of pathology is the region of the common carotid bifurcation and proximal internal carotid artery in the neck, but stenosis, ulceration, and/or occlusion also occur in the carotid siphon, distal internal carotid, and proximal middle cerebral arteries.

TIAs usually last from a few seconds to several minutes, and rarely last longer than 30 minutes (33). Occasionally, the duration may be up to 8 hours, which has been suggested as the upper limit for a TIA. The history may be of only one attack or several hundred, but most patients have had less than five attacks when first seen. Recurrent attacks are usually of the same general type (63). On rare occasion, a patient will present with syncopy, dizziness, or seizures.

TMB may be total or partial. The characteristic description is the sudden onset of a gray-black shade or curtain, gradually and painlessly descending or ascending to obscure all or part of monocular vision and then gradually recovering with the sensation that the shade is receeding. Some patients complain of a fog, blurriness, or blindness of one eye. Others will note one or a shower of specks of bright light or sparks that dart across the field of vision.

The most frequent THAs consist of numbness of the fingers followed in decreasing order of prevalence by speech disturbance, numbness and weakness of the hand and arm, weakness of the arm and leg, weakness of the hand, numbness and weakness of the arm and leg, and numbness of the face (31). When the history indicates that both TMB and THA have been present in the same patient, the TMB usually occurs first and the THA and TMB do not occur simultaneously (63).

The pathophysiology of the transient cerebral and ocular symptoms is unsettled. Fisher brought attention to the relationship between carotid occlusive disease and stroke, and it was thought that the major mechanism of stroke related to inadequate distal cerebral perfusion (30–32). Subsequently, more attention has been focused on the possible role of embolization from the carotid bifurcation to the intracranial vessels as a mechanism of stroke (6, 55, 64). It is likely that both factors play a role in causing symptoms.

The neurological examination in a patient with TIAs is usually normal. A bruit is sometimes heard over the neck. Careful auscultation over the entire course of the carotid artery from the clavicle to the angle of the jaw can often determine the point of maximum intensity. Bruits associated with internal carotid stenosis are usually localized in the mid-cervical region and are not heard in the low neck and chest. In general, the higher the pitch of the bruit, the tighter the stenosis, and a severe stenosis is suggested if the bruit extends into diastole. However, with a very tight stenosis, the bruit may become less intense and even disappear as the rate of blood flow is reduced. On occasion, platelet or cholesterol embolus may be seen in the retina.

A significant number of patients who have had a stroke will also have atheromatous occlusive disease. The distressing fact is that in a group of patients who developed a permanent moderate to severe neurological deficit due to carotid occlusion, 60% had a prior history of TIAs that might have led to preventive treatment; 20% were associated with a fluctuating or stepwise progression which might have allowed time for treatment, and 20% came on suddenly without warning (31). Clearly, careful attention must be paid to any patient who has a history of TIAs.

On examination, the patient who has had a stroke may also have a bruit. The neurological deficit will, of course, depend on the area of brain infarction. Occasionally, the only permanent deficit in a patient with carotid occlusive disease is impaired vision due to a retinal artery embolus.

Diagnostic Studies

Guidelines for Planning Studies

The patient with TIAs and a carotid bruit on the side appropriate to explain the symptoms should have digital subtraction angiography (DSA) and/or selective carotid angiography (Table 1.1). Non-invasive carotid studies are not needed. For the patient with a typical TMB and no bruit, angiography is also indicated. The patient with a THA and no bruit should have a computerized tomographic (CT) scan done first because an occasional patient with a tumor, especially a metastatic lesion, subdural hematoma, or aneurysm may present with TIAs. If the CT is not diagnostic, angiography is indicated. Angiography is also indicated when the clinical examination and non-invasive studies suggest significant carotid disease in patients who have presented with dizziness, syncope, or seizure.

For patients who have had an established stroke, a CT scan is usually done first to define the extent of the infarction, if any, and to exclude hemorrhage as a cause of the problem. When the history and examination suggest carotid occlusive disease, angiography is indicated. If the problem is an acute stroke with mild-to-moderate deficit or a fluctuating or progressive stroke, immediate angiography is done. The patient with a massive stroke with altered level of consciousness will have a CT scan but usually angiography is not done unless significant improvement occurs since these patients do not benefit from surgery.

Non-invasive tests have been useful in certain clinical situations including assessment of hemodynamic change and follow-up in patients with asymptomatic bruits (see Chapter 3), the study of patients with

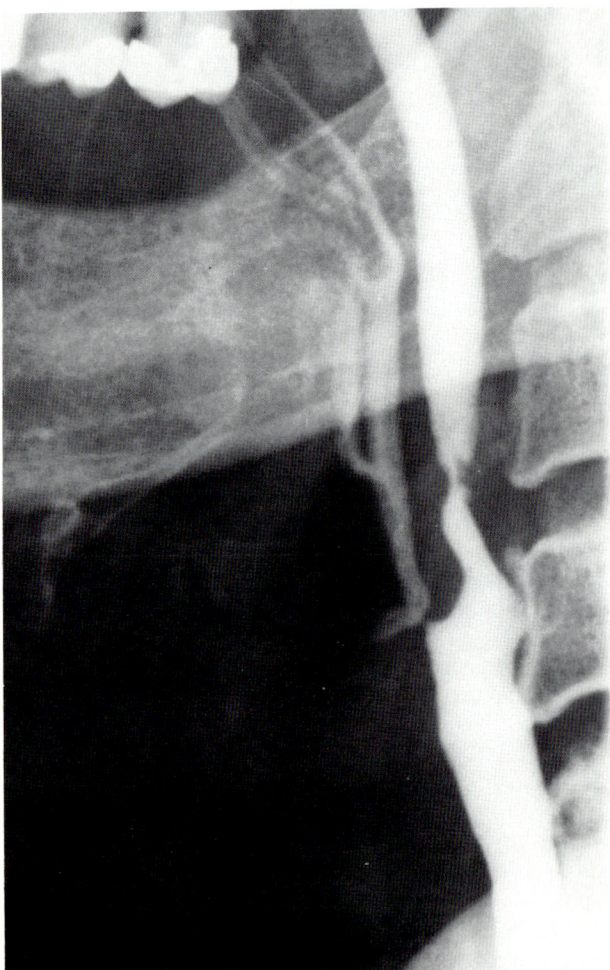

Figure 1.1 Measuring degree of stenosis. Lateral angiogram showing the carotid bifurcation with severe stenosis in the proximal internal carotid artery and markedly severe stenosis at the origin of the external carotid artery with reduced flow. Comment: We prefer to describe the degree of stenosis by measuring the lumen diameter at the narrowest point corrected for magnification, here 1.0 mm in the internal carotid artery. We have avoided using a percentage narrowing for description because it is often difficult to decide what value to use for the denominator. Here the widest diameter distal to the stenosis is 9 mm and the narrowest, 7 mm.

Table 1.1
Diagnostic Studies when Carotid Occlusive Disease is Suspected

Clinical Indication	Study
TIA (THA or TMB)	Angiography[a]
THA without bruit	CT, (?) angiography
Seizure, dizziness, syncope and bruit or + non-invasive tests	Angiography[a]
Completed stroke (moderate)	CT, (?) angiography
Completed stroke (severe with improvement)	CT, non-invasive tests[a]
Acute stroke (moderate)	Angiography[a], (?) CT
Acute stroke (severe)	CT, (?) angiography[a]
Asymptomatic bruit	Non-invasive tests[a]
Central retinal occlusion	Non-invasive tests[a]
Vague symptoms	Non-invasive tests

[a] DSA with improved resolution may eventually replace.

Atherosclerosis of Carotid Circulation

central retinal occlusion, evaluation of patients with atypical or vague symptoms and possible carotid disease, and some patients with established strokes. In the future, digital subtraction angiography (DSA) will likely replace many of these tests, but they will still be useful in patients where DSA is contraindicated, for initial screening and for follow-up evaluation of asymptomatic bruits.

Angiography

Angiography must include visualization of both carotid bifurcations, the intracranial carotid circulation, and in some patients, the vertebrobasilar system. The study is best done by retrograde femoral catheterization with selective carotid injection and serial films. In some cases, subtraction studies give additional information. Aortic arch injections usually do not clearly define the pathology and do not help in patient management (38). If there is significant disease in the distal aorta or its branches, catherization can be done through the right brachial or axillary artery.

What constitutes a significant degree of narrowing of the internal carotid artery on the angiogram? Most publications refer to a percentage narrowing of the internal carotid artery lumen. In many angiograms this percentage is hard to determine because the internal carotid diameter is not uniform (Fig. 1.1), and the distal artery may narrow when pressure is reduced (slim sign) (50) (Fig. 1.2). Therefore, we prefer to measure the lumen diameter in millimeters (mm) at the point of maximum narrowing with correction for magnification. In general, a residual internal carotid artery diameter of 2 mm represents at least a 70% narrowing of the lumen diameter. As the lumen narrows below this diameter, a hemodynamic change usually begins to occur in the artery distal to the stenosis (20). Another point to remember is that in some patients the severity of the stenosis (Fig. 1.3) or degree of ulceration (Fig. 1.4) may not be seen unless the area is visualized in two planes.

The vast majority of patients with TIAs and a carotid bruit will have a severe stenosis (<2 mm lumen diameter) on the angiogram. The stenosis may occur anywhere from the common carotid bifurcation to a point in the internal carotid artery 3–4 cm distal to the bifurcation, and narrowing may be short or long (Fig. 1.5 A to D). In a small number of patients with TIAs, an ulcer will be the principal pathology (Figs. 1.4 and 1.12). Some patients have both stenosis and ulceration (Fig. 1.6). A few have complete internal carotid occlusion.

It is important that serial films be done for up to 10–15 seconds. These films may demonstrate collateral flow in cases of severe internal carotid artery stenosis (Fig. 1.7) or occlusion (Fig. 1.8). One must be careful in evaluating intracranial occlusion or stenosis on a single injection when there is significant collateral circulation into the hemisphere because an

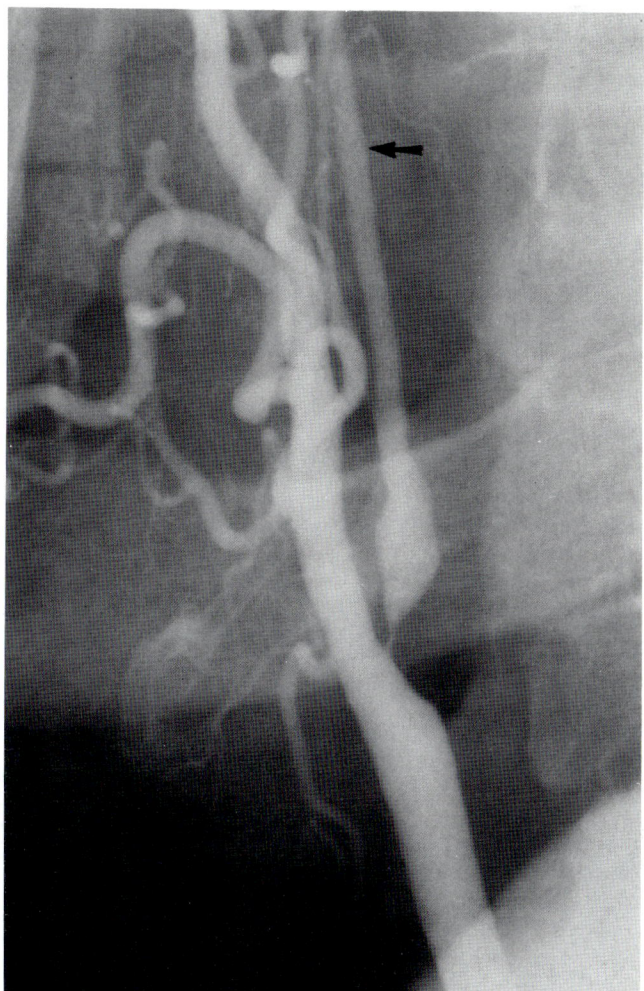

Figure 1.2 Carotid "slim" sign. Left carotid angiogram showing stenosis at the origin of the internal carotid artery. The stenosis is severe with a residual lumen diameter of less than 1 mm and a post-stenotic dilatation. The distal internal carotid artery is small (*arrow*) with a diameter less than the external carotid artery diameter, a finding noted when the pressure is reduced distal to the stenosis (slim sign). This sign does not indicate distal atherosclerosis or hypoplasia of the artery.

intraluminal defect may be due to washout (59). Late films may also show dye in an ulcer crater, indicating an area of stagnation and potential thrombus formation (Fig. 1.9). One may see varying degrees of retrograde flow down the internal carotid artery in patients with complete occlusion (Figs. 1.8 and 1.19B). There may be delayed flow through an area of severe stenosis ("pseudo-occlusion") or evidence of embolic occlusion of an anterior or middle cerebral branch.

In patients with internal carotid occlusion, the appearance of the proximal end does not accurately predict the age of the occlusion. In a report of patients with acute stroke and angiography done within 6 days of the onset, three configurations were found,

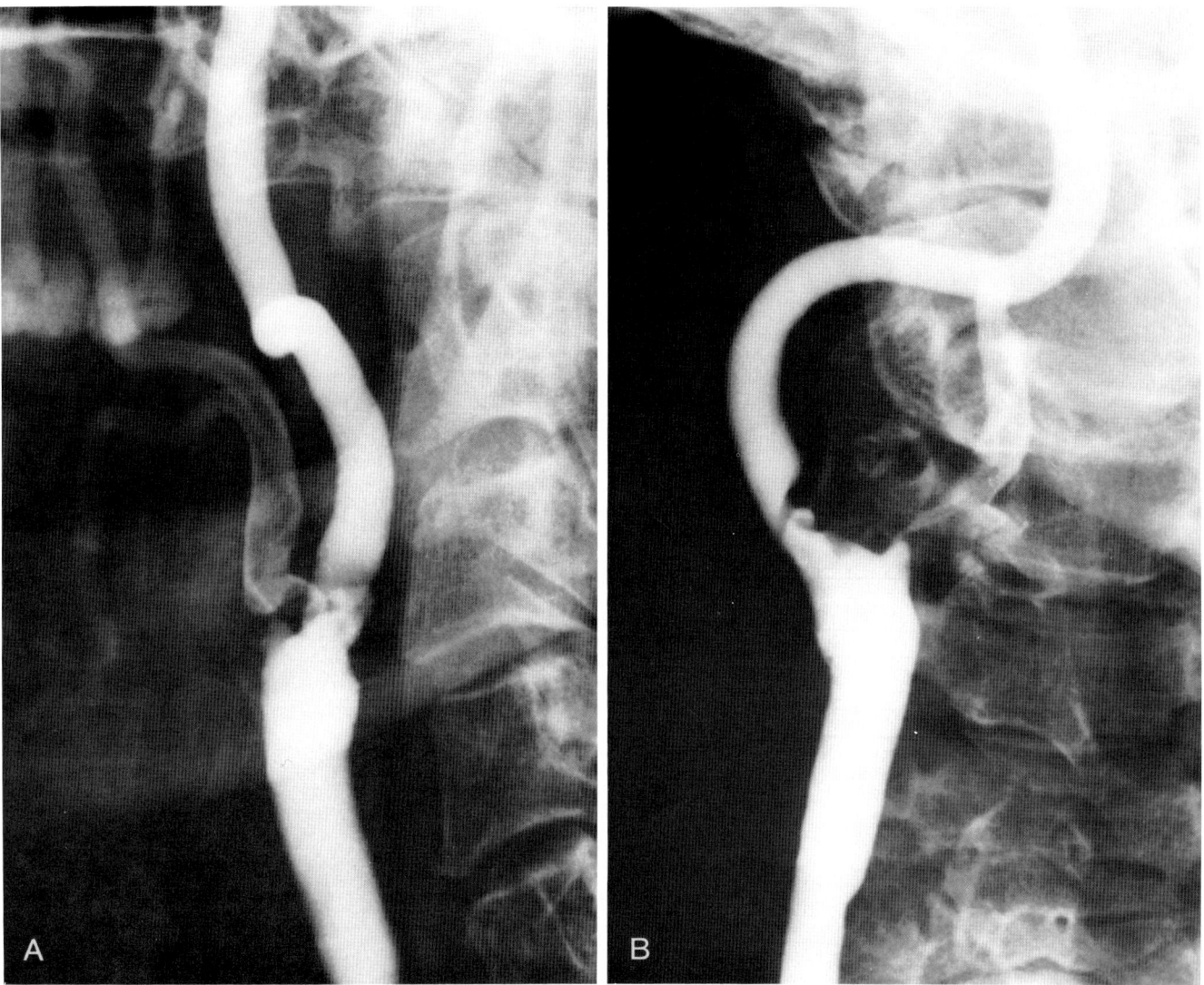

Figure 1.3 Need for two planes of view in some cases of stenosis. *A,* lateral angiogram of the carotid bifurcation showing severe stenosis and reduced flow at the origin of the external carotid artery and marked irregularity at the internal carotid origin. *B,* AP angiogram reveals the true degree of stenosis at the internal carotid artery origin.

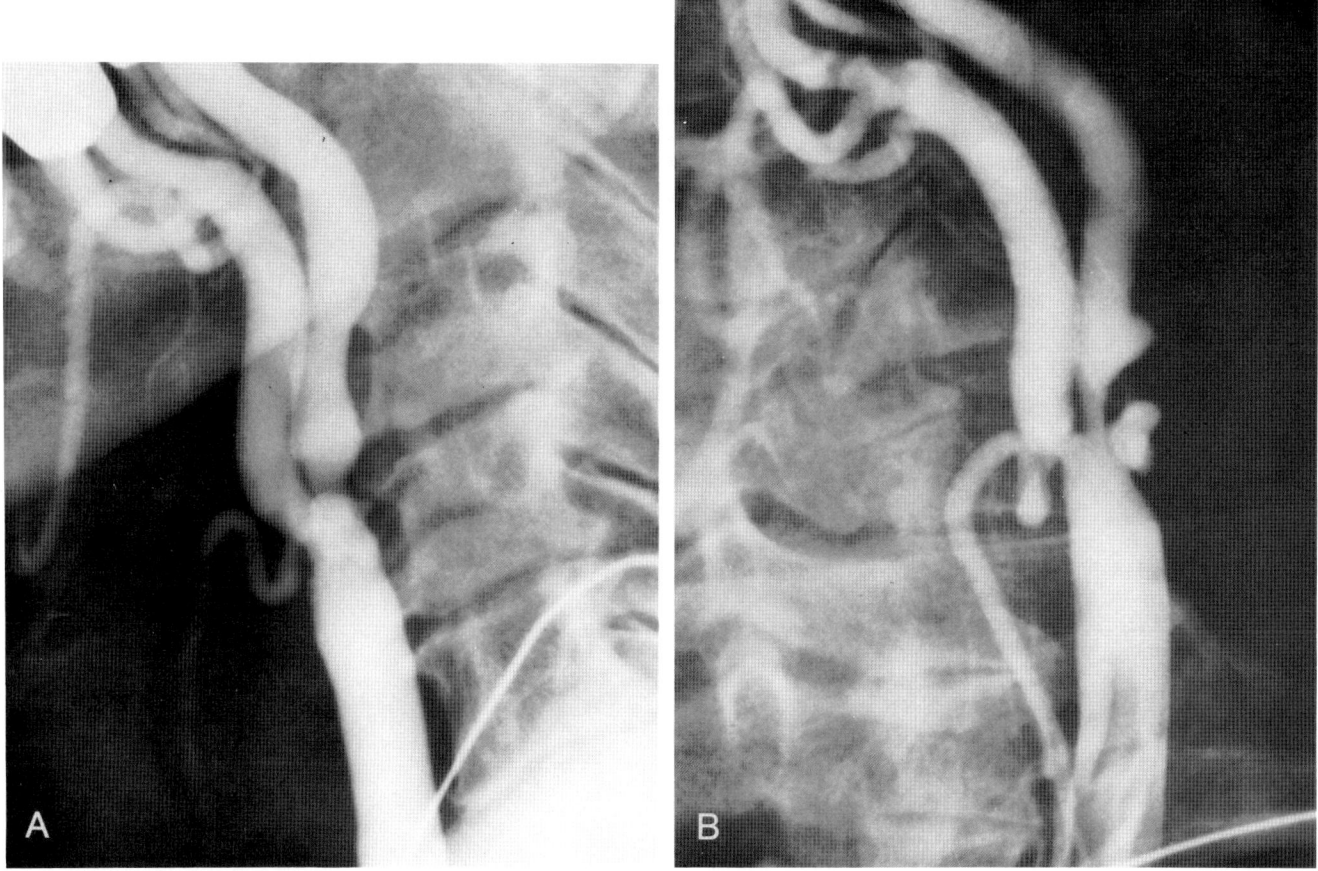

Figure 1.4 Need for two planes of view in some cases of ulceration and stenosis. *A*, lateral angiogram of carotid bifurcation does not show significant stenosis (diameter 5.0 mm) in the proximal internal carotid artery. Careful inspection reveals a double density at the bifurcation suggesting an ulcer. *B*, AP angiogram reveals that stenosis is 3 mm at narrowest point and a large ulcer crater is seen. Comment: The patient presented with episodes of weakness in the upper extremity. The true pathology is only apparent on the AP view.

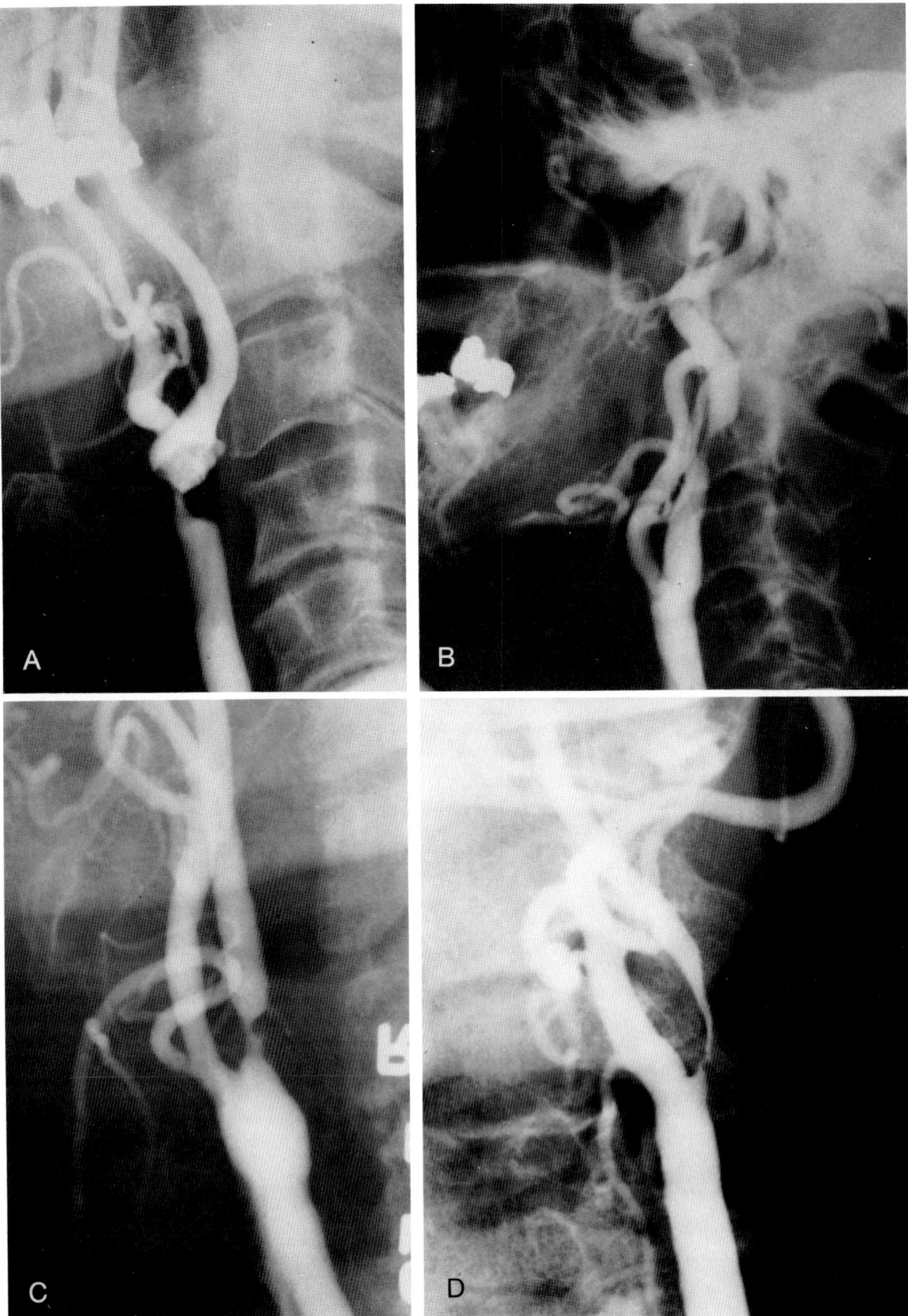

Figure 1.5 Varieties of ICA stenosis. Angiograms of carotid bifurcation. The stenosis may be located from the common carotid bifurcation (A) to a point 3–4 cm distal in the internal carotid artery (B). The length of the lesion may be short (C) or long (D). Comment: All of these patients presented with TIAs.

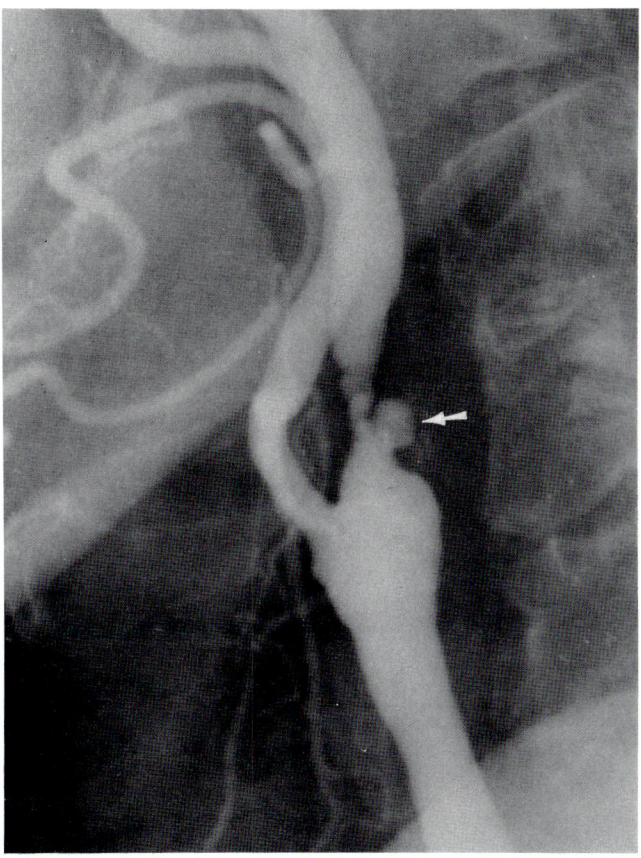

Figure 1.6 ICA stenosis and ulceration. Left carotid angiogram showing severe stenosis in the proximal internal carotid artery with associated large ulcer (*arrow*). Both the degree of the stenosis and the size of the ulcer are of concern. Comment: Patient presented with TIAs. At operation a thrombus was noted in the ulcer. The symptoms were relieved.

in descending order of frequency: a sharp pointed stump, virtual absence of the artery, and a rounded blunt stump (65).

In a consecutive series of patients who had angiography for TIAs, 37% had a severe stenosis (lumen <2 mm diameter) of the carotid bifurcation or proximal internal carotid artery; 12% had a complete internal carotid occlusion; 3% had severe stenosis distal to the bifurcation; 6% had moderate stenosis at the bifurcation (3–5 mm diameter lumen); 23% showed minimal stenosis at the carotid bifurcation (6–8 mm diameter lumen) and 19% had a normal carotid bifurcation and proximal internal carotid artery (63). A few patients with severe stenosis also had ulceration at the carotid bifurcation, and a few had intracranial branch occlusion. In the patients with a normal carotid bifurcation region, 22% had non-obstructive irregularity of the common carotid artery and 17% had intracranial branch occlusion. In the patients with minimal stenosis, 27% had ulcerative lesions and 20% intracranial branch occlusion. No correlation between most of the clinical features of the ischemic attack and a specific angiographic finding was noted. If a THA was longer than 60 minutes, there was more chance of finding a non-significant carotid stenosis and an intracranial branch occlusion suggesting an embolic cause for the problem. When the patient had both TMB and THA, a severe carotid stenosis was more likely.

The major deterrent to cerebral angiography is the risk of a lasting neurological complication. In the best hands, 0.5% serious complications can be anticipated, including ilio-femoral occlusion or cerebral infarction.

Digital Subtraction Angiography

A major step forward in the radiographic evaluation of patients with occlusive vascular disease has been the development of digital subtraction angiography (DSA) (14, 15, 28, 51, 73). The procedure has been made possible by developments in computer technology. Extracranial and intracranial vessels can be clearly visualized.

Prior to injection of contrast media, the head and neck are fluroscoped. The images are converted to digital data and stored. After intravenous injection of a bolus of contrast media, the region of interest is imaged and information is amplified, digitized, and

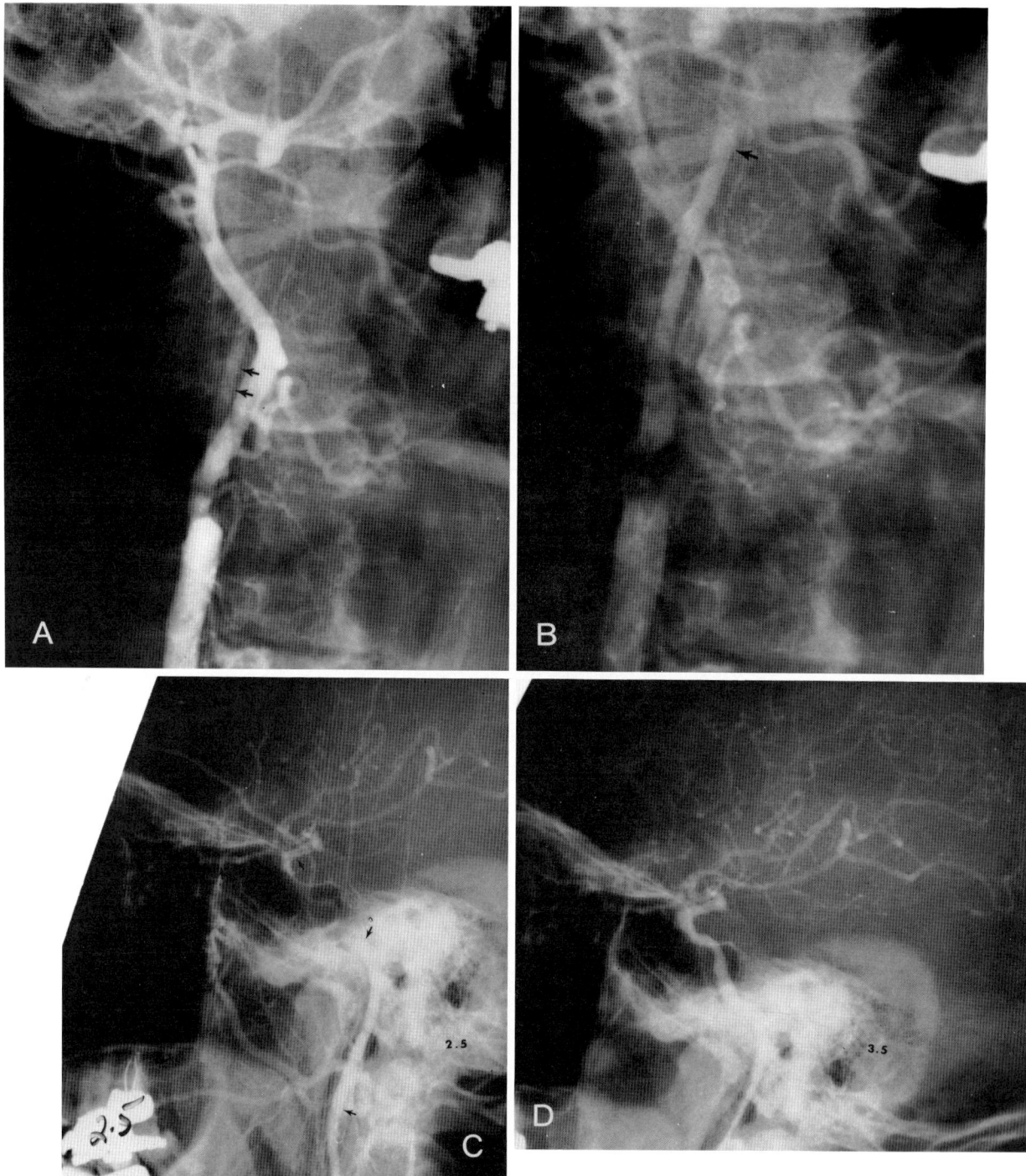

Figure 1.7 Importance of delayed films: slow ICA flow and ophthalmic collateral. *A,* the right internal carotid artery (*arrows*) fills slowly and faintly due to severe stenosis at its origin. Rapid, normal flow is seen in the external carotid artery. *B,* two seconds later, contrast in the internal carotid artery (*arrow*) is shown flowing upward as the external carotid opacification is clearing. *C,* an early film of the lateral cranial series shows opacification of the supraclinoid internal carotid artery and distal carotid siphon by ophthalmic artery collateral flow (*upper arrow*), prior to the arrival of contrast from delayed antegrade flow in the internal carotid artery (*lower arrows*). *D,* one second later, the internal carotid artery is completely opacified as the two streams of flow combine. Comment: This patient reported that 3 days before admission he had an episode of weakness in the left upper extremity and numbness in the left thigh. On the morning of admission he had severe weakness in the left foot for 30 minutes and in the left arm for several hours. Admission examination was normal and there was no right carotid bruit. Operation was done on an urgent basis a few hours after the angiogram. There was full recovery. (From Ojemann RG, Crowell RM, Roberson GH, Fisher CM: Surgical treatment of extracranial carotid occlusive disease, Ch. 14, in *Clinical Neurosurgery.* Baltimore, Williams & Wilkins, 1974, vol 22, with permission.)

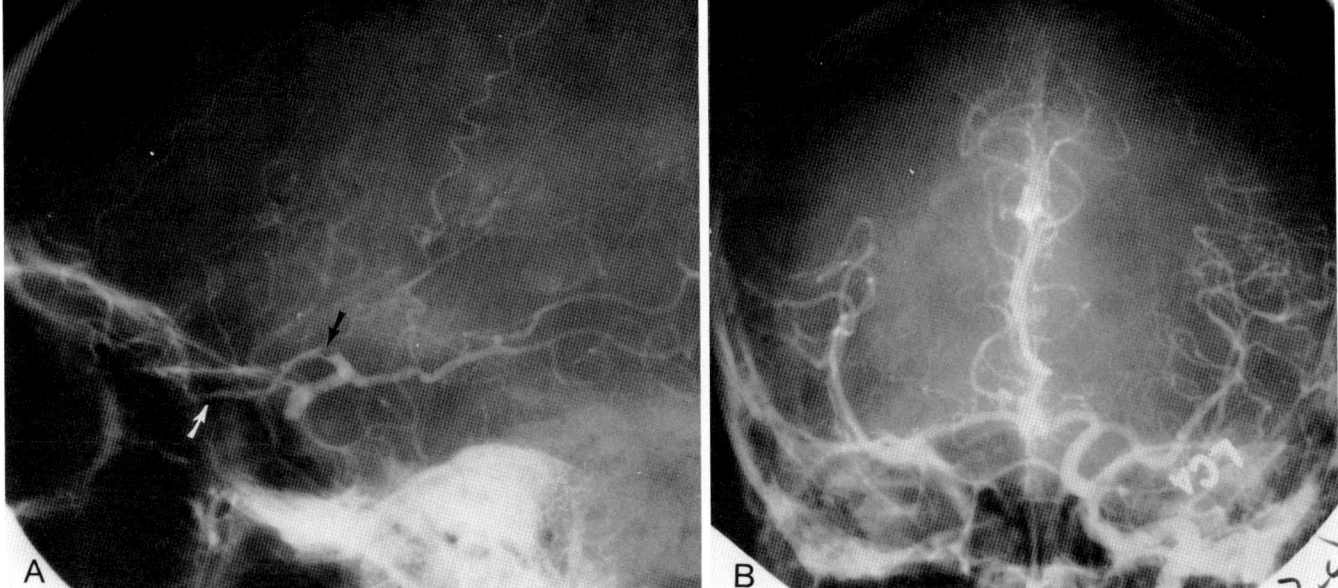

Figure 1.8 Internal carotid occlusion, collateral circulation, and intracranial "pseudo-stenosis." *A,* right carotid angiogram showed complete occlusion of the internal carotid artery at its origin. The distal internal carotid artery is supplied by collateral through the ophthalmic artery (*white arrow*). There is retrograde flow for a few millimeters to the distal end of the occlusion and filling of the posterior cerebral artery and faint filling of MCA branches. The *black arrow* points to a pseudo-stenosis due to washout from cross-circulation from the opposite side. *B,* left carotid injection shows cross-filling into both right anterior and middle cerebral arteries. Comment: Patient had history of TMB in the right eye followed by a mild stroke. The artery cannot be re-opened. Bypass graft is not indicated. The patient should be treated with anticoagulation to prevent emboli. Care must be taken in interpretation of a single angiogram film. Patients with the finding seen in Fig. 1.8A have been referred for bypass graft because of the presumed intracranial stenosis.

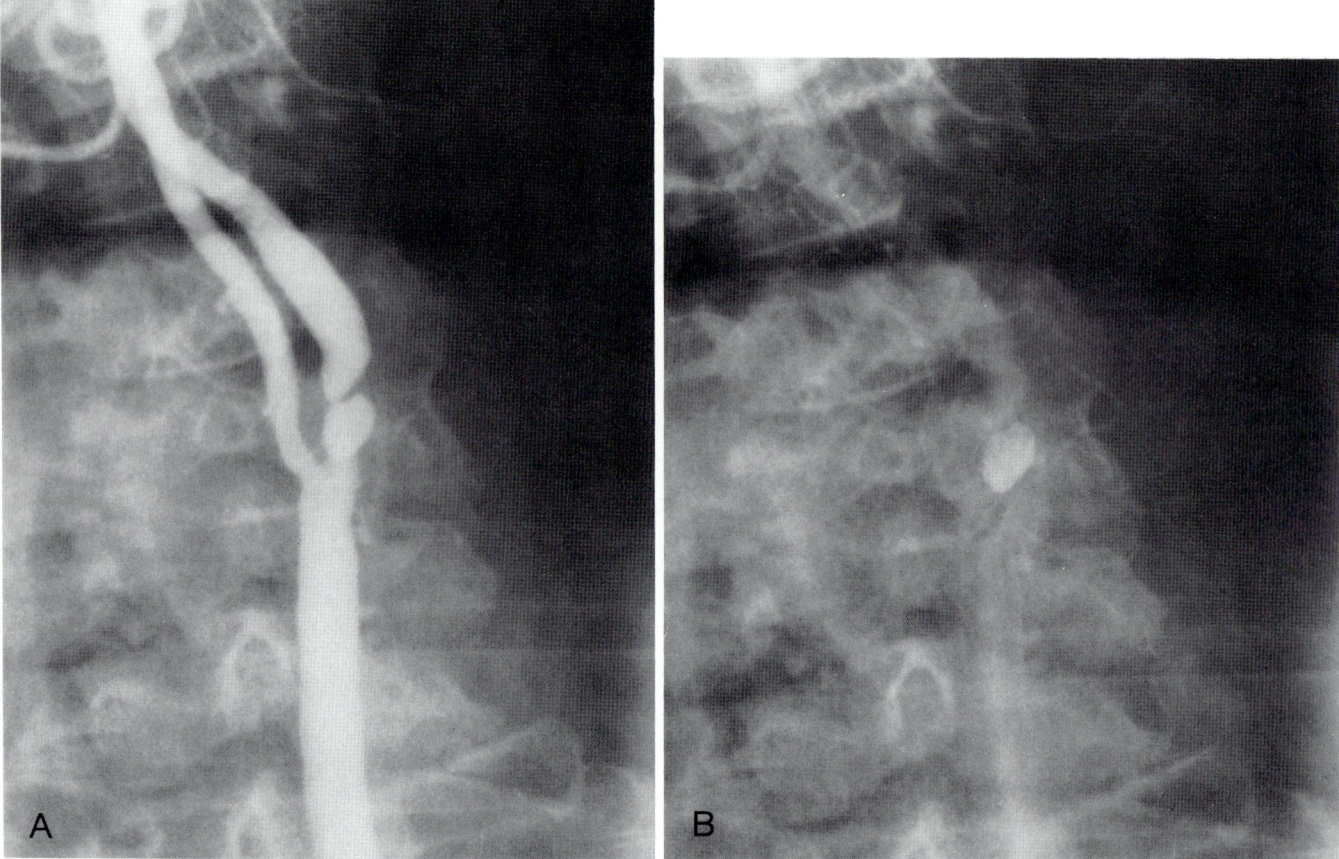

Figure 1.9 Delayed films highlight carotid ulceration. Angiogram of the carotid bifurcation. *A*, at the origin of the ICA, there is a pocket of dye suggesting an ulcer crater. Just distal to this is a severe stenosis. *B*, at 2.5 seconds after injection, the artery is faintly outlined but dye remains in the large ulcer crater. Comment: The patient presented with an episode of difficulty with speech, dizziness, and light-headedness. The endarterectomy speciman confirmed the angiogram findings. No further attacks occurred following the operation.

stored. The image obtained before injection is then subtracted and the DSA images displayed.

For each injection of Renografin-76, 40 ml is given at 12–18 ml/second. Up to five injections may be used if the blood urea nitrogen and creatinine are not elevated. For evaluation of the cervical region, left and right posterior oblique views are obtained. For intracranial studies, anteroposterior, lateral, and oblique views are recorded.

One study reported that the carotid bifurcation was clearly seen in 88% of the studies (51). Internal carotid artery ulceration, stenosis, and occlusion can be visualized (Fig. 1.10, *A* and *B*). Subclavian and vertebral artery stenosis have also been demonstrated. Major intracranial vessels can be seen in some patients and the procedure has been used to study postoperative superficial temporal artery (STA) to middle cerebral artery (MCA) bypass (22).

The inability to precisely define intracranial stenosis and to outline collateral circulation are problems with this technique. At the present time, conventional angiography is still recommended for evaluation of most patients with occlusive cerebrovascular disease. With the improvement in resolution which is likely to come, DSA may gradually supplant conventional angiography.

CT Scan

The CT scan is done to determine the presence and extent of infarction and to exclude other pathology. The characteristic appearance of an infarct is an area of low density with sharp margins, extending to the surface of the brain and tending to narrow medially (Fig. 1.11) (24, 58, 79). If the CT scan on a patient with stroke does not show pathology and angiography is normal, diagnostic possibilities include embolus from a cardiac source and lacunar disease. Pure motor or sensory transient ischemic hemispheral symptoms are characteristic of the lacunar stroke syndrome. A history of hypertension suggests this as a cause, but neither the CT scan or angiography will establish this diagnosis.

An infarct is usually not seen on CT for at least 24 hours and may become prominent over several days (Fig. 1.12). However, with improved spatial and contrast resolution of the new scanners, evidence of

Atherosclerosis of Carotid Circulation

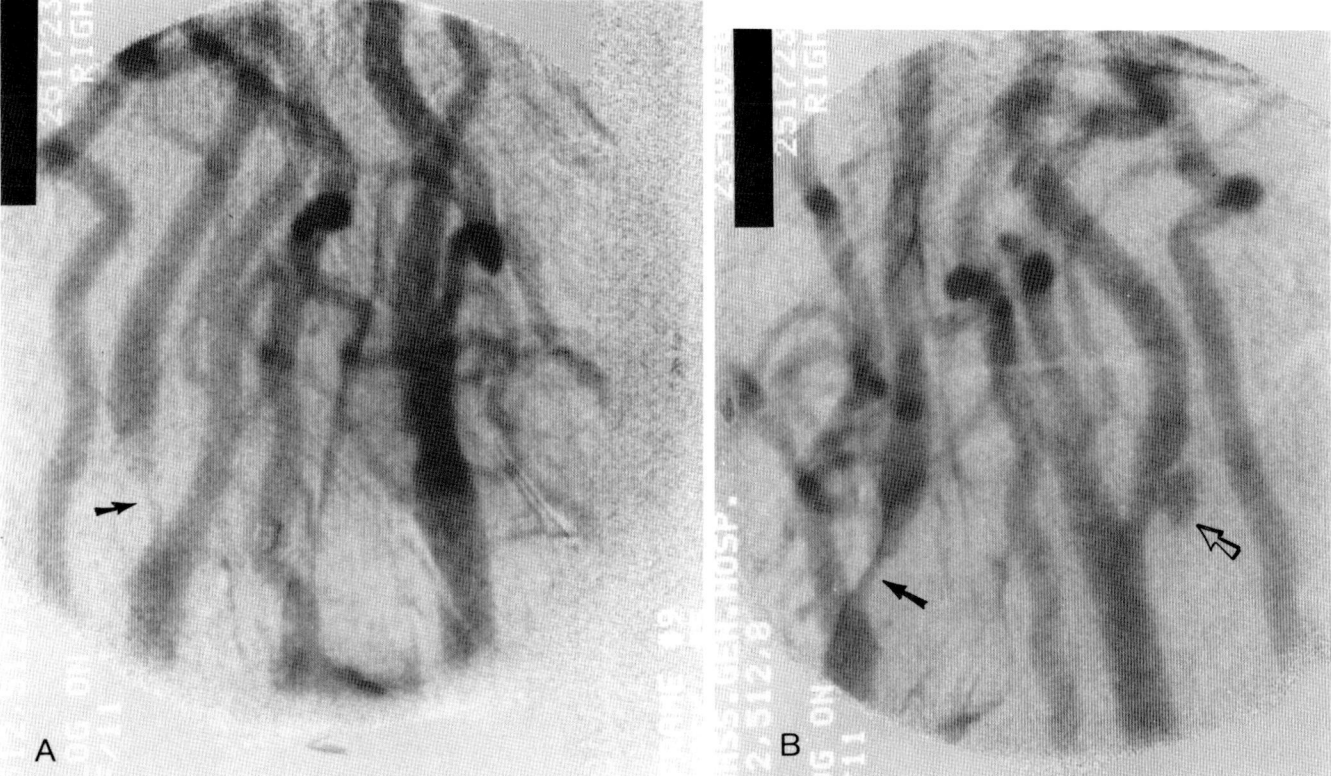

Figure 1.10 Stenosis and ulceration demonstrated by digital subtraction angiography. *A* and *B*, right and left oblique views. There is severe stenosis at the origin of the right internal carotid artery (*closed arrow*) and slight stenosis, but a large ulcer at the origin of the left internal carotid artery (*open arrow*).

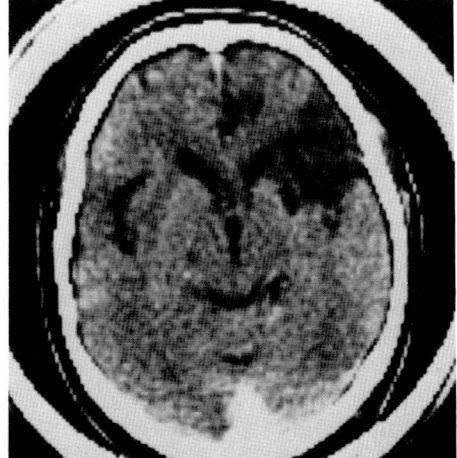

Figure 1.11 Cerebral infarction. This patient had a stroke several months prior to this scan. There is no enhancement. Note the characteristic appearance of an infarct with low density, sharp margins, triangular or quadrilateral shape, extending to the surface of the brain and a tendency to narrow medially.

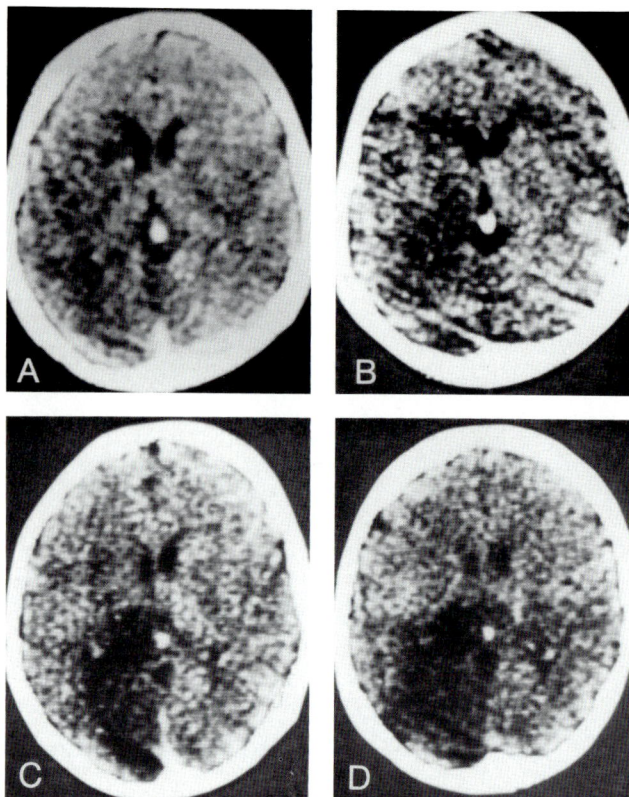

Figure 1.12 Serial CT scans following infarction in left posterior cerebral artery territory. *A*, day 1, slight low density noted. *B*, Day 2, more pronounced low density area seen. *C*, Day 4, sharply demarcated low density region is more prominent. *D*, Day 7, area of low density somewhat larger than seen on previous scan.

infarction was seen in 21 of 26 patients within 24 hours (77). Contrast enhancement of the area of the infarction occurs in some patients, usually within 1 to 4 weeks of the onset of clinical symptoms. However, enhancement may be seen as early as the first day or it may not appear until several months after the event. When there is enhancement, the area of infarction may revert to a non-enhanced appearance over several months, but on occasion it may persist indefinitely. In an occasional patient, contrast enhancement is the only manifestation of infarction and, therefore, both pre- and post-contrast scans should be done. There is no characteristic on the CT scan which will definitely establish the diagnosis of an infarct or its age. An enhanced infarct can be confused with glioma, metastatic tumor, or arteriovenous malformation. Other findings such as surrounding edema and a low density center may also be seen in recent infarcts.

Non-invasive Studies of Carotid Circulation

Over 20 non-invasive tests have been developed to assess carotid occlusive disease (Table 1.2). The use and limitations of these tests have been reviewed in

Table 1.2
Non-invasive Tests for Carotid Occlusive Disease

I. Indirect (Orbital circulation)
   A. Superficial
      Dynamic palpation of pulses
      Thermography
      Doppler ultrasonography[a]
   B. Deep
      Ophthalmodynamometry (ODN)
      Oculoplethysmography (OPG)[a]
      Oculotonography
II. Direct (carotid bifurcation)
      Bruit analysis
      Phonoangiography[a]
      Doppler imaging
      B scan imaging

[a] Combination provides 85–90% accuracy in detection of hemodynamically significant occlusive lesions.

detail (1, 2, 3, 16, 21, 22, 35, 44, 69). A few are useful in the evaluation of certain groups of patients as previously noted (Table 1.1), but many tests provide so little useful information that they are a waste of time and money. The useful tests give information about the presence of a hemodynamic lesion (Doppler ultrasonography and oculoplethysmography), analyze the bruit to determine the residual lumen diameter (phonoangiography), or image the artery with ultrasound (B-scan ultrasonography). A battery of six tests was reported to be 90% effective in identifying carotid stenosis with a residual lumen of 2 mm or less (1). The false-positive rate was 3–5%.

Phonoangiography gives the most useful information in evaluation of a carotid bruit (25, 45, 46, 49). Quantitative phonoangiography records the bruit, does a computer analysis, and plots the bruit intensity against frequency. The frequency with maximum intensity (break frequency) is proportional to the residual lumen diameter. The residual lumen diameter at the point of stenosis can be accurately estimated in about 90% of these patients. (25, 46). Serial studies over time can identify progressive stenosis (see Chapter 3). In addition, this test can be used to differentiate between bruits originating at the carotid bifurcation and those emanating from the thorax.

Other tests help determine if there is a hemodynamically significant lesion. Periorbital Doppler ultrasonography reveals the direction of flow in external carotid branches on the brow (2, 37, 53). Reversal of flow indicates reduced pressure in the internal carotid artery system. The test requires careful positioning of probes and can be influenced by external carotid stenosis. It is the best test for studying the superficial orbital circulation. Oculoplethysmography (OPG) measures the relative arrival time of the ocular pulse in each eye (44). A delay of greater than 20 ms is significant. This is the most useful test to study the deep orbital circulation. Results are difficult to interpret in 10–20% of patients because of technical artifacts. For internal carotid occlusion OPG is 95% accurate (3).

Ultrasound imaging records the acoustical impedence of tissues to construct a real-time tomographic image of the carotid bifurcation (16, 41, 49, 78). Difficulties in interpretation may be caused by calcification in the wall of the artery, a deep vessel, a high or low bifurcation, a thrombus being isodense with blood, and a severe stenosis mistaken for occlusion. The test may one day image carotid ulceration, but to date, many ultrasound images have provided disappointing resolution.

MANAGEMENT AND INDICATIONS FOR SURGICAL TREATMENT

Transient Ischemic Attacks (TIAs)

TIAs with Unilateral Carotid Stenosis and/or Ulceration

Carotid endarterectomy is usually indicated for the patient with TIAs and severe stenosis (lumen less than 2 mm in diameter), and/or severe ulceration in the common carotid bifurcation or proximal internal carotid artery (Figs. 1.1 to 1.6). These attacks are warnings of possible impending disaster. In 29 patients with persistent moderate-to-severe neurological deficits due to carotid occlusion, 60% had prior TIAs (31). Removal of the area of pathology not only stops the attacks but reduces the chance of future stroke. Our results suggest that for the patient with severe carotid stenosis and TIAs, carotid endarterectomy is associated with less risk than the natural history of the disease or the use of medical therapy. However, statistical proof of this fact has not been presented (7, 21).

If the angiogram shows severe stenosis with reduced flow in the internal carotid artery (Figs. 1.7 and 1.13), a thrombus in the lumen (Fig. 1.14), or if the clinical picture includes increasingly severe attacks in the preceding days, attention should be directed to doing the surgery as soon as possible. If there is going to be a delay of more than 12-24 hours, the patient should be heparinized.

If ulceration is found with a non-obstructive plaque, decision regarding endarterectomy or medical therapy will be made based on the severity of the lesion. In the past, carotid endarterectomy has been recommended for patients with TIAs who were found to have an area of ulceration, even though the lumen diameter was greater than 2 mm (Fig. 1.15). There is some evidence that shallow ulcer associated with non-obstructive artherosclerosis may have a very low risk of future stroke (47). Such patients may be treated with antiplatelet therapy and be followed by non-invasive tests. Should there be evidence of development of stenosis or should TIAs continue, then surgery is indicated. However, if the ulceration is deep (Figs. 1.6 and 2.37), or if dye remains in the ulcer crater on delayed films (Fig. 1.9), carotid endarterectomy is indicated. Evidence has been presented to suggest that deep and irregular ulceration may cause stroke in as many as 12.5% of cases per year (56).

Table 1.3 summarizes our results in 304 consecutive elective carotid endarterectomies done for carotid stenosis and/or ulceration in patients with TIAs. The mortality rate was 1%. The incidence of major strokes 1% and the incidence of minor strokes 1%. Virtually

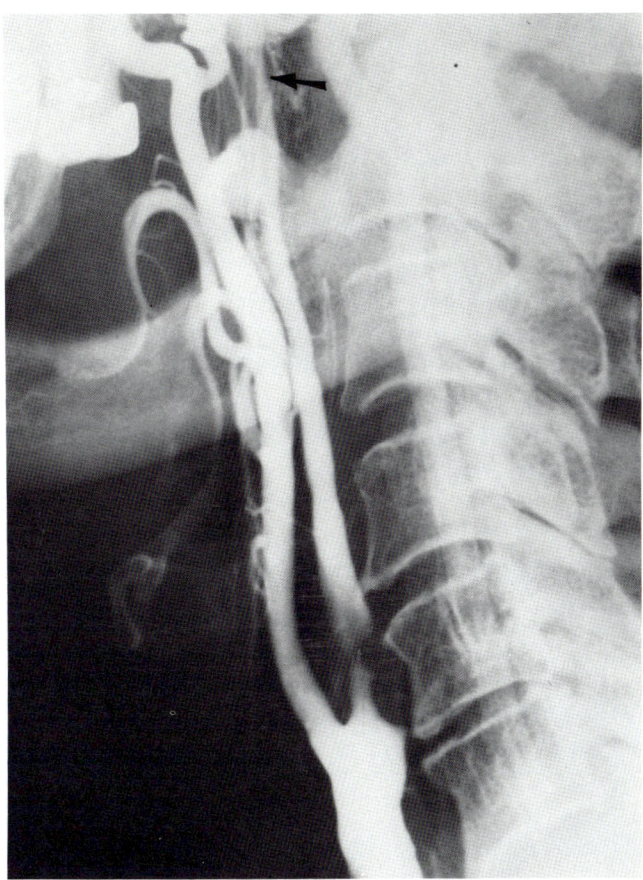

Figure 1.13 Severe internal carotid stenosis with delayed flow. Angiogram of carotid bifurcation region shows severe stenosis at the origin of the internal carotid artery with delayed flow beyond this area (*arrow*). The dye is less dense and the diameter smaller than that seen in the external carotid artery. Comment: The patient presented with TIAs. This is a worrisome situation because of ischemia, as well as possible occlusion or thrombus formation and embolus.

Table 1.3
Results of Elective Carotid Endarterectomy for Carotid Stenosis

	TIA	Stroke	Asymptomatic	Total
Operations	304	63	41	408
Mortality	3 (1%)	0	0	3 (0.7%)
Strokes				
Minor	3 (1%)	3 (4.7%)	0	6 (1.5%)
Major	3 (1%)	3 (4.7%)	0	6 (1.5%)

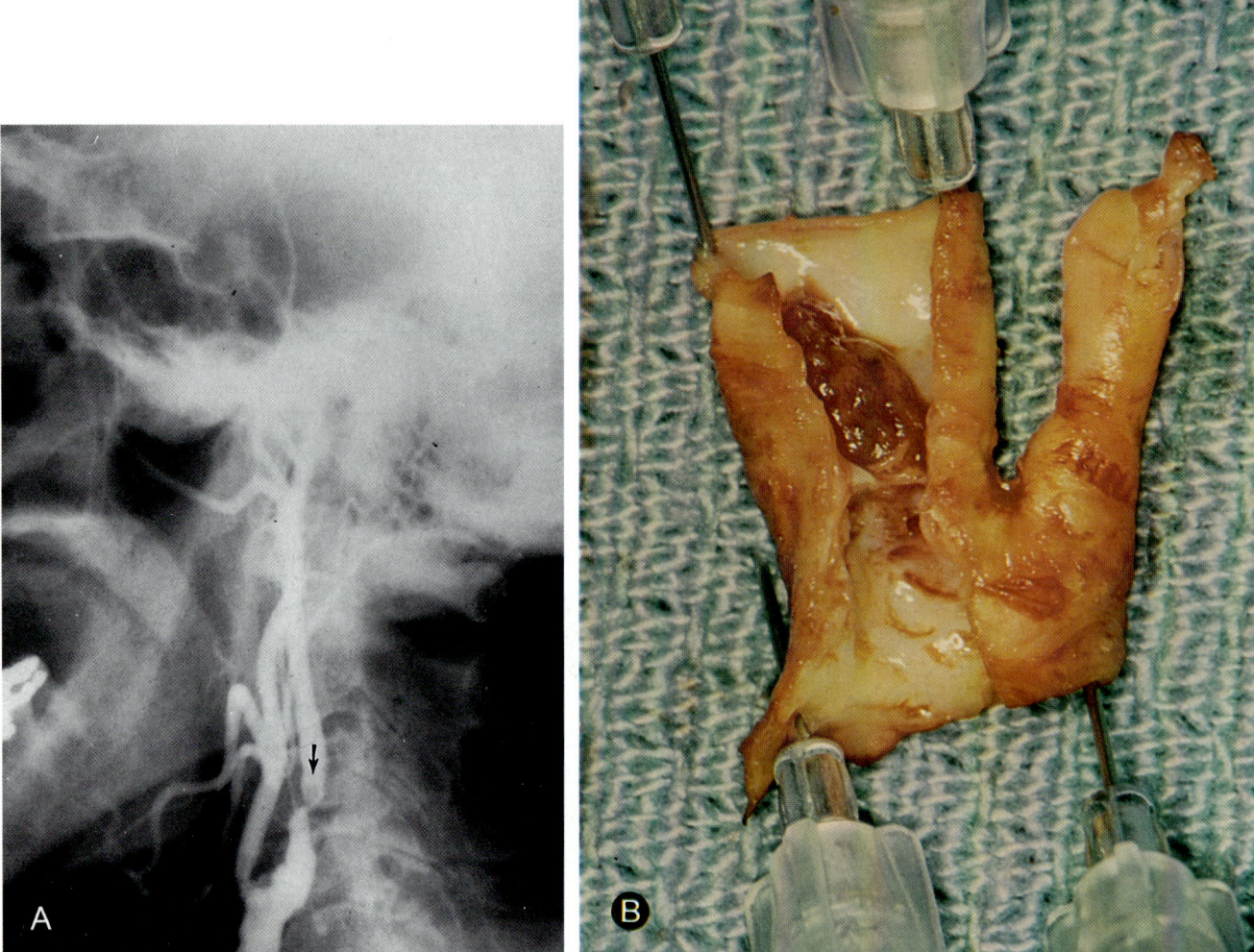

Figure 1.14 Stenosis with thrombus formation. *A*, angiogram of carotid bifurcation showing severe stenosis with thrombus projecting distally into the internal carotid lumen from the stenosis (*arrow*). Note that there is also slight delay in internal carotid flow with the superficial temporal artery filling ahead of the intracranial circulation. *B*, specimen removed at surgery. The thrombus is adherent to the distal end of the stenosis as it almost always is when present.

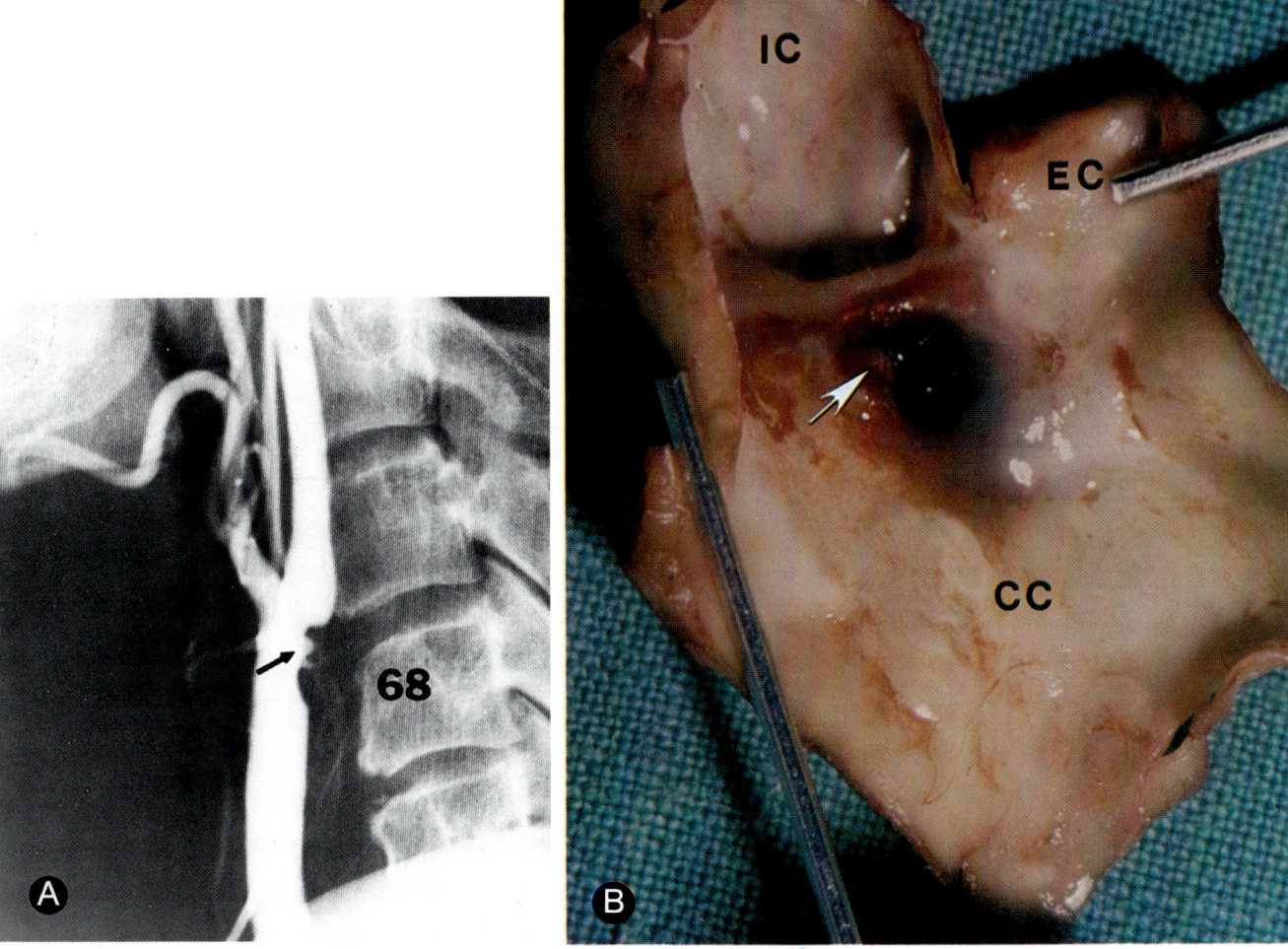

Figure 1.15 TIAs from ulcerated plaque with thrombus. A, angiogram of carotid bifurcation shows no significant stenosis, but there is a discrete ulceration (*arrow*) within a plaque along the posterior wall of the distal common and proximal internal carotid artery. B, atheromatous plaque removed intact at operation and then opened longitudinally on the anterior wall. CC, common carotid artery; EC, external carotid; IC, internal carotid artery. The *arrow* points to a thrombus in the well-circumscribed ulceration. Comment: The patient presented with THAs. There was no bruit. Neurological examination and non-invasive studies were normal. No further attacks were noted after surgery and follow-up angiogram 4 years later, when he had attacks referable to the opposite side, showed a normal artery. (From Ojemann RG, Crowell RM, Roberson GH, Fisher CM: Surgical treatment of extracranial carotid occlusive disease, Ch. 14, in *Clinical Neurosurgery.* Baltimore, Williams & Wilkins, 1974, vol 22, with permission.)

all the other patients returned to their previous level of activity free of attacks. Several other reports of patients who have had elective carotid endarterectomy for TIAs have documented a similar low morbidity and mortality rate in experienced hands (4, 8, 12, 20, 26, 27, 36, 60, 61, 75, 76). The presence of a significant medical risk factor slightly increases the morbidity and mortality (74). This is discussed in Chapter 2.

TIAs with Bilateral Carotid Stenosis

Occasionally, a patient may present with a history of TIAs related to both carotid arteries. More often, the patient is studied because of symptoms due to stenosis in one artery, and significant narrowing of the internal carotid artery is found on the opposite side. There may be bilateral carotid bruits. Angiography documents the pathology. Non-invasive studies (see page 12) may be necessary to help decide about the hemodynamic significance of the lesions.

Carotid endarterectomy is indicated for the hemodynamically significant lesions. When only one side is symptomatic, it is generally treated first unless the asymptomatic side has a tighter stenosis with a more severe hemodynamic lesion, as demonstrated by angiography and non-invasive tests (Fig. 1.16). If both sides are symptomatic, the side with the most severe hemodynamic lesion is operated first. The second side is usually done within 7 to 14 days. When the second stenosis is very severe, heparin therapy may be indicated until the second operation is done. The case illustrated in Fig. 1.17 indicates why these guidelines should be followed and emphasizes that TIAs and severe stenosis may be warnings of impending disaster.

TIAs with Ipsilateral Carotid Stenosis and Contralateral Carotid Occlusion

Most patients with this combination of lesions present with TIAs related to the internal carotid stenosis. Occasionally, patients will have had neurological symptoms related to the contralateral carotid occlusion. There may be a bruit localized over the carotid bifurcation region. The neurological examination is usually normal, but there may be a residual deficit if there was a stroke related to the carotid occlusion.

The indications for surgery are the same as for TIAs associated with unilateral carotid stenosis. The patient with a contralateral occlusion is more likely to have an EEG change and need a shunt at the time of the carotid clamping for the endarterectomy than is the patient with a normal contralateral internal caortid artery (60, 62). However, our experience, as well as that of others, is that there is no increase in neurological complications in this group (62, 66). It must be noted that no neurological complications were encountered in a series of 28 patients with this combination of lesions when no shunt was used, but we believe this is taking an unnecessary risk (61).

TIAs with Tandem Stenosis

No unusual clinical features are present in a patient with more than one lesion in the internal carotid artery. Angiography will show one area of stenosis in the carotid bifurcation or proximal internal carotid artery and another stenosis in the intracavernous or intracranial portion of the internal carotid artery (Fig. 1.18). The occurrence of this problem emphasizes the importance of complete angiography. Usually the stenosis in the neck is more severe than the distal lesion. If the stenosis in the neck is less than 2 mm, carotid endarterectomy is indicated for TIAs even if the distal lesion is also significantly stenotic. Postoperatively, a decision is made between anticoagulation or antiplatelet therapy and bypass graft. It is known that the establishment of a STA-MCA bypass graft in this circumstance may be followed by complete occlusion of distal carotid stenosis (19, 34). In general, our plan has been to use bypass surgery only if symptoms persist after carotid endarterectomy and medical treatment, unless the distal stenosis is very severe.

TIAs With Ipsilateral Internal Carotid Occlusion and the Problem of External Carotid Stenosis

TIAs can occur in the territory normally supplied by a completely occluded internal carotid artery (5, 9, 11, 42, 43, 60, 70). The cause of symptoms may be an embolus from the distal end of the occlusion, an embolus passing through the external carotid circulation from atheromatous stenosis of the external or distal common carotid artery, or from the stump proximal to the occlusion in the internal carotid artery, or a reduction of flow to the eye and/or cerebral hemisphere.

Angiography should include evaluation of the collateral circulation from the opposite carotid artery, and in many patients the vertebrobasilar circulation. Lateral serial films of the head and neck for several seconds help to determine the collateral flow and show how far down the internal carotid artery dye flows (60). This is important in deciding about the etiology of the symptoms and the probability of reopening the complete occlusion.

In a report of 35 patients (43), the angiographic visualization of the internal carotid artery (ICA) distal to the occlusion was categorized as follows: 1) no visualization of ICA; 2) visualization of ICA from posterior communicating artery distally; 3) visualization from ophthalmic artery distally; 4) retrograde flow to a point even with the floor of the sella turcia; 5) retrograde flow into carotid canal to near base of skull. None of the category 1 patterns could be reopened even with immediate surgery. In category 2 and 3, only six of 18 arteries could be reopened and

Atherosclerosis of Carotid Circulation

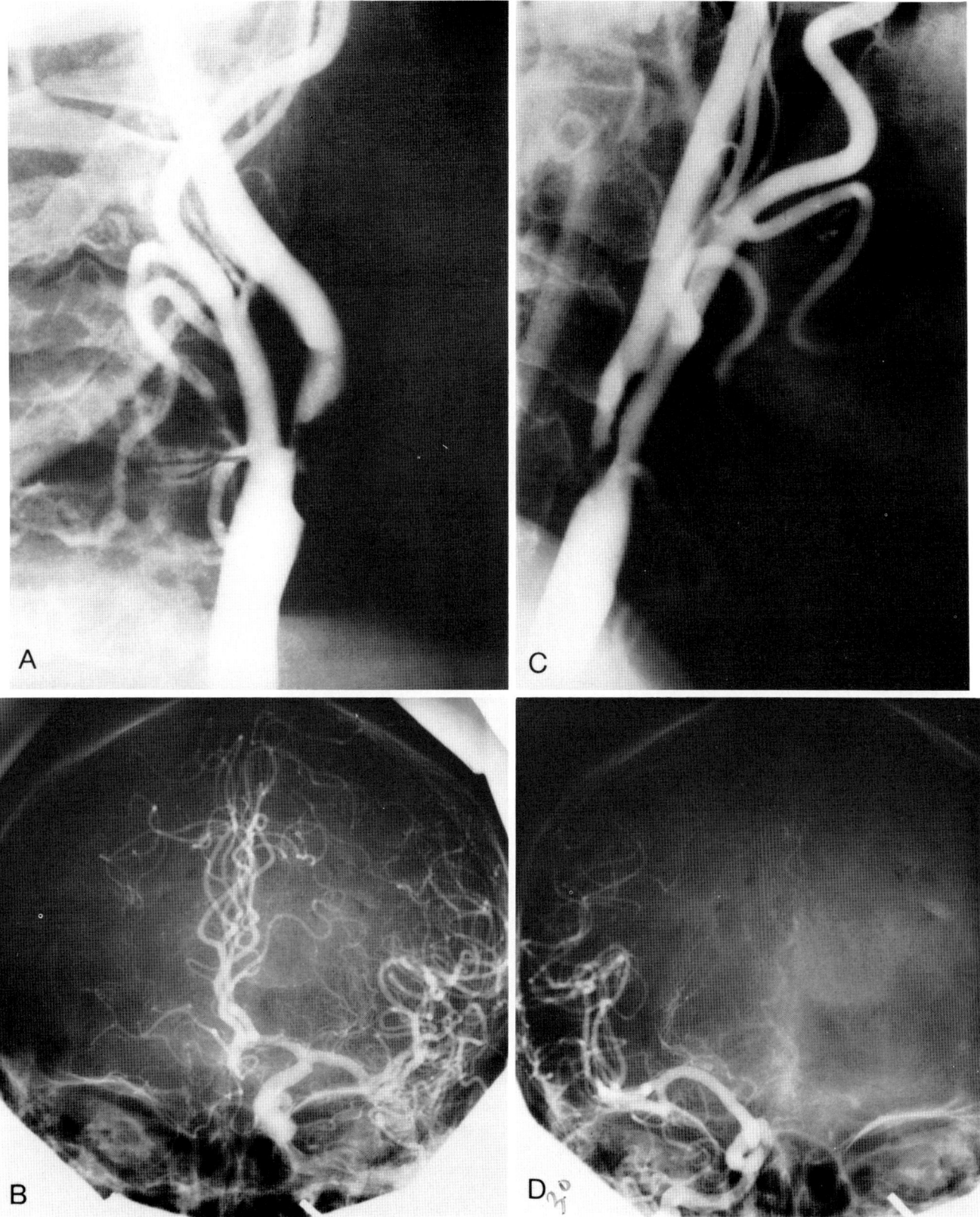

Figure 1.16 Bilateral carotid stenosis with unilateral TIAs. *A*, left carotid angiogram showing severe stenosis at the origin of the internal carotid artery. *B*, A-P view reveals that this left internal carotid artery supplies both anterior cerebral arteries with flow into the watershed area on the right. *C*, right carotid angiogram showing stenosis so severe that one can hardly see the dye going through. *D*, A-P view shows only slight filling of anterior cerebral complex. Comment: The patient presented with left brain THAs. The angiogram indicates that the most severely involved artery is the asymptomatic right side. The recommendation would be to do right carotid endarterectomy followed within a week by an operation on the left side.

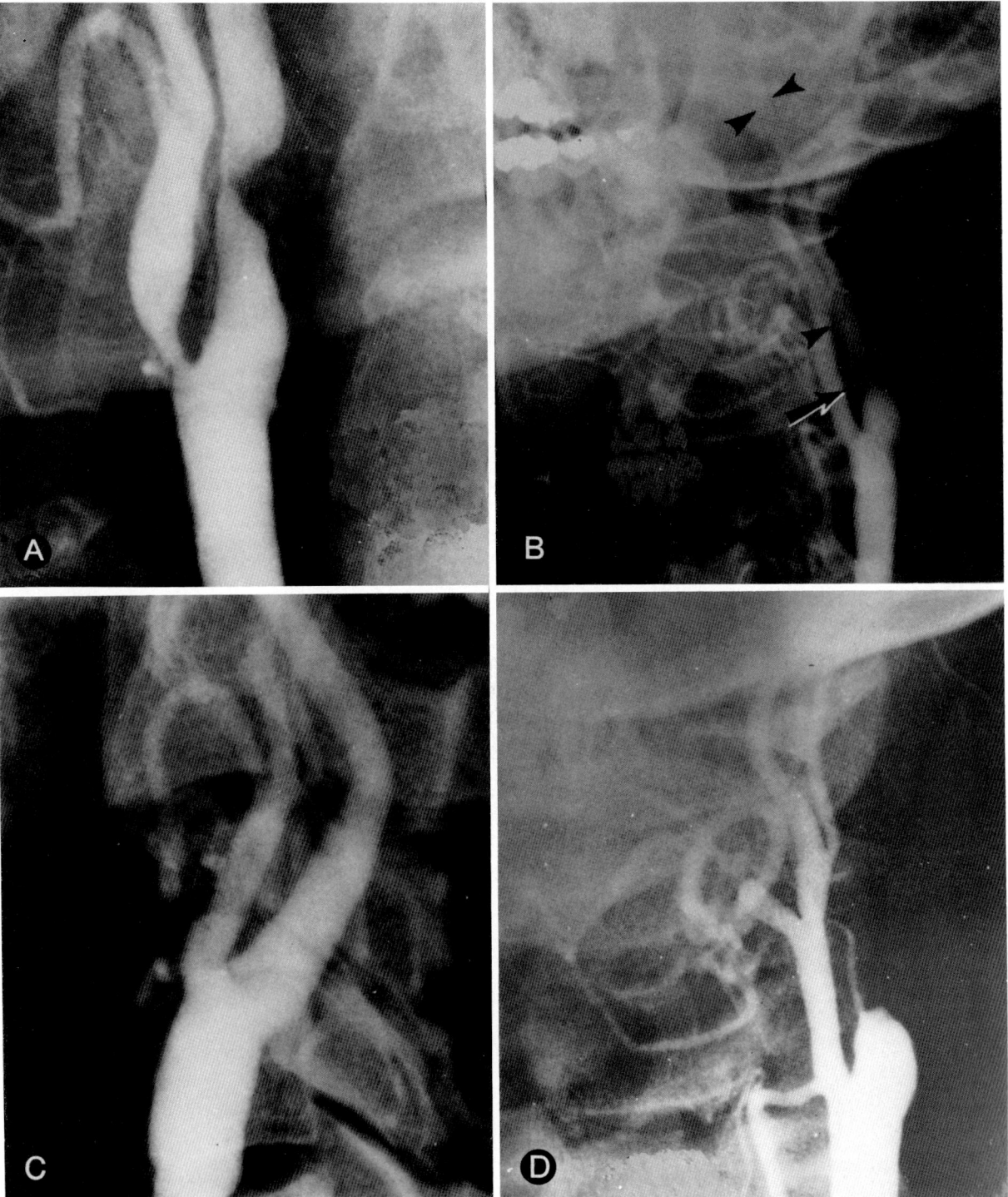

Figure 1.17 Bilateral carotid stenosis with bilateral TIAs: operate the tighter stenosis first. *A*, right carotid angiogram showing localized plaque on the posterior wall 2 cm above the bifurcation. Stenosis is also present in the external carotid artery. *B*, left carotid angiogram shows a more severe stenosis with reduced flow in the internal carotid artery. *C*, right carotid angiogram 1 month after operation showing normal restoration of both external and internal carotid lumens. The slight widening at the ends of the endarterectomy is normal. *D*, left carotid angiogram with complete occlusion of the internal carotid artery. Comment: The patient presented with a history of TIAs relative to the left carotid artery beginning 1 year before admission but none had occurred for 9 months. In the weeks before admission, TIAs relative to the right carotid circulation were noted. Bilateral carotid bruits were present and the examination was normal. This patient was seen early in our series and the most recent symptomatic side was operated. He then declined the second operation planned a week later. One month after operation, he developed a stroke related to the left hemisphere. (From Ojemann RG, Crowell RM, Roberson GH, Fisher CM: Surgical treatment of extracranial carotid occlusive disease, Ch. 14, in *Clinical Neurosurgery*. Baltimore, Williams & Wilkins, 1974, vol 22, with permission.)

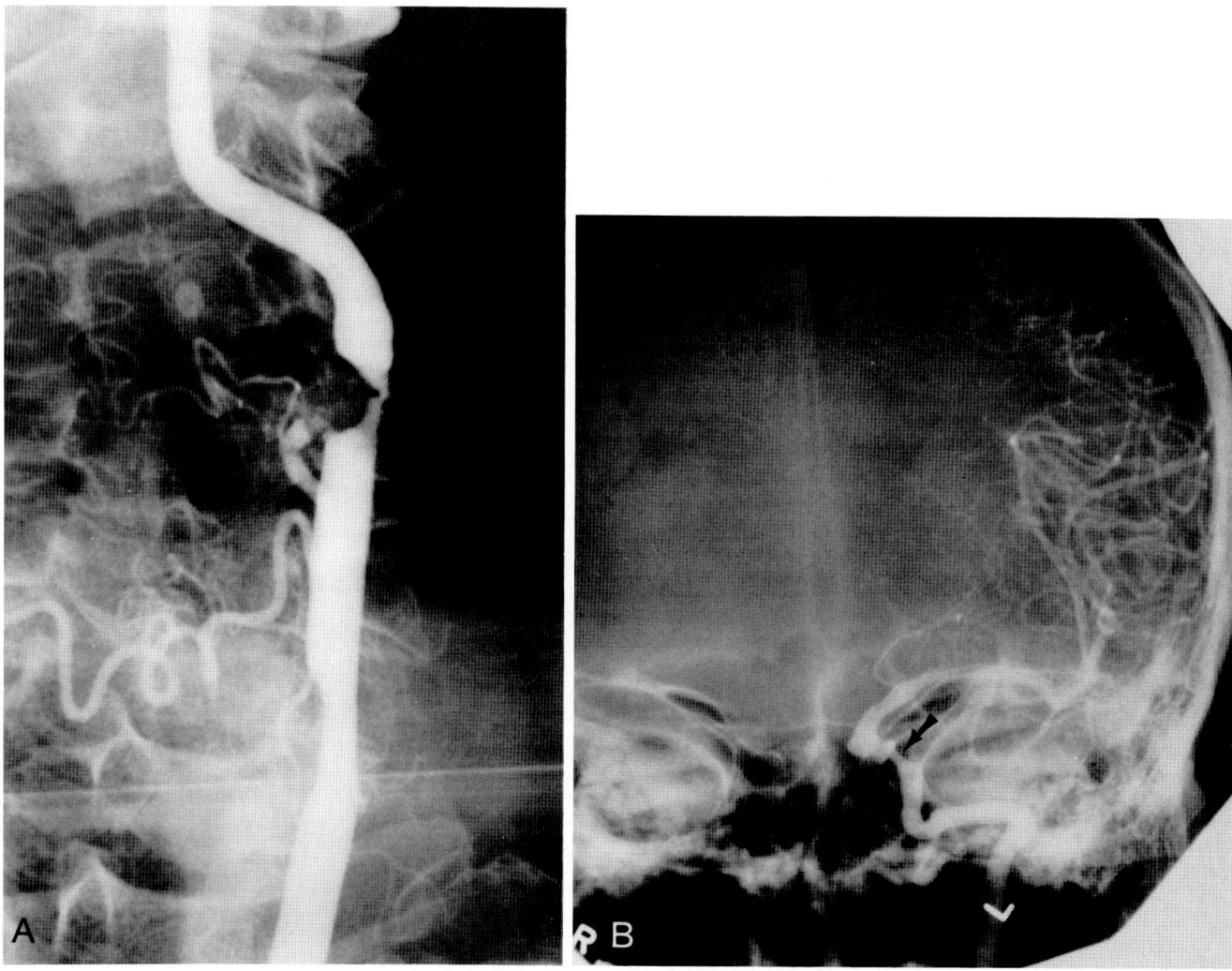

Figure 1.18 Tandem ICA stenosis. *A*, severe stenosis at the origin of the internal carotid artery (residual lumen 1 mm) with occlusion of much of external carotid artery. Slight narrowing in the common carotid artery is also noted. *B*, severe stenosis in the carotid siphon (*arrow*) with residual lumen of a little over 1 mm. Comment: Carotid endarterectomy is indicated to remove the severe stenosis at the origin of the internal carotid artery and to reopen the external carotid artery in case a STA-MCA bypass is needed in the future. After surgery, a program of medical therapy is started. In case of recurrent TIAs, STA-MCA bypass is performed.

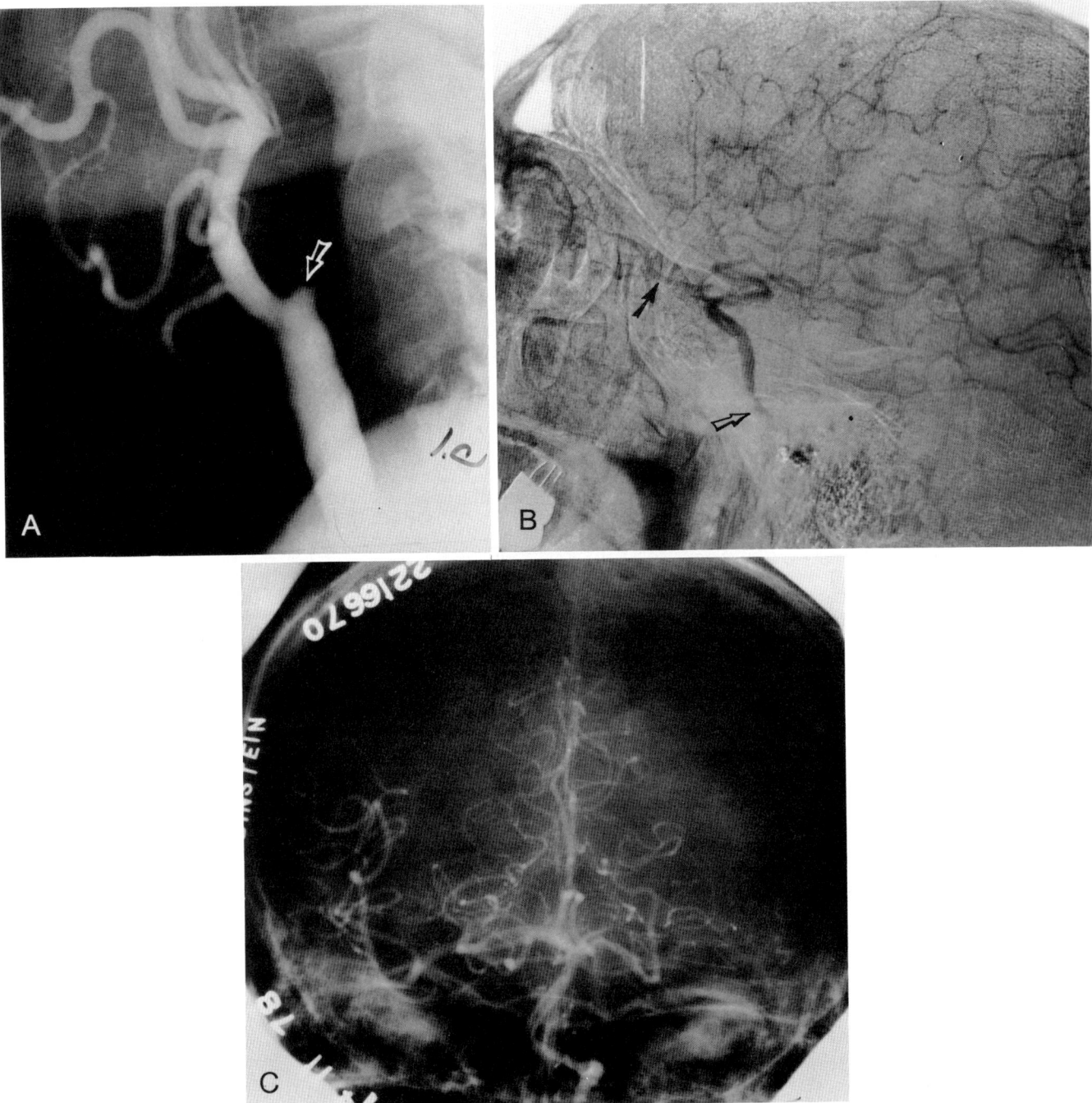

Figure 1.19 Reopening an internal carotid occlusion. *A,* complete occlusion of right internal carotid artery (*arrow*). *B,* subtraction lateral view several seconds after injection showing collateral flow through the ophthalmic artery (*solid arrow*) into the internal carotid artery with retrograde flow toward the base of the skull (*open arrow*). This finding means that there is a good chance of reopening the artery. *C,* good collateral flow into the right middle and anterior cerebral arteries from the vertebral injection. This collateral circulation does not protect the patient from possible serious neurological deficits due to emboli. Comment: Patient presented with right cerebral THA. Carotid endarterectomy restored right internal carotid artery flow; no TIAs occurred after operation.

Atherosclerosis of Carotid Circulation

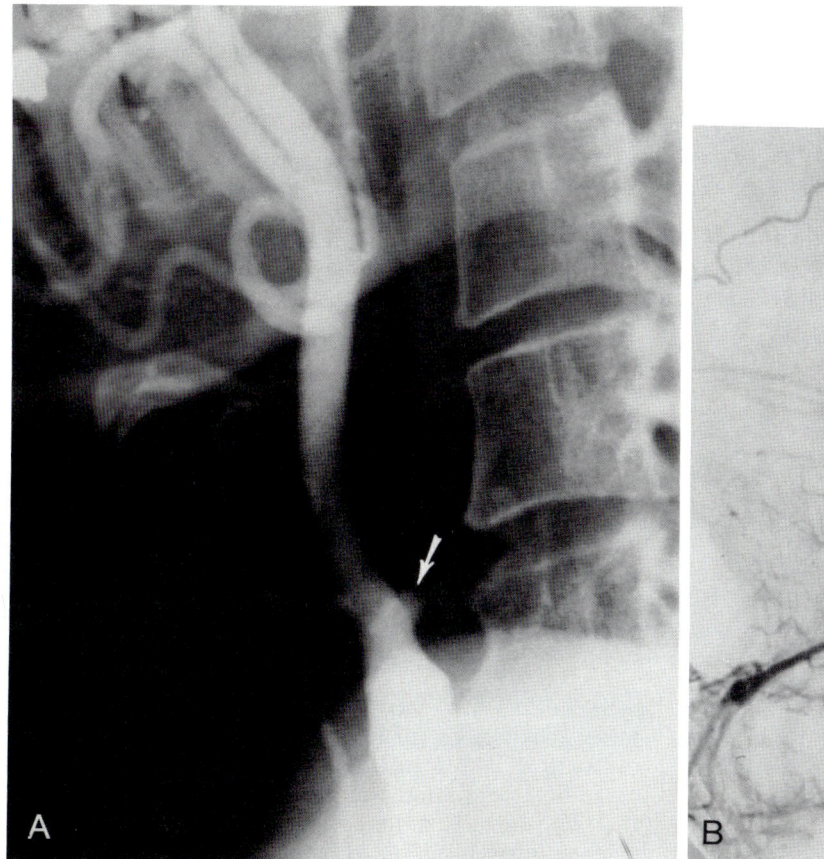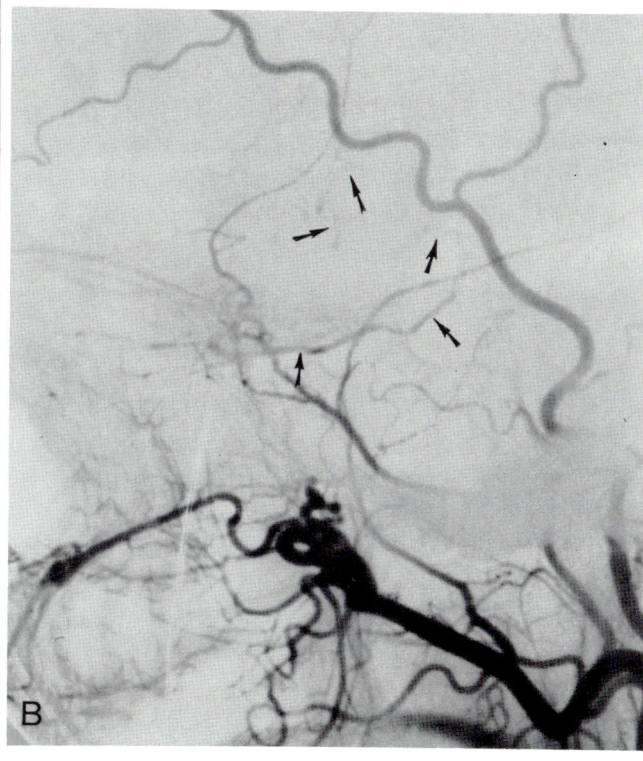

Figure 1.20 Proximal "stump" as source of embolus. *A*, angiogram of carotid bifurcation showing a small "stump" at the origin of the occluded internal carotid artery (*arrow*). *B*, a later film shows collateral flow through the ophthalmic artery into an ascending frontal-parietal branch of the middle cerebral artery (*arrows*). The patient continued to have TIAs characterized by transient dysphasia several months after a small stroke. Operation disclosed a friable thrombus in the origin of the occluded internal carotid artery. A thromboendarterectomy was done and the origin of the internal carotid artery was closed with a suture. No further symptoms were noted after operation.

five of the six were operated within 7 days of the occlusion. In category 4 patients, four of six were reopened and the two failures had been occluded 7 months and 3 years. All of the category 5 patients were reopened regardless of the time of occlusion (Fig. 1.19).

In two of our patients, angiography revealed an occluded internal carotid artery several weeks before we saw the patient (60). Re-evaluation of the x-rays with subtraction and repeat angiography was done because of continuing transient spells, and these revealed retrograde flow almost to the base of the skull. The arteries were reopened and the symptoms relieved. Others have reported similar cases (70). Even after a month of occlusion, there may be a reasonable chance of reopening the internal carotid artery if the occlusion does not extend too far distally (42, 43).

If the angiogram shows a significant proximal stump in the occluded internal carotid artery in the neck and external carotid to ophthalmic artery collateral, this may be the source of embolus and should be treated with endarterectomy (5) (Fig. 1.20). The evidence that emboli can pass through the external carotid collateral circulation has been summarized (11).

If there is atherosclerosis with stenosis and/or ulceration at the origin of the external carotid artery, this may also be the source of emboli and ischemia (9). In a report of 22 patients with internal carotid occlusion and external carotid collateral flow, 10 patients with no significant atherosclerotic narrowing or ulceration of the external carotid artery remained free of symptoms over 6 to 40 months (17). In the other 12 patients, delayed recurrent cerebral or retinal symptoms developed ipsilateral to the internal carotid occlusion, and all were found to have stenosis or ulceration involving the common and/or external carotid artery. Subsequently, 17 patients with amaurosis fugax were reported to have the same findings (18). Endarterectomy completely stopped the symptoms. Occasionally, opening of a severely stenotic external carotid artery may be helpful in halting the

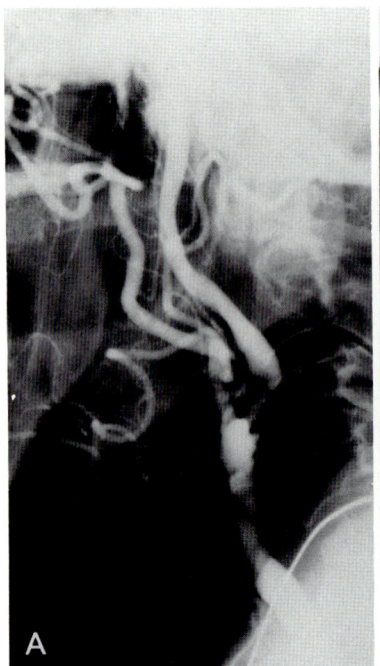
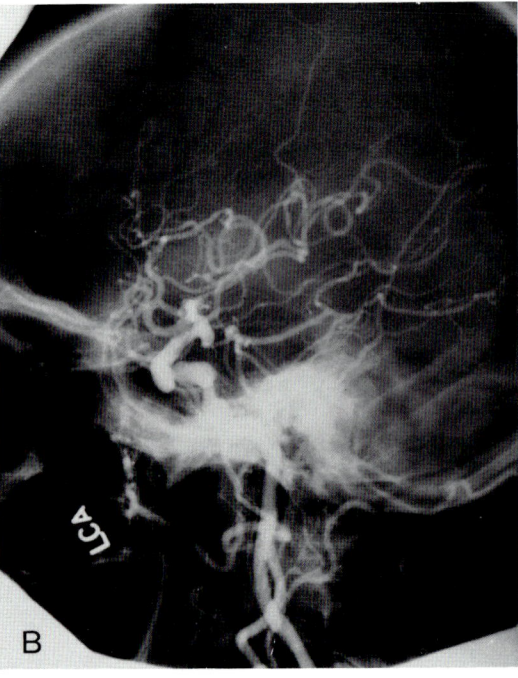

Figure 1.21 Carotid stenosis and vertebrobasilar TIAs. *A*, lateral angiogram of neck showing severe stenosis at the origin of the left internal carotid artery, as well as some disease in the common carotid artery. *B*, lateral angiogram of head showing filling of posterior cerebral and basilar arteries from the carotid circulation. Other films showed occlusion of both vertebral arteries. Comment: Patient presented with TIAs related to both the left middle cerebral and vertebrobasilar circulation. Carotid endarterectomy was done with a shunt. There were no further attacks.

progression of ischemic retinopathy. When the internal carotid artery is open, external carotid stenosis or occlusion does not cause significant clinical symptoms.

If the complete occlusion of the internal carotid artery extends into the carotid siphon, a decision has to be made between attempting to reopen the internal carotid artery, using anticoagulation or performing a bypass graft. In general, the artery cannot be reopened in patients with this angiographic finding, and unless it is an acute occlusion, we usually do not try to reopen the artery. Even if there is good collateral circulation, we have favored anticoagulation because of the risk of embolization (29).

Posterior Circulation TIAs with Carotid Stenosis

Occasionally, patients will present with posterior circulation TIAs secondary to carotid stenosis. Diagnosis is more difficult because of the diverse clinical presentations. The most characteristic symptoms of TIA in the vertebrobasilar circulation are diplopia, dysarthria, dizziness, and weakness or numbness of part or all of one or both sides of the body (33). Other manifestations include headache, staggering, veering to one side, blurred vision, blindness, ptosis, dysphagia, confusion, and memory lapse. Occasionally, patients will have both cerebral and vertebrobasilar TIAs.

When there is evidence of carotid artery disease either from physical examination or non-invasive studies in a patient with posterior circulation TIAs, angiography is indicated. This should include both the carotid and posterior circulation. Carotid endarterectomy is usually indicated if the angiogram shows: filling of the posterior cerebral artery via the stenotic internal carotid artery or filling of the posterior circulation from the internal carotid artery because of vertebral artery occlusive disease (Fig. 1.21), or a persistent hypoglossal or trigeminal artery (71). We have not been convinced that carotid endarterectomy will alter vertebrobasilar symptoms unless one of the conditions noted above is found on the angiogram, and this has also been the experience of others (52). When severe carotid stenosis is present with no filling of the posterior circulation from that artery, one considers the problem as an asymptomatic carotid stenosis. The optimal treatment for this lesion is correlated with management of the vertebrobasilar occlusive disease.

Intracranial Aneurysm with Carotid Stenosis

Severe internal carotid stenosis may be found in association with an intracranial aneurysm on the ipsilateral intracranial circulation (60). In patients with TIAs it is presumed that the stenosis is the cause of the symptoms, and relief of symptoms has usually followed endarterectomy. It is recognized, however, that the aneurysm can be the source of an embolus that causes the transient attack. Occasionally, asymptomatic carotid stenosis is found in a patient being studied for subarachnoid hemorrhage. A CT scan is usually done to be sure about the true size of the aneurysm. When the stenosis is asymptomatic, non-invasive carotid studies may be helpful in determining if the lesion is causing a hemodynamic change.

A review of 20 patients, from one institution, with extracranial stenosis and intracranial aneurysm, revealed that 15 had TIAs and an incidental aneurysm and five presented with symptoms referable to the aneurysm and were found to have asymptomatic

Atherosclerosis of Carotid Circulation

carotid stenosis (72). It was concluded that there was no additional risk in performing carotid endarterectomy in patients with asymptomatic aneurysm. However, there was considerable risk when endarterectomy was performed after subarachnoid hemorrhage (SAH), and it was recommended that the aneurysm be treated before the endarterectomy is performed in these patients.

Our own experience in a smaller series substantiates the conclusion that carotid endarterectomy can be performed safely in a patient with an asymptomatic aneurysm. A decision regarding treatment of the asymptomatic aneurysm is based on the guidelines discussed in Chapter 19. When there is SAH, priority must be given to treating the aneurysm. When surgery is indicated for both lesions, the two operations are usually done under the same anesthesia (Fig. 1.22). If the treatment of the aneurysm will likely require profound hypotension, a significant carotid stenosis should be treated, even if it is not symptomatic. If the stenosis is to be treated without exposing the aneurysm, intraoperative hypertension is avoided and a shunt used if necessary, with temporary heparinization during cross-clamping.

TIAs with Common Carotid Stenosis or Occlusion

Stenosis at the origin of the common carotid artery is rare and is not often a cause of transient ischemic attacks. More frequently the distal common carotid artery is involved at the bifurcation (Fig. 1.5A). Occasionally, significant stenosis may involve the midportion of the common carotid artery (Fig. 1.23). Occlusion of the common carotid artery may be due to retrograde thrombosis superimposed on the atherosclerosis at the carotid bifurcation or antegrade thrombosis from atherosclerosis at the origin of the artery from the aortic arch. In some of these patients, there may be continued circulation from the external to the internal carotid artery (Fig. 1.24). This circumstance or a trickle of antegrade flow via the common carotid artery is best seen in delayed films.

In a review of 12 patients with angiographic demonstration of common carotid occlusion, it was found that only three had hemispheric TIAs, one had a hemispheric stroke, while five had vertebrobasilar TIAs, and three were completely asymptomatic (67). There were often multiple vessels involved. In six of nine patients explored, both the external and internal carotid arteries were found to be open.

The indication for surgery is continuation of symptoms in spite of medical therapy. The operative technique is discussed in Chapter 2.

Established Stroke

Evaluation of patients who have had a stroke and have a neurological deficit will lead to the finding of carotid artery disease in a significant number. Often, carotid occlusive disease is suggested by the history. In a group of patients we treated who had suffered a stroke and were found to have carotid disease, more than half had a prior history of TIAs due to carotid stenosis which had not brought the patient to medical attention (20). In a group of 29 patients with a persistent neurological deficit following carotid occlusion, 60% had a prior history of TIAs, 20% were associated with a fluctuating or step-wise deficit, and 20% developed deficits suddenly without warning (31).

Since these patients are at risk for further stroke, they should be studied. A CT scan is done to define the extent of the infarction and to look for other pathology. In most patients, carotid angiography is indicated. To determine the collateral circulation it is important that serial films be obtained over about 15 seconds, especially if there is a complete occlusion.

In general, the presence of severe stenosis or a deep ulcer is an indication for surgical treatment. If the angiogram shows thrombus in the lumen, a stenosis so tight that flow is delayed, or circumstances where a carotid occlusion may be reopened, then surgery is performed promptly. In those patients with a recent stroke who are continuing to show improvement, and prompt surgery is not indicated from the angiogram, operation may be delayed to allow recovery from cerebral ischemia. How long one should delay has not been established. Some have advocated waiting several weeks to reduce the possible chance of postoperative brain hemorrhage (13). If the neurological deficit is mild, we would operate within a few days. If the deficit is moderate-to-severe, the patient will usually have CT evidence of an infarct. In this circumstance, we would wait 2-4 weeks to allow maximum recovery. Surgery can then be done safely as long as there is careful control of postoperative blood pressure.

The results in 63 consecutive patients with stroke who had carotid endarterectomies are summarized in Table 1.2. As expected, the risk of a major stroke is slightly higher than for patients with TIAs.

If the patient has had a massive stroke with a severe fixed deficit, evaluation may be limited to a CT scan. These patients cannot be helped by carotid endarterectomy. Angiography is done if significant improvement occurs.

An occasional patient will have a slowly progressive neurological deficit due to chronic cerebral ischemia (75). CT scan excludes an intracranial mass lesion. Angiography usually shows multiple vessel occlusions. A combination of endarterectomy and bypass procedures may need to be considered.

Acute Stroke

Laboratory experiments have demonstrated that focal cerebral ischemia is a progressive phenomenon which can be reversible in its early stages by restitution of blood flow (23). However, after several hours of ischemia, infarction becomes complete and restoration of blood flow has no beneficial effect.

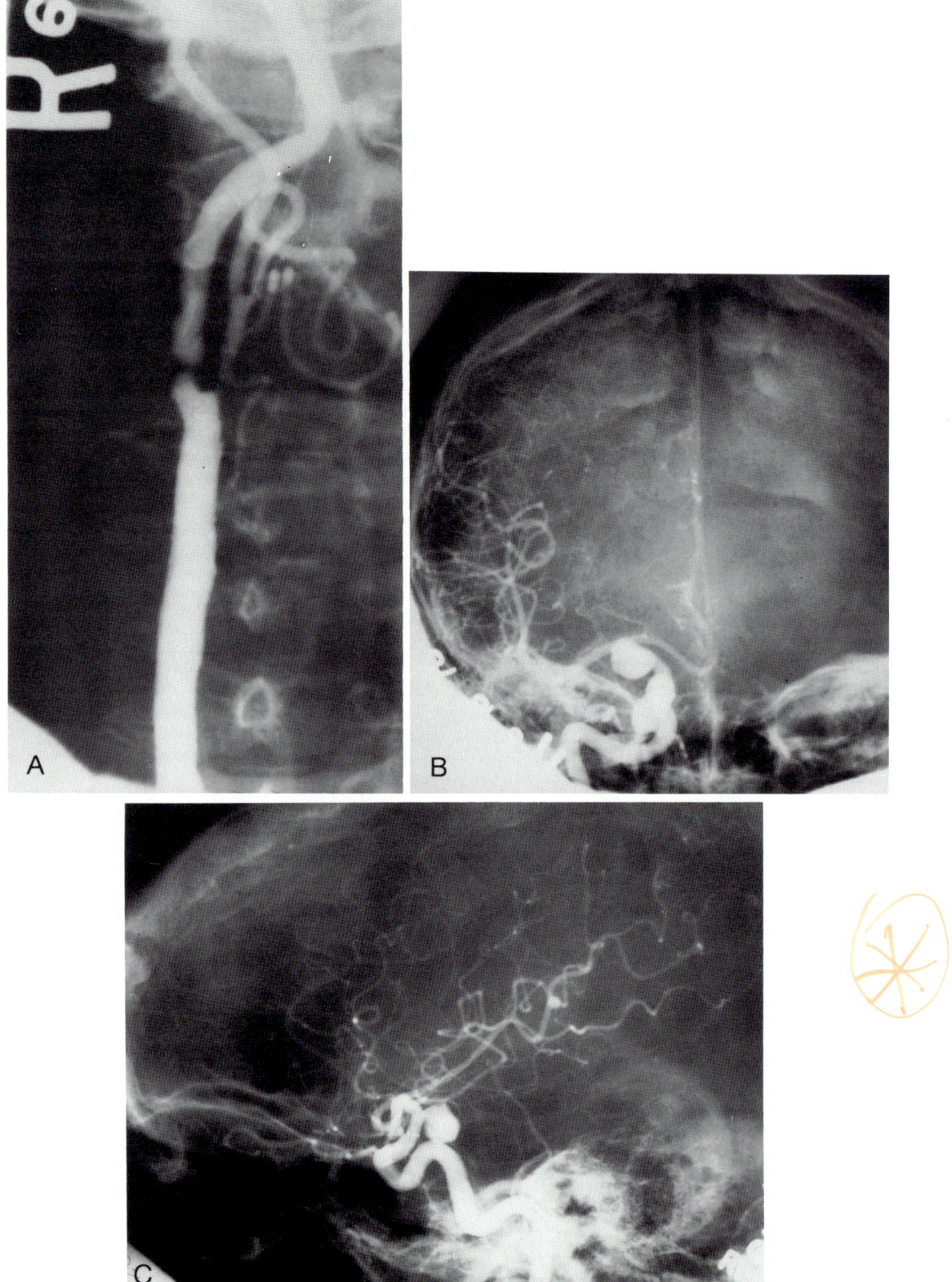

Figure 1.22 Intracranial aneurysm with carotid stenosis. *A*, right carotid angiogram showing severe stenosis at the origin of the internal carotid artery. *B* and *C*, A-P and lateral angiogram of the head revealing a large internal carotid-posterior communicating artery aneurysm. Comment: This patient presented with THAs. Her neurological examination was normal. There had been no symptoms referrable to the aneurysm. She was treated with carotid endarterectomy and intracranial microsurgical occlusion of the aneurysm under the same anesthesia.

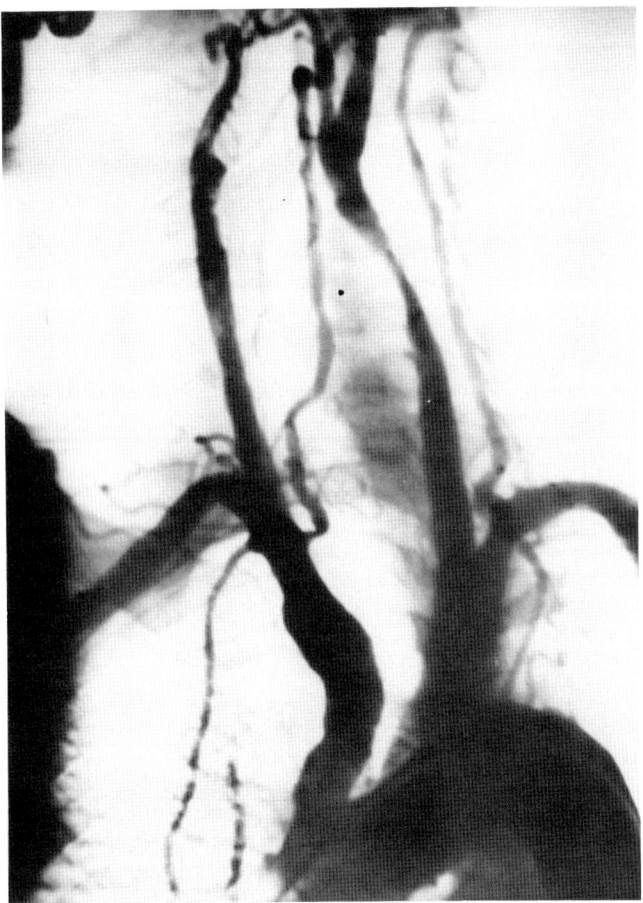

Figure 1.23 Stenosis of common carotid artery. Arch angiogram. Subtraction study showing stenosis in the common carotid artery. The patient had TIAs which ceased after operation.

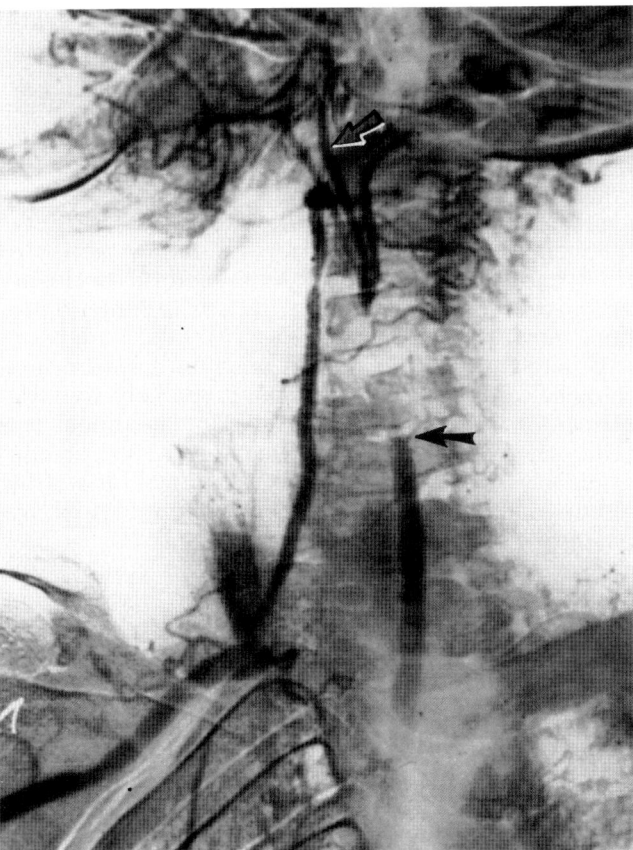

Figure 1.24 Common carotid occlusion. Right innominate artery injection. The subtraction study shows complete occlusion of the distal common carotid artery (*closed arrow*) with reconstitution of the internal carotid artery (*open arrow*) from the external carotid artery branches via thyrocervical and vertebral artery collateral flow. Comment: Operation revealed atherosclerosis at the carotid bifurcation with thrombosis. Flow was restored following surgery.

These data suggest that emergency carotid endarterectomy might be indicated in some clinical situations. Many clinicians have concluded that a patient with an acute ischemic stroke should be treated symptomatically and no attempt made to establish a diagnosis in the acute phases of the illness because of the concern of increased morbidity with angiography and surgery. However, some patients will have unstable neurological syndromes of mild-to-moderate degree which may progress to a severe disability without treatment. For such problems, we believe a diagnosis should be established at the time of admission, using whatever tests are indicated, and then a rational program of treatment instituted (61). This same approach has also been utilized by other centers with encouraging results in the surgical treatment of selected acute stroke patients (39, 40, 54, 57, 74).

A careful history and examination will lead to a correct diagnosis in a high percentage of patients. Almost every patient admitted with an acute stroke problem should have an ECG and immediate CT scan to differentiate between infarction and hemorrhage (10). Laboratory tests should include blood count, blood chemistries, and coagulation studies.

If the history and/or findings suggest carotid disease, then immediate angiography or, if available, digital subtraction angiography, should be done. This is especially important if the patient has had increasing TIAs in preceding days (crescendo TIAs), or the sudden onset of a mild-to-moderate neurological deficit with or without prior TIAs, or has a progressive or fluctuating deficit. TIAs which last more than 1 hour or TIAs involving face, arm, and leg are particularly worrisome and should be promptly investigated. If there is severe stenosis with delayed flow, thrombus in the lumen distal to the stenosis or carotid occlusion with reflux to the intrapetrous segment of the carotid artery, surgery should be done to allow maximum blood flow to ischemic brain tissue, prevent extension of a thrombus, and remove a source of embolization. A stenosis with residual lumen diameter greater than 2.0 mm (not hemodynamically significant), or ulceration in a plaque at the carotid bifurcation, suggests an embolus as the cause of the problem and the patient should be considered for anticoagulation. If an acute neurological deficit occurs with loss of a previously documented carotid bruit, emergency endarterectomy should be undertaken without CT scan or angiography. If there is careful control of postoperative blood pressure, we would not agree with the statement that "establishing flow and pressure during acute carotid occlusion accompanied by neurological deficits is likely to produce intracerebral hemorrhage" (10).

Where there is the sudden onset of a severe neurological deficit which persists, it is likely that significant infarction has occurred. This is almost certainly the case if there is a decreased level of consciousness. In this situation, restoration of blood flow either by emergency carotid endarterectomy or bypass graft has generally not been beneficial.

The indications for treatment in this group of patients are based on our experience with emergency carotid endarterectomy in 55 consecutive patients. The special surgical problems in dealing with complete internal carotid occlusion are discussed in Chapter 2. Table 1.4 correlates the outcome with preoperative status. Patients with crescendo TIAs had severe stenosis with either an intraluminal thrombus or marked reduction of flow in the distal internal carotid artery. Patients with mild-to-moderate neurological deficits may be stable or have progressing or fluctuating deficits. In our series of 36 patients with worrisome TIAs, acute mild-to-moderate deficit, or fluctuating stroke, 29 enjoyed excellent or good outcome. In this group there was one death; the patient had complete neurological recovery but then died of a cardiopulmonary complication. There were two occasions where the neurological deficit was worse after the operation, but there were also several spectacular recoveries in the immediate postoperative period after operation for both stenosis and occlusion. In another report of emergency carotid endarterectomy, seven patients with crescendo TIAs all made a full recovery and of 17 patients with stroke-in-evolution, none were worse, four were unchanged, 12 made a good recovery, and one died (54).

The correlation of surgical findings and outcome is striking with the finding that 18 of 21 patients with total occlusion and restoration of internal carotid flow showed improvement (Table 1.5). Only one of eight improved where occlusion could not be reopened. The time elapsed from the onset of symptoms to revascularization was usually under 24 hours, but an excellent result was reported as late as 36 hours after onset of symptoms. In other reports, it was possible to restore and maintain patency in patients who underwent surgery within 48 hours (42) and 86% of the arteries operated within 72 hours of the presumed onset of total occlusion (48). Long-term

Table 1.4
Results of Emergency Carotid Endarterectomy

Pre-Op Neurological Status	Outcome				Total
	Excellent	Good	Poor	Death	
TIAs	4	–	–	–	4
Mild deficit	2	2	–	–	4
Moderate deficit	7	14	6	1	28
Sudden severe deficit	1	5	6	7	19
Total	14	21	12	8	55

Table 1.5
Emergency Carotid Endarterectomy: Surgical Findings and Outcome

Findings	Outcome				Total
	Excellent	Good	Poor	Death	
Stenosis	8	11	4	3	26
Occluded (flow restored)	5	11	2	3	21
Occluded (flow not restored)	–	1	5	2	8
Total	13	23	11	8	55

prognosis was better in these patients than in those with persistent occlusion.

Patients with sudden severe deficits do not benefit from endarterectomy. Such patients typically have hemiplegia, aphasia if the dominant side is involved, and are drowsy. Only one such patient in our series did well with operation. In that case, flow was restored within 4 hours. Five of the seven deaths were related to extensive cerebral damage and two were due to myocardial infarction. These cases were done early in the series and we no longer operate on such patients.

On rare occasion, acute massive ischemic infarction with progressive signs of brain stem compression and failure to respond to medical therapy is treated with hemicraniectomy. We have done this in two patients with relief of pressure and eventual partial recovery of function. In a report of three patients, the factors that influenced undertaking this surgery were the relatively young age of the patient, involvement of the nondominant hemisphere, lack of systemic illness, and a positive attitude of the family (68).

REFERENCES

1. Ackerman RH: The relative effectiveness of six noninvasive tests for carotid disease. Neurology 26:379–380, 1976.
2. Ackerman RH: A perspective on noninvasive diagnosis of carotid disease. Neurology 29:615–622, 1979.
3. Ackerman RH: Non-invasive carotid evaluation. Stroke 11:675–678, 1980.
4. Baker WH: *Diagnosis and Treatment of Carotid Artery Disease.* Mount Kisco, New York, Futura, 1979.
5. Barnett HJM, Peerless SJ, Kaufmann JCE: "Stump" of internal carotid artery: A source for further cerebral embolic ischemia. Stroke 9:448–456, 1978.

6. Barnett HJM: The pathophysiology of transient cerebral ischemic attacks. Med Clin N Am 63:649–680, 1979.
7. Barnett HJM: Progress towards stroke prevention. Neurology 30:1212–1225, 1980.
8. Bland, JE, Lazar ML: Carotid endarterectomy without shunt. Neurosurgery 8:153–157, 1981.
9. Bogousslavsky J, Regil F, Hungerbuhler JP, Chrzanowski R: Transient ischemic attacks and external carotid artery. Stroke 12:627–630, 1981.
10. Buonanno F, Toole JF: Management of patients with established ("completed") cerebral infarction. Stroke 12:7–16, 1981.
11. Burnbaum MD, Selhorst JB, Harbison JW, Brush JJ: Amaurosis fugax from disease of the external carotid artery. Arch Neurol 34:532–535, 1977.
12. Callow AD: An overview of the stroke problem in the carotid territory. Am J Surg 140:181–191, 1980.
13. Caplan LR, Skillman J, Ojemann R, Fields WS: Intracerebral hemorrhage following carotid endarterectomy: A hypertensive complication? Stroke 9:457–460, 1978.
14. Chilcote WA, Modic MT, Pavlicek WA, Little JR, Furlan AJ, Duchesneau PM, Weinstein MA: Digital subtraction angiography of the carotid artery: A comparative study in 100 patients. Diagn Radiol 139:287–395, 1981.
15. Christenson PC, Ovitt TW, Fisher HD III, Frost MM, Nudelman S, Roehrig H: Intravenous angiography using digital videosubtraction: Intravenous cervicocerebrovascular angiography. Am J Neuroradiol 1:379–386, 1980.
16. Cooperberg PL, Robertson WD, Fry P, et al: High-resolution real-time ultrasound of the carotid bifurcation. J Clin Ultrasound 7:13–17, 1979.
17. Countee RW, Vijayanathan T: External carotid artery in internal carotid artery occlusion. Angiographic, therapeutic and prognostic considerations. Stroke 10:450–460, 1979.
18. Countee RW, Vijayanathan T, Chavis P: Recurrent retinal ischemia beyond cervical carotid occlusions. J Neurosurg 55:532–542, 1981.
19. Crowell RM: Direct Brain Revascularization, in Schmdek H, Sweet W (eds): *Current Technique in Operative Neurosurgery* (in press).
20. Crowell RM, Ojemann RG: *Extracranial Cerebrovascular Disease*, Chapt 28, in Hoff JT (ed): *Practice of Surgery*. Philadelphia, Harper and Row, 1981.
21. Crowell RM, Ojemann RG, Kistler JP: Asymptomatic carotid bruit, in Thompson RA, Crowell RM (eds): *Advances in Neurology*. New York, Raven Press (in press).
22. Crowell RM, Kistler JP, Ojemann RG, Thompson RA: Noninvasive techniques in cerebrovascular disease. Clin Neurosurg (in press).
23. Crowell RM, Olsson Y, Klatzo I, Ommaya A: Temporary occlusion of the middle cerebral artery in the monkey: Clinical and pathological observations. Stroke 1:439–448, 1970.
24. Davis KR, Ackerman RH, Kistler JP, Mohr JP: Computed tomography of cerebral infarction: Hemorrhage, contrast enhancement and time of appearance. Comput Tomogr 1:71–86, 1977.
25. Duncan GW, Gruber JO, Dewey CF, Meyers GS, Lees RS: Evaluation of carotid stenosis by phonoangiography. N Engl J Med 293:1124–1128, 1975.
26. Easton JD, Sherman DG: Stroke and mortality rate in carotid endarterectomy: 228 consecutive operations. Stroke 8:565–568, 1977.
27. Ennix CL Jr, Lawrie GM, Morris GC Jr, Crawford ES, Howell JF, Reardon MJ, Weatherford SC: Improved results of carotid endarterectomy in patients with symptomatic coronary disease: An analysis of 1546 consecutive carotid operations. Stroke 10:122–125, 1979.
28. Ergun DL, Mistretta CA, Kruger RA, Riederer SJ, Shaw CG, Carbone DP: Computerized fluoroscopy technique in non-invasive cardiovascular imaging. Radiology 132:739–742, 1979.
29. Finklestein S, Kleinman GM, Cuneo R, Baringer JR: Delayed stroke following carotid occlusion. Neurology 30:84–88, 1980.
30. Fisher CM: Occlusion of the internal carotid artery. Arch Neurol Psychiat 69:346–377, 1951.
31. Fisher CM: Clinical syndromes in cerebral thrombosis, hypertensive hemorrhage, and ruptured saccular aneurysm. Clin Neurosurg 22:117–147, 1975.
32. Fisher CM: The natural history of carotid occlusion, in Austin GM (ed): *Microneurosurgical Anastomoses for Cerebral Ischemia*. Springfield, Illinois, Charles C Thomas 1976, pp 194–201.
33. Fisher CM, Dalal PM, Adams RD: Cerebrovascular disease and stroke syndrome. in Harrison TR, et al (ed): New York, McGraw-Hill, 1962.
34. Furlan AJ, Little JR, Dohn DF: Arterial occlusion following anastomosis of the superficial temporal artery to middle cerebral artery. Stroke 11:91–95, 1980.
35. Gee W, Oller DW, Wylie EJ: Non-invasive diagnosis of carotid occlusion by ocular pneumoplethysmography. Stroke 7:18–21, 1976.
36. Giannotta SL, Dicks RE III, Kindt GW: Carotid endarterectomy: technical improvements. Neurosurgery 7:309–312, 1980.
37. Ginsberg MD, Greenwood SA, Goldberg HI: Noninvasive diagnosis of extracranial cerebrovascular disease: Oculoplethysmography-phonoangiography and directional Doppler ultrasonography. Neurology 29:623–631, 1979.
38. Goldstein SJ, Fried AM, Young B, Tibbs PA: Limited usefulness of aortic arch angiography in the evaluation of carotid occlusive disease. Neurosci Res 2:559–564, 1981.
39. Goldstone J, Moore WS: Emergency carotid artery surgery in neurologically unstable patients. Arch Surg 111:1284–1291, 1976.
40. Goldstone J, Moore WS: A new look at emergency carotid artery operations for the treatment of cerebrovascular insufficiency: Current Concepts of Cerebrovascular Disease. Stroke 9:599–602, 1978.
41. Gompels BM: High definition imaging of carotid arteries using a standard commercial ultrasound "B" scanner. Br J Radiol 52:608, 1979.
42. Hafner CD, Tew JM: Surgical management of the totally occluded internal carotid artery: A ten-year study. Surgery 89:710–717, 1981.
43. Hugenholtz H, Elgie RG: Carotid thromboendarterectomy: A reappraisal. Criteria for patient selection. J. Neurosurg 53:776–783, 1980.
44. Kartchner MM, McRae LP: Noninvasive evaluation and management of the "asymptomatic" carotid bruit. Surgery 82:840–847, 1977.
45. Kistler JP, Lees RS, Friedman J, Pessin M, Mohr JP, Roberson GS, Ojemann RG: The bruit of carotid stenosis versus radiated basal heart murmurs: Differentiation by phonoangiography. Circulation 57:975–981, 1978.
46. Kistler JP, Lees RS, Miller A, Crowell RM, Roberson G: Correlation of spectral phonoangiography and carotid angiography with gross pathology in carotid stenosis. N Engl J Med 305:417–419, 1981.
47. Kroener JM, Dorn PL, Shoor PM, Wickbom IG, Bernstein EF: Prognosis of asymptomatic ulcerating carotid lesions. Arch Surg 115:1387–1392, 1980.
48. Kusunoki T, Rowed DW, Tator CH, Lougheed WM: Thromboendarterectomy for total occlusion of the internal carotid artery: A reappraisal of risks, success rate and potential benefits. Stroke 9:34–38, 1978.
49. Lees RS, Kistler JP: Carotid phonoangiography, in Bernstein EF (ed): *Noninvasive Diagnostic Techniques in Vascular Disease*. St. Louis, CV Mosby, 1978, pp 187–194.
50. Lippman HH, Sundt TM Jr, Holman CB: The post stenotic carotid slim sign; spurious internal carotid hypoplasia. Mayo Clin Proc 45:762–767, 1970.
51. Little JR, Furlan AJ, Modic MT, Bryerton B, Weinstein MA: Intravenous digital subtraction angiography: Application to cerebrovascular surgery. Neurosurgery 9:129–136, 1981.
52. McNamara JO, Heyman A, Silver D, Mandel ME: The value of carotid endarterectomy in treating transient cerebral ischemia

of the posterior circulation. Neurology 27:682–684, 1977.
53. Maroon JC, Campbell RL, Dyken ML: Internal carotid artery occlusion diagnosed by Doppler ultrasound. Stroke 1:122–127, 1970.
54. Mentzer RM Jr, Finkelmeier BA, Crosby IK, Welions HA Jr: Emergency carotid endarterectomy for fluctuating neurologic deficits. Surgery 89:60–66, 1981.
55. Mohr JP, Caplan LR, Milski JM, Goldstein RJ, Duncan GW, Kistler JP, Pessin MS, Bleich HL: The Harvard cooperative stroke registry: A prospective registry. Neurology 28:754–762, 1978.
56. Moore WS, Malone JM, Boren C, Roon AJ, Goldstone J: Asymptomatic ulcerative lesions of the carotid artery: natural history and effect of surgical therapy compared. Stroke 10:96, 1979.
57. Najafi H, Javid H, Dye WS, Hunter JA, Wideman FE, Julian OC: Emergency carotid thromboendarterectomy. Arch Surg 103:610–613, 1971.
58. Norton GA, Kishore PRS, Lin J: CT contrast enhancement in cerebral infraction. Am J Roentgenol 131:881–885, 1978.
59. Ojemann RG: Comment on paper. Little JR, Sawhyn B, Weinstein M: Pseudo-tandem stenosis of the internal carotid artery. Neurosurgery 7:577, 1980.
60. Ojemann RG, Crowell RM, Roberson GH, Fisher CM: Surgical treatment of extracranial carotid occlusive disease. Clin Neurosurg 22:214–263, 1975.
61. Ott DA, Cooley DA, Chapa L, Coelho A: Carotid endarterectomy without temporary intraluminal shunt. Arch Surg 191:708–714, 1980.
62. Patterson RH Jr: Risk of carotid surgery with occlusion of the contralateral carotid artery. Arch Neurol 30:188–189, 1974.
63. Pessin MS, Duncan GW, Mohr JP, Poskanzer DC: Clinical and angiographic features of carotid transient ischemic attacks. N Engl J Med 296:358–362, 1977.
64. Pessin MS, Hinton RC, Davis KR, Duncan GW, Roberson GH, Ackerman RH, Mohr JP: Mechanisms of acute carotid stroke. Ann Neurol 6:245–252, 1979.
65. Pessin MS, Duncan GW, Davis KR, Hinton RC, Roberson GH, Mohr JP: Angiographic appearance of carotid occlusion in acute stroke. Stroke 11:485–487, 1980.
66. Phillips MR, Johnson WC, Scott RM, Vollman RW, Levine H, Nabseth DC: Carotid endarterectomy in the presence of contralateral carotid occlusion. The role of EEG and intraluminal shunting. Arch Surg 114:1232–1239, 1979.
67. Podore PC, Rob CG, DeWeese JA, Green RM: Chronic common carotid occlusion. Stroke 12:98–100, 1981.
68. Rengachary SS, Batnitzky S, Morantz RA, Arjunan K, Jeffries B: Hemicraniectomy for acute massive cerebral infarction. Neurosurgery 8:321–328, 1981.
69. Sandok BA: Non-invasive techniques for diagnosis of carotid artery disease. Stroke 9:427–429, 1978.
70. Shucart WA, Garrido E: Reopening some occluded carotid arteries. J Neurosurg 45:442–446, 1976.
71. Stern J, Correll JW, Bryan N: Persistent hypoglossal artery and persistent trigeminal artery presenting with posterior fossa transient ischemic attacks. Report of two cases. J Neurosurg, 49:614–619, 1978.
72. Stern J, Whelan M, Brisman R, Correll JW: Management of extracranial carotid stenosis and intracranial aneurysm. J Neurosurg 51:147–150, 1979.
73. Strother CM, Sackett JF, Crummy AB, Lilleas FG, Swiebel WJ, Turnipseed WD, Javid M, Mistretta CA, Kruger RA, Ergun DL, Shaw CG: Clinical applications of computerized fluoroscopy. Radiology 136:781–783, 1980.
74. Sundt TM Jr, Sandok BA, Whisnant JP: Carotid endarterectomy. Complications and preoperative assessment of risk. Mayo Clin Proc 50:301–306, 1975.
75. Sundt TM Jr, Sharbrough FW, Piepgras DG, Kearns TP, Messick JM Jr, O'Fallon WM: Correlation of cerebral blood flow and electroencephalographic changes during carotid endarterectomy. With results of surgery and hemodynamics of cerebral ischemia. Mayo Clin Proc 56:533–543, 1981.
76. Thompson JE, Garrett WV: Peripheral arterial surgery. N Engl J Med 302:491–503, 1980.
77. Wall SD, Brant-Zawadzki M, Jeffrey RB, Barnes B: High frequency CT findings within 24 hours after cerebral infarction. Am J Neuroradiol 2:553–557, 1981.
78. White DN, Curry GR: Color-coded Differential Doppler ultrasonic scanning system for the carotid bifurcation: Results on 486 bifurcations angiographically confirmed. Excerpta Medica, Amsterdam, 1978, pp 238–249.
79. Wing SD, Norman D, Pollock JA, Newton TH: Contrast enhancement of cerebral infarcts in computed tomography. Radiology 121:89–92, 1976.

Chapter 2 CAROTID ENDARTERECTOMY

PREOPERATIVE EVALUATION

Many patients with carotid atherosclerosis have significant medical risk factors. These include the presence of symptomatic coronary artery disease, myocardial infarction within 6 months, severe peripheral arterial disease, rheumatic heart disease, congestive heart failure, severe hypertension (blood pressure more than 180/110 mm Hg), chronic obstructive pulmonary disease, diabetes, hyperlipidemia, and obesity. Previous publications have documented that the operative risks are higher in these patients (12, 36). In one report involving patients who were neurologically stable but had significant medical risk factors, the morbidity and mortality rate was 7%, primarily related to cardiac disease (36).

All patients who are being considered for operation for carotid occlusive disease are evaluated with a complete blood count, blood sugar, blood urea nitrogen, serum electrolytes, clotting studies (prothrombin time (PT), partial thromboplastin time (PTT), and platelet count), electrocardiogram (ECG), and chest x-ray. Blood cholesterol and triglycerides are also checked.

When there is a question about cardiac reserve, treadmill ECG test is indicated. Inability to adequately perform this test is a relative contraindication to surgery. A history of myocardial infarction within 6 months or evidence of overt left ventricular failure are contraindications to the exercise stress testing and strong but not absolute contraindications to surgery. Preoperative pulmonary function tests are obtained in patients with pulmonary dysfunction.

Many patients will be on several drugs for treatment of the diseases noted above. In general these drugs are continued. Patients receiving diuretic medication should have serum potassium checked prior to operation and any deficiency should be treated. It is important that severe hypertension be treated since the incidence of postoperative hypertension and morbidity is higher in this group (41). This is particularly true for those patients who have an associated cerebral infarction and are at risk to develop a cerebral hemorrhage (5).

Indications for intraoperative monitoring with a pulmonary artery catheter include failed treadmill ECG or stress test, left ventricular failure, a recent myocardial infarction, severe mitral valvular disease, and persistent angina after a coronary artery bypass. Patients with symptomatic heart block undergo placement of a temporary intravenous pacer.

In a group of over 400 carotid endarterectomies, we found 86 patients who were judged to have evidence of increased cardiopulmonary risk (9a). They underwent 95 endarterectomies. Coronary artery disease was the most common risk factor being present in 72 patients, with previous coronary bypass surgery in five, serious arrhythmias in two, and previous cardiac arrest during anesthetic induction in one. The other risk factors were chronic obstructive pulmonary disease in nine and rheumatic valvular disease in five patients. Recognition of these factors, careful preoperative evaluation and preparation, an experienced anesthesia team, and well-staffed intensive care unit have made it possible to keep the morbidity and mortality low in this group (about 4%).

Several reports indicate that patients who have symptomatic carotid stenosis, as well as severe coronary artery disease, and who are candidates for myocardial revascularization, should have both operations done under the same anesthesia to reduce the risk of coronary occlusion (12, 32). In one report, it was found that the perioperative mortality up to 30 days after operation was 1.5% in 1306 consecutive endarterectomies done in 1026 patients without symptomatic coronary artery disease (12). Those patients with significant cardiac symptoms were divided into two groups. In one, 85 carotid endarterectomies performed in 77 patients without prior coronary by-pass operation had a perioperative mortality of 18.2%. In the other group, 155 operations in 135 patients who were treated with either prior coronary artery by-pass (84 patients) or simultaneous carotid endarterectomy and coronary artery bypass (51 patients) had an operative mortality of only 3%. However, if the carotid stenosis or occlusion is asymptomatic in a patient who is to have coronary or peripheral arterial reconstruction, there is reported to be no increased risk of stroke, and prophylactic or simultaneous carotid endarterectomy is usually not indicated (1, 6, 13, 42, 43).

ANESTHETIC MANAGEMENT

Preoperative medication is kept to a minimum because of the fragile cardiovascular state of many of these patients. We prefer general endotracheal anesthesia. This technique provides good airway control, maintenance of normal arterial blood gases, maximum patient comfort, optimal surgical exposure, and some protection against cerebral ischemia.

As soon as the patient arrives in the operating

room, blood pressure is recorded, a peripheral intravenous (IV) infusion is started, and an intra-arterial cannula is inserted percutaneously into the radial artery for direct blood pressure recording and for blood gas measurement. If there is any indication of low blood volume or hypotension, central venous pressure (CVP) is recorded and the patient is given fluid or colloid to raise the CVP to 8–10 cm of water. A vasopressor IV infusion is prepared, usually with 10 mg of phenylephrine hydrochloride in 250 ml of saline, and administered as needed through a pediatric microdrop set to maintain an adequate blood pressure. Electroencephalogram (EEG) electrodes are attached to the scalp and ECG leads are placed. All patients receive prophylactic antibiotics.

After preoxygenation, the anesthesia is induced slowly during continuous monitoring of BP, ECG, and EEG. We aim for smooth induction, light levels of anesthesia, and rapid emergence to permit prompt assessment of the postoperative neurological status. The two major anesthetic combinations used are: 1) narcotic and muscle relaxant plus nitrous oxide and oxygen, and 2) halothane plus nitrous oxide and oxygen. During the procedure, arterial blood gas measurements are done frequently to assure adequate ventilation and to maintain the arterial pCO_2 in the range of 36–40 mm/Hg. Blood replacement is usually not necessary. Of major importance for successful results is a team approach to the surgical and anesthetic management of these cases.

When monitoring with a pulmonary artery catheter is indicated, critical information for blood and drug management is provided. A slow infusion of nitroglycerin (1 μg/kg/min as a solution of 30 mg/250 ml normal saline) is used in many patients with stable angina. Nitroglycerine generally reverses ST segment elevation and any increase in pulmonary artery pressure.

BRAIN PROTECTION AND MONITORING

The best method of maintaining adequate cerebral circulation during the operation is to combine the benefits of general anesthesia with the maintenence of adequate blood volume and a normal or slightly elevated arterial pressure. At the time of carotid clamping for the endarterectomy, the arterial pressure is elevated to an average systolic level of 170 mm mercury (Hg) if there is no cardiac contraindication. In the normal brain, constant cerebral blood flow is maintained by autoregulation over a wide range of arterial pressures. However, in areas of focal cerebral ischemia, autoregulation of blood flow may be lost and flow becomes passively dependent on the perfusion pressure and blood volume.

The most effective method of monitoring the intracranial circulation during the time of clamping for the carotid endarterectomy is continuous EEG recording with a full set of leads from both sides of the head (4, 7, 9, 26, 29, 34). If the EEG shows minor slowing and/or a slight decrease in voltage, usually nothing needs to be done. The surgeon must check and be sure the BP is being maintained over 170 mm Hg if there is no cardiac contraindication. In most patients with significant EEG abnormality, the change occurs soon after the arteries are occluded and comes on over a period a few seconds to less than a minute (Fig. 2.1). When this occurs, a shunt should be placed promptly (see page 43).

A high degree of correlation has been found between cerebral blood flow measurements during carotid occlusion and changes in the EEG (34, 38). The critical cerebral blood flow (flow required to maintain a normal EEG) was approximately 30% (15 ml/100 gm per min) of normal flow (50 ml/100 gm per min). The degree of EEG change reflected the severity of flow reduction. This change was reversed with placement of a shunt which was done if the flow was less than 18 to 20 ml/100 gm per min. Our clinical experience confirms these findings. In a consecutive series of 173 elective operations for carotid stenosis, 10 patients showed a significant change in EEG tracing at some point following carotid occlusion (29). In four, further elevations of blood pressure resulted in improvement in the EEG, but six patients required a shunt. All 10 patients recovered with no neurological deficit. The EEG will not tell you if an embolus has occluded a perforating artery, but it will tell you if the hemisphere needs more blood. Other methods have been advocated for monitoring, including measurement of stump pressure and sampling of jugular venous pCO_2, but these tests have not been reliable (24, 29).

The question of whether a temporary shunt is indicated during carotid endarterectomy has been the subject of several articles. Some surgeons routinely use a shunt for cerebral protection (16, 19, 40, 41, 44). Other surgeons report that a shunt is not needed and some believe monitoring is not necessary (3, 14, 30). Still others use a shunt when monitoring indicates a need for it (29, 37). The use of a shunt carries with it a possible risk of embolization and injury to the distal intima, although we have not seen this, and it does make the technical removal of the distal end of the plaque in the internal carotid artery a little more difficult. But we should ask, "Why take any chance?" Everything should be done to reduce the morbidity of the operation to as low a level as possible. Every patient should be monitored. In only a small percentage of patients will a shunt be needed, but when it is indicated, it should be used.

In some patients the surgeon will know preoperatively that a shunt will be needed. These include patients where the vertebrobasilar circulation depends on the carotid artery (Fig. 1.21) or where there are multiple occlusions of major extracranial vessels. It should also be remembered that one can stop the operation if circumstances warrant. Such would be the case when the EEG changes are severe and a

Carotid Endarterectomy

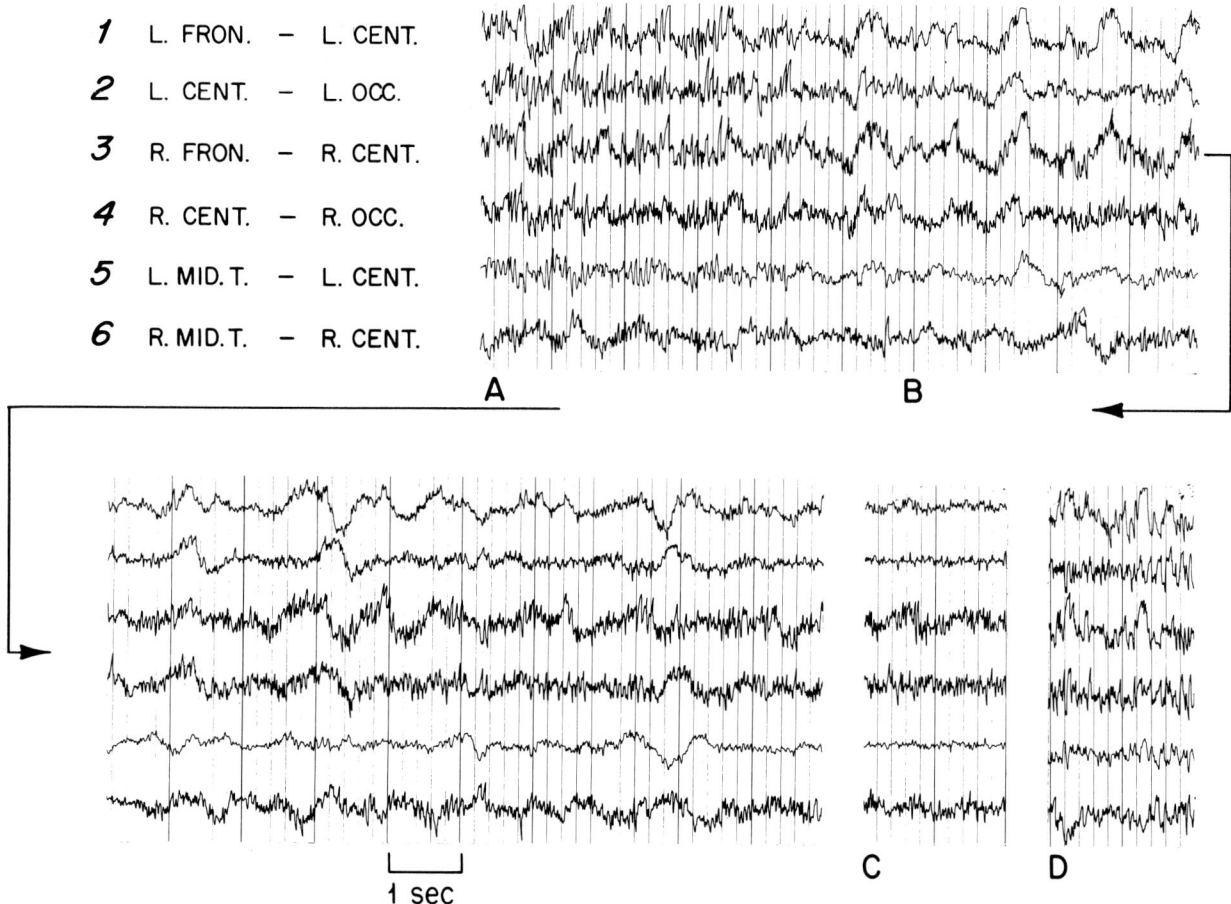

Figure 2.1 EEG recording during carotid endarterectomy. At (*A*), the carotid circulation is occluded. BP is 170–180 mm Hg systolic. By 6 seconds (*B*), definite slowing and reduced voltage are noted in the left side recordings (*lines 1, 2,* and *5*). The changes are more pronounced over the next several seconds. At one minute (*C*), the left mid-temporal to central tracing is almost flat (*line 5*). One minute after insertion of the shunt, a normal record is restored (*D*).

shunt is technically difficult to place because of tortuosity or other reason. In such patients, medical therapy can be reassessed and a bypass operation considered.

OPERATIVE TECHNIQUE

Since the original report of our operative approach, we have gradually revised and refined the technique (9, 29). The patient is placed in the supine position with a thyroid bag inflated under the shoulders. The head is slightly extended and turned away from the side of the operation. The entire operation is done using a headlight and magnifying loupes.

Figure 2.2 outlines the setup in the operating room for a left carotid endarterectomy. The important points to note are: 1) the nurse stands directly opposite the surgeon, 2) the EEG is where the surgeon can see the tracing if necessary, and 3) the anesthesiologist has full access to the head and right arm.

It is important to mark the incision beginning along the anterior border of the sternocleidomastoid muscle. Just below the level of the angle of the jaw the incision should be curved over the muscle posteriorly and superiorly toward the mastoid process (Fig. 2.3A). This will allow maximum exposure to the base of the skull beneath the parotid gland and helps avoid retraction on the lower branch of the facial nerve near the angle of the jaw.

After the skin incision is made, the platysma is incised. The external jugular vein is ligated, small transverse cervical nerves divided, and the great auricular nerve identified at the upper end of the exposure (Fig. 2.3B). This nerve, which usually crosses the upper portion of the incision just beneath the platysma muscle, is preserved, if possible, thus avoiding unpleasant numbness of the ear.

Dissection is continued along the anterior border of the sternocleidomastoid muscle (Fig. 2.4). Self-retaining retractors are used to aid the exposure. The medial blades must be kept on the subcutaneous tissue and platysma. If they are placed too deeply against the paratracheal muscles, the recurrent laryngeal nerve may be injured.

The internal jugular vein is identified just medial

32 Surgical Management of Cerebrovascular Disease

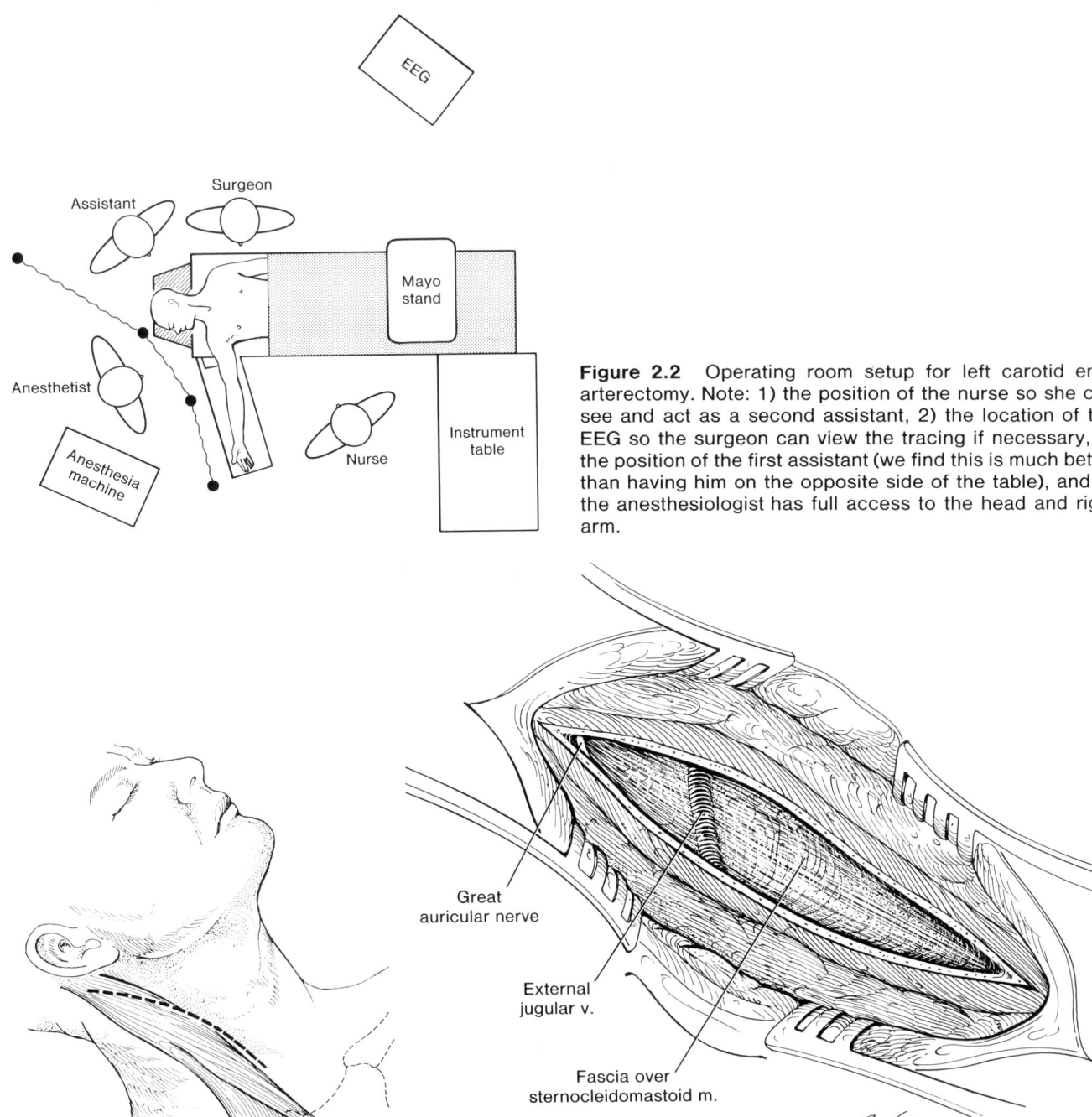

Figure 2.2 Operating room setup for left carotid endarterectomy. Note: 1) the position of the nurse so she can see and act as a second assistant, 2) the location of the EEG so the surgeon can view the tracing if necessary, 3) the position of the first assistant (we find this is much better than having him on the opposite side of the table), and 4) the anesthesiologist has full access to the head and right arm.

Figure 2.3 Carotid endarterectomy. Skin incision and initial exposure. A, note that the upper end of the incision curves over the sternomastoid muscle toward the mastoid process. B, the skin incision has been made and the platysma incised in line with the anterior border of the sternocleidomastoid muscle.

Carotid Endarterectomy

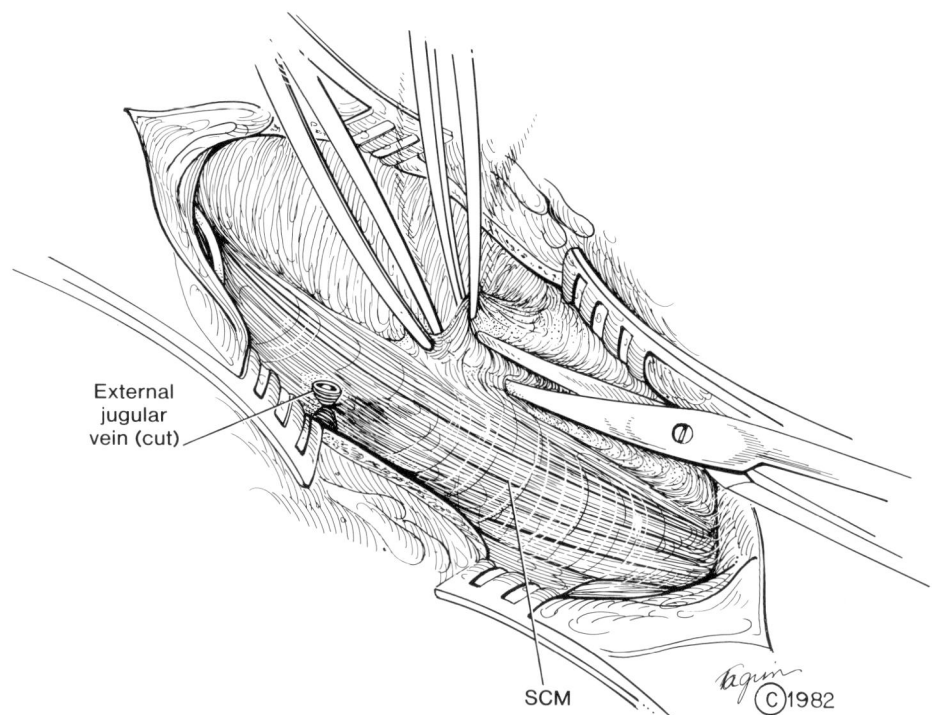

Figure 2.4 Carotid endarterectomy. Opening of fascia along anterior border of sternocleidomastoid muscle.

and deep to the sternocleidomastoid muscle (Fig. 2.5). The dissection then extends along the medial border of the internal jugular vein, ligating medial draining branches as necessary. The most prominent of these is usually the common facial vein. The descendens hypoglossi nerve is often seen in the tissue just medial to the internal jugular vein and overlying the common carotid artery. This nerve is reflected medially.

The common carotid artery is exposed medial to the internal jugular vein in the lower part of the incision (Fig. 2.6). A tape is placed around this vessel which maintains its exposure and facilitates the further dissection. On rare occasions, the vagus nerve lies anteriorly on the common carotid artery and one must be alert for this possibility.

The dissection is then extended superiorly along the medial border of the internal jugular vein (Fig. 2.7). The descendens hypoglossi nerve is kept medially and leads one to the hypoglossal nerve, which may swing low into the neck across the carotid bifurcation or lie high beneath the edge of the posterior belly of the digastric muscle. Often it lies just beneath the common facial vein and may be adherent to this vessel. In some patients, nerve branches will come around the lateral side of the common carotid artery to enter the descendens hypoglossi nerve. Usually these branches are from the cervical plexus, but on rare occasion they seem to come from the vagus nerve. In most cases, they can be divided to allow the descendens hypoglossi nerve to be reflected medially. However, if the branch is large or is coming from the vagus nerve, the descendens hypoglossi nerve is divided close to the hypoglossal nerve and the branch from the vagus nerve is reflected laterally.

To give adequate exposure, it may be necessary to remove a group of lymph nodes which are commonly present over the region of the carotid bifurcation. When the carotid bifurcation is exposed, the region of the carotid sinus is blocked with lidocaine hydrochloride to avoid hypotension and carotid sinus reflex bradycardia (Fig. 2.7). Care is taken to leave the region of the distal common carotid artery, carotid bifurcation, and proximal internal carotid artery adherent to the posterior tissue. This avoids undue manipulation of the area reducing the possibility of dislodging an embolus, lessening the chance of carotid sinus stimulation, and avoiding possible injury to the superior laryngeal nerve.

The distal internal carotid artery is carefully exposed staying in the tissue plane between the hypoglossal nerve or descendens hypoglossi nerve medially and the internal jugular vein laterally (Fig. 2.8). If one follows these guidelines, the distal internal carotid artery can be nicely exposed. As the hypoglossal nerve swings medially, an arterial branch often comes across the inner side of the curve of the nerve and passes posteriorly. This fairly constant sternocleidomastoid artery, often accompanied by a vein, is ligated. The hypoglossal nerve and, if necessary, the descendens hypoglossi nerve are gently reflected medially with a soft rubber band tape. If the carotid bifurcation is located high in the neck,

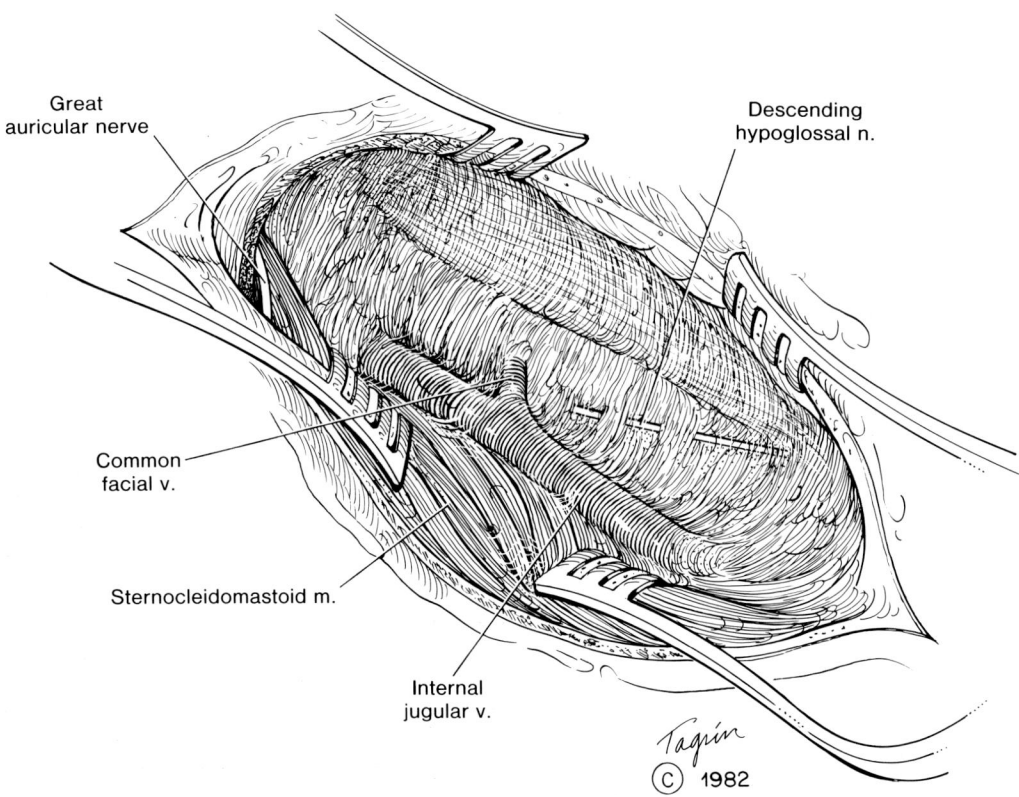

Figure 2.5 Carotid endarterectomy. The anterior border of the SCM muscle has been retracted laterally and the anterior and medial aspect of the internal jugular vein brought into view.

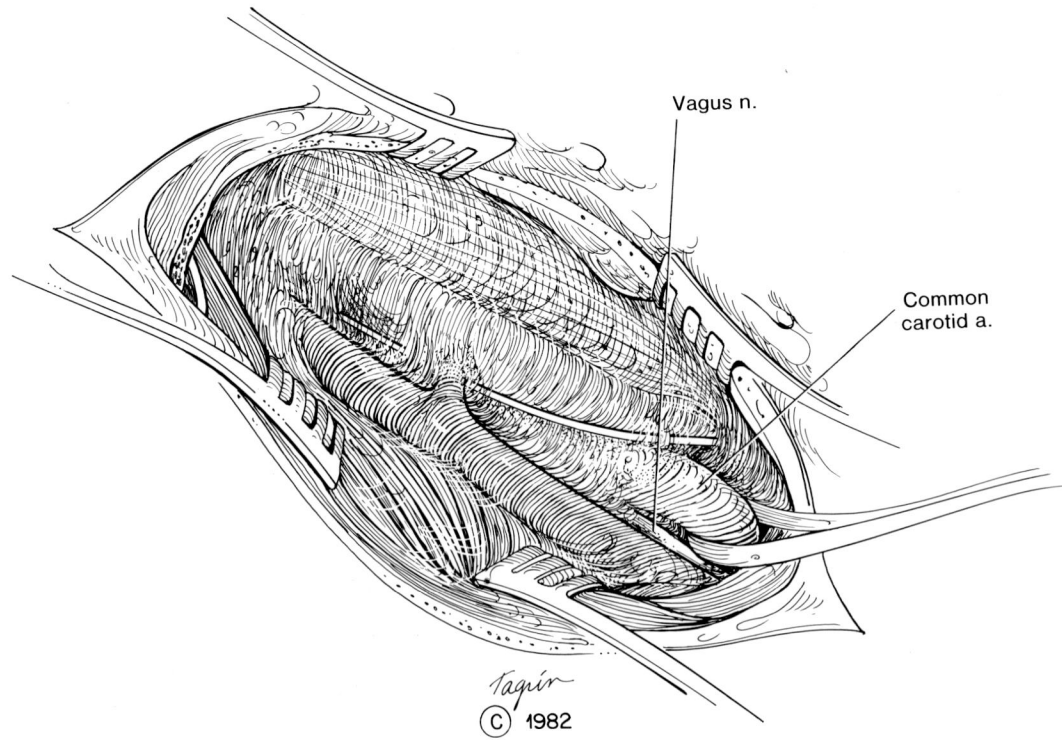

Figure 2.6 Carotid endarterectomy. The proximal common carotid is exposed and a tape passed around it.

Carotid Endarterectomy

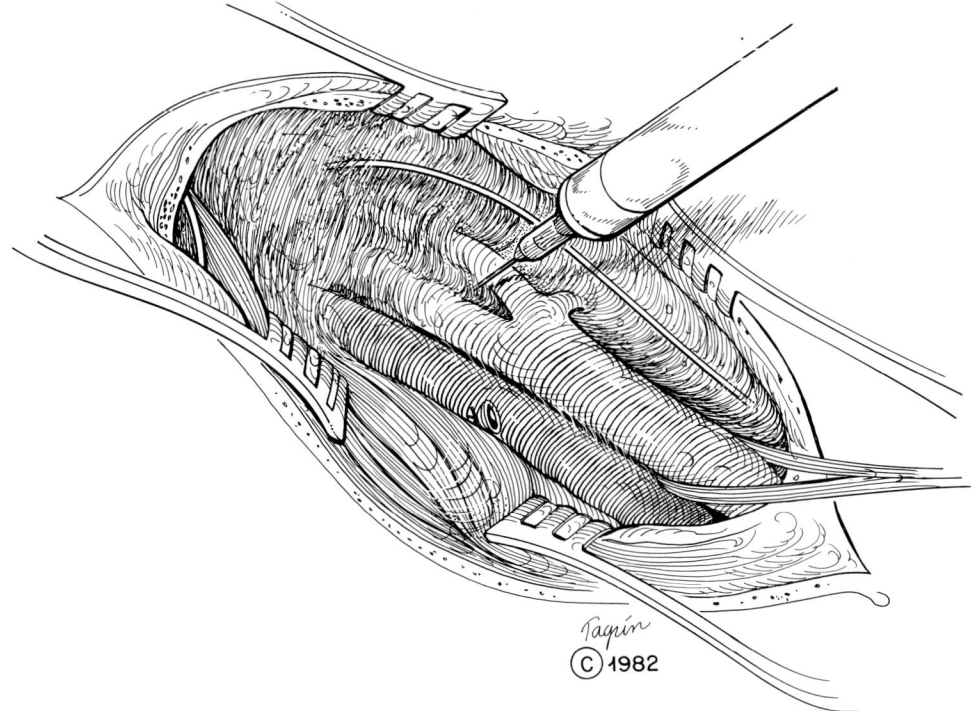

Figure 2.7 Carotid endarterectomy. The bifurcation of the common carotid artery has been exposed by staying along the medial border of the internal jugular vein and reflecting the descending hypoglossal nerve medially. The region of the carotid sinus is blocked with lidocaine hydrochloride.

dissection is carried along the medial border of the internal jugular vein and beneath the parotid gland. It may be necessary to retract the posterior belly of the digastric muscle. Rarely will it need to be divided. On occasion, the occipital artery must be divided to free the hypoglossal nerve in order to expose the distal internal carotid artery.

The superior thyroid artery is identified on the medial wall of the distal common or proximal external carotid artery and a tape placed around it (Fig. 2.9). The external carotid artery is exposed to the level of the first major branching of this vessel and a tape placed at this point. If the angiogram shows an ascending pharyngeal artery coming off the region of the bifurcation, this will have to be separately exposed and controlled. The exposure of the distal internal carotid artery is carried to a point at least one centimeter above the distal end of the plaque. In the many patients, the atheromatous plaque extends several millimeters further up the posterior wall of the internal carotid artery than it does the anterior wall. Great care is taken in exposing this vessel to avoid any undue pressure or manipulation of the artery. The vagus nerve may be closely adherent to the posterior wall of the artery; occasionally it will be lateral or anterior to the artery. It must be carefully dissected free before placing the tape around the vessel. A second tape is placed around the common carotid artery several millimeters distal to the original tape, and tourniquets are placed on this tape, as well as on the internal carotid artery tape in case a shunt is needed.

When hemostasis has been obtained, the patient is given an intravenous bolus of 7000 units of heparin. If the blood pressure is not already elevated with the anesthetic technique being used, a phenylepherine hydrochloride drip may be necessary to raise the blood pressure to at least 170 mm Hg systolic. The EEG is monitored continuously. The surgeon should check to be sure that the shunt tubing is available (see page 43).

The common carotid artery is then occluded with an appropriate vascular clamp being careful to avoid injury to the underlying vagus nerve (Fig. 2.10). We prefer to use medium and long straight Heifetz aneurysm clips to occlude the other arteries, but on occasion a large internal or external carotid artery will require the use of a small bulldog clamp. Because of its size, it is advantageous to use the Heifetz clip on the internal carotid artery for it can be placed several millimeters more distally on the artery. Care must also be taken to avoid injury to the vagus nerve at this point because it lies in the tissue just behind the internal carotid artery. The clip on the external carotid artery is placed as far distally as possible, usually at or just below the first major bifurcation.

A longitudinal incision is made in the distal common carotid artery with a #15 knife blade (Fig. 2.11). The incision is carried through the wall of the artery until the shiny yellow surface of the atheromatous

36   Surgical Management of Cerebrovascular Disease

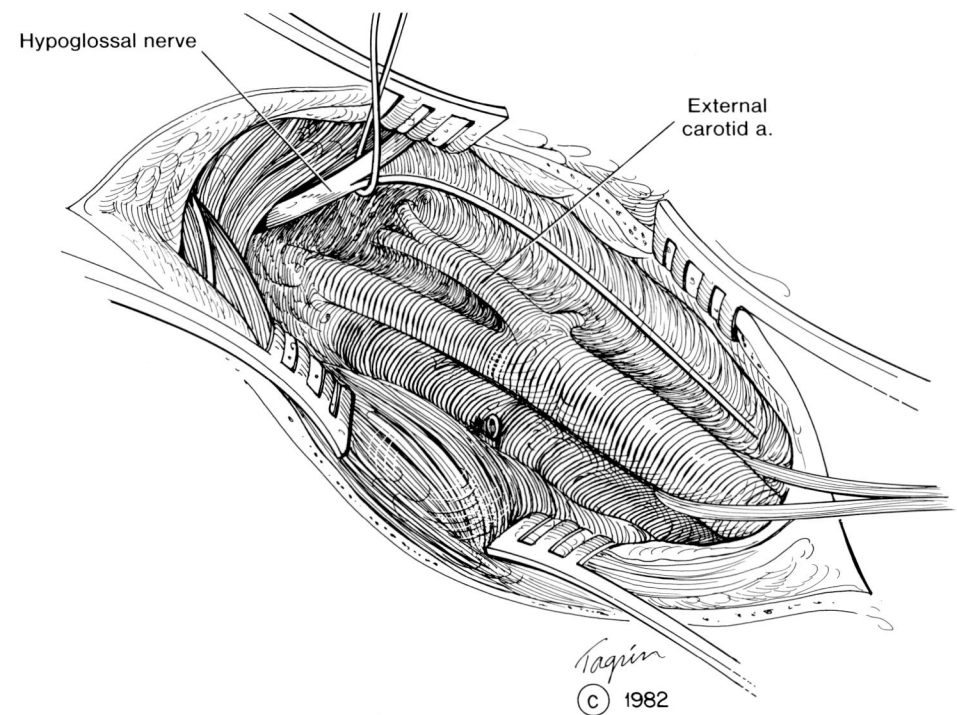

Figure 2.8   Carotid endarterectomy. The internal carotid, external carotid, and superior thyroid arteries have been isolated.

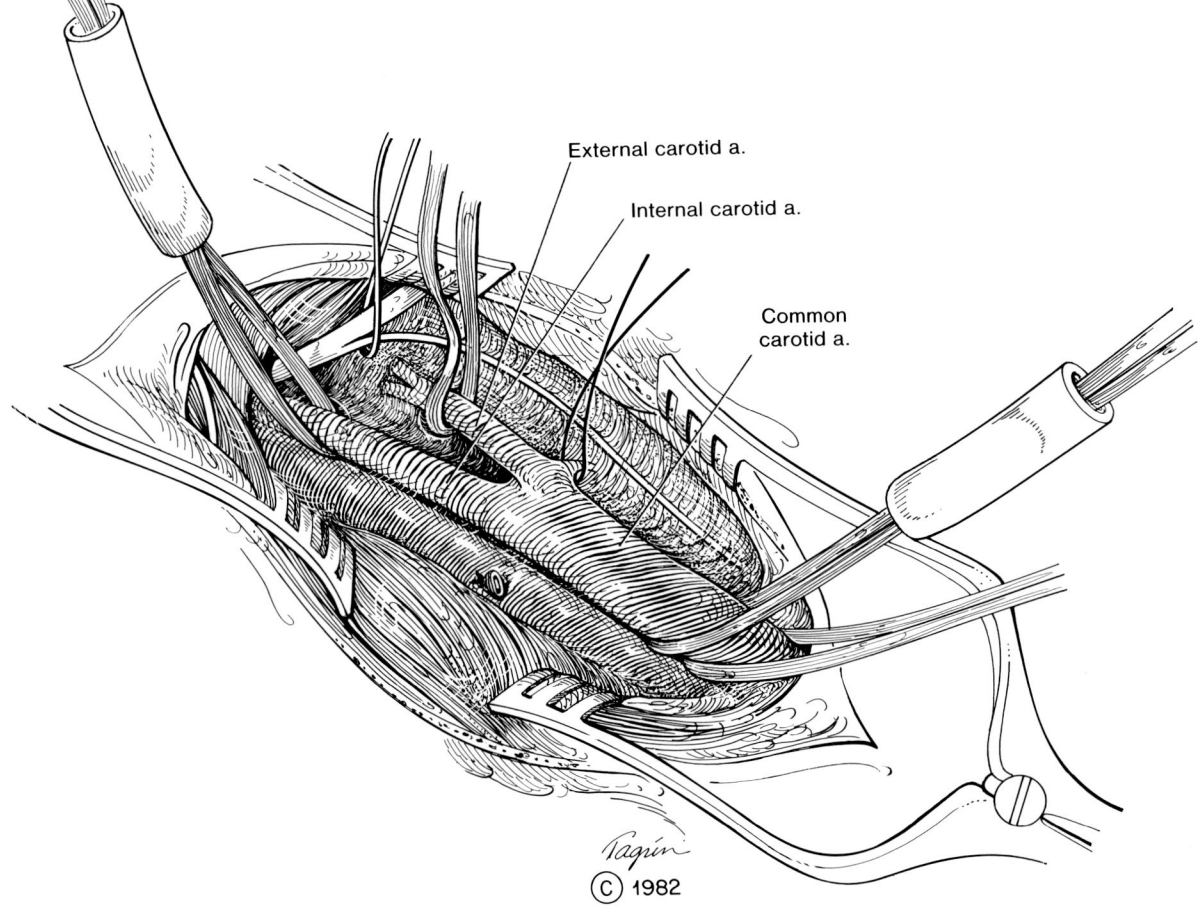

Figure 2.9   Carotid endarterectomy. Appropriate tapes and tourniquets have been placed.

Carotid Endarterectomy

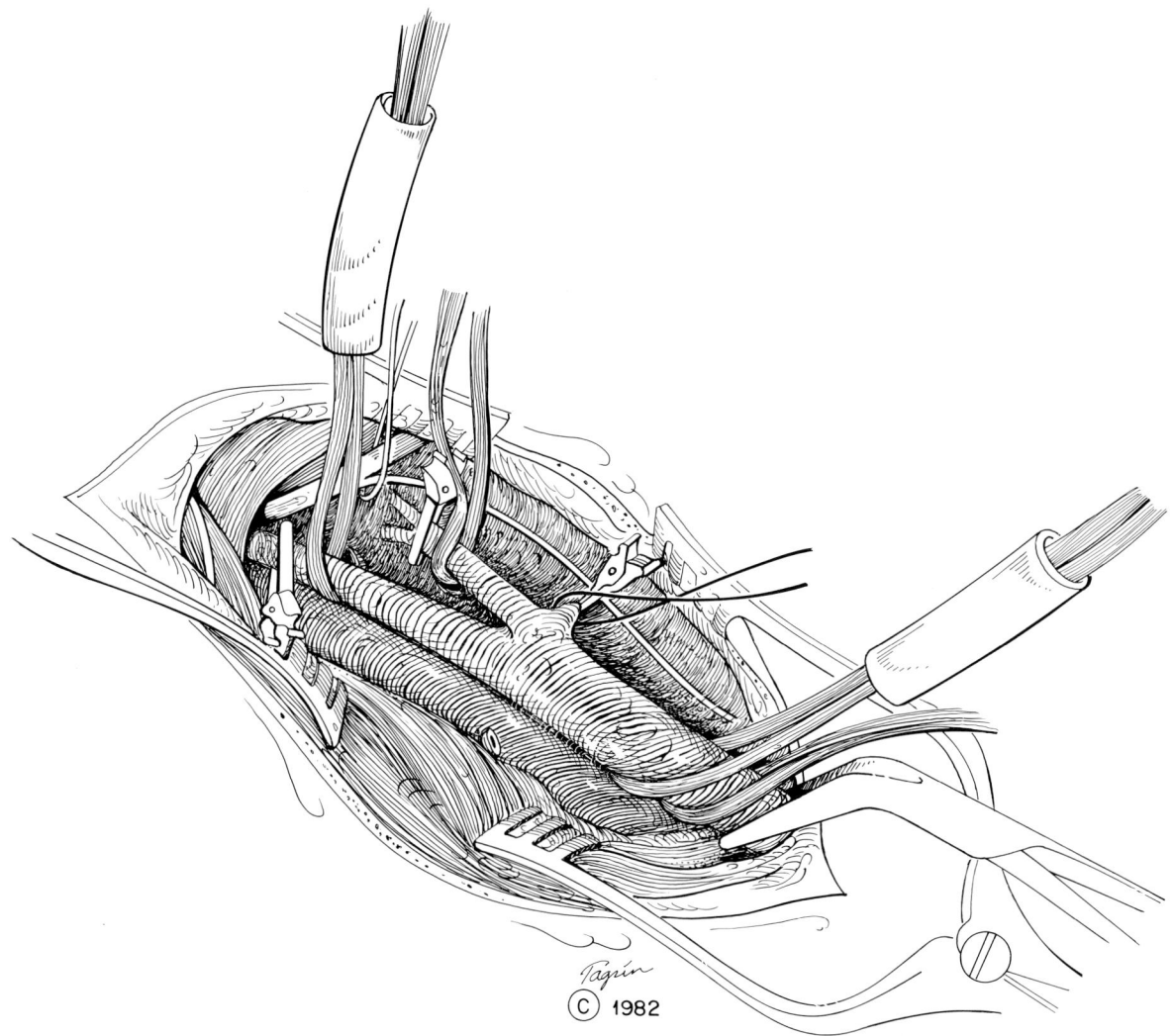

Figure 2.10 Carotid endarterectomy. The circulation has been occluded. Heifetz clips are used on the distal vessels when possible.

plaque is seen. A Penfield #4 dissector is then used to separate the plane between the atheroma and outer arterial wall (Fig. 2.12). Often the atheroma is adherent to a relatively thin outer wall at the bifurcation. It is best to separate the plaque for a few millimeters and then extend the incision with Potts scissors before attempting further dissection (Fig. 2.13). The distal end of the incision extends up the internal carotid artery to approximately the distal end of the plaque. The proximal extent of the incision can be estimated from the angiogram. The incision usually does not need to be more than 1–2 cm below the bifurcation. A thin layer of atheromatous plaque will usually extend proximally in the common carotid artery and does not need to be of concern as long as one is proximal to the stenosis.

The atheromatous plaque is then carefully separated from the outer arterial wall in the common carotid artery with a Penfield dissector. A right angled clamp is placed around the plaque and the plaque is cut off sharply at the proximal end of the arteriotomy in the common carotid artery with a #15 knife blade (Fig. 2.14). If the cut across the plaque reveals a residual area of stenosis, the incision is extended as far proximal as is necessary. The plaque is kept intact and is removed first from the origin of the superior thyroid artery and the proximal external carotid artery (Fig. 2.15). In some patients it is necessary to temporarily open the clamp on the external carotid artery to remove the plaque which may extend quite far distally. Once this removal has been accomplished, the atheroma is carefully dissected from the outer wall of the internal carotid artery which, on occasion, may be exceedingly thin. Usually there is a very clean dissection plane. Great care is taken as the distal end of the plaque is reached. With gentle traction on the intact plaque, the wall of the internal carotid artery can be slightly everted and the dissection carried distally pushing the media away from the plaque until normal intima is reached (Fig.

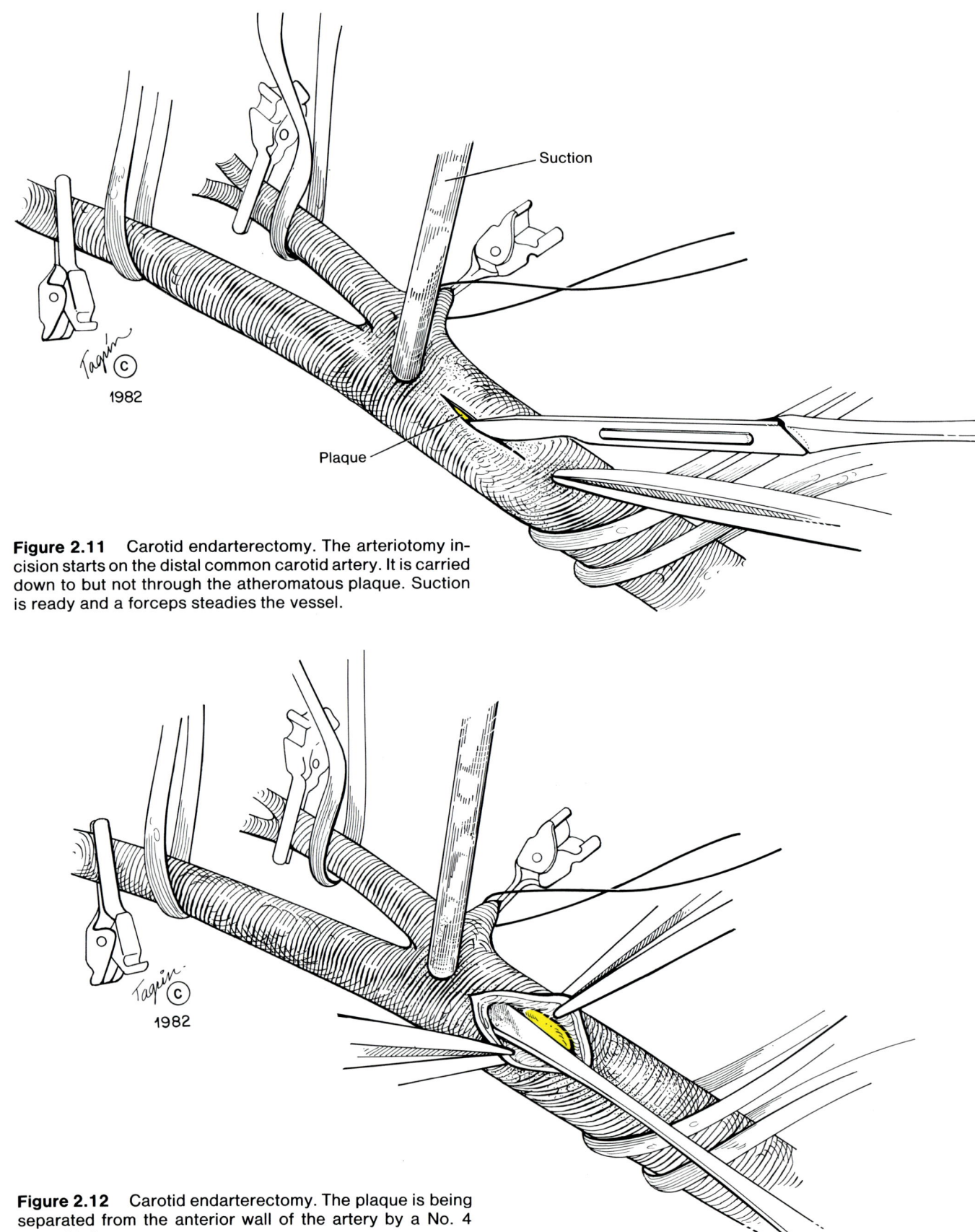

Figure 2.11 Carotid endarterectomy. The arteriotomy incision starts on the distal common carotid artery. It is carried down to but not through the atheromatous plaque. Suction is ready and a forceps steadies the vessel.

Figure 2.12 Carotid endarterectomy. The plaque is being separated from the anterior wall of the artery by a No. 4 Penfield dissector.

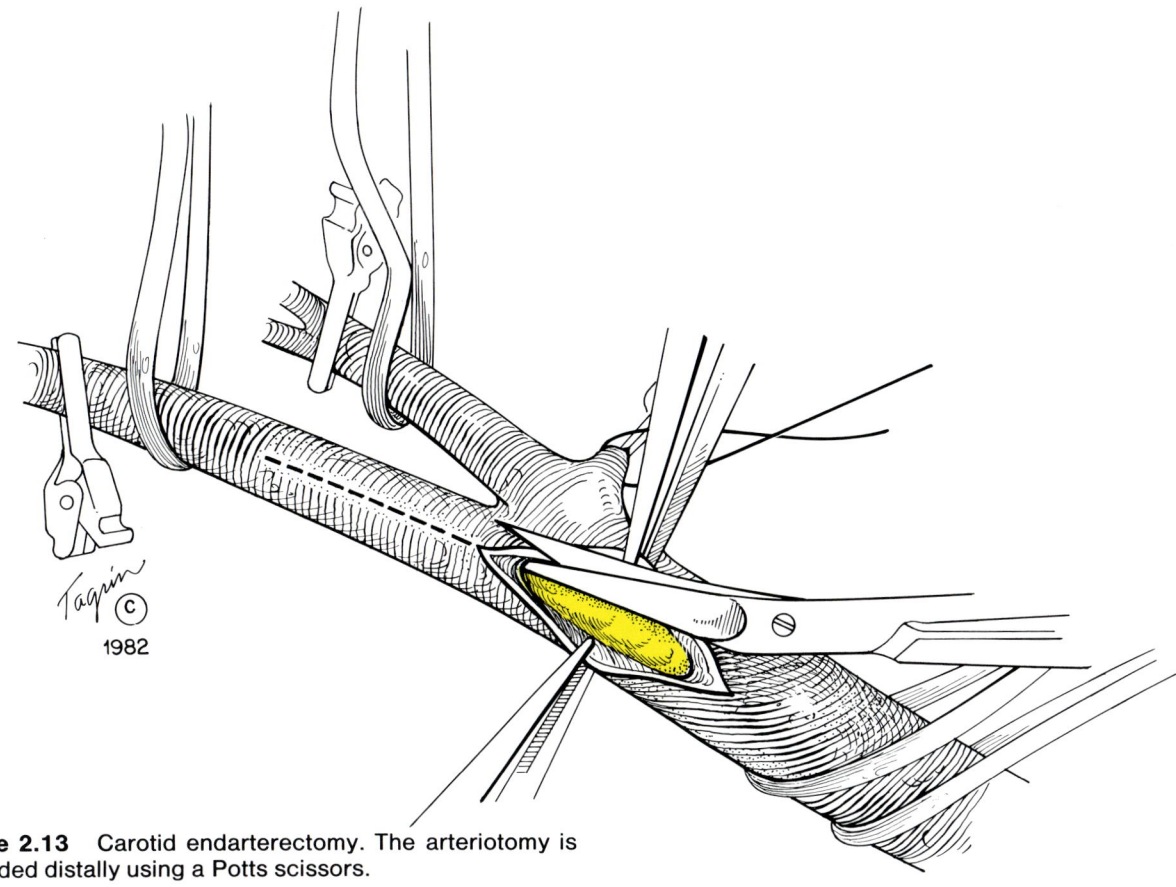

Figure 2.13 Carotid endarterectomy. The arteriotomy is extended distally using a Potts scissors.

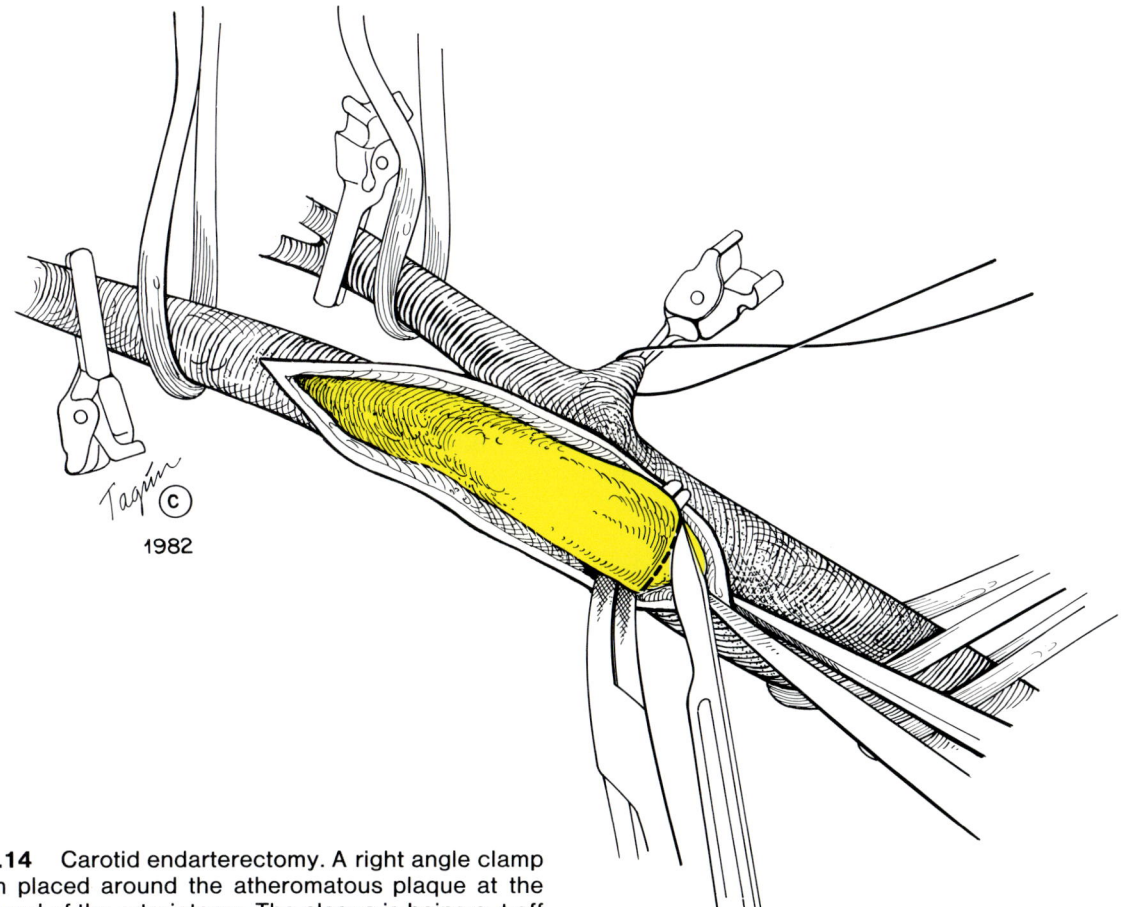

Figure 2.14 Carotid endarterectomy. A right angle clamp has been placed around the atheromatous plaque at the proximal end of the arteriotomy. The plaque is being cut off sharply with a No. 15 knife blade.

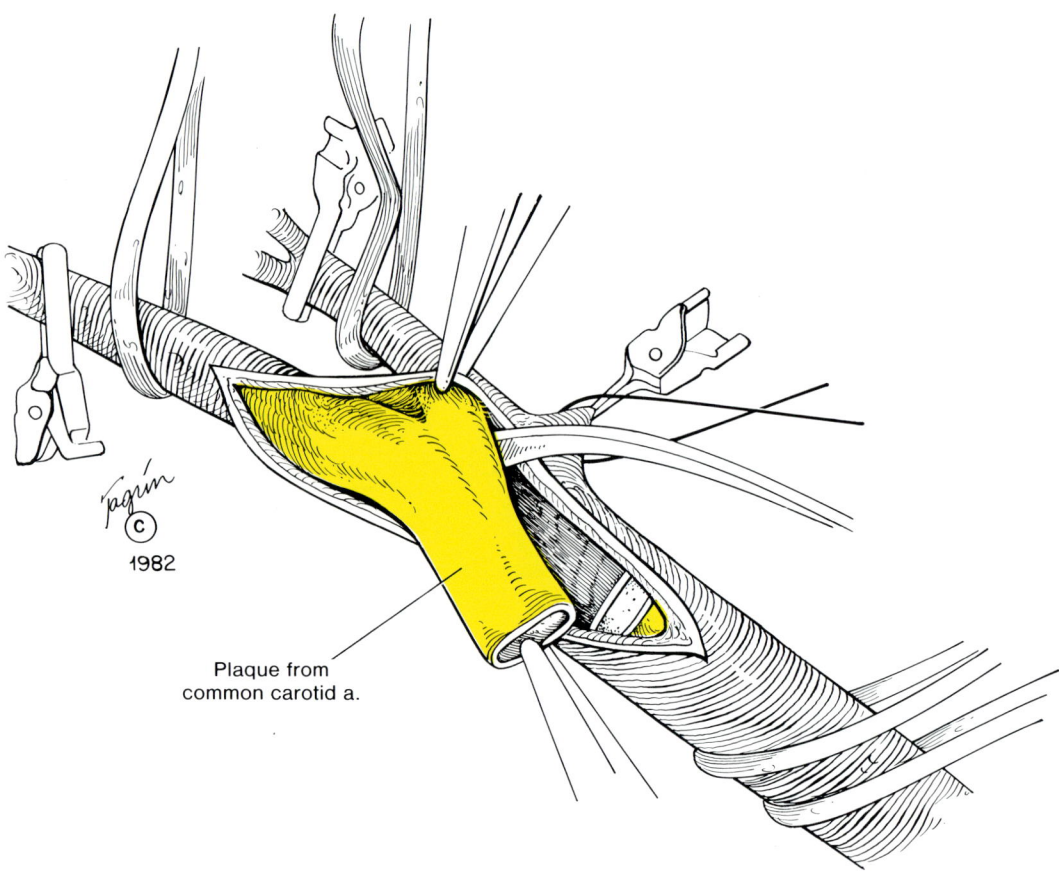

Figure 2.15 Carotid endarterectomy. The plaque has been separated from the outer wall of the common carotid artery and is now being removed from the origin of the external carotid artery.

2.16). Usually the plaque will extend distally several millimeters further along the posterior wall of the artery. Care must be taken to remove this portion of the atheroma. Once the plaque has been separated, it usually breaks away cleanly at the junction with normal intima and does not leave an intimal flap. Only on rare occasions is it necessary to suture a distal intima flap (Fig. 2.17). The intima adjacent and beyond the distal end of the plaque is usually of normal thickness and firmly adherent to the media. Occasionally, a very thin sheet of atheromatous material may extend distally in the internal carotid artery but does not cause stenosis or ulceration. The area of the endarterectomy is irrigated with heparinized saline and inspected with the help of the headlight and magnification. There are almost always some loose fragments adherent to the wall which are picked up with a fine forceps or baby intestinal clamp and removed by peeling them in a circumferential fashion. A final inspection is made of the distal end of the internal carotid artery by visualizing the area directly using a headlight and fine suction.

The arteriotomy is then closed with continuous 5-0 Prolene suture beginning at the distal end of the arteriotomy on the internal carotid artery and progressing down onto the common carotid artery (Fig. 2.18). It is important that the sutures be placed just inside the cut edge and not more than a millimeter apart. Magnification helps in placing these small sutures. Just before the final sutures are placed, back flow is allowed from both the external and internal carotid arteries so that air and any debris are flushed out of the area of the endarterectomy (Fig. 2.19). If the back flow is poor, the arteriotomy is reopened and the problem corrected. In this situation there may be an intimal flap or narrowing at the distal end of the suture line. When the closure is completed, a rubber dam is placed over the suture line and held with gentle pressure on a sponge. Blood flow is allowed first into the external carotid artery to wash out any further residual debris and then into the internal carotid artery. Bleeding from the suture line is usually not a problem and is easily controlled by gentle pressure on the rubber dam. One should not be in any hurry to close small areas of leak from the suture line since most will clot with gentle pressure and patience. Occasionally, an area of persistent bleeding requires control by bringing across a flap of periarterial tissue or utilizing a small piece of muscle. Unless the hemorrhage persists, one should avoid placing additional sutures into the arteriotomy incision. By utilizing magnifying loupes, the arterial su-

Carotid Endarterectomy

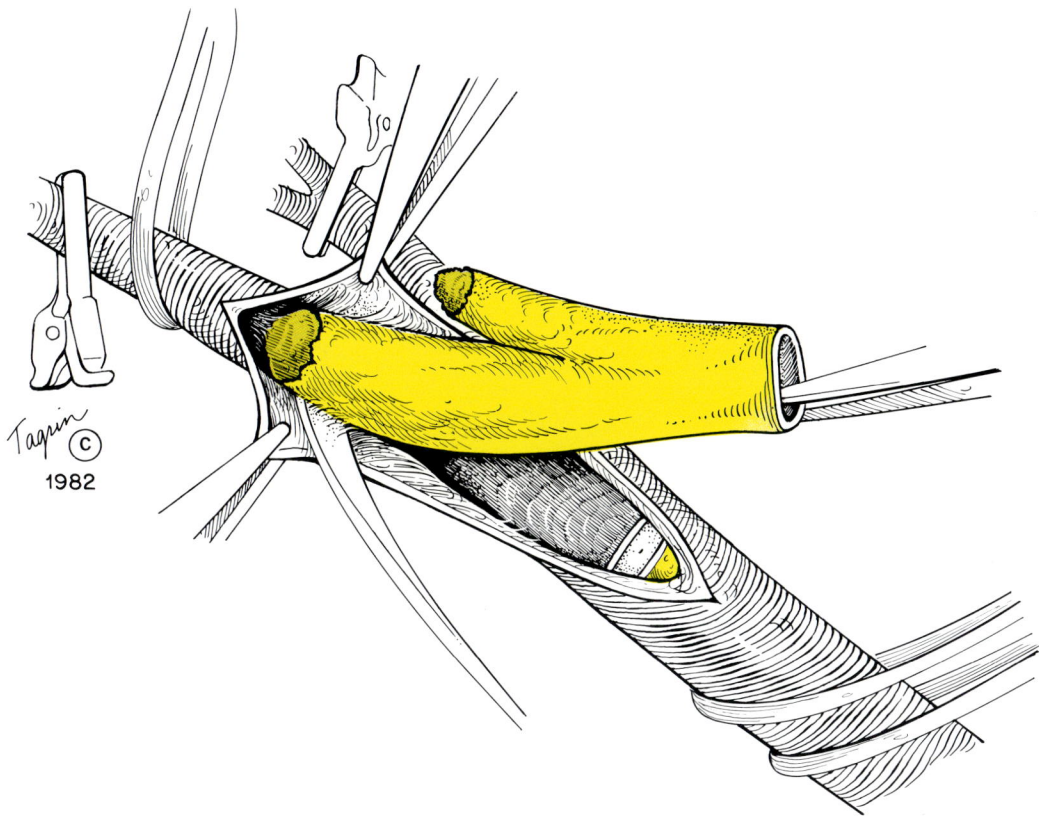

Figure 2.16 Carotid endarterectomy. The plaque is being removed from the internal carotid artery. Often the plaque may extend several millimeters farther distally on the posterior wall of the internal carotid artery.

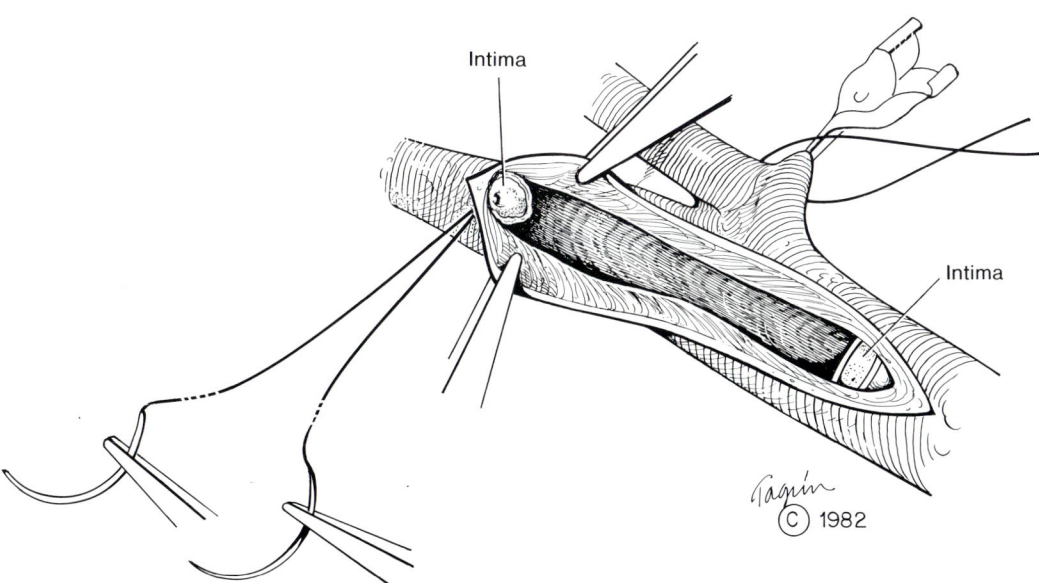

Figure 2.17 Carotid endarterectomy. Placement of sutures to tack down the distal intimal flap on the rare occasion when it is needed. Care must be taken not to place the two ends of the sutures too far apart to avoid constricting the lumen.

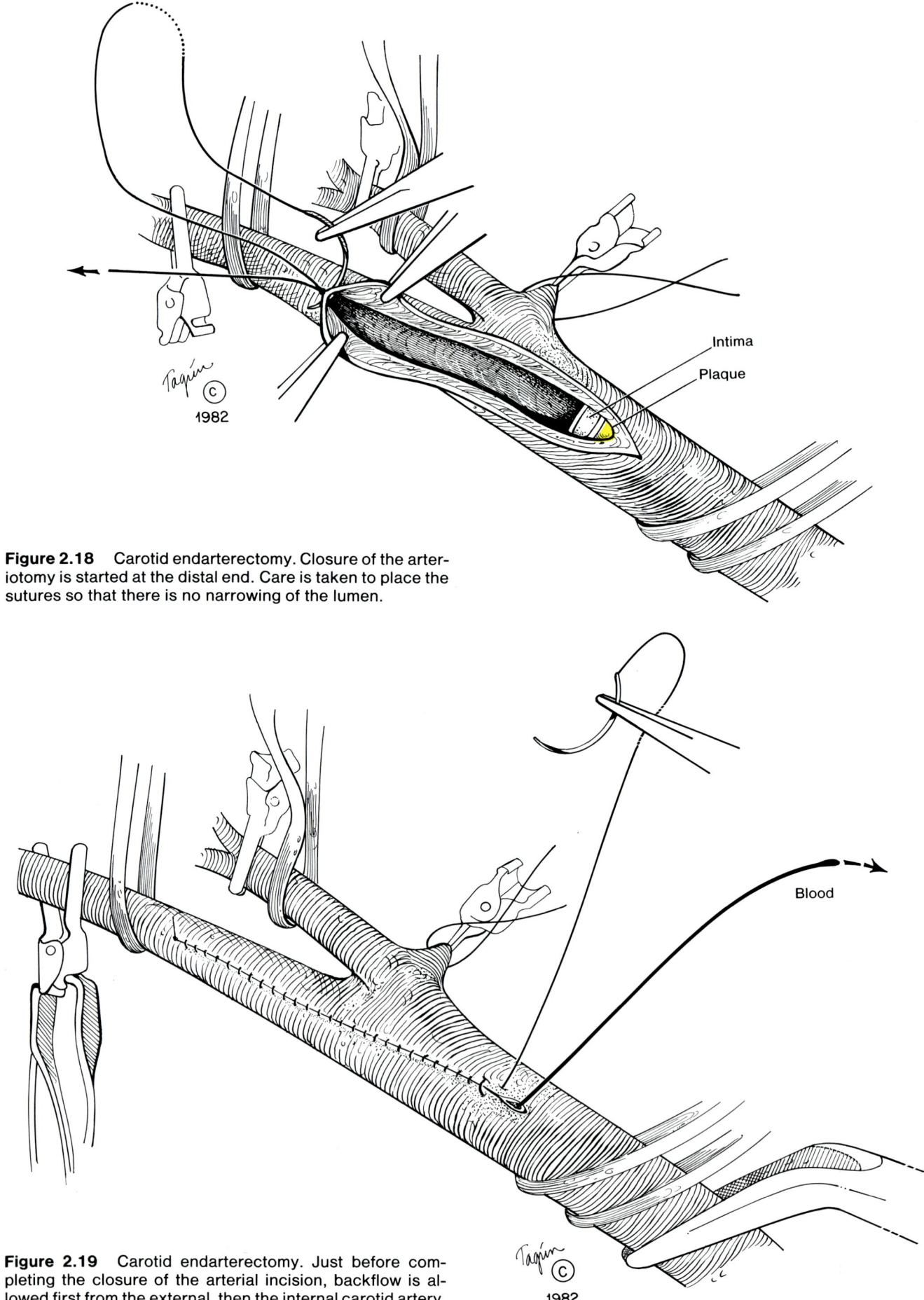

Figure 2.18 Carotid endarterectomy. Closure of the arteriotomy is started at the distal end. Care is taken to place the sutures so that there is no narrowing of the lumen.

Figure 2.19 Carotid endarterectomy. Just before completing the closure of the arterial incision, backflow is allowed first from the external, then the internal carotid artery.

Carotid Endarterectomy

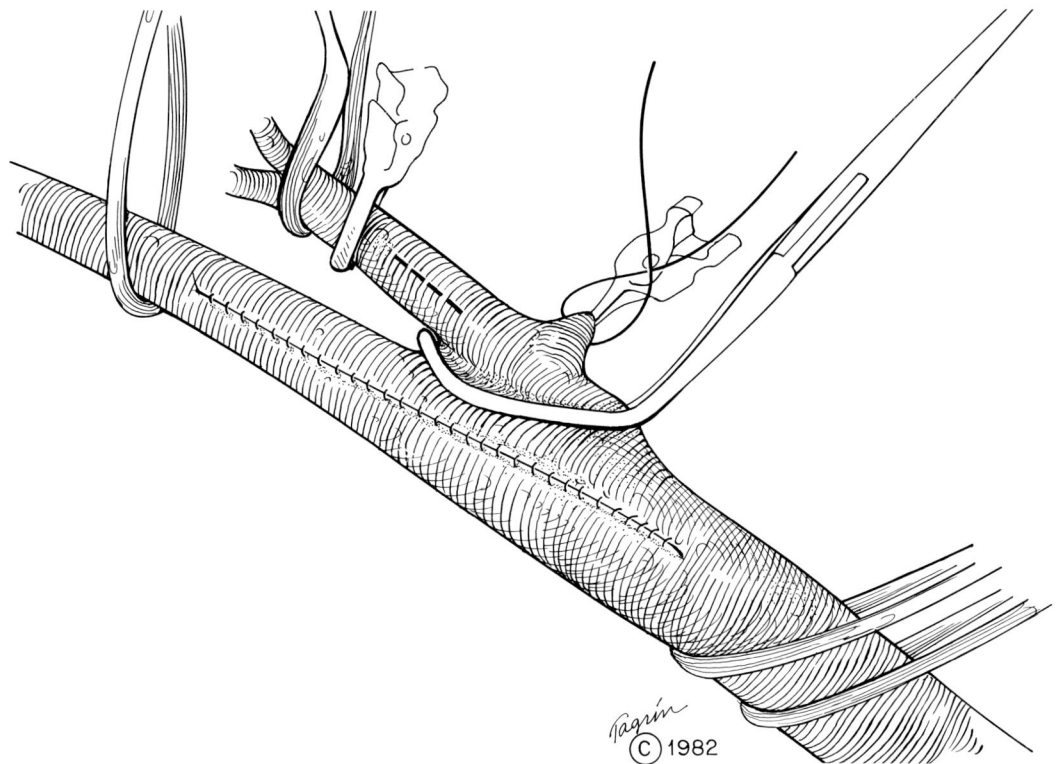

Figure 2.20 Carotid endarterectomy. Clamps have been placed so that, if there is a thrill in the external carotid artery after the endarterectomy, an incision can be made in the artery for inspection while allowing flow in the internal carotid artery.

tures can be carefully placed during the initial exposure, resulting in the reconstruction of a normal caliber lumen.

Once flow has been reestablished, the arteries are gently palpated. If there is a thrill in the internal carotid artery, the clamps are replaced and the artery reopened to correct the problem. If one is concerned about narrowing of the internal carotid lumen, a patch can be used. We use either a Dacron patch or a vein graft, using the saphenous vein from the ankle (see page 44). If there is a thrill in the external carotid artery, the vessel is occluded, maintaining internal carotid flow and a separate incision is made on the proximal external carotid artery (Fig. 2.20). Usually a flap of intima is the cause of the problem.

At this point a decision must be made regarding reversal of the heparin. In the past we have partially reversed the heparin by giving 30–40 mg of Protamine sulfate intravenously. However, there may be some advantage to not reversing the heparin since this may protect against thrombus formation, particularly during the first hours after the closure (38). Therefore, if hemostasis is complete, no Protamine is given.

When hemostasis has been obtained, the operative wound is irrigated with a Bacitracin solution. The platysma and subcutaneous tissue are then closed with absorbable suture material and the skin with a continuous 5-0 nylon. Some surgeons prefer to leave a drain deep to the platysma for 12–24 hours. This should always be done when anticoagulation is being continued in the immediate postoperative period. We prefer to use a medium Hemovac for the drain, finding it to be much more effective than the Penrose drain. Prophylactic antibiotics are continued until the drain is removed.

SPECIAL TECHNICAL PROBLEMS

Use of a Shunt

We use the Argyle carotid shunt catheters. The advantage of these sterile polyethylene catheters is that the surgeon has four sizes (8, 10, 12, 14 French) immediately available which are the correct length (15 cm) and have smooth ends. A suture is tied around the mid portion of the catheter to serve as a marker, to be sure the tube has not slipped, and to help with the removal of the shunt.

After arterial clamps and clips are placed, a rapid arteriotomy incision is made including the plaque, starting a few millimeters more proximally on the common carotid artery than one would normally start, and extending the incision a few millimeters more distally on the internal carotid artery (Fig. 2.21). The shunt tube is first passed distally into the internal carotid artery visualizing the intima so that a flap is not dissected by the tip of the catheter. A tourniquet gently snugs the arterial wall around the shunt. The shunt is checked to be certain there is satisfactory backflow of blood. The catheter is temporarily occluded and then passed proximally into the common

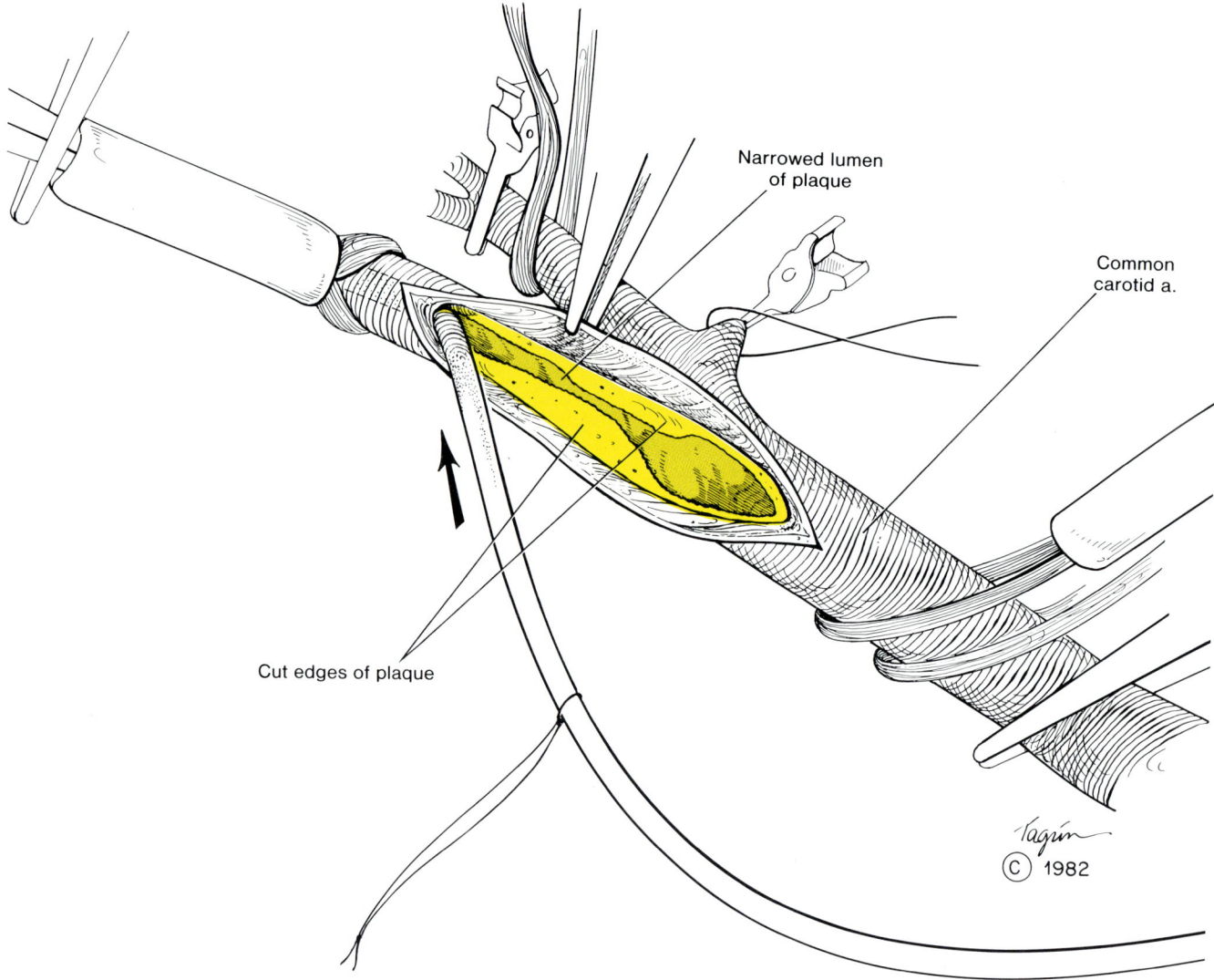

Figure 2.21 Carotid endarterectomy: placement of a shunt. The shunt is first passed distally into the internal carotid artery.

carotid artery and the tourniquet is tightened (Fig. 2.22). The clamp is removed from the shunt catheter. The catheter usually remains outside the lumen at this point (Fig. 2.23). The plaque can then be dissected and removed as previously described. The shunt tube is then placed in the lumen. Occasionally, the distal catheter must be temporarily removed (with cross-clamping) to complete removal of the plaque. Approximately two-thirds of the arteriotomy incision is then closed in the usual fashion with a continuous suture beginning on the internal carotid artery. A second suture is then started at the proximal end of the arteriotomy on the common carotid artery and is sutured distally to within 2 mm of the previously placed suture. The catheter is then clamped and removed. Sometimes this is facilitated by utilizing two fine clamps and cutting the catheter between them. As the catheter is removed, bleeding is controlled initially with a tourniquet and then occluding clamps are placed on the common and internal carotid arteries. The closure of the arteriotomy is then completed, the sutures are tied, and the remainder of the operation is done as previously described.

Insertion of a Patch Graft

With the routine use of magnification (loupes) for the endarterectomy, we have found that in most cases the arterial incision can be closed with a continuous 5-0 Prolene running suture. When the internal carotid artery appears to be too small for satisfactory closure or it appears that closure will compromise the lumen, there is no hesitation in using a patch graft. In most patients with recurrent stenosis, a patch graft is used because of scar formation in the wall of the artery. Some surgeons use a patch routinely (38).

The patch graft can be made from either a saphe-

Carotid Endarterectomy

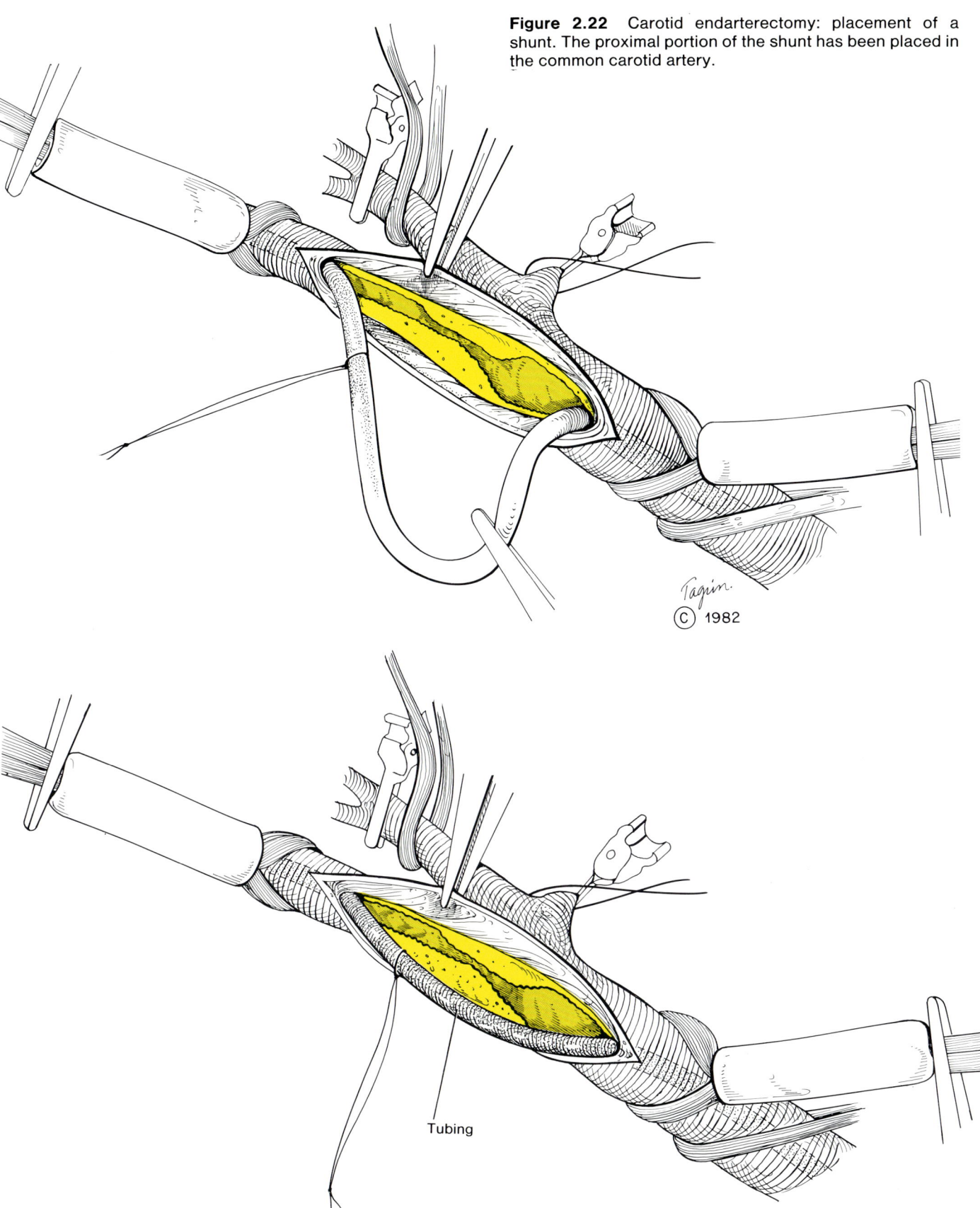

Figure 2.22 Carotid endarterectomy: placement of a shunt. The proximal portion of the shunt has been placed in the common carotid artery.

Tubing

Figure 2.23 Carotid endarterectomy: placement of a shunt. The shunt tube has been positioned so that the endarterectomy can be done.

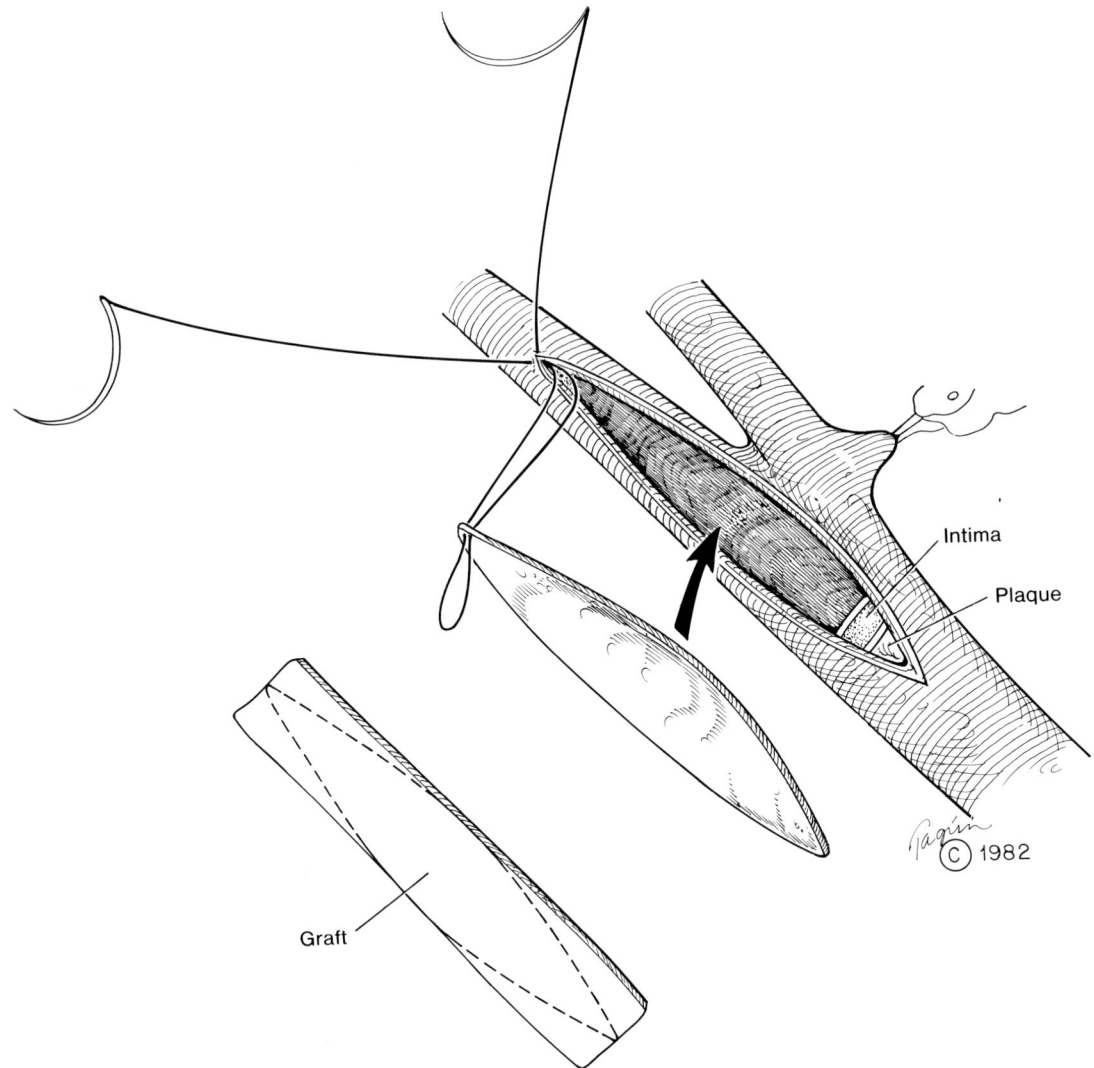

Figure 2.24 Carotid endarterectomy: insertion of patch graft. The graft has been cut as outlined. The first sutures are placed at the distal end of the arteriotomy.

nous vein taken from the ankle or a preclotted knitted Dacron patch. We usually use the latter, and if there is any possibility that a patch might be needed, the Dacron is preclotted before giving systemic heparin. The patch is cut to fit the arteriotomy as illustrated (Fig. 2.24). The graft is usually 6–8 mm in width in the central portion and tapers to a rounded point at each end. Double-armed sutures of 5-0 Prolene are used at each end. One arm of the suture is placed through one end of the graft from outer to inner surface and then carefully placed at the distal end of the arteriotomy from inside the lumen to the outer wall. The other arm of the suture is placed in a similar fashion very close to the first and the suture is then tied. The final length of the graft is then determined and another double armed suture is placed in a similar fashion at the proximal end of the graft (Fig. 2.25). One of the sutures is then used for a continuous closure on each side of the graft (Fig. 2.26). The closure is done so that the knot can be tied away from the end of the graft. Just before completing the closure, backflow is allowed as is done in the usual endarterectomy closure.

Stenosis at C2 Level

Occasionally, the carotid bifurcation will be quite high in the neck or the stenosis will be localized at the C2 level (Fig. 2.27). This finding does not preclude carotid endarterectomy.

By using the full upper extent of the incision as outlined, staying on the sternomastoid muscle beneath the parotid gland and following the plane between the internal jugular vein laterally and the hypoglossal nerve medially, the internal carotid artery can be exposed to the C1 level well above the stenosis. It may be necessary to divide the occipital artery and retract or at times even divide the posterior belly of the digastric muscle.

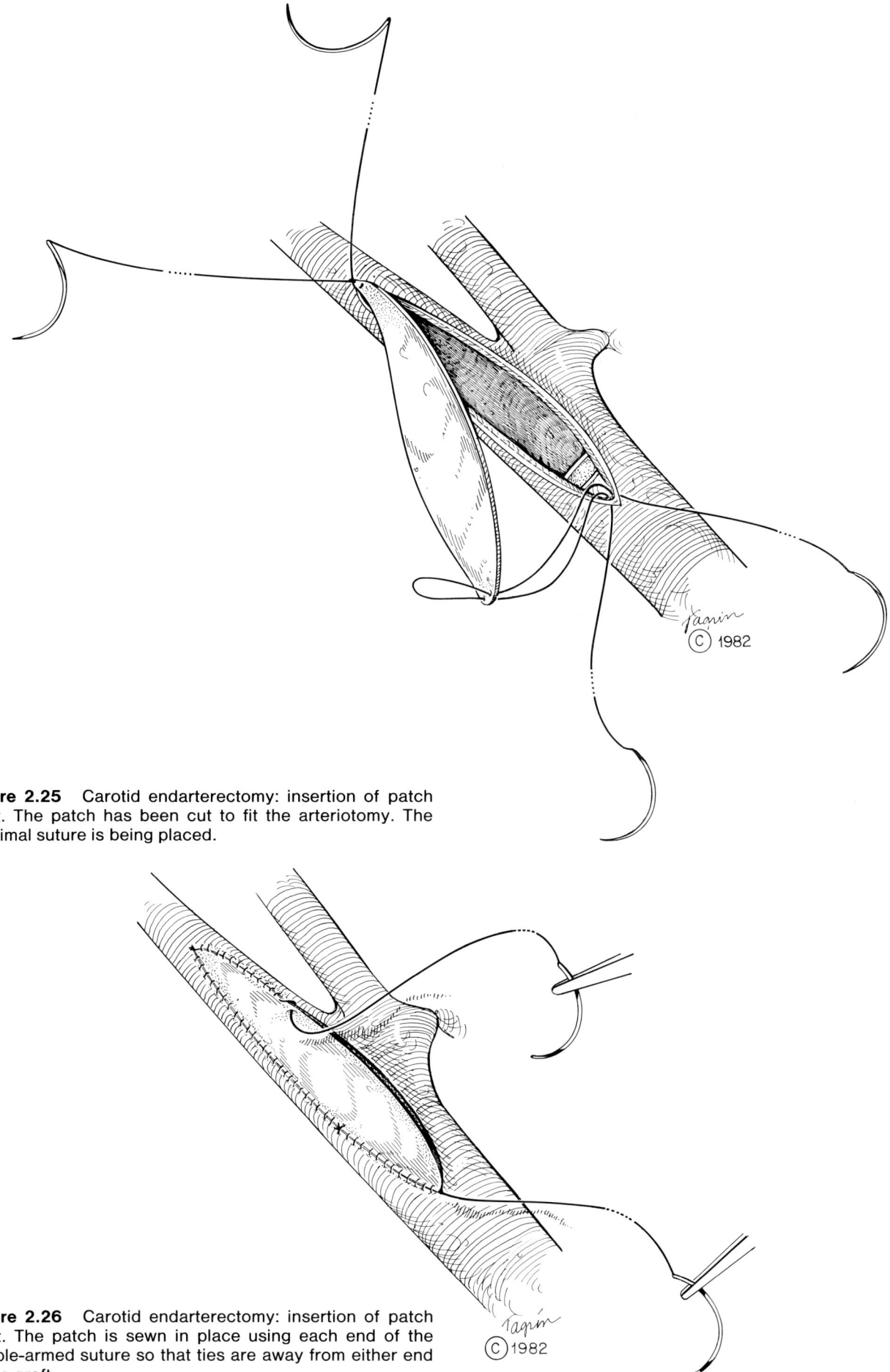

Figure 2.25 Carotid endarterectomy: insertion of patch graft. The patch has been cut to fit the arteriotomy. The proximal suture is being placed.

Figure 2.26 Carotid endarterectomy: insertion of patch graft. The patch is sewn in place using each end of the double-armed suture so that ties are away from either end of the graft.

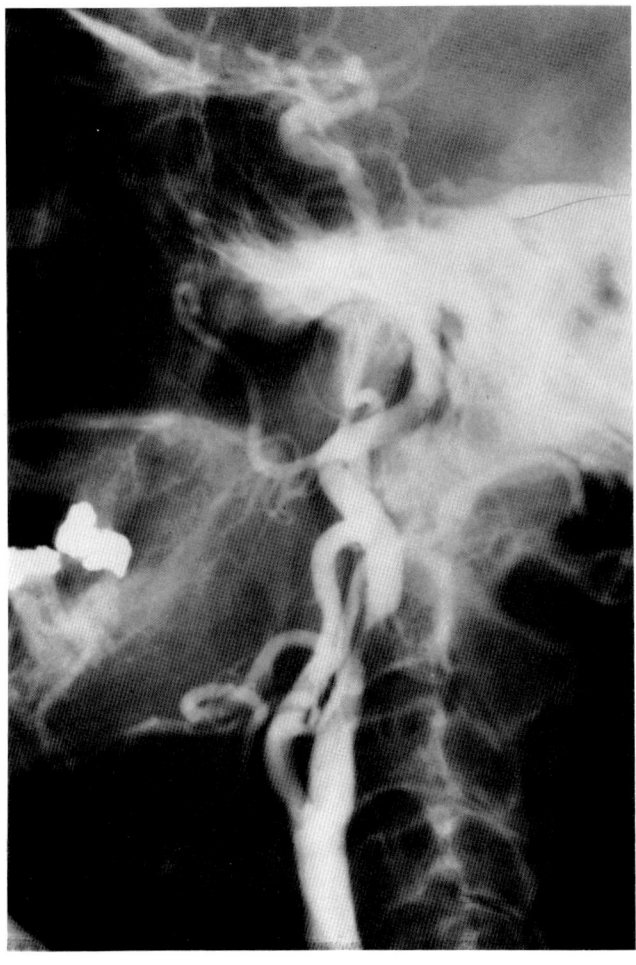

Figure 2.27 Internal carotid stenosis localized at the C2 level. Occasionally, atherosclerosis can cause localized stenosis 3–4 cm distal to the bifurcation. The finding of a lesion at the C2 level does not preclude surgery. Good exposure can be obtained by following the techniques outlined.

Abnormal Arterial Anatomy

In a small number of patients there may be a significant loop of the extracranial internal carotid artery distal to the stenosis (Fig. 2.28, A and B). Care must be taken in dissection of these loops because postoperative kinking can occur with occlusion and resultant infarction (29). We try to leave the loop adherent to the posterior periarterial tissue to avoid this problem. Usually, one will need to dissect the artery distal to the loop to place the controlling tape because the atheroma may extend right up to the proximal part of the curve (Fig. 2.29). Should the loop become mobile, it may be held in place by periarterial sutures or a place made for it. In one patient, a large loop was positioned in a plane dissected under the internal jugular vein.

Unusual arterial anatomy may be found. In three patients in our series, a branch arose from the internal carotid artery approximately 1.0 cm distal to its origin. This was likely a persistent hypoglossal artery. The vessel was occluded by atheromatous plaque and was not seen on the angiogram. A large ascending pharyngeal artery may arise from the anterior part of the bifurcation. In one patient, a superior thyroid artery originated from the lateral aspect of the common carotid artery and passed medially across the bifurcation (Fig. 2.30). The internal carotid artery arose medially and then turned beneath the external carotid artery to assume a more normal lateral position.

In some patients with severe carotid stenosis, the distal internal carotid artery is quite small in diameter due to reduced intravascular pressure. This has been described as the "slim" sign on the angiogram. (Fig. 1.2) (25a). The artery tends to dilate almost immediately when normal pressure is restored. It should not be mechanically dilated. Occasionally a patch graft is needed, but usually with the use of magnification the arteriotomy can be closed primarily.

Complete Internal Carotid Artery Occlusion

When the angiogram indicates complete internal carotid occlusion, changes in the operative approach may be indicated. If the operation is being done as an emergency for acute neurological deficit, every effort is made to expedite the surgery. Great care is taken to avoid hypotension. In the majority of patients a thrombus will be found, but in a few the

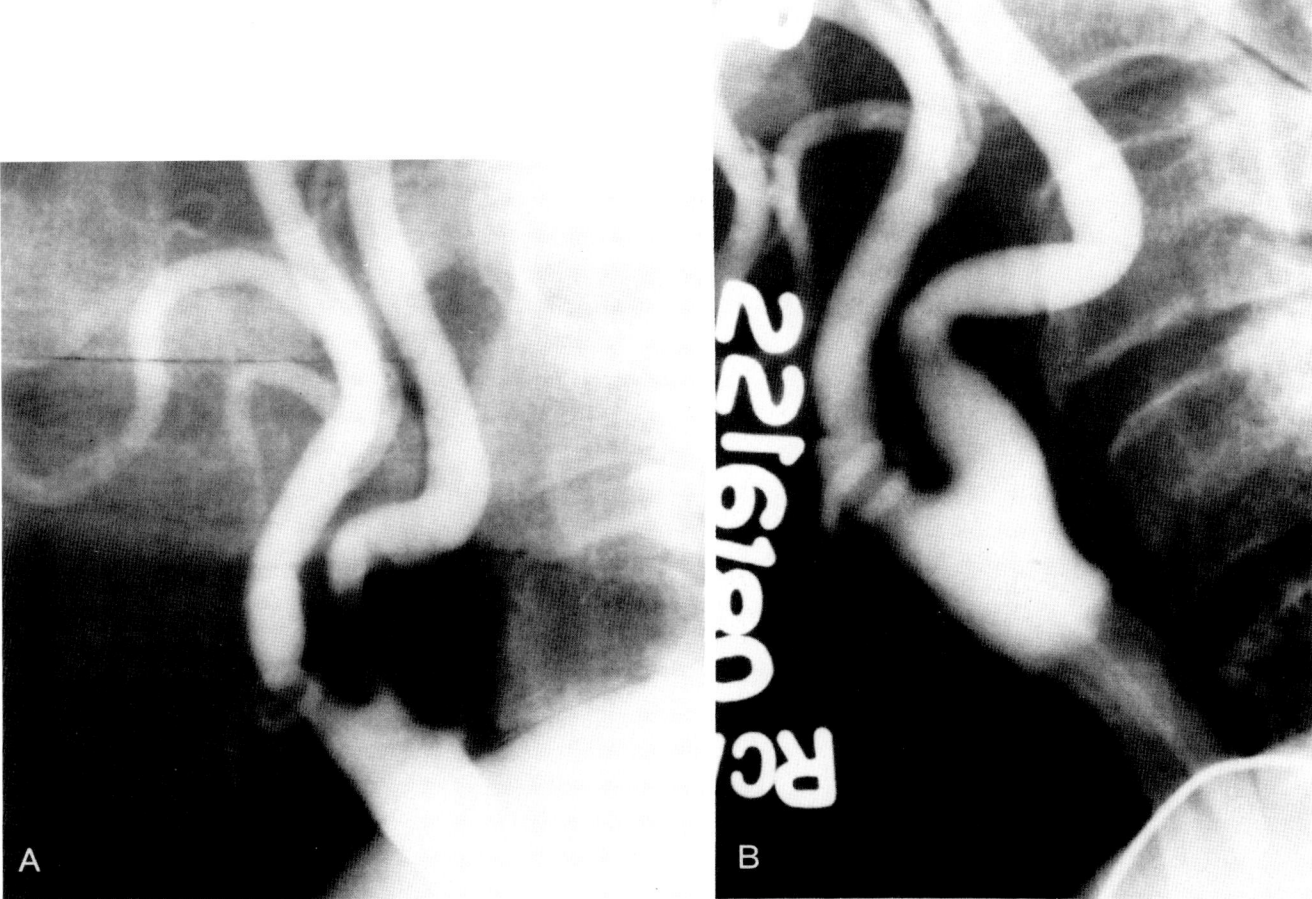

Figure 2.28 Loop in the internal carotid artery. *A*, angiogram of bifurcation shows such severe stenosis at the origin of the internal carotid artery that only a minute thread of dye can be seen. A prominent loop in the internal carotid artery is also apparent and atheroma extends beyond the first curve. *B*, postoperative angiogram showing restoration of normal lumen. There is slight narrowing at the proximal loop.

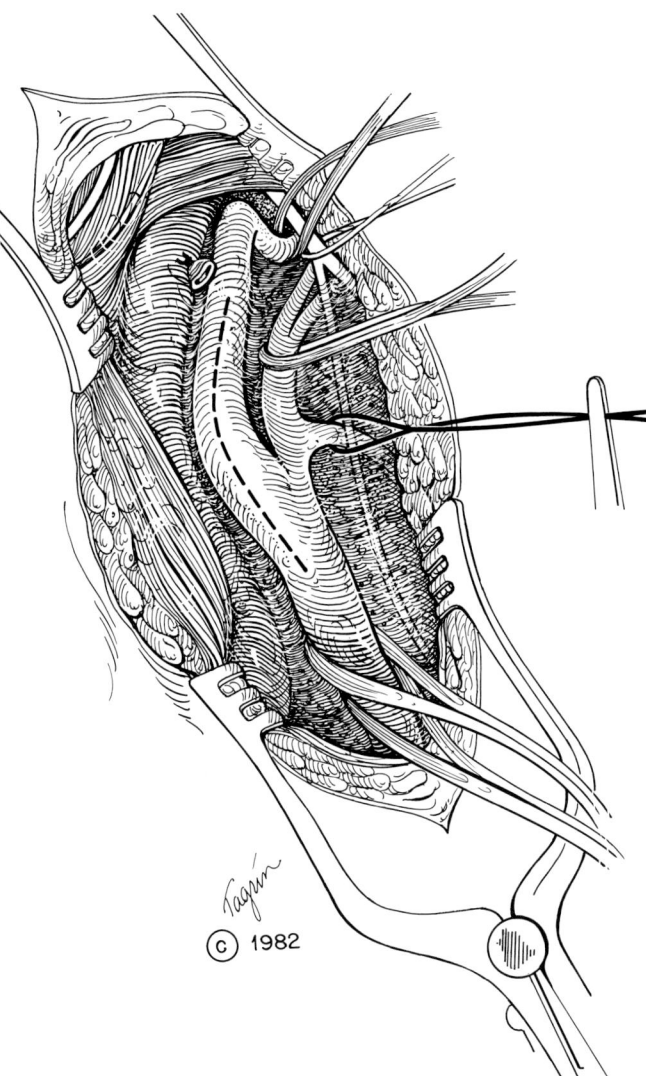

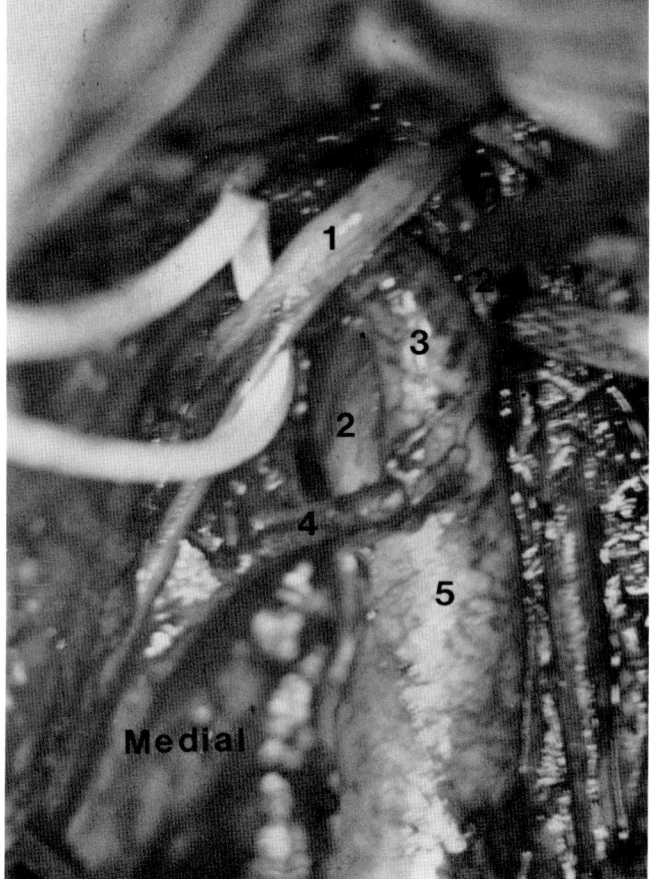

Figure 2.29 Loop in the internal carotid artery: operative exposure. When a significant loop is present in the internal carotid artery beyond the stenosis, that portion of the artery distal to the loop must be exposed and care taken not to disturb anymore of the artery than is necessary.

Figure 2.30 Unusual anatomy in region of the left carotid bifurcation. There is reversal of the normal origin of the internal and external carotid arteries. *1,* hypoglossal and descendens hypoglossal nerves. *2,* internal carotid artery arising medially and then passing behind. *3,* the external carotid artery which originates laterally and then turns medially. *4,* superior thyroid artery arising from lateral wall of *5,* distal common carotid artery and then passing across the bifurcation to go medially. (From Ojemann RG, Crowell RM, Roberson GH, Fisher CM: Surgical treatment of extracranial carotid occlusive disease, Ch. 14, in *Clinical Neurosurgery.* Baltimore, Williams & Wilkins, 1974, vol 22, with permission.)

Carotid Endarterectomy

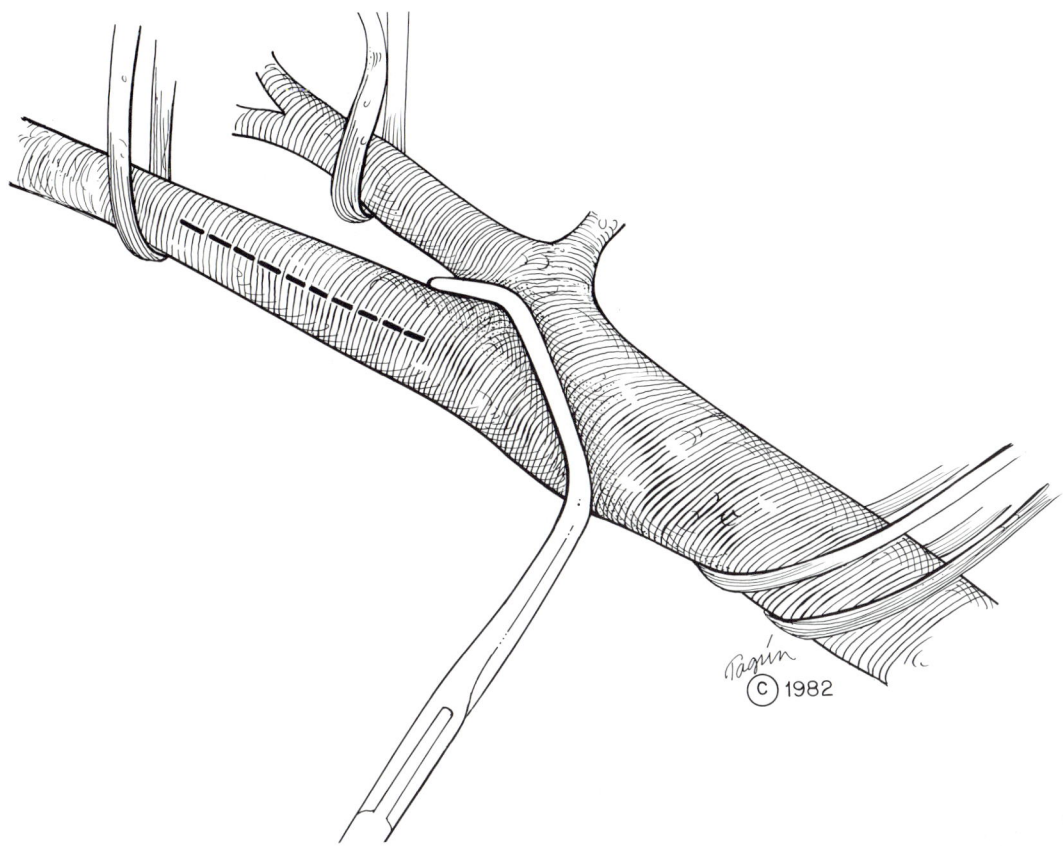

Figure 2.31 Complete internal carotid occlusion. A Satinsky clamp has been placed across the carotid bifurcation to maintain blood flow in the external carotid artery while the internal carotid artery is being reopened.

lumen of the internal carotid artery will be open distal to the atheromatous plaque (21). In many of these patients, there will be good backflow, but in some there will be a further obstruction distally. If there is a long-standing occlusion, the artery may be a firm fibrous cord and no further procedures are indicated.

An incision is made on the internal carotid artery distal to the plaque without occluding the common and external carotid arteries, and an attempt is made to remove the thrombus. If the thrombus can be removed and backflow established, the endarterectomy is done as described. In some patients with complete occlusion of the internal carotid artery, the external carotid artery may supply significant collateral flow to the brain. Flow can be maintained in the external carotid artery by the application of a Satinsky clamp across the bifurcation at the origin of the internal carotid artery (Fig. 2.31) or a common-external carotid artery shunt.

Certain techniques may help in opening the completely occluded artery. If a thrombus is encountered in the internal carotid artery, an effort is made to withdraw it gradually with forceps using a hand-over-hand technique. Thrombi as long as 20 cm have been removed (Fig. 2.32). If this technique fails, a smooth-ended suction catheter is introduced into the internal carotid lumen until resistance is felt. Suction is then applied and this may withdraw the thrombus. If this method fails, a Fogarty #3 catheter is passed gently as far as the base of the skull, inflated, and withdrawn (17). Care is required to avoid injuring the distal internal carotid artery with subsequent development of a carotid-cavernous fistula (10). Measurements on the angiogram from the internal carotid bifurcation to the base of the skull may help in determining the safe length of catheter which may be inserted. A single lateral intraoperative angiogram with 10 cc of Renograffin 70 via an Argyle shunt catheter is recommended to document restoration of flow without intimal flap or distal thrombus. If good backflow with satisfactory angiography cannot be achieved, the internal carotid artery is doubly ligated with 0 silk. When flow is reestablished, anticoagulation should be continued in the postoperative period (25). Heparin at 500 units per hour is recommended for 12 hours, then full heparinization to maintain a partial thromboplastin time of about 50 seconds.

External Carotid Stenosis

If it is thought that external carotid stenosis is the cause of symptoms and the occluded internal carotid cannot be opened, an incision is made on the common carotid artery and extended onto the external carotid

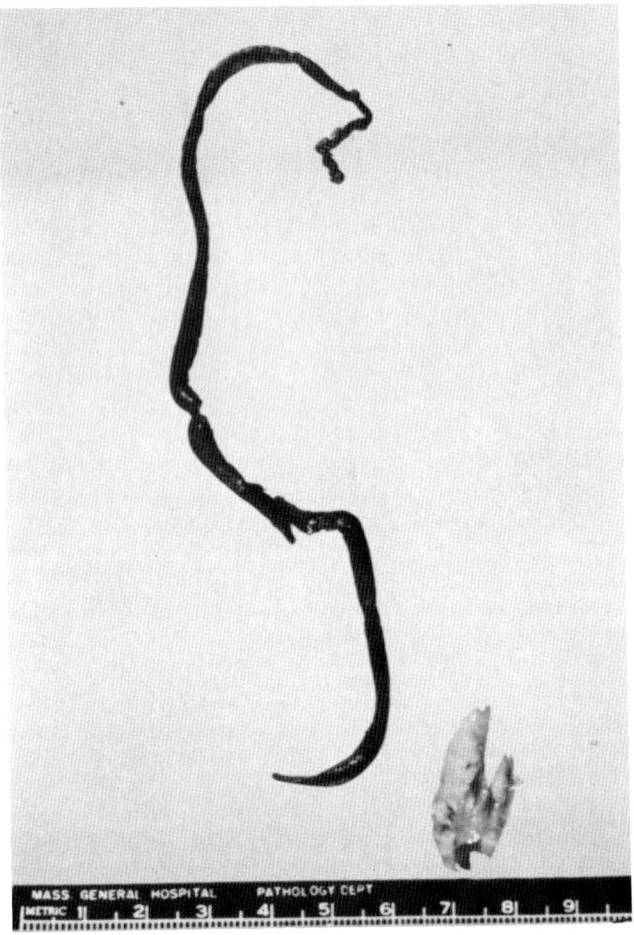

Figure 2.32 Removal of thrombus from internal carotid artery. Angiography showed a complete occlusion of the internal carotid artery. By carefully withdrawing the thrombus using forceps and with the help of back pressure from the collateral circulation, this long thrombus was removed and flow reestablished (courtesy of Dr. Charles Poletti).

artery (20). Endarterectomy should be done in the usual fashion being sure to obliterate the origin of the internal carotid artery. If the external carotid collateral is crucial for cerebral circulation, a shunt may be needed. Removal of the external carotid stenosis in association with the endarterectomy for internal carotid stenosis may require a separate incision in the external carotid artery (22).

When a proximal stump in the internal carotid artery is thought to be the source of the embolus, the operative procedure is an endarterectomy of the carotid bifurcation to include the distal common and proximal external carotid arteries. Exclusion of the stump of the proximal internal carotid artery is done by either oversewing the origin of the artery or obliteration by a large metallic clip to give a smooth lumen (2, 18) (Fig. 2.33).

Common Carotid Artery Stenosis and Occlusion

Occlusion of the common carotid artery is usually due to one of two atheromatous lesions. The plaque either involves the distal common carotid artery and/or both the external and internal carotid artery with development of a retrograde thrombus, or the atheromatous plaque is located at the origin of the common carotid artery and antegrade thrombus develops. The former circumstance is more common.

The problem should be initially approached as one would for a carotid endarterectomy. If inspection of the distal common carotid artery and bifurcation region reveals significant atheromatous plaque, this plaque is removed, and if this appears to be the site of the occlusion with retrograde thrombus, a thrombectomy is done. Careful dissection identifies the plane between the organized thrombus and the arterial intima. The thrombus is divided and a smooth, large endarterectomy stripper is passed over the thrombus in the plane between the thrombus and the intima (Fig. 2.34). The stripper is advanced down the lumen and usually following several gentle passes the thrombus will be freed and the thrombotic core is pushed out by the head of arterial pressure. A Fogarty catheter may then be used to be sure the lumen is clean. The closure than follows the procedure described for carotid bifurcation endarterectomy, being sure to allow flow first up the external carotid artery. On rare occasions, the occlusion will involve only the distal common carotid artery (Fig. 2.12).

If the initial exploration of the carotid bifurcation

reveals a thrombus in the common carotid artery without significant atheromatous occlusion in the region of the carotid bifurcation, there is likely to be atheromatous occlusion at the origin of the common carotid artery. This occurs more frequently on the left side. At this point partial thrombectomy is done. The common carotid artery is occluded to exclude the proximal thrombus. If it is deemed advisable to restore circulation to this artery, a bypass graft is done from the subclavian artery, from a point distal to the vertebral artery, to the common carotid artery. Although only a small number of cases have been reported, this procedure seems preferable to doing a sternotomy and trying to reconstruct the origin of the common carotid artery.

Occasionally, symptomatic stenosis may involve the mid-portion of the common carotid artery (Fig. 1.23). Usually, this is treated with endarterectomy. One patient has been reported where catheter dilatation of a proximal carotid stenosis was done during distal bifurcation endarterectomy (24). There were no complications.

POSTOPERATIVE MANAGEMENT
Medical Therapy

Following completion of surgery, the patient's vital signs and neurological functions are monitored carefully in the recovery room. Systolic blood pressure is generally maintained in the range of 110–150 mm Hg, with efforts to avoid both hypotension and hypertension. If hypotension develops, the ECG is checked. Mild hypotension will usually respond to administration of fluid or colloid. The phenylephrine drip is available if needed. If the hypotension does not immediately respond to volume replacement, a CVP is inserted. If the CVP is maintained in the range of 5–10 cm with judicious utilization of fluid, this problem will generally resolve (39). On occasion, bradycardia may develop, and administration of atropine may be necessary. Bradycardia and hypotension may be the result of increased pressure waves reaching the carotid sinus receptors after removal of the plaque (39). The blood pressure and pulse usually return to normal level within a few hours.

Control of postoperative hypertension is also important and there is a significant incidence of this problem (5, 41). In one series, the incidence of neurological morbidity was higher in those patients with severe hypertension (41). Patients who develop postoperative systolic readings which are persistently maintained above 170 mm require treatment with rapid-acting intravenous antihypertensive medication. We have utilized either trimethaphan camsylate, sodium nitroprusside or nitroglycerine infusions until long-acting antihypertensive medications such as propanolol or hydralazine become effective. We have encountered intracerebral hemorrhage with postoperative hypertension, as previously reported, but since the institution of careful postoperative blood pressure control, this complication has been rare (5, 29).

Intravenous nitroglycerine is also used to control EKG changes. Sublinguinal nitroglycerine is given for angina.

Generally we have not utilized anticoagulation except in the circumstance when dissection was difficult, the endarterectomy plane seemed roughened, the plaque was particularly long, or a complete occlusion had been reopened. Heparin is used in a dose of 500 units/hour for the first 12 hours then is increased to keep the PTT at about 50 seconds. A special circumstance where anticoagulation should probably be continued occurs when the patient has an asymptomatic middle cerebral stenosis or a severe contralateral internal carotid stenosis. In one patient, occlusion of a previously asymptomatic opposite middle cerebral stenosis led to a neurological deficit (Fig. 2.35). If anticoagulation is used, a drain should be placed at the time of surgery and left for 24–48 hours. We prefer a medium Hemovac.

In the postoperative period, the management of risk factors is emphasized. This program aims to halt the progression of generalized atherosclerosis and prevent recurrence of carotid stenosis. If indicated, an attempt is made to reduce weight. Hypertension diabetes mellitus and hypertriglyceridemia or hypercholesterolemia are treated. In almost all cases, antiplatelet medication is given and is usually started the morning after surgery if there is no wound hematoma.

Angiography

Postoperative angiography usually is not done. Reports of angiography in the early postoperative period have documented a number of abnormal findings including flaps, roughness, stenosis, forceps marks, corrugation, filling defects, and superior thyroid, external carotid, and internal carotid artery occlusion. However, many of the arteries showing an irregular wall will become smooth in later angiograms, and in general the endarterectomized arteries remain patent and smooth for many years (33).

Even though the risks of postoperative angiography are small, we have not felt this risk was warranted. Most of the changes demonstrated do not lead to reoperation. Many surgeons now continue low-dose heparin in the postoperative period and most patients receive antiplatelet therapy. We have reserved angiography for those patients who have unexplained neurological deficit in the postoperative period or who have a postoperative bruit that is found on noninvasive studies to be hemodynamically significant (see "Complications").

We have had the opportunity to study 39 operated arteries with delayed angiography months to years after the endarterectomy. One group of patients so

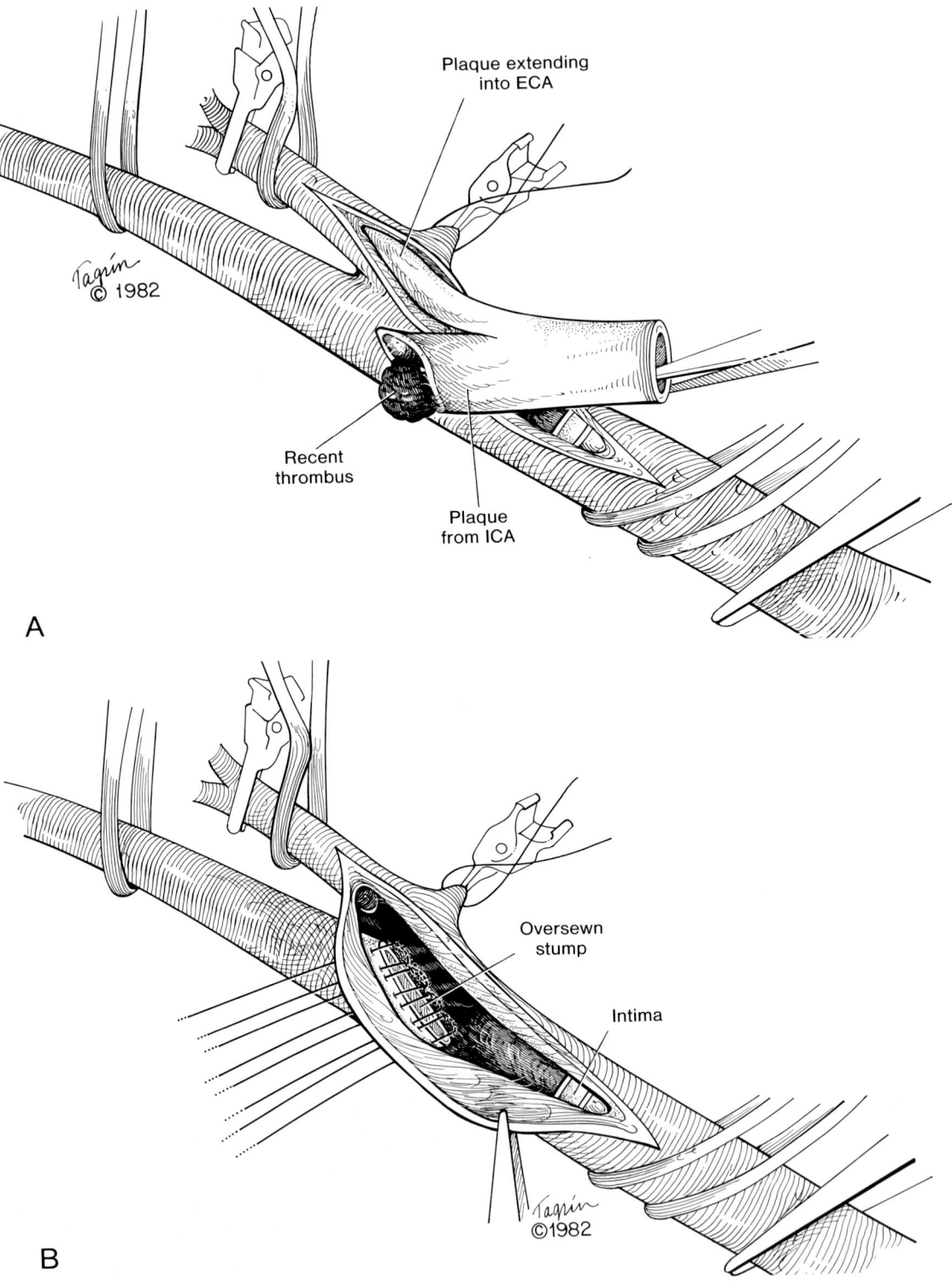

Figure 2.33 Endarterectomy for stump embolus. *A*, endarterectomy is performed by making the arteriotomy incision onto the external carotid artery and removing a portion of the thrombus from the proximal internal carotid artery. *B*, interrupted mattress sutures are placed across the origin of the internal carotid artery to obliterate the stump and give a smooth internal lumen. *C*, closure is completed as shown. *D*, operative specimen showing the thrombus in the stump of the internal carotid artery projecting into the lumen of the common carotid artery.

Carotid Endarterectomy

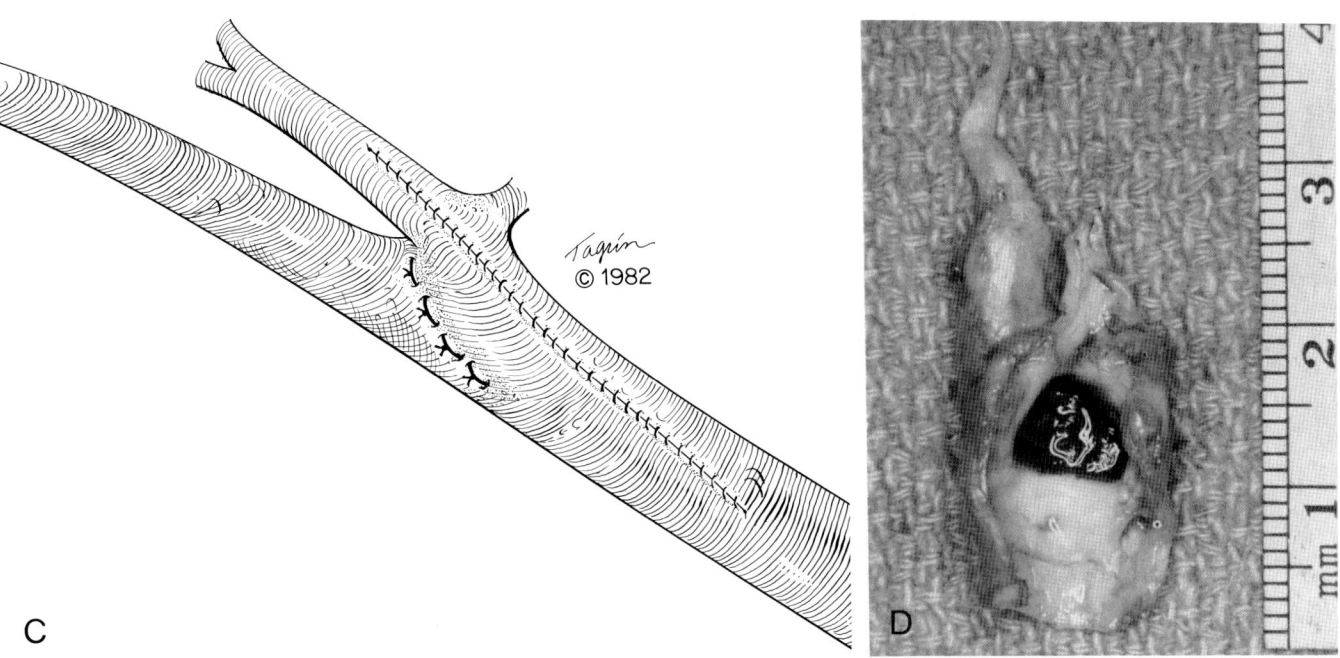

Figure 2.33 (*C* and *D*)

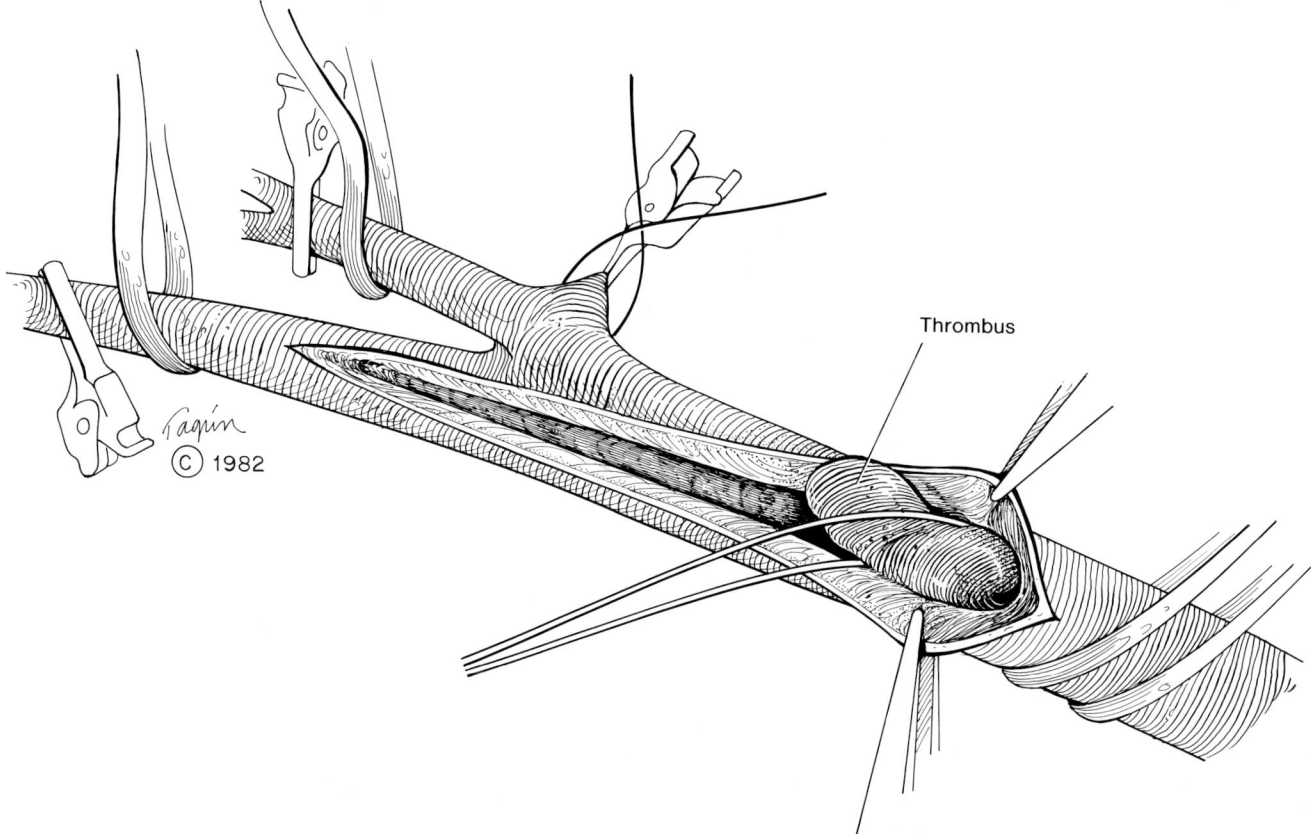

Figure 2.34 Common carotid artery occlusion with retrograde thrombus. A carotid endarterectomy has been performed as described. An endarterectomy stripper is being passed around the thrombus.

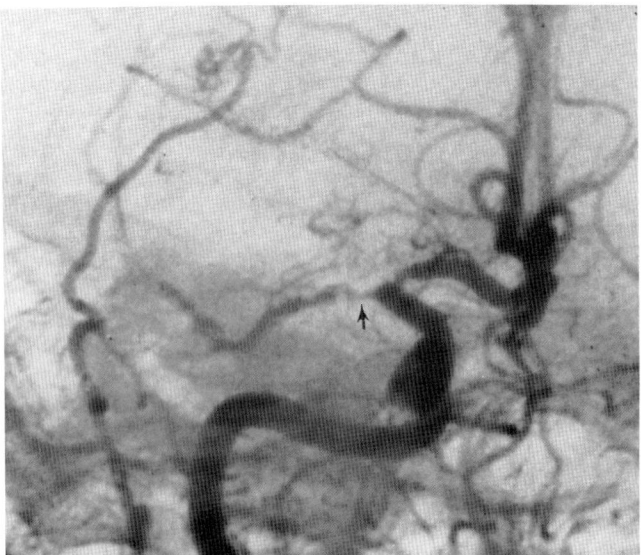

Figure 2.35 Symptomatic internal carotid stenosis and asymptomatic contralateral middle cerebral stenosis. Severe stenosis at the origin of the middle cerebral artery (*arrow*) is associated with delayed flow. This lesion was asymptomatic until 5 days after carotid endarterectomy on the opposite side. (From Ojemann RG, Crowell RM, Roberson GH, Fisher CM: Surgical treatment of extracranial carotid occlusive disease, Ch. 14, in *Clinical Neurosurgery.* Baltimore, Williams & Wilkins, 1974, vol 22, with permission.)

studied was done because of recurrent neurological symptoms in the territory of the operated artery. Most of these patients showed recurrent stenosis, although a normal vessel or minor irregularities were also occasionally found (see page 60). In the second group of patients studied because of neurological symptoms in the territory of another intracranial vessel, most of the operated internal carotid arteries were patent and smooth with a few showing only minor irregularities (Figs. 1.17 and 2.28B). Occasionally, external carotid stenosis or occlusion was found (Fig. 2.36).

POSTOPERATIVE COMPLICATIONS
Neurological
Cerebral Ischemia

The EEG electrodes are left on the patient until he or she awakens in the recovery room. If a neurological deficit is found as the patient awakens and significant EEG change has occurred, the patient is returned immediately for exploration of the artery. If the deficit is present with no change in the EEG, the patient is immediately investigated with a measurement of retinal artery pressure and a CT scan to look for hemorrhage. If these are normal, angiography is done (Fig. 2.37). If there is any question about the status of the operated artery, it is reexplored. If studies show the endarterectomy site is normal, blood volume and blood pressure are maintained and a decision is made regarding anticoagulation. If the neurological deficit is mild and non-progresive, the same non-invasive tests are done, but usually no abnormality is found. In such patients it is assumed that an embolus was dislodged sometime during the dissection.

If the patient develops a neurological deficit after initial good recovery, this change may mean occlusion at the site of the operation. If the superficial temporal pulse is lost or the retinal artery pressure is reduced, the patient should be taken immediately to the operating room to ascertain the status of the artery. In other cases, an angiogram is done. The usual reason for postoperative carotid occlusion is a residual plaque or intimal flap, but occasionally the problem may be associated with an unrecognized hypercoagulable state. As digital subtraction angiography is improved, it may be the procedure of choice to rapidly evaluate these postoperative neurological problems.

Transient Ischemic Attacks

A small number of patients will have one or more transient ischemic episodes in the postoperative period. Usually it is a single attack, but if there are more than one they usually occur within the first 10–14 days after surgery. This symptom does not usually signify a serious problem in the operated artery. None of our patients who experienced this problem went on to have a stroke.

Non-invasive studies are done to ascertain whether there is a hemodynamic lesion. If a bruit is present, a phonoangiogram is also done. A significant abnormal finding would lead to an angiogram. In our experience, most patients will not have evidence of stenosis. They are treated with antiplatelet or anticoagulant therapy. If TIAs persist, angiography is indicated and will usually demonstrate a lesion that needs reoperation (33).

Intracerebral Hemorrhage

Early in our series, a typical hypertensive hemorrhage occurred in the basal ganglia 4 days after surgery when blood pressure was 200/100 mm Hg (29). Since that time, careful control of postoperative hypertension has reduced the incidence of this complication. However, even with mild elevation in blood pressure, a hemorrhage may occasionaly occur (Fig. 2.38). This problem is also of concern in patients who have had previous cerebral infarction when postoperative heparin or antiplatelet therapy is used (40).

Seizure

On rare occasion a seizure may occur. Presumably this is related to an embolus occluding a small cortical artery (45). Appropriate anticonvulsant treatment is given.

Carotid Endarterectomy

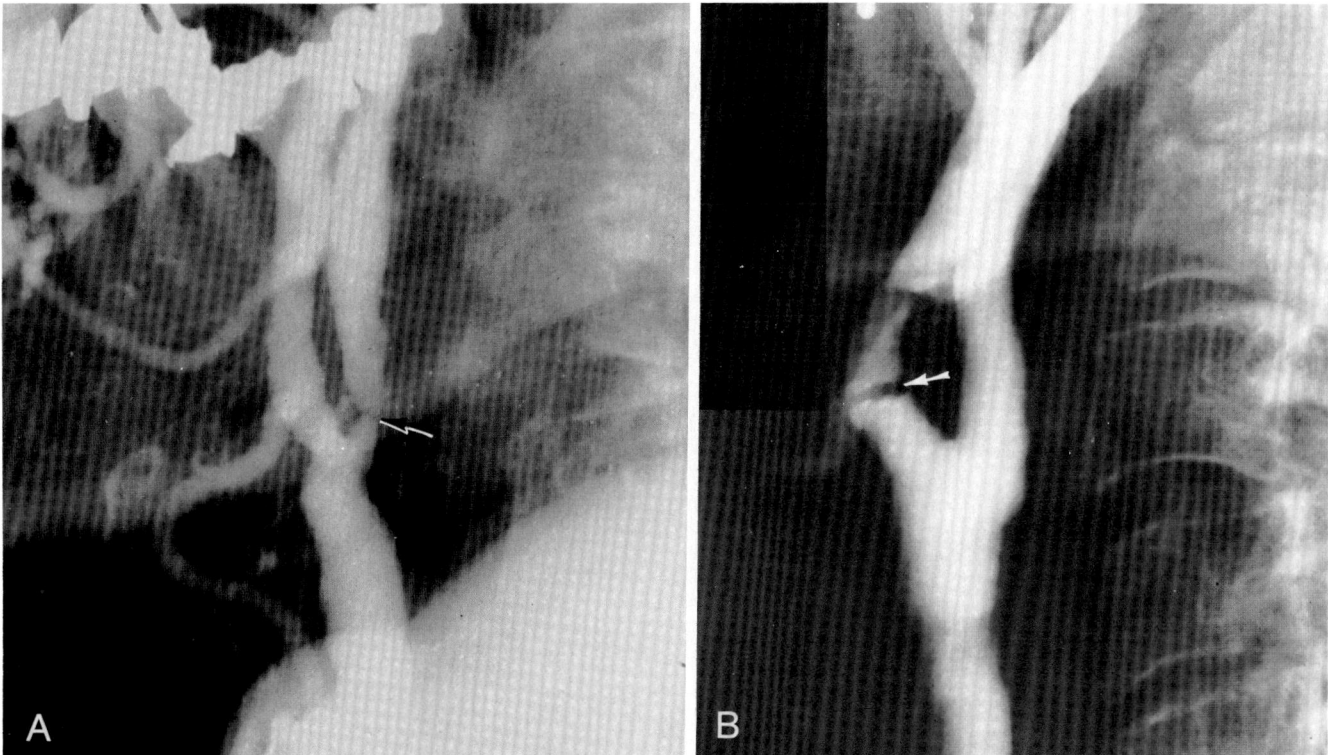

Figure 2.36 Postoperative angiography: A, preoperative angiogram showing stenosis in the proximal internal carotid artery (*arrow*). B, angiogram 2 years later. The internal carotid artery is smooth and has a normal caliber. A sharply localized narrowing is seen in the external carotid artery (*arrow*). Comment: The patient was studied for symptoms in the opposite cartoid artery. The slight widening in the common carotid artery where the plaque was cut off is normal. The external carotid lesion is probably due to a flap of atheroma and intima left at the time of the endarterectomy.

Headache

In the postoperative period, the patient may complain of significant unilateral headache in the retrobulbar, frontal, or temporal region. Blood pressure is usually normal and the pain is not like that noted in the face, jaw, or neck with internal carotid dissection. The symptom responds to mild analgesics and usually subsides in a few days. No serious sequlae have been related to this symptom in our patients.

In a report of 50 patients (57 endarterectomies), 24 had postoperative headaches encompassing the entire spectrum of vascular headaches: nonspecific diffuse headaches, severe hemicranias, cluster headaches, chronic paroxysmal hemicranias, and carotidynia (28). The frequency and severity of headaches in our series was much less.

Cranial Nerve Injury

Facial Nerve (Mandibular Branch)

If the incision is carried too near the angle of the jaw or retraction is too vigorous, the mandibular branch of the facial nerve can be stretched causing weakness of the lower lip. This is an annoying problem which causes a cosmetic change and may make the patient drool from the corner of the mouth. Spontaneous recovery almost always occurs (19). We have avoided this problem by curving the incision away from the angle of the jaw toward the mastoid process (Fig. 2.3A) and by being careful with placement of the self-retaining retractors.

Vagus Nerve

Injury to the vagus or recurrent laryngeal nerve with vocal cord paresis has been reported to occur in about 1% of patients undergoing carotid endarterectomy (29, 46). Traction or pressure on the nerve is the usual cause. As noted in the discussion of operative technique, the vagus nerve can lie on the anterior surface of the common carotid artery and may be encountered early in the dissection. Another area where the nerve is susceptible to injury is in dissection of the internal carotid artery where it may closely adhere to the artery. Direct injury to the recurrent laryngeal nerve may occur if the retraction blades are placed too deeply in the medial aspect of the incision. On rare occasion, a branch will come off the vagus nerve high in the neck and either run separately or join the descendens hypoglossi nerve. This branch must be saved.

There is nothing that can be done about the loss of vocal cord function. A majority of patients will show spontaneous recovery within a year (19). The problem is particularly crucial if bilateral operations are

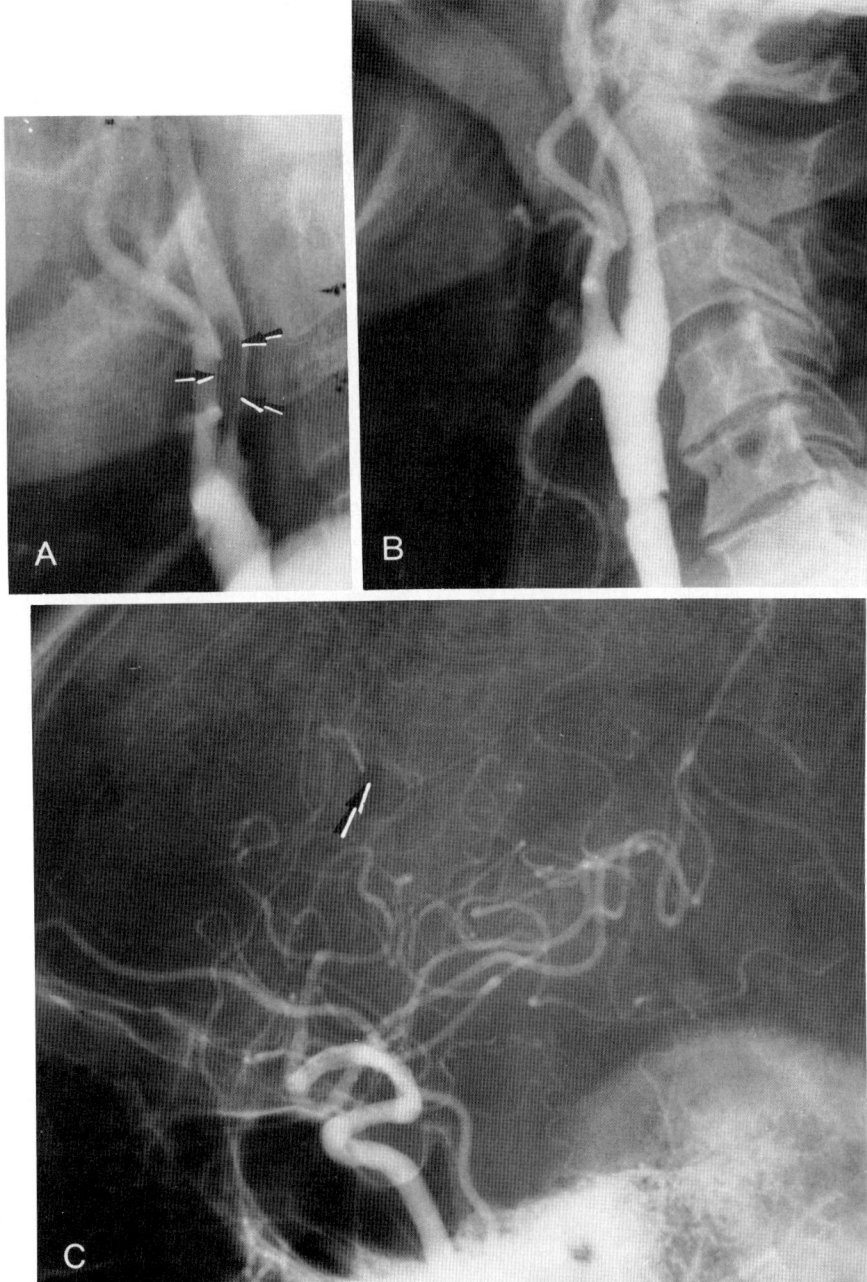

Figure 2.37 Emergency operation for Intraluminal thrombus: intraoperative cerebral embolization. *A*, preoperative left carotid angiogram. There is severe stenosis and, in addition, the irregular distal shadow (*arrows*) in the internal carotid artery suggests an intraluminal thrombus which was found at surgery. There is also reduced flow in the internal carotid artery as shown by reduced density of dye compared to the external carotid artery. *B*, postoperative angiogram showing restoration of normal internal carotid artery. There is slight constriction at the proximal end of the endarterectomy which is not significant. *C*, postoperative lateral angiogram of head showing embolus in a distal middle cerebral branch (*arrow*). After heparinization, the patient recovered to a mild deficit. Comment: In spite of careful dissection, occasionally an embolus will be dislodged and cause a postoperative neurological deficit. There has been some discussion as to how long one should wait before operating on a patient with an intraluminal thrombus. Some have advocated treatment with heparin for several days to allow more organization of the thrombus so there would be less chance of an embolus breaking off. However, we believe the risk of spontaneous embolus or thrombosis is high in such patients and operation should be done promptly.

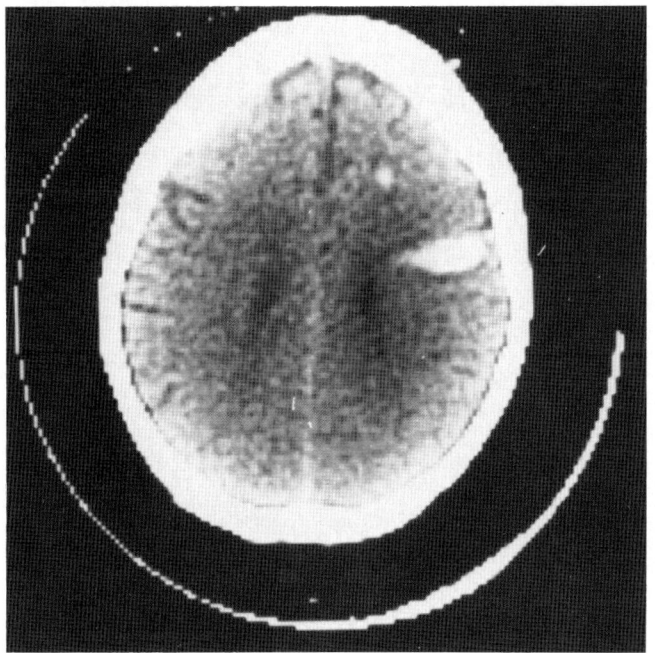

Figure 2.38 Small intracerebral hemorrhage after carotid endarterectomy. This 60-year-old man had a 6-month history of right TMB and a 3-week history of episodes of left hemiparesis. The neurological examination was normal. A right carotid bruit was present. Right carotid endarterectomy was done. His course was uncomplicated with systolic blood pressure ranging from 140–160 mm. Five days after operation, he developed sudden headache, thickness of speech, and mild left facial and left upper extremity weakness. CT scan shows the small subcortical hemorrhage. Noninvasive carotid studies were normal. He made a full recovery.

planned. If it is essential to do the opposite carotid endarterectomy following this complication, appropriate planning for tracheotomy is necessary should a bilateral weakness develop.

Superior Laryngeal Nerve

Dissection posterior to the carotid bifurcation may injure the superior laryngeal nerve. Trauma to this nerve may cause some relaxation of the ipsilateral vocal cord manifested by easy fatigability of the voice and impairment in phonation at a high pitch. Fortunately, the injury is usually asymptomatic. In one report where injury of the nerve was found on examination, four of five patients had no symptoms (19).

Hypoglossal Nerve

This complication is generally avoided by following the steps outlined in "Operative Technique." When it does occur, it is usually due to excessive traction on the nerve. Nothing need be done. Usually there are no symptoms. A majority of the patients will have a spontaneous recovery within a few months (19).

Cardiopulmonary

These complications have been reduced by following the guidelines discussed under "Preoperative Evaluation" and "Postoperative Management." Nitroglycerine given IV is used to control EKG change. Sublingual nitroglycerine is used for angina. Hypertension and hypotension are treated as discussed on page 53.

Wound Infection

Most infections have been superficial and are due to staphyococcus aureus. They respond to the usual measures of opening the incision, irrigation, and antibiotics and allowing the wound to close secondarily. If the infection is deep, an angiogram should be done to check for a false aneurysm.

Wound Hematoma

Some patients will have significant swelling of the wound. This may be due to either hematoma or a lymph collection. If there is no problem with the airway, nothing need be done. The swelling will gradually subside over a few weeks. However, if the trachea is shifted and the airway compromised, the patient should be reintubated and returned to the operating room. A Hemovac drain has been effective in reducing the incidence of neck hematoma.

False Aneurysm

We have not encountered this problem, but it has been reported (11). The diagnosis should be considered when a patient develops a late wound infection or has evidence of what appears to be a persistent hematoma or swelling in the neck. The recommended treatment is excision of the aneurysm with repair of the wall of the artery using a saphenous vein graft.

THE PATHOLOGY OF CAROTID ENDARTERECTOMY SPECIMENS

Dr. C. Miller Fisher examined 40 endarterectomy specimens removed, when possible, in one piece (29). These specimens were serially sectioned at eight microns after being fixed in formalin and embedded in parafin. Various stains were used, with phosphotungstic acid hematoxylin being the chief one. The 40 cases were classified clinically as follows:

TIAs	13
TIAs with superimposed stroke	14
Stroke without prodomatus	6
Stepwise or progressive stroke	2
Asymptomatic	5

In the 35 cases that were symptomatic, the main occluding mass was an atheromatous plaque in 75%, hemorrhage into a plaque in 15%, and a fibrin mass on the plaque in 10%.

Hemorrhage dissecting into a plaque from the lumen was common and appeared to be the mechanism by which an ulcer crater was produced rather than by primary hemorrhage deep within the plaque. No fewer than 60% of the 35 symptomatic cases showed hemorrhage into the main plaque. In only one-third of these did it add significantly to the mass of occluding tissue, but in some cases it furnished the nidus for the deposition of a mural thrombus that finally occluded the lumen. In these interpretations, it was assumed that the hemorrhage into the plaque was not the result of surgical manipulation.

The mural thrombus superimposed on the atheromatous plaque varied in size and contributed in varying degrees (10–80%) to the stenosis of the residual lumen. It might be anticipated that the mural thrombus would be deposited in a somewhat haphazard way in relation to the plaque and probably in multiple areas. There was as a rule, however, only one mural thrombus and it regularly lay at the point of greatest narrowing or within one millimeter of this area (Fig. 2.39). In the group of 13 patients with only TIAs, the lumen was narrowed to 1 × 2 mm or less in 12 cases. In the exception, the residual lumen was 4 × 4 mm and had an ulceration 1.5 mm wide, 2.5 mm deep, and 3.2 mm axially which contained a fibrin platelet mural thrombus in the depth of the crater (Fig. 2.40). The ulceration was probably the result of the blood dissecting into the shallow atheromatous plaque. Of the 12 severely stenosed cases, five had a mural thrombus containing platelet material, five had a fibrin mural thrombus without platelets, and two had no mural thrombus at all.

In 10 of the 14 patients with TIAs and stroke, the lumen was occluded. In two it was narrowed to a fraction of a millimeter, in one there was hemorrhage into the plaque, and in one a fibrin mural thrombus may have served as a source of a middle cerebral embolism. In eight patients with stroke with or without step-wise progression, the lumen was totally occluded by recent fibrin platelet material.

In five asymptomatic patients, all of whom had the opposite carotid artery operated for symptoms, the lumen ranged from 1–3 mm in diameter and no mural thrombus was present.

In two cases of recurrent carotid stenosis approximately 4 years after operation, microscopic examination disclosed unusually abundant local fibrous connective tissue proliferation jutting into the lumen. There was little evidence of fatty deposition in the connective tissue, and any role of lipid in the reaction was not obvious.

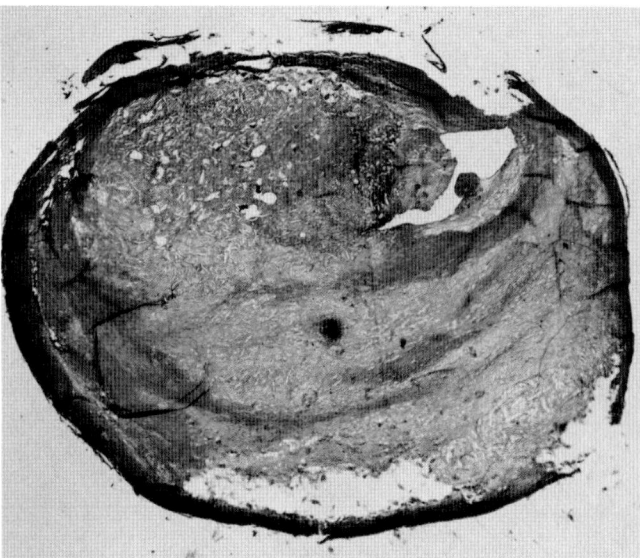

Figure 2.39 Mural thrombus. Cross-section of endarterectomy specimen, PTAH stain. At the point of maximum narrowing, a small mural thrombus is projecting into the lumen. This is the usual location when a mural thrombus is found.

RECURRENT STENOSIS

Incidence and Pathology

Recurrent stenosis occurs in a small percentage of patients who have had carotid endarterectomy. There seem to be three groups of patients in which this problem arises:
1. Patients in whom surgical technique has contributed to the problem (15). This includes:
   a. Failure to remove the distal tongue of the plaque
   b. Narrowing of the lumen during the arteriotomy closure
   c. Damage to the intima by vascular clamps
2. Patients who have a tendency to excess scar formation
3. Patients in whom a combination of fibrosis, recurrent atherosclerosis, and, at times, associated thrombus formation develops

Symptomatic stenosis may recur within a few months of the operation. This usually relates to one of the problems in surgical technique or to the thickened fibrosis of the arterial wall which is grossly and histologically distinct from the typical atherosclerotic plaque. Fortunately, this tendency to excess scar formation is a rare happening. Recurrent stenosis that occurs after 2 years usually has significant atheroma, as well as fibrosis.

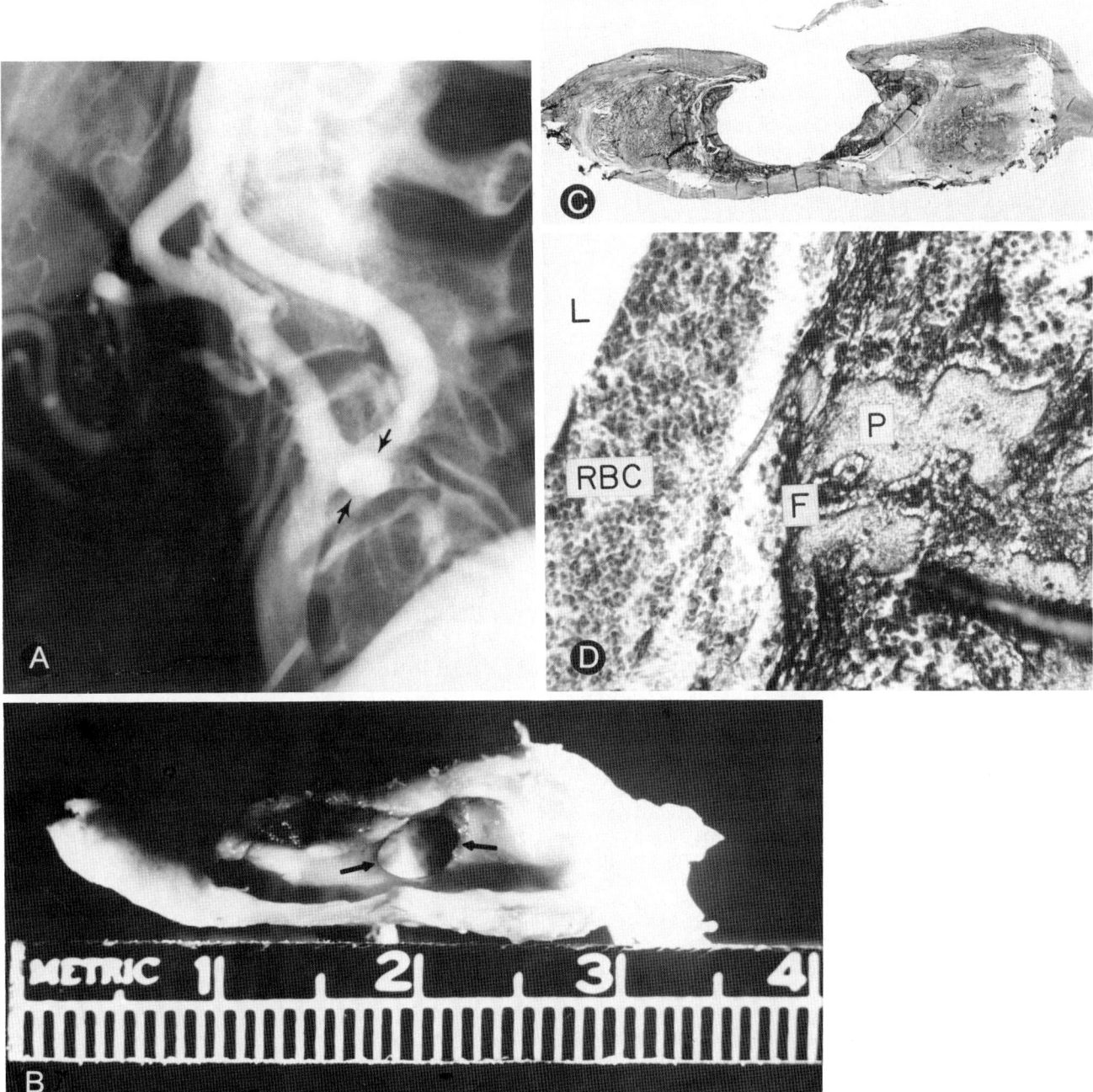

Figure 2.40 Ulcerated plaque. *A,* left carotid angiogram showing a large, round ulcer crater (*arrows*) within a plaque at the origin of the internal carotid artery. *B,* the endarterectomy specimen was removed intact and opened longitudinally, demonstrating a large undermining cavity in the plaque (*arrows*). *C,* microscopic section of plaque demonstrating large undermining cavitation. *D,* wall of ulcer showing fibrin (*F*) platelet material (*P*) and red blood cells (*RBC*) at surface adjacent to lumen (*L*). (From Ojemann RG, Crowell RM, Roberson GH, Fisher CM: Surgical treatment of extracranial carotid occlusive disease, Ch. 14, in *Clinical Neurosurgery.* Baltimore, Williams & Wilkins, 1974, vol 22, with permission.)

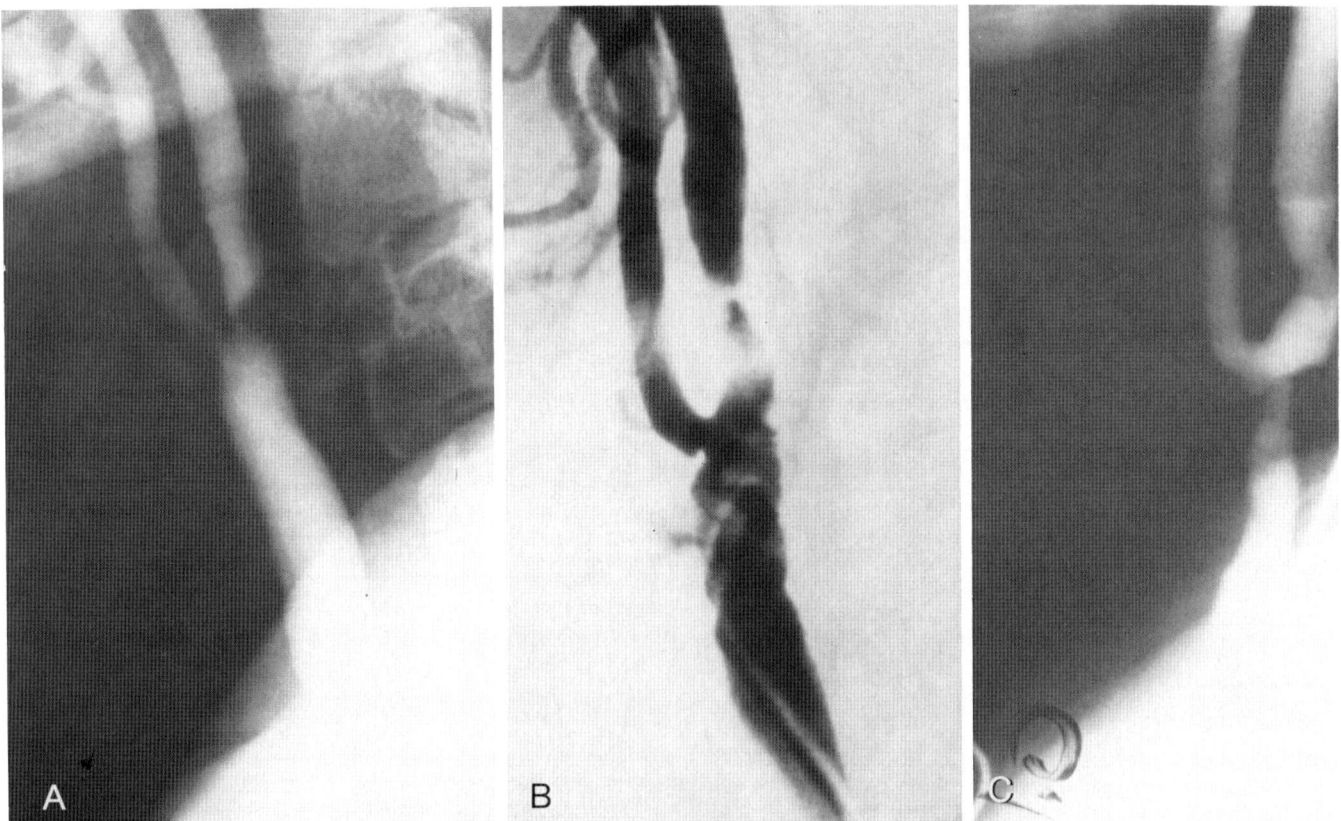

Figure 2.41 Restenosis after carotid endarterectomy. Left carotid angiograms. *A*, patient presented with TMB and THA (tingling right hand). Angiogram shows severe stenosis at origin of left internal carotid artery. Carotid endarterectomy was done with satisfactory postoperative course. *B*, 6 years later, THA followed by TMB. Severe stenosis at distal end of endarterectomy. Carotid endarterectomy done. The plaque in the common carotid artery was fibrotic with irregular islands of atheromatous plaque. More marked atheroma was present in the internal carotid artery with an associated thrombus. Primary closure done without a patch. *C*, 3 years after the second operation, THA (numbness and tingling right upper extremity). The angiogram now shows narrowing and irregularity in the distal common carotid artery and slight narrowing in the internal carotid. Carotid endarterectomy done. The plaque consisted of fibrous tissue with endothelium, but in the distal common carotid artery extending to the origin of the external and internal carotid arteries was a collar of yellowish atheromatous tissue measuring approximately 1.0 cm in longitudinal dimension and encircling the inner lumen of the vessel. At the distal end of this material at the origin of the internal carotid artery was a small thrombus. In the external and internal carotid arteries was found only scar tissue with endothelium. Because of the fibrous tissue and narrowed caliber of the artery, a Dacron patch graft was placed. Postoperative course was satisfactory.

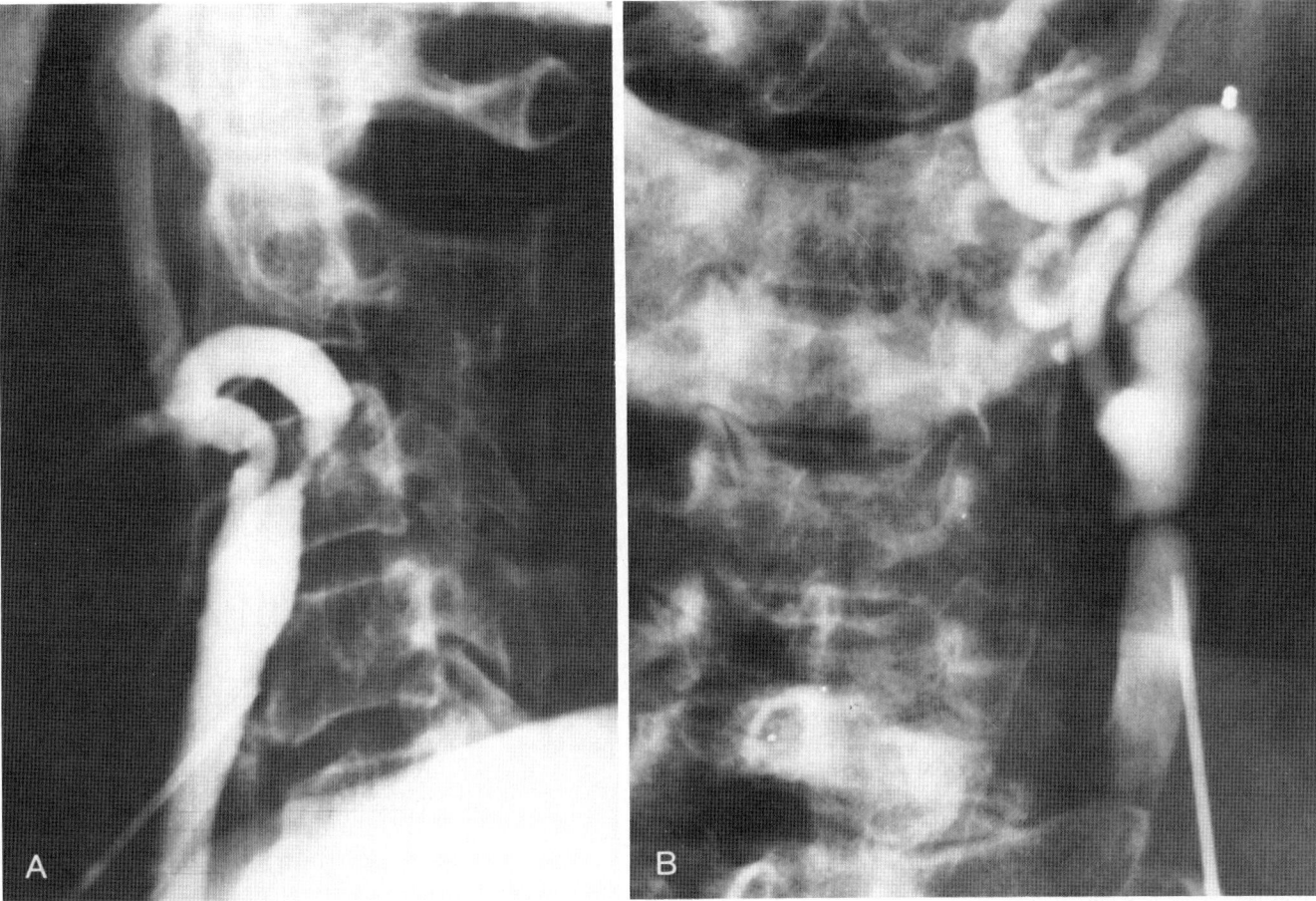

Figure 2.42 Restenosis by fibrous web. *A*, initial angiogram shows stenosis at the origin of the internal carotid artery. There is also a prominent loop in the proximal internal carotid artery. *B*, angiogram 4 years later shows normal internal carotid artery but a web at site of the proximal edge of the endarterectomy. Comment: Patient presented with recurrent TIAs. A localized area of thickened intima with fibrosis was found at operation. (From Ojemann RG, Crowell RM, Roberson GH, Fisher CM: Surgical treatment of extracranial carotid occlusive disease, Ch. 14, in *Clinical Neurosurgery*. Baltimore, Williams & Wilkins, 1974, vol 22, with permission.)

Restenosis within 24 months of carotid endarterectomy was found in 3.6% of 361 operations (8). The average time for recognition of the recurrence was 12 months with a range of 5 to 24 months. In another report, intimal fibrosis was the predominent finding in the first postoperative year and atheroma was seen only in recurrent stenosis more than 2 years after the original operation (35).

In our series, recurrent symptomatic stenosis developed in 12 patients. One patient developed bilateral and another unilateral restenosis twice (Fig. 2.41). Except for one progressive asymptomatic bruit, all patients came to attention because of recurrent TIAs. The interval between operations and symptoms ranged from 1 to 6 years. The patient with the earliest lesion had thickening of the entire arterial wall due primarily to fibrosis with no evidence of atheroma over a longitudinal distance of 3–4 cm. She had a tendency for keloid formation in other scars. Other findings in patients who had operations within 3 years of the original surgery included a fibrous web-like diaphragm at the proximal end of the endarterectomy with thickened intima and little atheroma, and a thin layer of multiple plaques of atheroma in a thickened, scarred intima with a small associated thrombus. Patients seen 3 years after operation had an atheromatous deposit in the thickened, scarred intima causing various degrees of narrowing and often associated with a superimposed thrombus. In two cases of recurrent symptomatic stenosis seen approximately 4 years after operation, angiography showed a narrow shelf-like obstruction (Fig. 2.42). Microscopic examination disclosed unusually abundant local fibrous connective tissue proliferation projecting into the lumen. Fatty deposition was relatively minor.

Technical Points

The operation is often difficult because of the dense periarterial scar and the fibrosis of the vessel wall. Great care is required to avoid injury to the internal jugular vein, vagus, and hypoglossal nerves. The thickened intima is often densely adherent to the outer arterial wall, particularly in the region of the previous suture line. It is, therefore, usually wise to make a new incision to start the arteriotomy. It is also more difficult to get a "clean" removal in the distal internal carotid artery. Most patients have some thickening of the arterial wall due to fibrosis and it is usually necessary to use a patch graft to repair the artery.

REFERENCES

1. Barnes RW, Marszalek PB: Asymptomatic carotid disease in the cardiovascular surgical patient: Is prophylactic endarterectomy necessary? Stroke 12:497-500, 1981.
2. Barnett HJM, Peerless SJ, Kaufmann JCE: "Stump" of internal carotid artery: A source for further cerebral embolic ischemia. Stroke 9:448-456, 1978.
3. Bland JE, Lazar ML: Carotid endarterectomy without shunt. Neurosurgery 8:153-157, 1981.
4. Callow AD: An overview of the stroke problem in the carotid territory. Am J Surg 140:181-191, 1980.
5. Caplan LR, Skillman J, Ojemann R, Fields WS: Intracerebral hemorrhage following carotid endarterectomy: A hypertensive complication? Stroke 9:457-460, 1978.
6. Carney WI, Stewart WB, DePinto DJ, Mucha SJ, Roberts B: Carotid bruit as a risk in aortoiliac reconstruction. Surgery 81:567-570, 1977.
7. Chiappa KH, Burke SR, Young RR: Results of electoencephalographic monitoring during 367 carotid endarterectomies. Use of a dedicated minicomputer. Stroke 10:381-388, 1979.
8. Cossman D, Callow AD, Stein A, Matsumoto G: Early restenosis after carotid endarterectomy. Arch Surg 113:275-278, 1978.
9. Crowell RM, Ojemann RG; Extracrannial cerebrovascular disease, in Hoff JT (ed): Practice of Surgery. Philadelphia, Harper and Row, 1981. Chapt. 28.
9a. Crowell RM, Ojemann RG, Lee RS, deBros F, Sundaram P: Carotid endarterectomy in high risk patients with cardiopulmonary disease. Stroke 12:123, 1981.
10. Davie JC, Richardson R: Distal internal carotid thromboembolectomy using a Fogarty catheter in total occlusion. J Neurosurg 27:171-177, 1967.
11. Ehrenfeld WK, Hays RJ: False aneurysm after carotid endarterectomy. Arch Surg 104:288-291, 1972.
12. Ennix CL Jr, Lawrie GM, Morris GC Jr, Crawford ES, Howell JF, Reardon MJ, Weatherford SC: Improved results of carotid endarterectomy in patients with symptomatic coronary disease: An analysis of 1546 consecutive carotid operations. Stroke 10:122-125, 1979.
13. Evans WE, Cooperman M: The significance of asymptomatic unilateral carotid bruits in preoperative patients. Surgery 83:521-522, 1978.
14. Ferguson GG, Gamache FW, Blume WT, Farrar JK: Monitoring during carotid endarterectomy. Further evidence that an internal shunt is not necessary. Neurosurgery 7:285, 1980.
15. French BN, Rewcastle NB: Recurrent stenosis at site of carotid endarterectomy. Stroke 8:597-605, 1977.
16. Giannotta SL, Dicks RE III, Kindt GW: Carotid endarterectomy: Technical improvements. Neurosurgery 7:309-312, 1980.
17. Hafner LD, Tew JM: Surgical management of the totally occluded internal carotid artery: A ten-year study. Surgery 80:710-717, 1981.
18. Hertzer NR: External carotid endarterectomy. Surg Gynecol Obstet 153:186-190, 1981.
19. Hertzer NR, Feldman BJ, Beven EG, Tucker HM: A prospective study of the incidence of injury to the cranial nerves during carotid endarterectomy. Surg Gynecol Obstet 151:781-784, 1980.
20. Hodosh RM, Boone SC: Neurological manifestations of external carotid artery disease. Clin Neurosurg 28:384-406, 1981.
21. Hugenholtz H, Elgie RG: Carotid thromboendarterectomy: A reappraisal. Criteria for patient selection. J Neurosurg 53:776-783, 1980.
22. Karmody AM, Shah DM, Monoco VJ, Leather RP: On surgical reconstruction of the external carotid artery. Am J Surg 136:176-180, 1978.
23. Kelly JJ, Callow AD, O'Donnell TF, McBride K, Ehrneberg B, Korwin S, Welch H, Gembarowicz RM: Failure of carotid stump pressure. Its incidence as a predictor for a temporary shunt during carotid endarterectomy. Arch Surg 114:1361-1366, 1979.
24. Kerber CW, Cromwell LD, Loehden OL: Catheter dilatation of proximal carotid stenosis during distal bifurcation endarterectomy. Am J Neurorad 1:348-349, 1980.
25. Kusunoki T, Rowed DW, Tator CH, Lougheed WM: Thromboendarterectomy for total occlusion of the internal carotid artery: A reappraisal of risks, success rate and potential benefits. Stroke 9:34-38, 1978.
25a. Lippman HH, Sundt TM Jr, Holman CB: The poststenotic carotid slim sign; spurious internal carotid hypoplasia. Mayo Clin Proc 45:762-767, 1970.
26. Matsumoto GH, Baker JD, Watson CW, Gleucklich D, Callow AD: Electroencephalographic surveillance as a means of extending operability in high risk carotid endarterectomy. Stroke 7:554-559, 1976.
27. McKay RD, Sundt TM Jr, Michenfelder JD, Gronert GA, Messick JM, Sharbrough FW, Piepgras DG: Internal carotid artery stump pressure and cerebral blood flow during carotid endarterectomy. Modification by halothane, enflurone and innover. Anesthesiology 45:390-399, 1976.
28. Messert B, Black JA: Cluster headache, hemicrania and other head pains: Morbidity of carotid endarterectomy. Stroke 9:559-562, 1978.
29. Ojemann RG, Crowell RM, Roberson GH, Fisher CM: Surgical treatment of extracranial carotid occlusive disease. Clin Neurosurg 22:214-263, 1975.
30. Ott DA, Cooley DA, Chapa L, Coelho A: Carotid endarterectomy without temporary intraluminal shunt. Ann Surg 191:708-714, 1980.
31. Owens ML, Atkinson JB, Wilson SE: Recurrent transient ischemic attacks after carotid endarterectomy. Arch Surg 115:482-486, 1980.
32. Rice PL, Pifarre R, Sullivan HJ, Montoya A, Bakhos M: Experience with simultaneous myocardial revascularization and carotid endarterectomy. J Thorac Cardiovasc Surg 79:922-925, 1980.
33. Schutz H, Fleming JFR, Awerbuck B: Arteriographic assessment of carotid disease. Ann Surg 171:509-521, 1970.
34. Sharbrough FW, Messick JM Jr, Sundt TM Jr: Correlation of continuous electroencephalograms with cerebral blood flow measurements during carotid endarterectomy. Stroke 4:674-683, 1973.
35. Stoney R, String T: Recurrent carotid stenosis. Surgery 80:705-710, 1976.
36. Sundt TM Jr, Sandok BA, Whisnant JP: Carotid endarterectomy. Complications and preoperative assessment of risk. Mayo Clin Proc 50:301-306, 1975.
37. Sundt TM Jr, Sharbrough FW, Trautmann JC, Gronert GA: Monitoring techniques for carotid endarterectomy. Clin Neurosurg 22:199-213, 1975.
38. Sundt TM Jr, Sharbrough FW, Piepgras DG, Kearns TP, Messick JM Jr, O'Fallon WM: Correlation of cerebral blood flow and electroencephalographic changes during carotid endarterectomy. With results of surgery and hemodynamics of cerebral ischemia. Mayo Clinic Proc 56:533-543, 1981.
39. Tarlov E, Schmidek H, Scott RM, Wepsic JG, Ojemann RG: Reflex hypotension following carotid endarterectomy: Mechanism and management. J Neurosurg 39:323-327, 1973.
40. Thompson JE: Surgery for Cerebrovascular Insufficiency, Stroke: With Special Emphasis on Carotid Endarterectomy. Springfield, Illinois, CC Thomas, 1968.
41. Towne JB, Bernhard VM: The relationship of postoperative

hypertension to complications following carotid endarterectomy surgery. Surgery 88:575–580, 1980.
42. Treiman RL, Foran RF, Shore EH, Levin PM: Carotid bruit: Significance in patients undergoing an abdominal aortic operation. Arch Surg 106:803–805, 1973.
43. Turnipseed WD, Berkoff HA, Belzer FO: Postoperative stroke in cardiac and peripheral vascular disease. Ann Surg 192:365–368, 1980.
44. Whittemore AD: Carotid endarterectomy. An alternative approach. Arch Surg 115:940–942, 1980.
45. Wilkinson JT, Adams HP Jr, Wright CB: Convulsions after carotid endarterectomy. JAMA 244:1827–1828, 1980.
46. Wylie EJ, Ehrenfeld WK: *Extracranial Occlusive Cerebrovascular Disease: Diagnosis and Management.* Philadelphia, WB Saunders, 1970.

Chapter 3 ASYMPTOMATIC CAROTID BRUIT

ETIOLOGY

The increased awareness that stroke might be preventable has led to the frequent finding on routine physical examination of an asymptomatic bruit over the lateral neck. Such bruits often reflect turbulent blood flow in the proximal internal carotid artery due to localized atherosclerosis with stenosis. However, cervical bruits may be caused by a variety of other pathological conditions (Table 3.1) (13).

Bruits due to atheroma are produced by turbulent jets of blood just distal to the stenosis (20). This turbulent flow is related to the residual flow rate in the most stenotic segment which in turn is related to the residual lumen diameter and length of the stenosis. For a bruit to occur, there must be more than 70% reduction in the cross-sectional area of the lumen of the artery; the diameter must, therefore, be reduced more than 50% (6). Because of the difficulty in estimation of percentage diameter reduction from angiographic films, it is more practical and reliable to estimate the residual lumen diameter in millimeters. Bruits generally occur when the residual lumen diameter is 2 mm or less, but when residual lumen diameter falls below 1 mm (impending occlusion), the bruit often diminishes in intensity (20).

NATURAL HISTORY

Because cervical bruits due to atherosclerosis can be caused by varying degrees of stenosis within the internal carotid artery and may or may not be associated with ulceration and may progress at varying rates, the natural history of these conditions is as variable as the underlying anatomic configurations. There is evidence that stenosis may be progressive in some patients and lead to hemodynamic insufficiency or distal embolization (4, 17). Angiographic selection criteria have the advantage of precision in anatomic diagnosis, but most clinical studies are highly selected. Series based on criteria developed by non-invasive diagnostic techniques are significantly less precise in anatomic diagnosis though broader populations of patients may be surveyed. Epidemiological studies may be population-based and prospective in their data gathering. However, such investigations generally rely on auscultation for a diagnosis and the anatomic precision is less satisfactory.

Given the restrictions of these types of data, it is not surprising that varying results are reported for patients with asymptomatic bruits (Table 3.2). These reports have been recently summarized (10). Some reports suggest that the natural history of an asymptomatic bruit is relatively benign. Wolf et al. investigated, in prospective fashion, asymptomatic bruits in the population of patients comprising the Framingham Study (35). Among 245 patients, five developed strokes relevant to the apparent carotid stenosis over a period of 12 years for a stroke rate of 0.16% per year. Multiple examiners documented the bruits and precise characteristics were not specified. Heyman et al. reported on a series of 72 patients followed for an average of 6 years (15). Three strokes clearly relevant to the artery with the bruit were recorded for a stroke rate of 0.7% per year. In that study, one single observer recorded the various bruits, the specific characteristics of which were clearly defined. On the other hand, Thompson et al. followed 138 selected patients with asymptomatic carotid stenosis documented by angiography (32). Over an average follow-up period of 4 years, the stroke rate was 4.5% per year. An ominous natural history was also suggested by Kartchner and McRae who found that 13 of 78 patients with hemodynamically significant carotid stenosis developed stroke in a 2-year follow-up period for an average stroke rate of 8.3% per year (19).

Sources of clinical data other than follow-up of asymptomatic bruit have provided indirect evidence that this condition may lead suddenly to a significant neurological deficit. Fisher studied 50 cases of internal carotid occlusion (14). Eight patients (16%) were asymptomatic and 13 (26%) experienced TIAs or mild stroke with good recovery, but 29 cases (58%) suffered moderate to severe neurological deficit which was incapacitating. In the cases with frank stroke, 60%

Table 3.1
Differential Diagnosis of Cervical Bruit

Internal carotid artery stenosis
External carotid artery stenosis
Internal carotid artery dissection
Internal carotid artery kink
Fibromuscular dysphasia
Subclavian or innominate artery stenosis
Radiated cardiac murmur
High flow state
   Intracranial AVM
   Carotid cavernous fistula
   Hyperthyroidism
Venous hum

Table 3.2
Risk of Stroke in Patients with Asymptomatic Carotid Bruit/Stenosis

Author	Subjects	Test	No. of Patients	% Strokes per Year	Follow-up Period (years)
Wolf (35)	Population	Auscultation	245	0.2	12
Heyman (15)	Population	Auscultation	72	0.7	6
Humphries (16)	2nd side[a]	Angiography	168	0.9	2.5
Thompson (32)	Selected	Angiography	138	4.5	4
Kartchner (19)	Selected	Non-invasive	78	8.3	2

[a] Asymptomatic carotid studied at the time of angiographic evaluation of a contralateral symptomatic carotid lesion.

had TIAs but 40% experienced no warning attacks of any sort. Similar findings were found by Pessin et al. where 64 patients with acute carotid stroke had documentation of prior TIAs in 54%, but in the other 46%, stroke came as a "bolt from the blue" with no clinical warning to permit therapeutic intervention prophylactically (26). It is likely that many of these patients had a bruit prior to having neurological symptoms.

At the present time there is no way to predict what the outcome will be in any given asymptomatic patient. Furthermore, to await the occurrence of warning TIAs to identify the patient at risk means settling for a potentially unacceptable outcome in about 30% of the cases where the stenosis is hemodynamically significant. These data support the position that management of asymptomatic carotid stenosis may be critical in reducing stroke (23).

Another problem related to defining the natural history of the asymptomatic bruit is the asymptomatic internal carotid ulcer. These lesions have commonly been regarded as benign (21). However, Moore et al. have presented evidence suggesting deep and irregular lesions may cause stroke in as many as 12.5% of cases per year (24).

CLINICAL EVALUATION

Various strategies have been devised for the evaluation and treatment of a patient with an asymptomatic carotid bruit. Some physicians have advised careful follow-up (16) while others have proposed antiplatelet therapy (5) or carotid endarterectomy (13, 32). Since the natural history has not been defined and various diagnostic and treatment protocols have been applied to selected patients, results cannot be reliably compared. Recent work has focused on the role of non-invasive diagnostic tests in providing guidelines for treatment of these patients (12, 29). Bruits associated with internal carotid stenosis are usually localized in the mid-cervical region and are not heard in the low neck and chest. The character of the bruit is also important. The higher the pitch of the bruit, the tighter the stenosis (11). High-pitched bruits extending into diastole are particularly important because they usually indicate tightly stenotic lesions with residual lumen diameters less than 2 mm. When the residual lumen becomes less than 1 mm, the bruit may diminish in intensity (20).

When the presence of an asymptomatic bruit in the region of the carotid bifurcation is established, non-invasive studies are ordered (see page 12). When the non-invasive tests suggest a hemodynamically significant internal carotid stenosis, angiography is the most reliable method of assessing the pathology in the carotid bifurcation region. In the future, the use of digital subtraction angiography may replace both non-invasive studies and angiography in the initial evaluation of asymptomatic carotid bruits.

INDICATIONS FOR TREATMENT

Reliable guidelines for management of asymptomatic carotid bruit have not been established. Consequently, controversies exist as to the value of antiplatelet or anticoagulant therapy and the indications for carotid endarterectomy. Evidence has been presented that antiplatelet therapy in patients with TIAs may diminish the subsequent frequency of stroke, at least for males (5). No data is available on the impact of antiplatelet therapy on the eventual stroke rate in patients with asymptomatic bruit (13). Anticoagulation with coumadin has long been utilized to prevent stroke, but its efficacy in patients with TIAs has not been proven (4). The advantage for patients with asymptomatic bruit has not been established and many physicians would be hesitant to prescribe this drug which has significant complications.

Several authors have recommended carotid endarterectomy for patients with asymptomatic bruit (18, 22, 31, 33). It must be pointed out that, to date, statistical evidence has not been presented that carotid endarterectomy improves the eventual outcome for patients with asymptomatic carotid stenosis. Reports of surgical treatment of asymptomatic patients include those of Thompson (32), two strokes in 167 operations for asymptomatic bruit (1.2%), and Moore (24), no complications in 78 operations for asymptomatic carotid ulcer. In our own experience, no complications were noted in 41 operations (Table 3.3) (25). A few of our patients demonstrated progressive stenosis on serial non-invasive studies. In all cases, the residual carotid lumen was 2 mm or less on angiography. We have not been impressed that patients with carotid bruits associated with residual lumen greater than 2 mm are at a greater risk for having a stroke and, therefore, have not offered end-

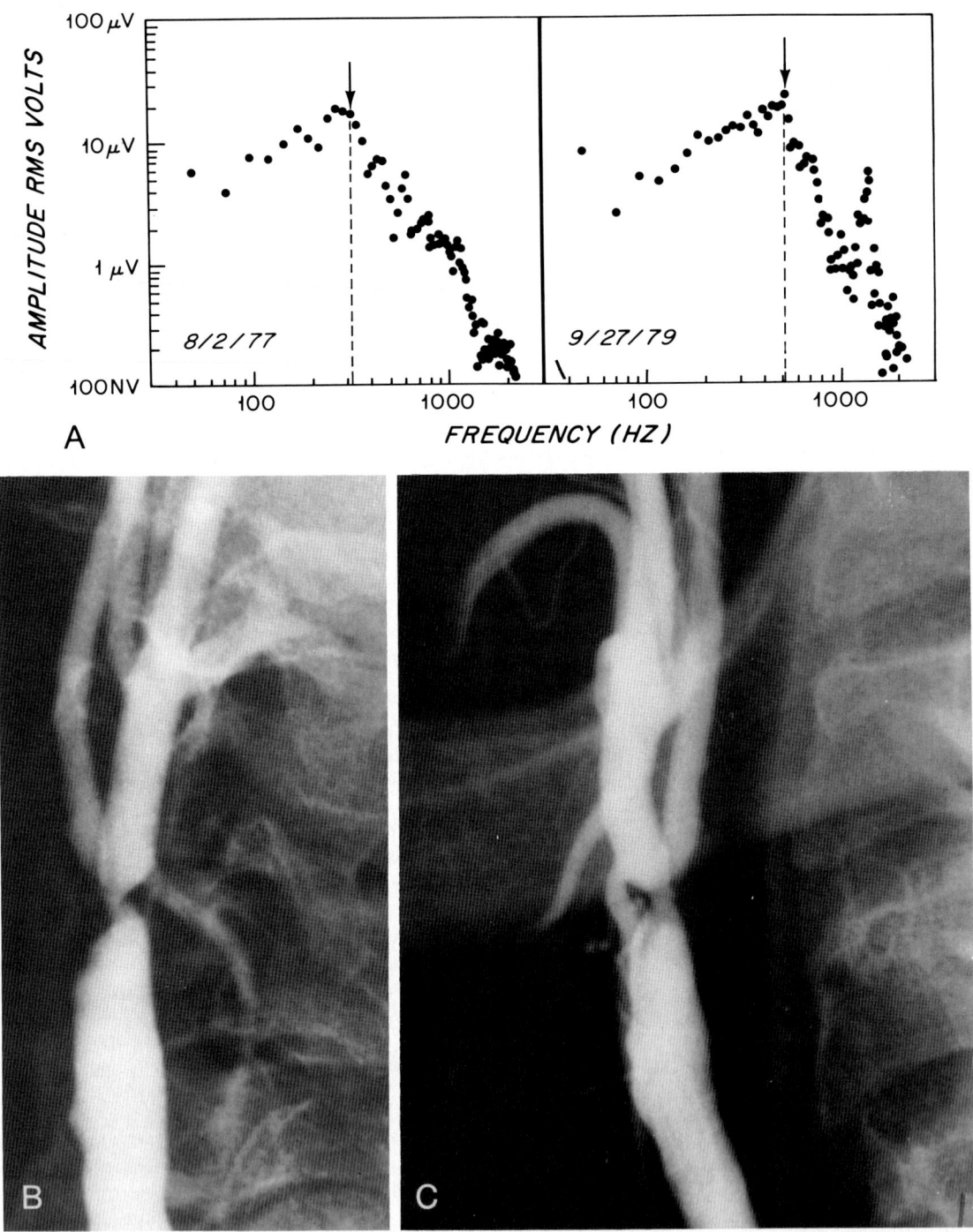

Figure 3.1 Asymptomatic bruit studied by phonoangiography. A, the phonoangiogram shows the sound spectrum of a left carotid bifurcation bruit with a break frequency of approximately 230 Hz. The calculated residual lumen diameter is 1.5 mm. The phonoangiogram 25 months later shows a break frequency of 510 Hz consistent with a residual lumen diameter of 1 mm (courtesy of Dr. Philip Kistler, MGH). B and C, the left carotid angiogram (AP and lateral) taken at the time of the second phonoangiogram in A shows a stenotic lesion of the left carotid bifurcation, but the residual lumen diameter is difficult to assess. D, cross-section of the plaque removed at operation, at the point of maximal stenosis, from the patient shown in A and B. Note that the residual lumen diameter is 1 mm.

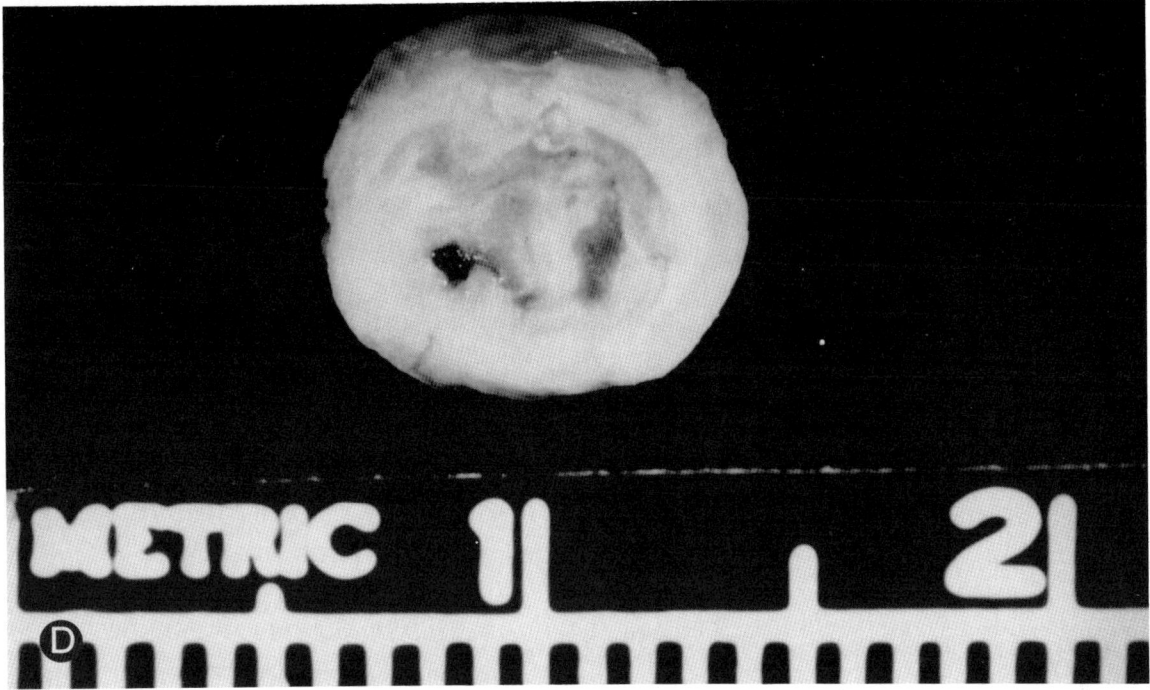

Figure 3.1 (D)

Table 3.3
Risk of Carotid Endarterectomy for Asymptomatic Bruit, Stenosis or Ulceration

Author	Number of Patients	Stroke	Death	Total Risk
Thompson	167	2	0	1.2%
Moore	78	0	0	0
Authors	41	0	0	0

Table 3.4
Risk of Stroke during Major Surgery in Patients with Asymptomatic Bruit

Three series reported a total of 1,082 patients (8, 12, 33)
- Perioperative stroke rate........1%
- None of 167 patients (15.4%) with asymptomatic bruit had a stroke

arterectomy to this category of patient. Fields has suggested that endarterectomy can be recommended for asymptomatic carotid stenosis only if the complication range is less than 1% (13). It has been emphasized that the complication rate can be minimized when the operator is experienced, carries out the procedure frequently, and utilizes standard and meticulous technique (28). In addition, careful perioperative medical management, particularly in regard to the cardiac status and control of hypertension in the postoperative period, has been shown to minimize risk (6, 8, 24, 26, 30).

Other authors, notably Humphrey, have suggested that patients with asymptomatic carotid stenosis be followed until the appearance of TIAs (16). The patient then is in a category where the risk of possible cerebral infarction is clearly greater than the risk of surgery but, as noted, this leaves a large group of patients at risk who do not have warning attacks before the stroke.

At the present time, we recommend angiography in those medically stable patients with an asymptomatic carotid bruit who have a hemodynamically significant lesion or show definite evidence of progression of the stenosis on non-invasive studies. This usually means that the residual lumen diameter is 2 mm or less. Angiography usually confirms this finding and surgery is recommended. In the future, digital subtraction angiography will be used when a significant lesion is suspected because of a bruit. Figure 3.1 illustrates the problem in a patient who had evidence of progressive worsening of the stenosis. If the non-invasive tests do not define a hemodynamic lesion and the clinical assessment of the bruit is not worrisome, it is recommended that the patient be followed and the non-invasive tests be repeated in 4 to 6 months.

Another question to consider is whether there is an increased risk of stroke in patients with asymptomatic carotid occlusive disease who are to have major surgery. In reviewing the significance of the presence of an asymptomatic carotid bruit in patients undergoing major vascular operative procedures, three reported series studied 1082 patients (8, 12, 33) (Table 3.4). The perioperative stroke rate was 1% and none of the 167 patients (15.4%) with an asymptomatic carotid bruit suffered a postoperative stroke. Other reports based on non-invasive studies conclude that there is no direct relationship between the presence of a carotid bruit, the severity of carotid disease, and the incidence of perioperative stroke (3, 34). Therefore, prophylactic carotid endarterectomy may not be indicated in this group of patients. However, we believe that when there is a severe stenosis at the internal carotid origin causing a marked hemodynamic change, carotid endarterectomy should be considered.

REFERENCES

1. Ackerman RH: A perspective on noninvasive diagnosis of carotid disease. Neurology 29:615-622, 1979.
2. Ackerman RH: Non-invasive carotid evaluation. Stroke 11:675-678, 1980.
3. Barnes RW, Marszalek PB: Asymptomatic carotid disease in the cardiovascular surgical patient: Is prophylatic endarterectomy necessary? Stroke 12:497-500, 1981.
4. Barnett HJM: Progress towards stroke prevention. Neurology 30:1212-1225, 1980.
5. Barnett HJM, et al: A randomized trial of aspirin and sulfinpyrazone in threatened stroke. The Canadian Cooperative Study Group. N Engl J Med 299:53-59, 1978.
6. Brewster DC, Schlaen HH, Raines JK, Abbott WM, Darling RC: Rational management of the asymptomatic carotid bruit. Arch Surg 113:927-930, 1978.
7. Caplan LR, Skillman J, Ojemann R, Fields WS: Intracerebral hemorrhage following carotid endarterectomy: A hypertensive complication? Stroke 9:457-460, 1978.
8. Carney WI, Stewart WB, DePinto DJ, Mucha SJ, Roberts B: Carotid bruit as a risk in aortoiliac reconstruction. Surgery 81:567-570, 1977.
9. Crowell RM, Ojemann RG: Extracranial Cerebrovascular Disease, chapt 28, in Hoff JT (ed): Practice of Surgery. Philadelphia, Harper and Row, 1981.
10. Crowell RM, Ojemann RG, Kistler JP: Asymptomatic Carotid Bruit, in Thompson RA, Crowell RM (eds): Advances in Neurology. New York, Raven Press (in press).
11. David TE, Humphries AW, Young JR, Beven EG: A correlation of neck bruits and atherosclerotic carotid arteries. Arch Surg 107:729-731, 1973.
12. Evans WE, Cooperman M: The significance of asymptomatic unilateral carotid bruits in preoperative patients. Surgery 83:521-522, 1978.
13. Fields WS: The asymptomatic carotid bruit—operate or not? Stroke 9:269-271, 1978.
14. Fisher CM: The Natural History of Carotid Occlusion, in Austin GM (ed): Microneurosurgical Anastomoses for Cerebral Ischemia. Springfield, Illinois, C C Thomas, 1976, pp 194-201.
15. Heyman A, Wilkinson W, Heyden S, Helms MJ, Bartel AG, Karp HR, Tyroler HA, Hames CG: Risk of stroke in asymptomatic persons with cervical arterial bruits—a population study in Evans County, Georgia. N Engl J Med 302:838-841, 1980.
16. Humphries AW, Young JR, Santilli PH, Beven EG, deWolfe VG: Unoperated, asymptomatic significant internal carotid artery stenosis: A review of 182 instances. Surgery 80:695-698, 1976.
17. Javid H, Ostermiller WE, Hengesh JW, Dye WS, Hunter JA, Najafi H, Julian OC: Natural history of carotid bifurcation atheroma. Surgery 67:80-86, 1970.
18. Javid H, Ostermiller WE, Hengesh JW, Dye WS, Hunter JA, Najafi H, Julian OC: Carotid endarterectomy for asymptomatic patients. Arch Surg 102:389-391, 1971.
19. Kartchner MM, McRae LP: Noninvasive evaluation and management of the "asymptomatic" carotid bruit. Surgery 82:840-847, 1977.
20. Kistler JP, Lees RS, Friedman J, Pessin M, Mohr JP, Roberson GH, Ojemann RG: The bruit of carotid stenosis versus radiated basal heart murmurs. Differentiation by phonoangiography. Circulation 57:975-981, 1978.
21. Kroener JM, Dorn PL, Shoor PM, Wickbom IG, Bernstein EF: Prognosis of asymptomatic ulcerating carotid lesions. Arch Surg 115:1387-1392, 1980.
22. Lefrak EA, Guinn GA: Prophylactic carotid artery surgery in patients requiring a second operation. South Med J 67:185-189, 1974.
23. Mohr JP: Transient ischemic attacks and the prevention of strokes. N Engl J Med 299:93-95, 1978.
24. Moore WS, Malone JM, Boren C, Roon AJ, Goldston J: Asymptomatic ulcerative lesions of the carotid artery—Natural history and effect of surgical therapy compared. Stroke 10:96, 1979.
25. Ojemann RG, Crowell RM, Roberson GH, Fisher CM: Surgical treatment of extracranial carotid occlusive disease. Clin Neurosurg 22:214-263, 1975.
26. Pessin MS, Hinton RC, Davis KR, Duncan GW, Roberson GH, Ackerman RH, Mohr JP: Mechanisms of acute carotid stroke. Ann Neurol 6:245-252, 1979.
27. Robertson JT: A neurosurgical approach to the therapy of extracranial occlusive disease. Clin Neurosurg 23:1-11, 1976.
28. Robertson JT, Watridge CB: The surgical management of extracranial and intracranial occlusive disease. Med Clin N Am 63:681-693, 1979.
29. Sandok BA: Non-invasive techniques for diagnosis of carotid artery disease. Stroke 9:427-429, 1978.
30. Sundt TM, Jr, Sandok BA, Whisnant JP: Carotid endarterectomy: Complications and preoperative assessment of risk. Mayo Clin Proc 50:301-306, 1975.
31. Thompson JE, Patman RD, Persson AV: Management of asymptomatic carotid bruits. Am Surg 42:77-80, 1976.
32. Thompson JE, Patman RD, Talkington CM: Asymptomatic carotid bruit: long-term outcome of patients having endarterectomy compared with unoperated controls. Ann Surg 188:308-316, 1978.
33. Treiman RL, Foran RF, Shore EH, Levin PM: Carotid bruit: significance in patients undergoing an abdominal aortic operation. Arch Surg 106:803-805, 1973.
34. Turnipseed WD, Berkoff HA, Beizer FO: Postoperative stroke in cardiac and peripheral vascular disease. Ann Surg 192:365-368, 1980.
35. Wolf PA, Kannel WB, McNamara PM, Dawber TR: Asymptomatic carotid bruits and risk of stroke: The Framingham Study. Stroke 10:96, 1979.

Chapter 4 SUPERFICIAL TEMPORAL ARTERY TO MIDDLE CEREBRAL ARTERY BYPASS GRAFT

INDICATIONS FOR SURGERY

Superficial temporal artery-middle cerebral artery (STA-MCA) anastomosis was developed to bypass areas of occlusive disease that are not amenable to direct surgery. It was first performed by Donaghy and Yasargil in 1967 using microsurgical techniques (10, 40, 41). Refinements in technique have included the use of interrupted sutures for greater precision (27), use of the angular branch of the MCA for maximum flow (5), and linear incision over the STA to avoid scalp flap necrosis (28).

The therapeutic role of STA-MCA bypass has not been fully defined. In Table 4.1 are listed the clinical problems and angiographic findings that have been used as indications for this procedure. Studies of regional cerebral blood flow and metabolism have been reported to assist in defining the indications for operation (15, 31).

The procedure carries a low risk and in selected cases appears to diminish the incidence of TIAs (5, 6, 10, 27, 28, 38, 40, 41). The impact of bypass surgery on subsequent cerebral ischemia and infarction is more difficult to determine. Our own experience shows that delayed stroke can occur in spite of a satisfactorily functioning bypass graft and that late strokes can occur which seem unrelated to bypass surgery. A cooperative randomized controlled study, The International Extracranial-Intracraial Bypass Study, is working to clarify the indications for STA-MCA bypass (4, 24). It is hoped that the results of this study, which will be made available in the next several years, will indicate the effect of bypass grafting on cerebral ischemia and infarction and better define the indications for this procedure.

Bypass graft seems helpful in preventing ischemia when planned internal carotid artery (ICA) occlusion is done for a giant ICA aneurysm in the presence of poor collateral supply (2, 13, 33, 37, 40). Since some patients tolerate carotid occlusion without bypass, the precise role of bypass in this setting has not yet been fully defined.

The use of emergency STA-MCA bypass grafting has been assessed and the reports from the literature indicate mixed results (7, 9). In most reported cases, the conditions have been far from ideal with a long delay between onset of symptoms and surgery or the presence of occlusive material in the lenticulostriate branches. Emergency direct cerebral revascularization is a rational concept which awaits several technical developments. These include a test for tissue viability to identify reversible cases, a method to extend the period of reversibility until blood flow is restored, and a technique for revascularization to decrease the time of surgery and increase the immediate volume of blood flow.

The role of bypass surgery remains uncertain for several other conditions including amaurosis fugax with ICA occlusion (22), moya moya syndrome (1, 21), chronic cerebral ischemia (18, 19), and dementia secondary to multiple cerebrovascular occlusions (11).

Our experience with 50 grafts in 45 patients has been reported (9). Patency has been high (92%), serious complications infrequent (4%), with no deaths directly attributable to surgery. Indications for surgery and similar results have been reported by others (5, 6, 10, 27, 28, 29, 36, 38, 40, 41).

PREOPERATIVE EVALUATION

The preoperative medical evaluation is similar to that described for carotid endarterectomy. The key-

Table 4.1
Tentative Indications for STA-MCA Bypass

Presentation	Angiography	Comment
TIAs	ICA occlusion	Good indication if TIAs continue
	Siphon stenosis	Natural history dangerous
	MCA stenosis	Medical Rx may be better
Giant aneurysm	(Planned) ICA occlusion	Indicated in some cases, but some may not require bypass. CBF studies may help guide selection.
Dementia, generalized hypoperfusion	Multiple occlusions, poor collateral	Anecdotal data; some patients may improve
Moya moya syndrome	Multiple occlusions, cloud-like collateral	Anecdotal data. Future strokes may be diminished in some
"Slow stroke"	ICA occlusion	Only anecdotal data; some patients may improve with bypass
Amaurosis fugax	ICA stenosis or occlusion	Conflicting reports regarding future strokes; medical Rx may be better
Fixed stroke	ICA occlusion	Anecdotal data suggest occasional patients may improve, (?) protection
Acute stroke	ICA (or MCA) occlusion	Anecdotal data; no striking improvement

stone for planning a bypass operation is three-vessel angiography to deliniate cerebrovascular occlusions, collateral circulation, and potential bypass vessels. Delayed films in some cases may show reconstitution of the carotid siphon with reflux to the upper cervical ICA, a sign which suggests the carotid occlusion may be opened surgically. Multiple filling defects in MCA branches suggest embolic occlusions which probably cannot be helped by STA-MCA anastomosis. Poor collateral circulation to a symptomatic hemisphere suggests a hemodynamic mechanism. Careful study of the angiogram usually permits identification of the best vessels for anastomosis. Failure to opacify MCA branches by collateral routes need not imply lack of a suitable recipient branch for the operation. The larger STA branch, usually the frontal, is selected, and when this is less than 1 mm in diameter, the occipital artery may be chosen instead. In the setting of a tiny STA and a proximally branching occipital artery, a short vein graft may be interposed between the STA or the occipital artery and the MCA recipient branch. Studies of regional cerebral blood flow and metabolism may help establish the indications for revascularization.

If the patient is on heparin, this is stopped at least 8 hours prior to operation. Many patients are on aspirin and/or dypyridamole. Generally, we prefer to stop these drugs several days before operation. However, some surgeons prefer to maintain antiplatelet therapy through the operative period. This does increase the risk of intraoperative oozing which may require platelet transfusion for hemostatsis. Antihypertensive medication is maintained. Diphenylhydantoin is begun the day before surgery to insure prophylactic blood levels of this anticonvulsant medication in the immediate postoperative period.

ANESTHESIA

Premedication is kept to a minimum. The patient's legs are wrapped with Ace bandages. General endotrachael anesthesia is used; usually halothane is chosen or a balanced technique with nitrous oxide, Innovar, and a muscle relaxant. Controlled ventilation is preferred to maintain the arterial pCO2 in the range of 35–40 torr. Precordial electrodes provide continuous EKG monitoring. Arterial blood pressure is monitored continuously with a radial artery catheter. Infusions of colloid, phenylephrine, or nitroprusside maintain blood pressure in the normal range for the individual patient during induction and surgery. Oxacillin is administered prior to incision and for 24 hours postoperatively in divided doses of 2 g every 6 hours.

OPERATIVE TECHNIQUE

Positioning

Prior to the induction of anesthesia, the operative area is shaved and the STA course marked with a marking pen because the pulse may be harder to delineate after induction. The patient lies supine with the head turned to the opposite side. The table is flexed slightly to bring the head above heart level. A small roll serves to elevate the shoulder on the operative side. The head is flexed and held in the three-point skeletal fixation headrest (Mayfield-Kees). The operating table may need to be tilted with the "side" adjustment to bring the temporal squama parallel to the floor.

Instruments

Several microsurgical instruments are essential for this operation. The Zeiss operating microscope is preferred with a 250-mm objective, 160-mm angled oculars, and 12.5X high-eye point eye pieces. The steroscopic binocular observer tube is attached to the microscope via the small beam-splitter. The assistant is positioned on the left (for a right-handed surgeon) to allow free access by the scrub nurse to the surgeon's dominant hand. A No. 5 Dumont jeweler's forceps adapted for bipolar coagulation is needed for precise hemostasis near bypass vessels. A similar forceps and a Heifetz curved scissors serve well to prepare the small arteries for anastomosis. Kleinert-Kees miniature clips are ideal for temporary occlusion of cortical arteries with minimal trauma. A 10-mm straight Heifetz clip is satisfactory for temporary occlusion of the STA origin. Miniature Gelpi retractors are helpful in maintaining satisfactory exposure. A curved Heifetz microscissors is used to fashion the cortical arteriotomy. Fine silastic tubing (0.025 inch outside diameter) serves as an MCA stent during surgery. The anastomosis is performed with a curved 8-inch Rhoton needle holder and 9-0 monofilament nylon suture on a BV-6 needle (Ethicon).

Incision

Before shaving and preparation of the scalp, the STA course is scratched into the skin over the previous pen marking. The position of the MCA recipient branch is determined from the angiogram and is likewise marked. In general, we prefer linear incisions in contrast to a scalp flap (Figs. 4.1 and 4.2). Linear incisions permit rapid STA preparation and avoid some scalp necrosis which may occur with a flap. One or two linear incisions may be needed, depending on the STA branch selected and occasionally on the MCA branch chosen. Most frequently, the frontal branch of STA and the angular branch of MCA are the largest and thus the best arteries available for anastomosis (Fig. 4.1A). The angular branch may be used with safety even on the dominant hemisphere. Occasionally, the posterior branch of STA (Fig. 4.1B) or a frontal branch of MCA will be selected for bypass (Fig. 4.1C). When a pterional or other approach to an intracranial aneurysm may be needed in conjunction with a bypass, a modified flap as shown in Figs. 4.1D or 4.1E may provide exposure for all contemplated surgical procedures. Although

STA-MCA Bypass Graft

—— Artery
---- Skin incision
.... Craniotomy

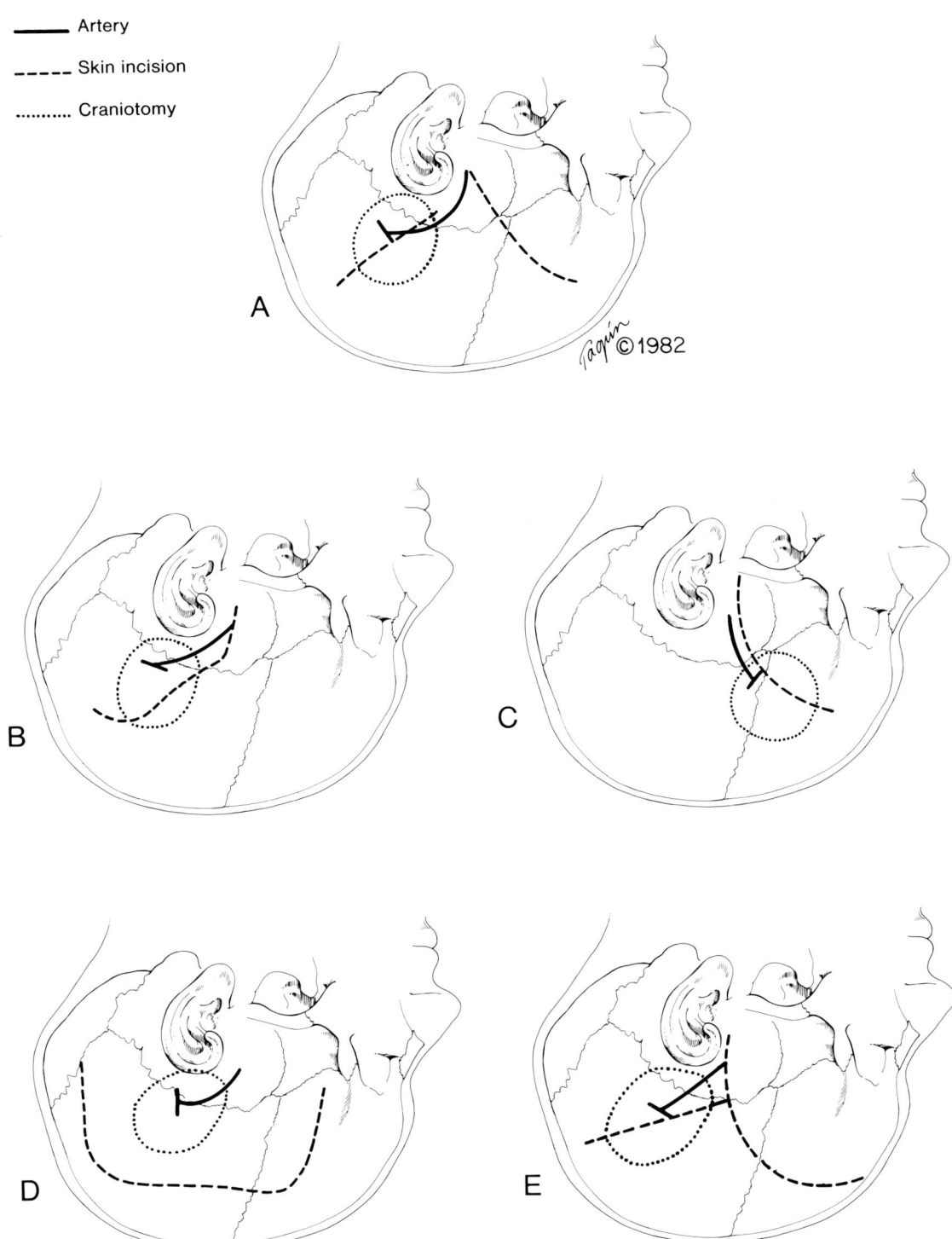

Figure 4.1 Scalp incisions. Several different approaches are used, depending on the suitability of donor and recipient vessels and on possible need for other intracranial surgery. *A*, two linear "cutdown" incisions. This is the most commonly used approach. It permits quick access to the largest arteries, usually the frontal branch of STA and angular branch of MCA, and avoids scalp edge necrosis. *B*, single posterior "cutdown" incision. A useful approach if the parietal branch of the STA is larger. *C*, single anterior "cutdown" incision. Uncommon, but can be used if the frontal branch of the MCA is selected. *D*, horseshoe flap which may be helpful if the status of STA and MCA branches is uncertain since it gives a wide field to search out the best vessels. Be sure to keep the base of the devascularized flap broad to avoid skin edge necrosis. *E*, combination STA-MCA bypass with craniotomy flap. Useful for approach to anterior circulation aneurysm (or tumor) where additional collateral blood supply is desired.

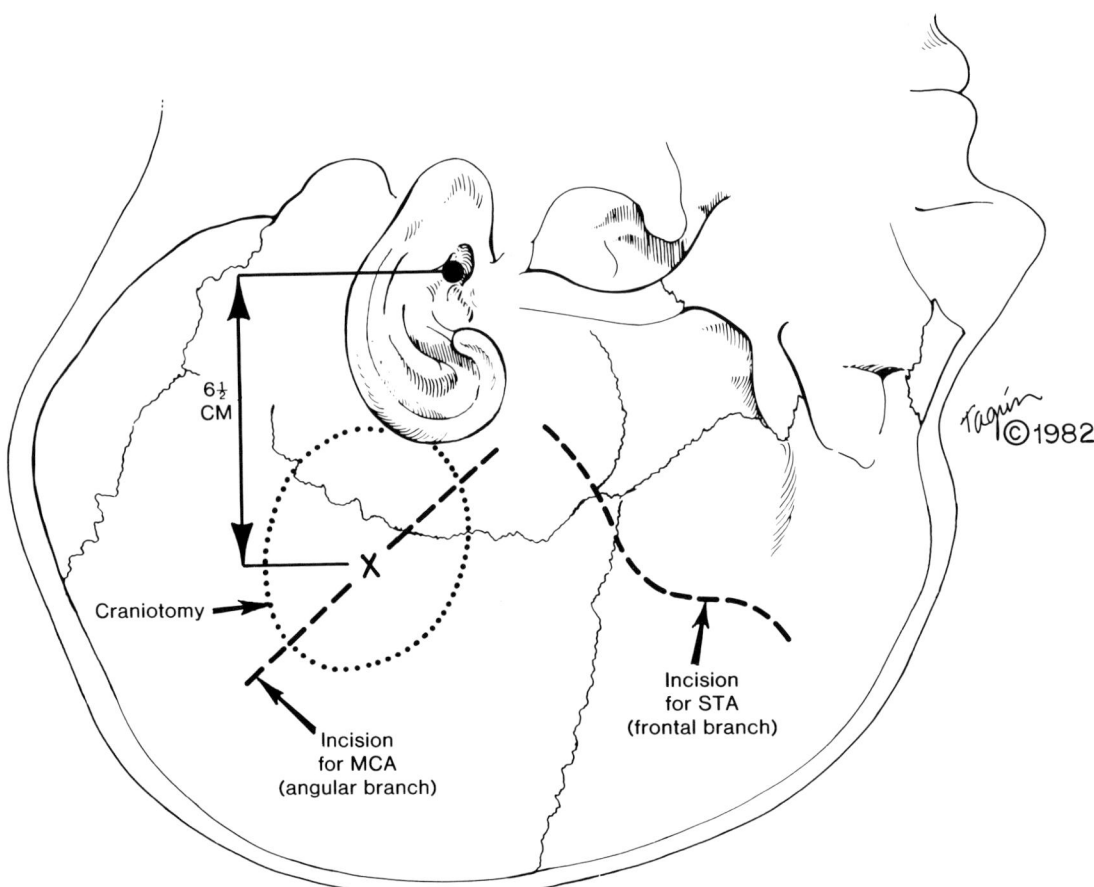

Figure 4.2 Linear incisions. This common approach provides rapid access to the donor and recipient arteries which are usually the largest; the frontal branch of the STA and the angular branch of the MCA. Shaving and marking the STA branch prior to anesthesia helps localize the vessel which may be elusive after induction. The posterior incision crosses a point about 6.5 cm rostral to the external auditory meatus; this overlies the posterior Sylvian fissure where the angular artery emerges. Keeping the incisions separate helps avoid scalp edge necrosis.

one might anticipate ischemia at the tips of the scalp flaps as in Fig. 4.1E, we have not experienced this problem.

The initial incision is made over the STA with the microscope at 10X (Fig. 4.2). The surgeon's arms are supported on either side with portable Mayo stands. The seated surgeon and assistant link arms to provide comfortable access for all four hands into the operative site. Subcutaneous injection of local anesthetic is omitted. The initial incision with a No. 15 blade is made over the distal STA down to the subcutaneous fat to avoid injury to the STA trunk. Then the surgeon and assistant elevate the scalp tissue with Adson forceps, and the plane just superficial to STA is developed with Metzenbaum scissors (Fig. 4.3). When the proper plane is chosen, the STA is readily exposed over an 8–10 cm length.

STA Preparation

Small scalp flaps, about 1 cm wide, are elevated on each side of the STA (Fig. 4.4). The adventitia is incised with a No. 15 knife blade approximately 2 mm to each side of the STA and down to the temporalis fascia. Small bleeders are coagulated with bipolar cautery away from the STA. Branches larger than 0.5 mm are divided between 6-0 silk ligatures. To facilitate this dissection, the surgeon uses a knife and forceps and the assistant uses a sucker and bipolar cautery. A few spreading movements with the Metzenbaum scissors develop a plane between STA and temporalis fascia, thus completing isolation of the vessel (Fig. 4.5). After exposure of the MCA recipient branch (described below), the STA is prepared. Satisfactory STA graft length is determined. This is usually 8 cm and includes a bit of extra length to facilitate suturing of the back wall. The artery is then occluded with a Heifetz clip and is divided (Fig. 4.6). Heparinized saline is flushed into the STA via a #20 Medicut catheter. This irrigation flushes out blood and helps identify bleeders for coagulation. When a large proximal side branch is available, an irrigation catheter may be tied into the branch to permit intermittent STA irrigation during anastomosis and bypass pressure measurement after completion of the graft (Fig. 4.7).

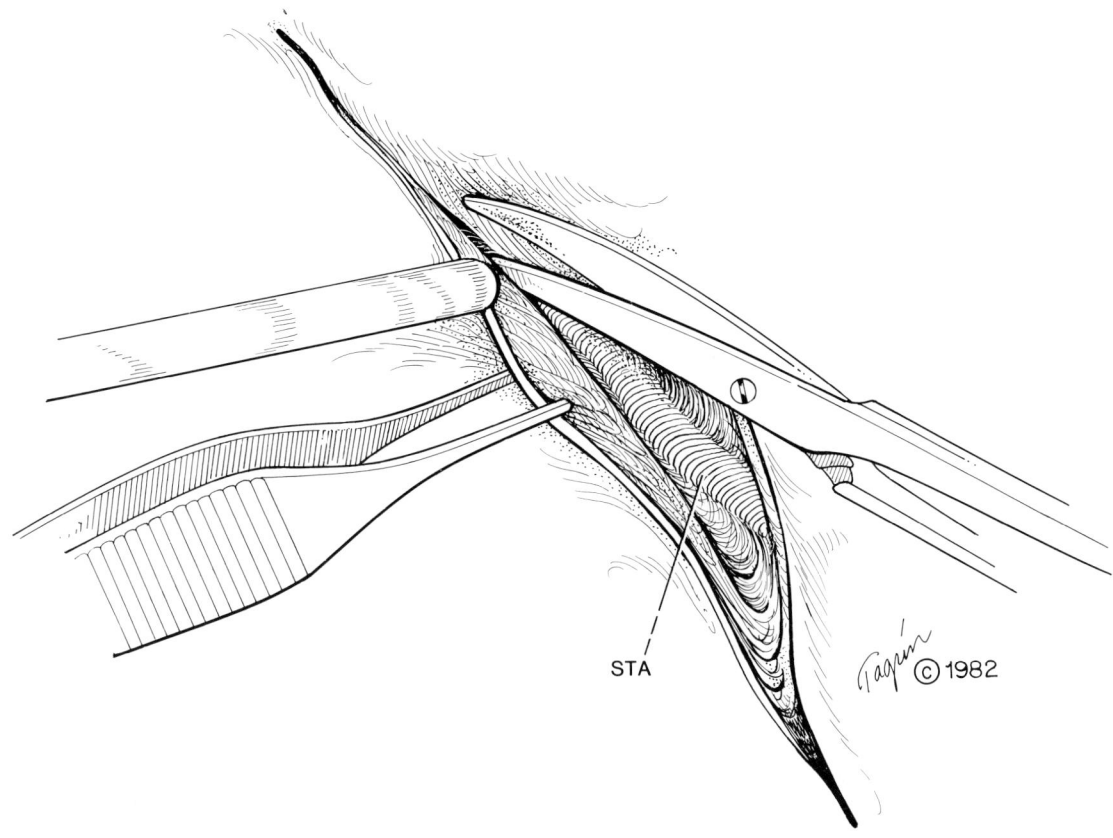

Figure 4.3 "Cutdown" incision over the STA branch. A #15 blade is used to incise the skin superficially. Then skin is elevated from the STA with forceps, and Metzenbaum scissors cut adventitia and overlying soft tissues.

The tip of the STA is then freed of adventitia over a 1 cm length. The tip is beveled in a fish-mouth fashion to maximize the anastomotic opening (Fig. 4.8). If the intima should separate from the muscularis, a second effort at beveling usually is associated with adherance of the two layers of the artery. After the STA tip is prepared, flow is measured by letting the artery bleed into a beaker for a specific length of time (Fig. 4.9). The artery is again flushed with heparinized saline.

In some patients, the STA segment must be led from one incision to another. A tunnel is prepared by blunt dissection between galea and temporalis fascia. The STA tip is pulled through the tunnel with a terminal silk tie. Twists and kinks in the STA segment are carefully avoided. When a flap technique is used (Fig. 4.1 D and E), the STA is isolated from adventitia by sharp dissection down to fat and hair follicles where a plane is established superficial to the vessel.

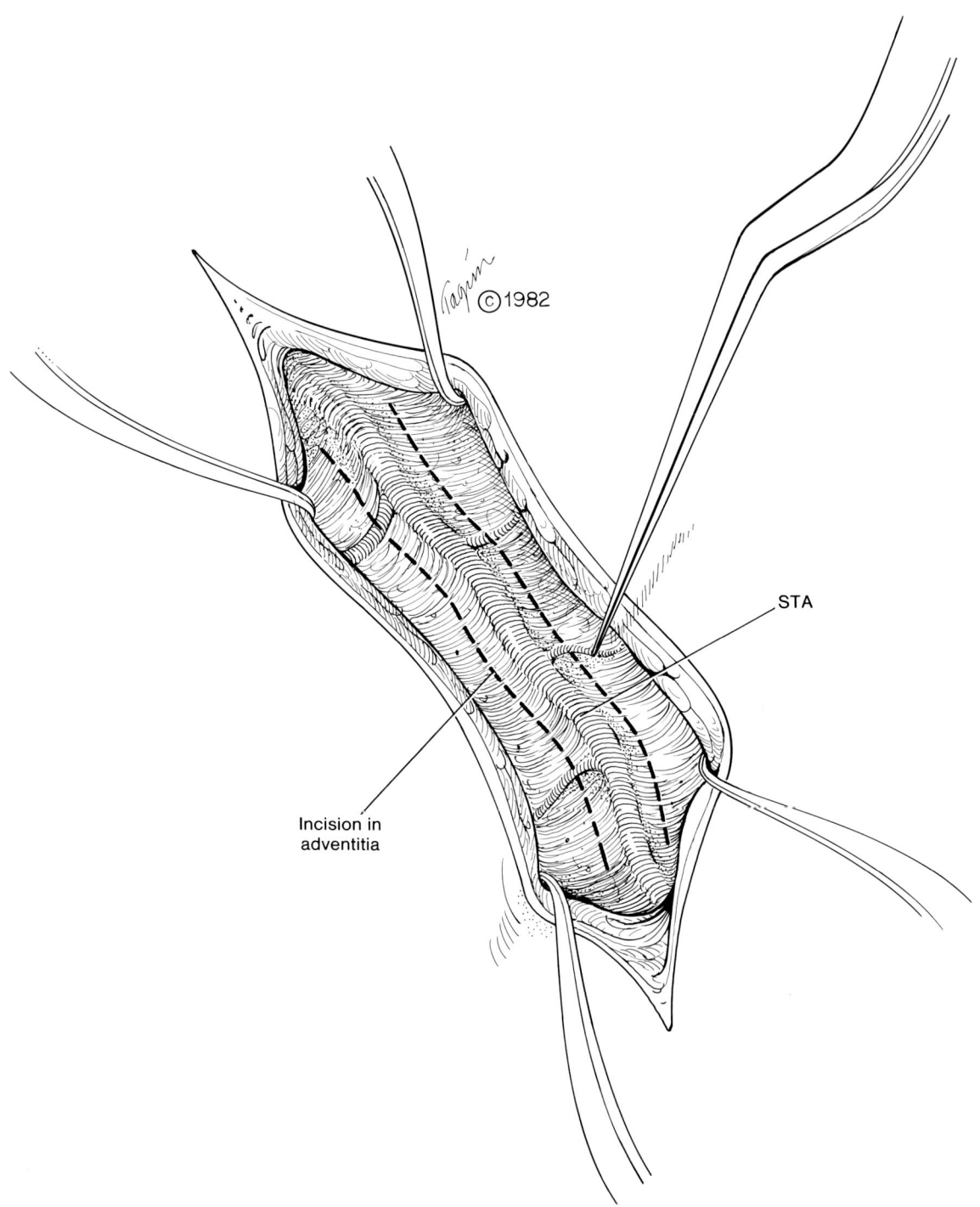

Figure 4.4 Exposure of STA. After the incision is complete, miniature Gelpi retractors are placed. Small side branches are coagulated with bipolar cautery; large ones are divided between 6-0 ligatures.

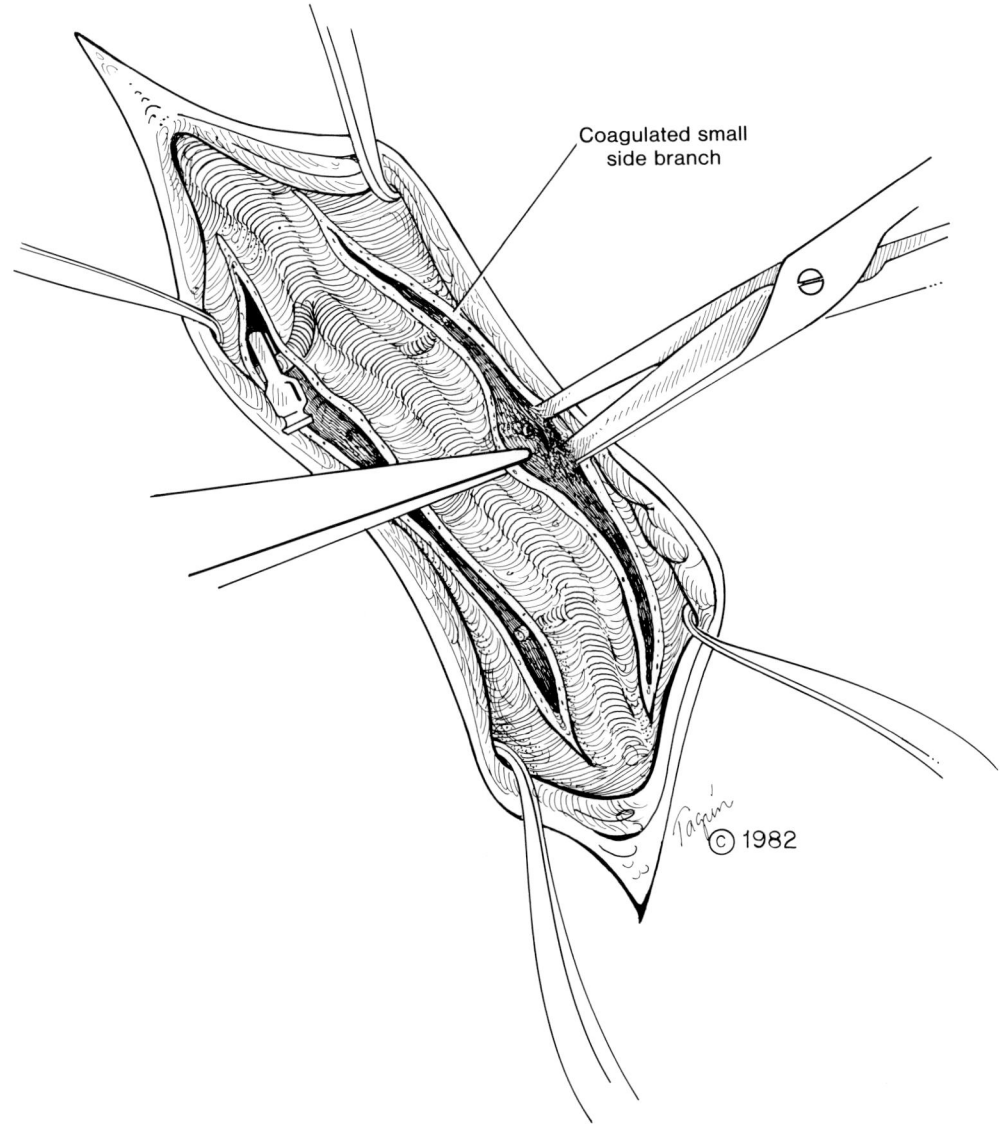

Figure 4.5 Isolation of STA. With a #15 blade, the adventitia is incised down to temporalis fascia. Scissors develop the plane between the vessel and deep fascia. The largest proximal side branch is clipped and preserved with adequate length to receive an irrigation catheter.

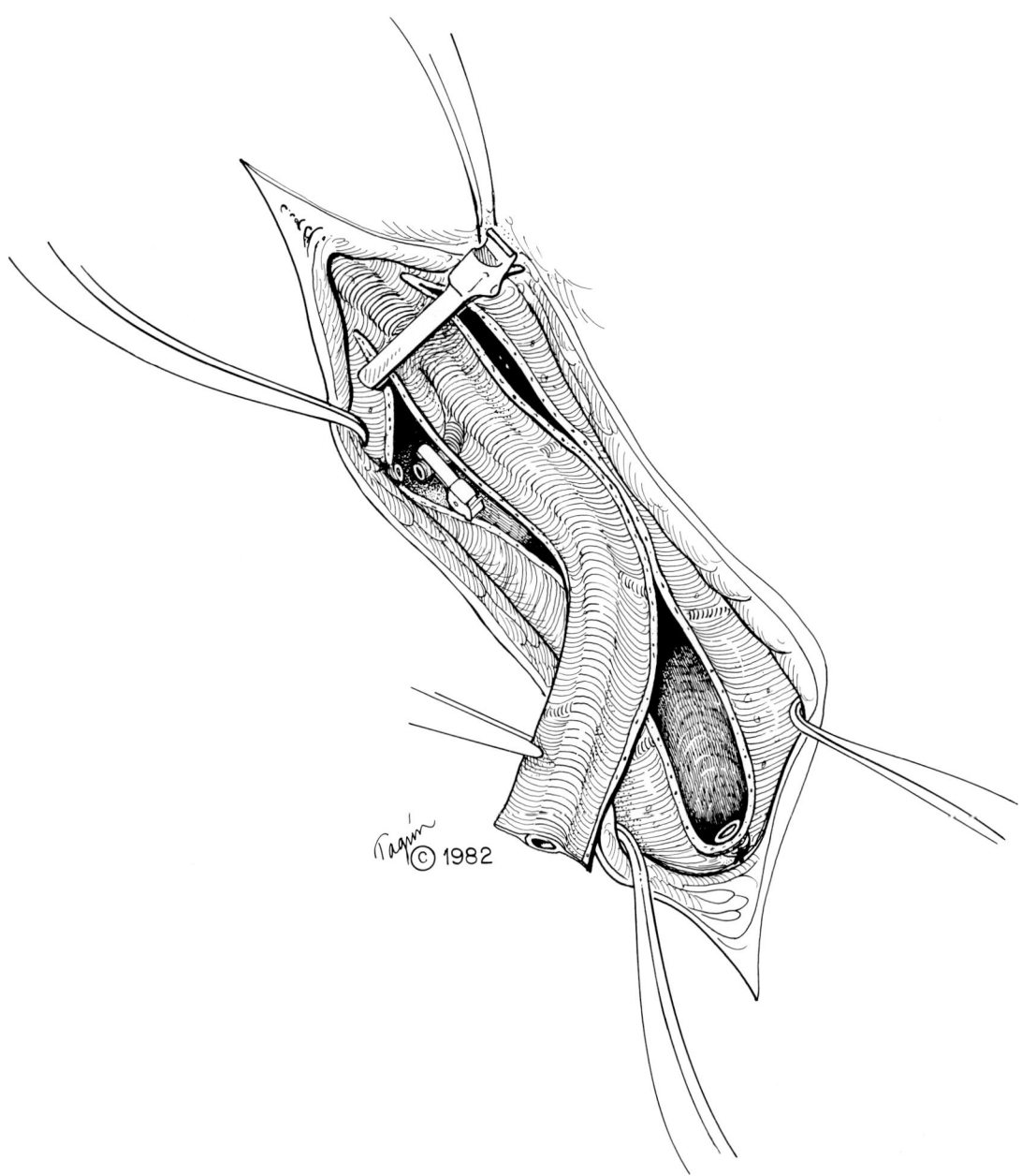

Figure 4.6 Preparation of STA. After checking to be sure the length is adequate, the STA is clipped proximally, cross-cut distally, and irrigated with heparanized saline.

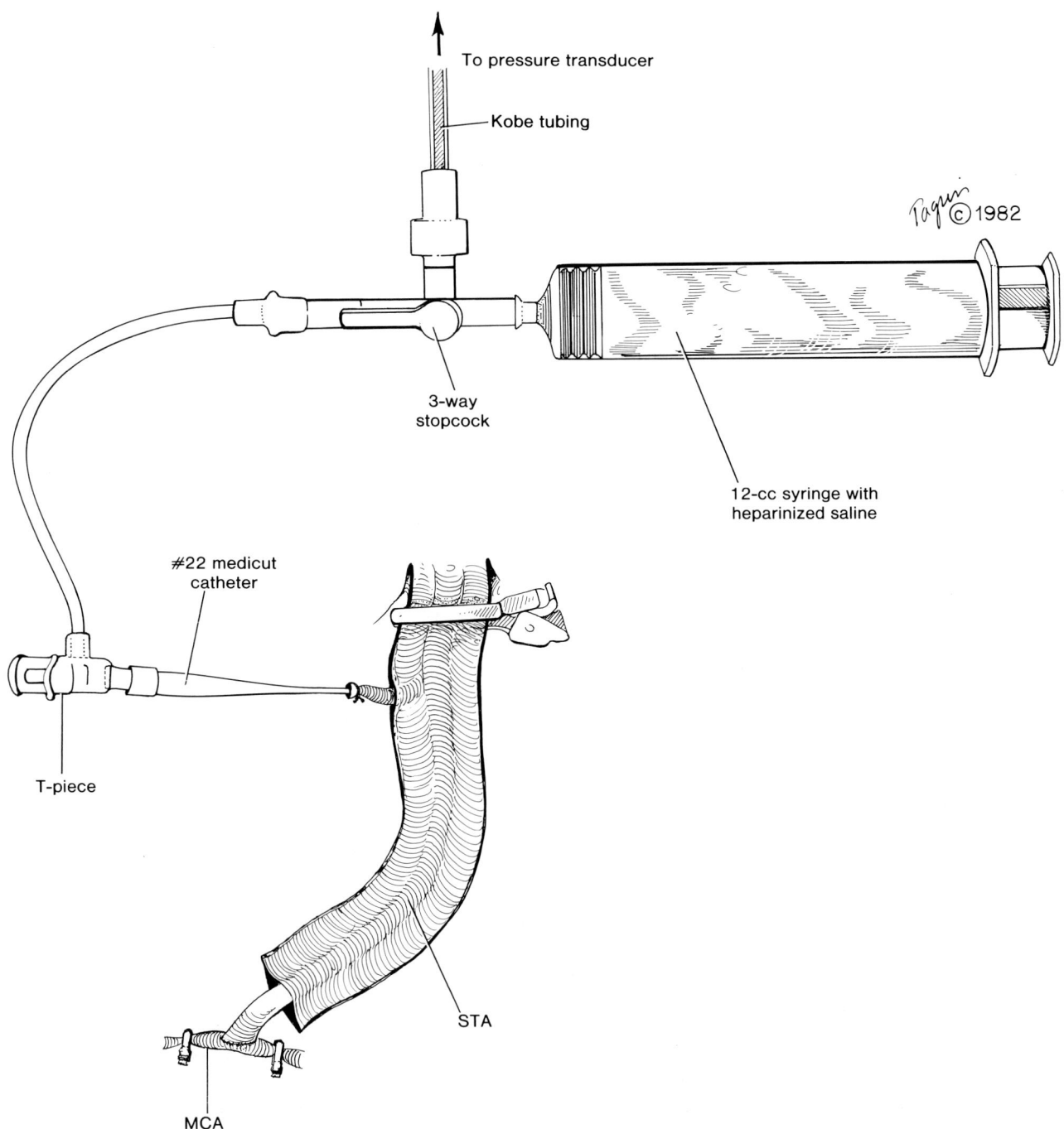

Figure 4.7 Side catheter into graft. Cannulation of a large proximal branch permits frequent irrigation with heparinized saline. Suture line leaks may be identified before restoring blood flow. The side catheter may also be used to measure pressure in the STA or in the MCA.

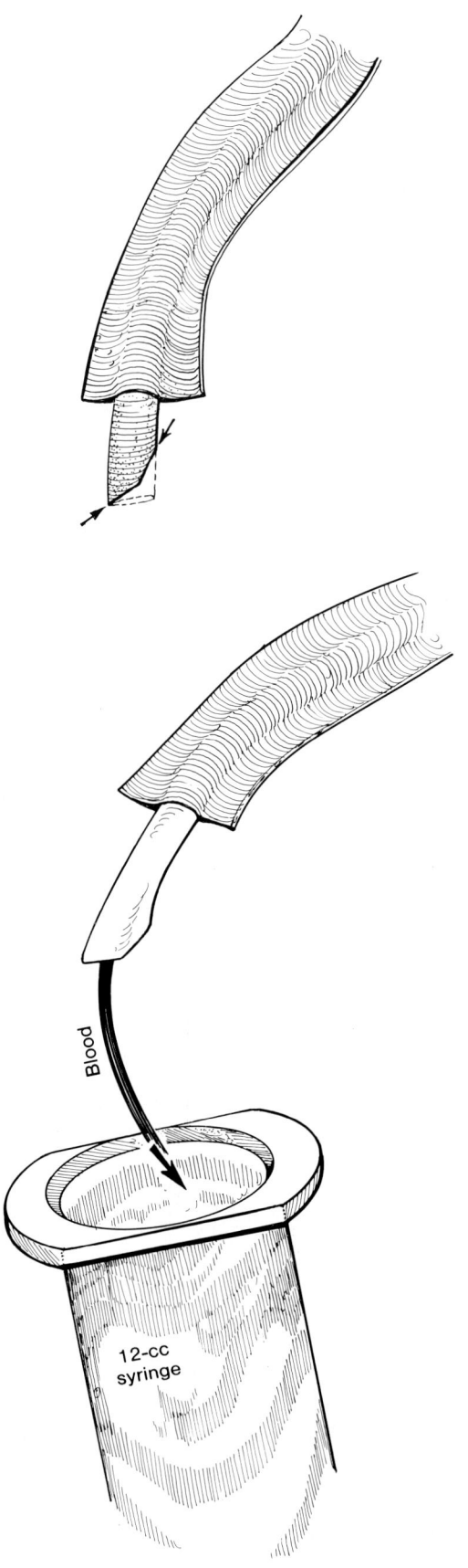

Figure 4.8 Preparation of STA tip. The distal tip is freed of adventitia and fish-mouthed for maximum ostium. We find two snips with straight microscissors effective. The lumen is checked for an intimal flap.

Figure 4.9 Measurement of STA flow. Flow into a 12-cc syringe is measured to gauge maximum immediate graft flow delivery from the graft.

STA-MCA Bypass Graft

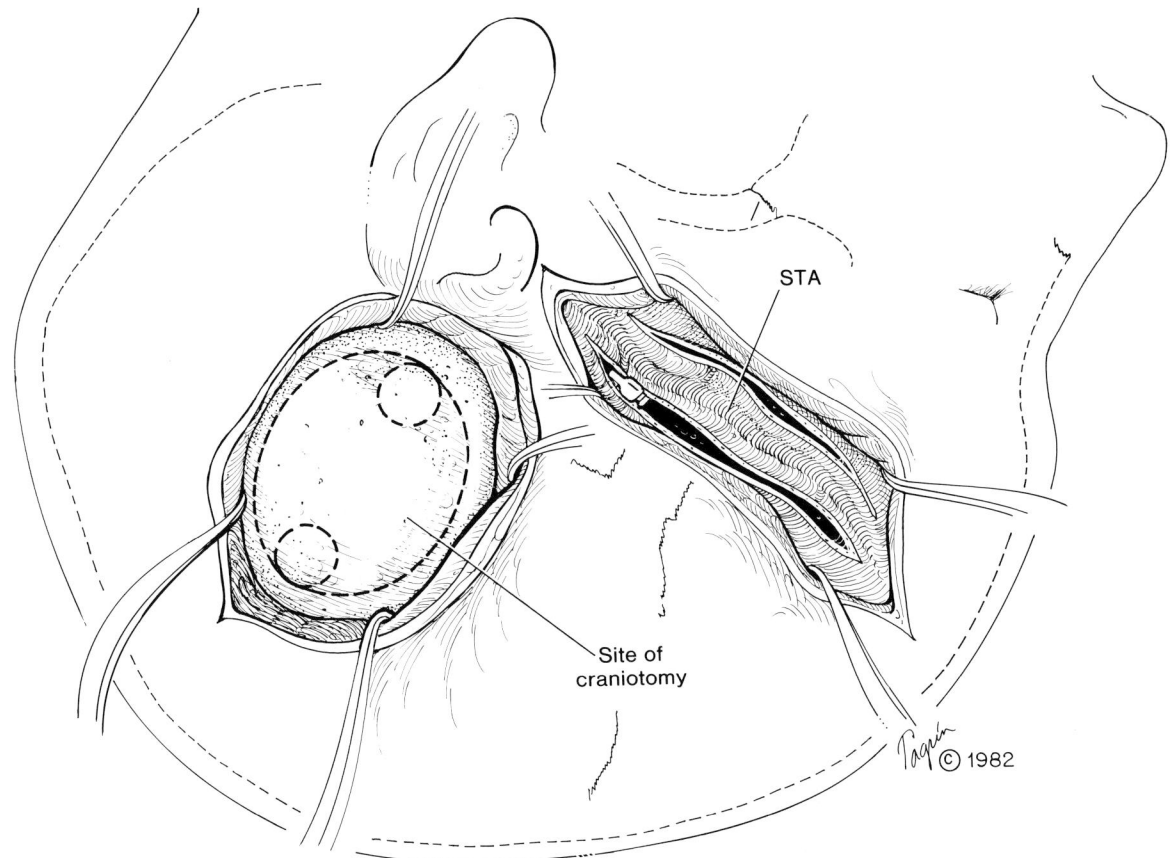

Figure 4.10 Craniotomy. The posterior wound is deepened by cutting cauterization down to bone. A small craniotomy is fashioned with the drill and craniotome. The anterior burr hole will serve to pass the graft. The exposure must be low enough to demonstrate temporal branches.

MCA Preparation

Generally the angular branch of the MCA is used, lying about 6.5 cm rostral to the external auditory canal. When the frontal STA is used, the angular branch is exposed through a separate incision (Fig. 4.1A). Temporalis muscle is opened with cutting cautery which also can be used to elevate the periosteum. When a frontal branch of the MCA is to be used, an incision and exposure in this area are employed as shown in Fig. 4.1C. When an aneurysm approach via a bone flap is anticipated, as in Fig. 4.1E, the scalp flaps will be raised as shown, but the incision through temporalis muscle is best made from the proximal STA to the assumed location of angular artery in order to facilitate routing of the graft prior to closure.

A small craniotomy flap, about 7 cm in diameter, is fashioned over the recipient artery with the power drill and craniotome (Fig. 4.10). We have found this method faster and safer than either craniectomy or trephine. Bone edges are waxed and the dura opened in a cruciate fashion. Additional bone may be removed if no suitable recipient branch is identified. When a suitable vessel is exposed, three drill holes are made in the bone edge for eventual bone flap replacement and dural to pericranial sutures are placed.

Employing 25X magnification, the arachnoid next to the MCA is cut with microscissors (Fig. 4.11). Tiny side branches may be coagulated with the bipolar cautery on low power and cut as needed to prepare a 1 cm length of artery. Generally, one or two larger side branches can be preserved by using temporary clips. A strip of rubber dam is placed under the MCA to protect cortex.

Final preparation of the MCA is achieved at 25X magnification with the prepared STA tip in full view. Kleinert-Kees clips are placed on the MCA branch at least 8 mm apart. A slender oval arteriotomy, the same length as the STA tip width, is made in the MCA with one or two snips of the microscissors (Fig. 4.12). The vessel is irrigated with heparinized saline. A stent of fine silastic tubing is inserted into the vessel.

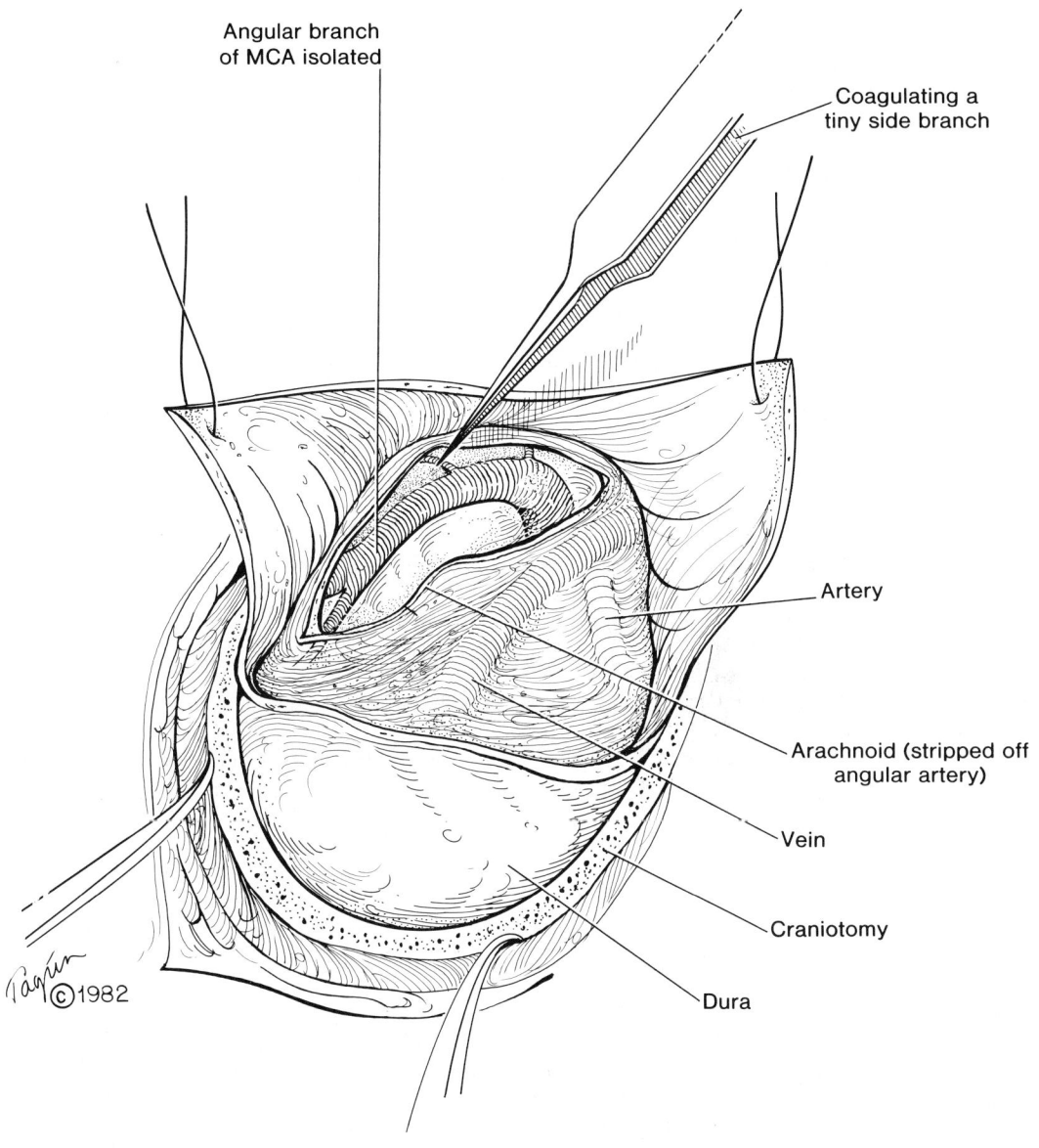

Figure 4.11 Exposure of cortical artery. After placement of dural-pericranial tenting sutures, the dura is opened just enough to expose a suitable recipient artery. Under 25X, arachnoid over the vessel is opened sharply. To obtain a 10-mm segment for anastomosis, one or two tiny side branches may be coagulated and cut.

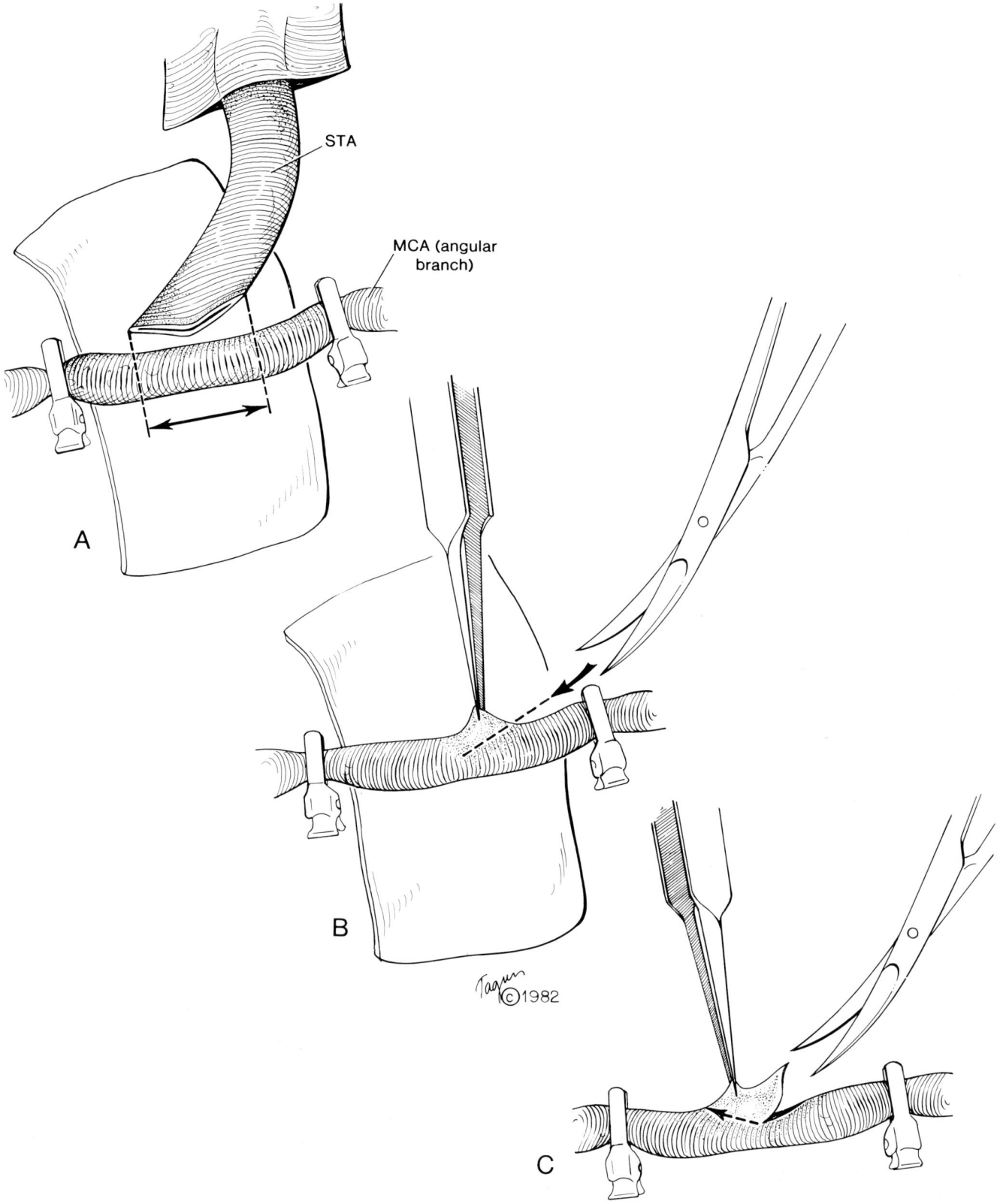

Figure 4.12 Preparation of MCA. A rubber dam is slipped under the vessel to protect the brain. Kleinert-Kees clips are placed (*A*). With the corresponding STA ostium adjacent, the MCA ostium is cut with curved microscissors (*B*). No. 5 jeweler's forceps elevate the segment for excision, and two snips provide a smooth edge (*C*). We prefer an ostium about half as wide as the vessel with a length that is 2½ times the vessel width.

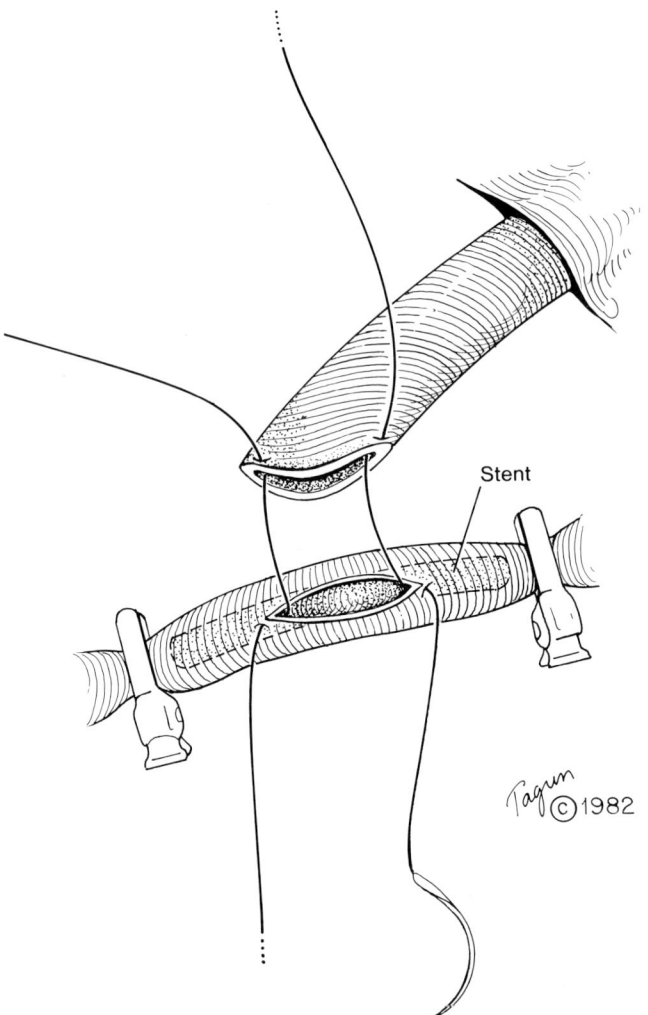

Figure 4.13 Corner stitches. 9-0 monofilament nylon is used. The distal tip is sutured first. If there is a tendency to an intimal flap in the STA, an in-to-out suture on this vessel is safest. If there is a discrepancy between wall lengths, it should be corrected prior to anchoring the second corner. After corner stitches are in, a fine silastic stent is introduced to prevent injury to back wall.

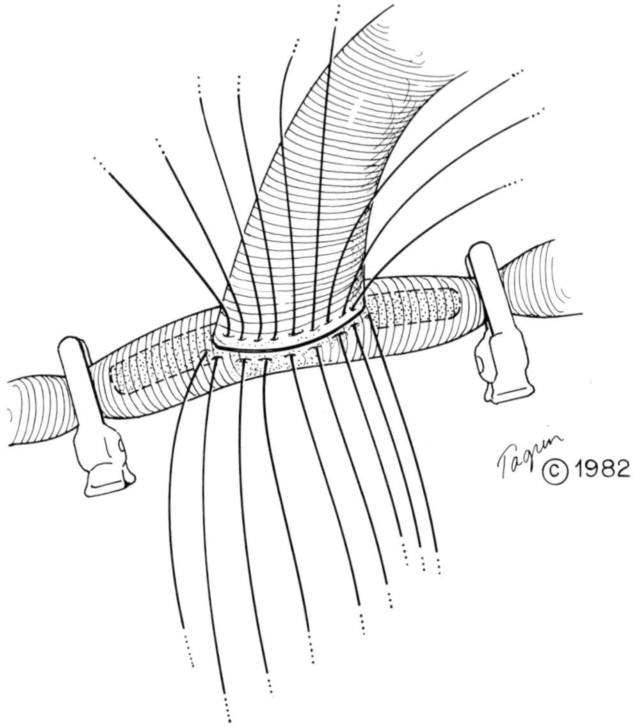

Figure 4.14 Front wall sutures. These are laid in separately without tying until all are placed. Bites are slightly thicker on the STA. Sutures are slightly closer together near the corners where it is most apt to leak. About seven sutures will be needed between the corner stitches.

Anastomosis

The STA tip is positioned against the MCA opening with the tip aimed backward toward the MCA origin to promote flow throughout the MCA territory. A needle holder and jeweler's forceps are used to place interrupted 9-0 nylon sutures in each corner (Fig. 4.13). Forceps are used primarily as a counter pressor during suturing, and the vessel wall is handled as little and as gently as possible. Squeezing the intima is particularly avoided. An additional six to eight interrupted sutures are placed in the front wall (Fig. 4.14) and these are tied down after all have been placed to give maximum accuracy. Bites are a bit larger on the STA side to promote slight eversion and intima-to-intima apposition. Sutures must accurately include STA intima which may be thickened and separated from muscularis. In-to-out passage of the needle through STA is recommended when an intimal flap threatens. Sutures are placed slightly closer together near the corner where leaks are more common. Keeping the area dry facilitates suture handling. Keeping the needle in view on the rubber dam minimizes time lost in searching.

The STA is reflected aside to reveal the back wall of the anastomosis. The front wall suture line is inspected from inside to confirm accurate suture placement. Then, six to eight interrupted sutures are

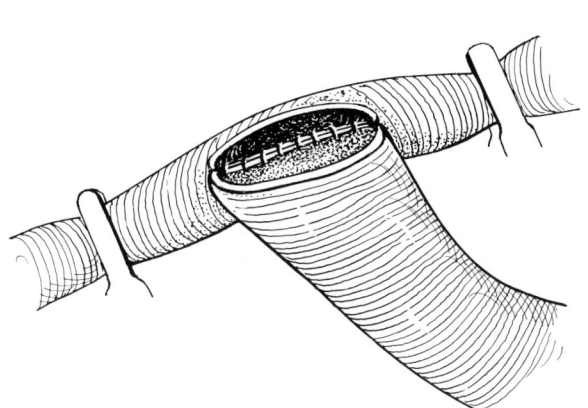

Figure 4.15 Back wall sutures. The front wall is checked from interiorly to correct problems. Back wall sutures are placed just like the front wall sutures.

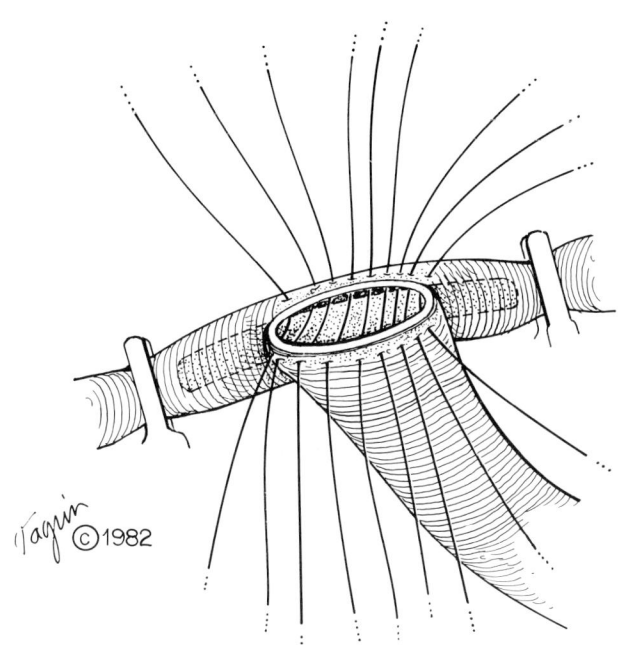

Figure 4.16 Stent removal. After all back wall sutures are placed (but not tied), the stent is gently removed.

used to complete the back wall (Fig. 4.15). Before the last two sutures are tied, the stent tube is gently removed and the three vascular limbs opened briefly to check flow and expel air (Fig. 4.16). Final sutures are tied down.

The distal MCA clip is removed first and then the proximal. Utilizing 25X magnification, the suture line is inspected for leaks. A major area of leak requires a stitch; suture line ooze will stop without additional sutures. The rubber dam is folded over the suture line, and a cottonoid provides pressure for 1–2 minutes. In some cases, a collar of gelfoam may secure suture line hemostasis. Finally, the STA clip is removed to begin augmented cerebral blood flow. One may measure graft pressures when a suitable side branch of STA has been cannulated. Graft flow may also be estimated with an electromagnetic flow probe, but great care must be exercised to avoid injury to the STA by the flow probe.

Closure

The dura is loosely approximated with 4-0 sutures. A Gelfoam pledget covers the exposed dura and surrounds the distal STA segment. After the graft is routed smoothly and without kinking, the bone flap is trimmed with rongeurs to avoid contact with the STA and then wired in place (Fig. 4.17). The temporalis muscle and fascia are approximated as separate layers with interrupted 3-0 coated Vicryl. Great care is taken to avoid compression of the graft. The wound is irrigated with Bacitracin solution and closed with 3-0 interrupted coated Vicryl to the galea and continuous nylon to the skin. When scalp edge viability is in question, closure using interrupted 5-0 nylon without tension offers the best chance of avoiding necrosis. A small dressing is applied together with a warning sign against pressure and a mark to indicate the point to check for pulse in the superficial temporal artery.

POSTOPERATIVE MANAGEMENT AND COMPLICATIONS

Blood pressure is carefully monitored with the aid of a radial artery catheter and is maintained in the normal range of the individual patient with infusions of colloid, pressors, or nitroprusside. Patients are gradually mobilized after 48 hours and blood pressure controlled with oral agents as needed. Diphenylhydantoin (300 mg/day) is used. Aspirin (300 mg) and Dipyridamole (25 mg) are given twice daily for 6 months. Careful management of risk factors continues indefinitely.

If the patient is not doing well in the immediate postoperative period, CT scan is performed, and if this does not clarify the problem, then angiography is done.

Major complications of this procedure include intra-operative graft thrombosis, graft thrombosis with either acute or late stroke, subdural hematoma, and intracerebral hemorrhage (8, 17, 26, 40, 41). Less se-

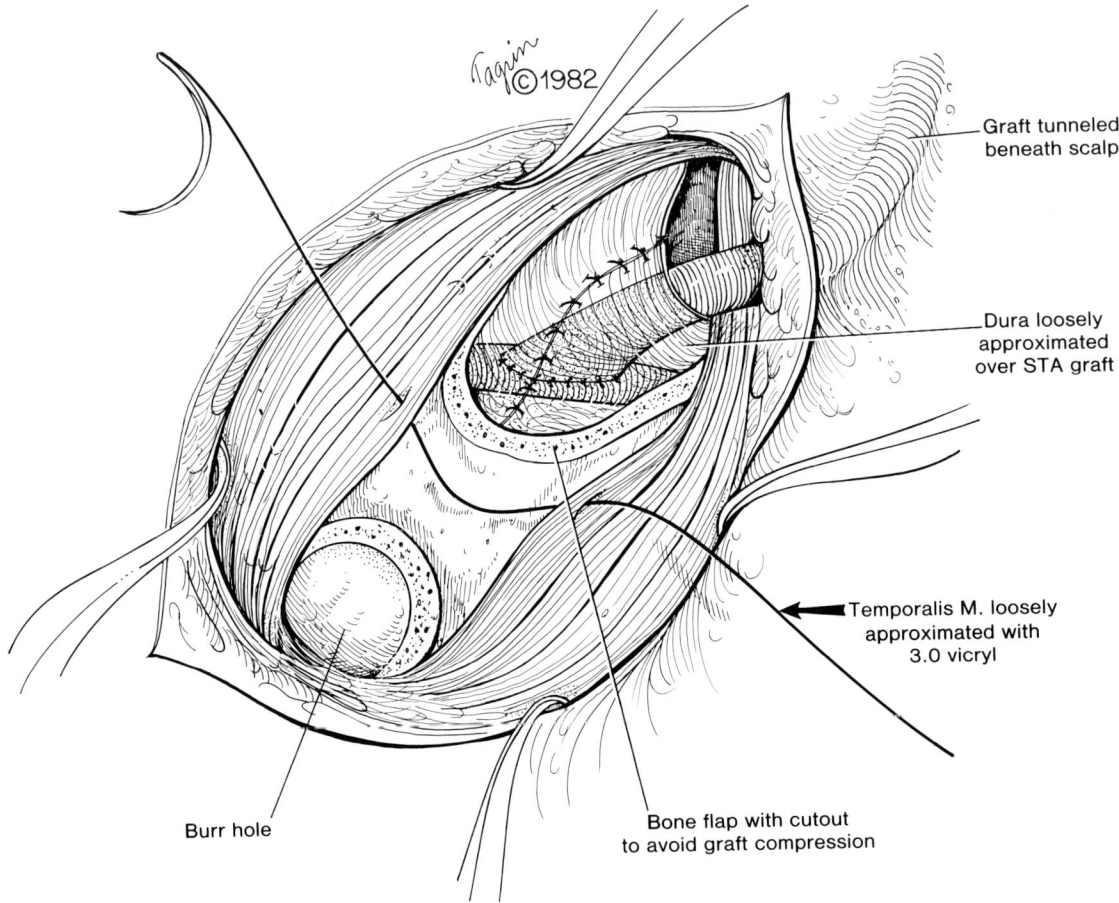

Figure 4.17 Closure. The graft is routed without kink or compression. The dura is loosely approximated without compression of the graft. The bone flap is replaced, with a cutout to avoid touching the graft. Muscle and fascia are brought together loosely with the graft piercing these as anteriorly as possible.

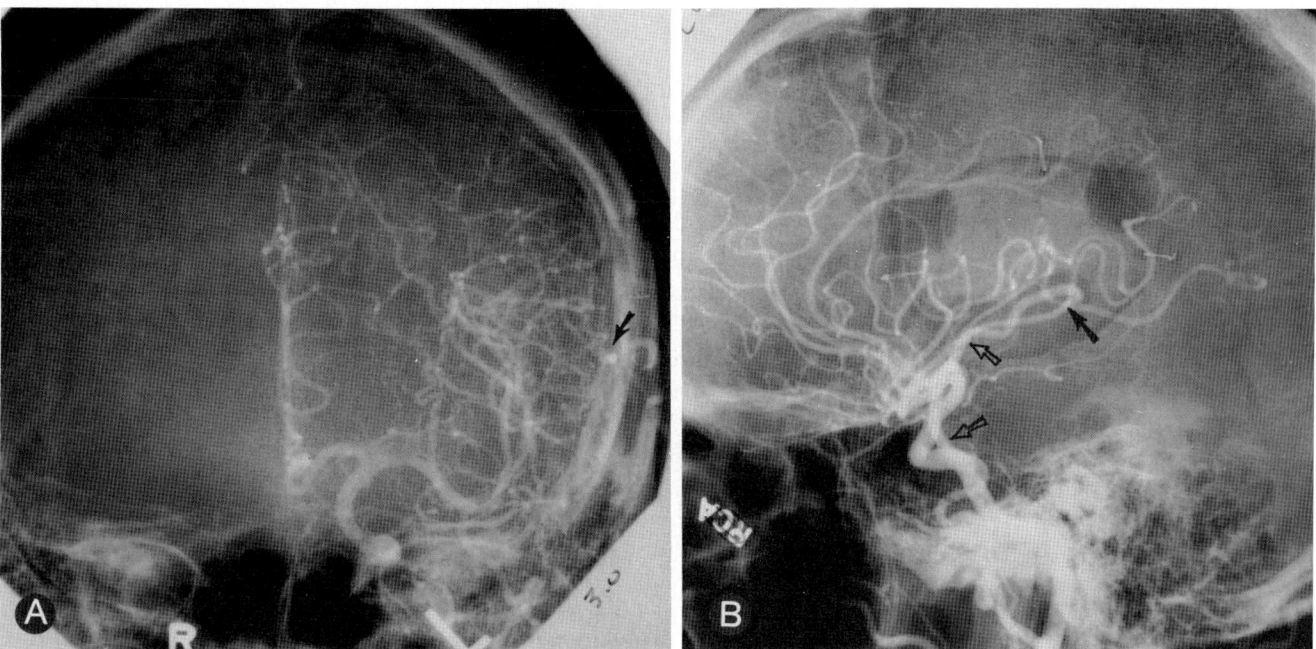

Figure 4.18 STA-MCA bypass for MCA stenosis. *A,* the AP angiogram shows the area of stenosis in the proximal middle cerebral artery. The site of the STA-MCA anastomosis is shown (*closed arrow*). *B,* the lateral angiogram shows the large STA (*open arrows*) and the site of the anastomosis (*closed arrow*). Comment: Severe episodes of dysphasia ceased after surgery.

rious complications include transient neurological worsening, wound infection, seizures, scalp edge necrosis, and myocardial ischemia.

When intraoperative thrombosis is noted, a check for technical errors is done, but in our experience when this problem occurred, a hypercoaguable state was found with spontaneous aggregation of platelets and the occlusion could not be reopened. The early postoperative occlusion usually relates to a technical error in performing the procedure.

In the uncomplicated patient, angiography is performed in one week to assess patency of the anastomosis. Patency in our series was documented angiographically in 45 of 49 grafts studied (Figs. 4.18 and 4.19). Technical errors led to thrombosis in two cases. In one, the first in the series, insufficient attention was paid to the course of the graft through the muscle and bone. Compression of the graft by these structures led to asymptomatic thrombosis. In the other patient, the STA segment was cut too short and there was tension on the suture line. Although an initial angiogram showed only minor irregularity at the anastomotic site, occlusion occurred 3 months later and was associated with a mild stroke. In two other cases, intraoperative thrombosis occurred without neurological sequlae.

Delayed strokes can occur despite a functioning bypass graft. This happened in three of our cases. In two, occlusion of a previously markedly stenotic intracranial internal carotid artery occurred after surgery. Mild strokes resulted in both these cases despite improved filling of MCA via the graft, as compared with the immediate postoperative studies. In the other case, a mild stroke occurred in the face of a functioning graft and poor collateral circulation. We have observed internal carotid occlusion once without symptoms. In these cases, STA-MCA bypass may have promoted ICA occlusion, protected against infarction, or both. Complete occlusion of distal carotid stenosis following establishment of STA-MCA bypass graft has also been reported by others (12, 26).

Occasionally, a patient will continue to have TIAs following a bypass procedure. This may indicate that the mechanism of ischemia is other than postulated preoperatively. For example, following ICA occlusion, the mechanism of TIAs may be external carotid artery stenosis or distal stump embolization rather than a hemodynamic problem and, therefore, a bypass could be ineffectual. Alternatively, the bypass may be occluded, providing no additional collateral circulation to the brain. Another possibility is the inducement of occlusion in a previously stenotic internal carotid artery as discussed in the previous paragraph. In order to evaluate the precise mechanism and symptomatology in this situation, cerebral angiography is required. In one of our patients, episodes of numbness in the left face presumably related to severe distal ICA stenosis persisted following su-

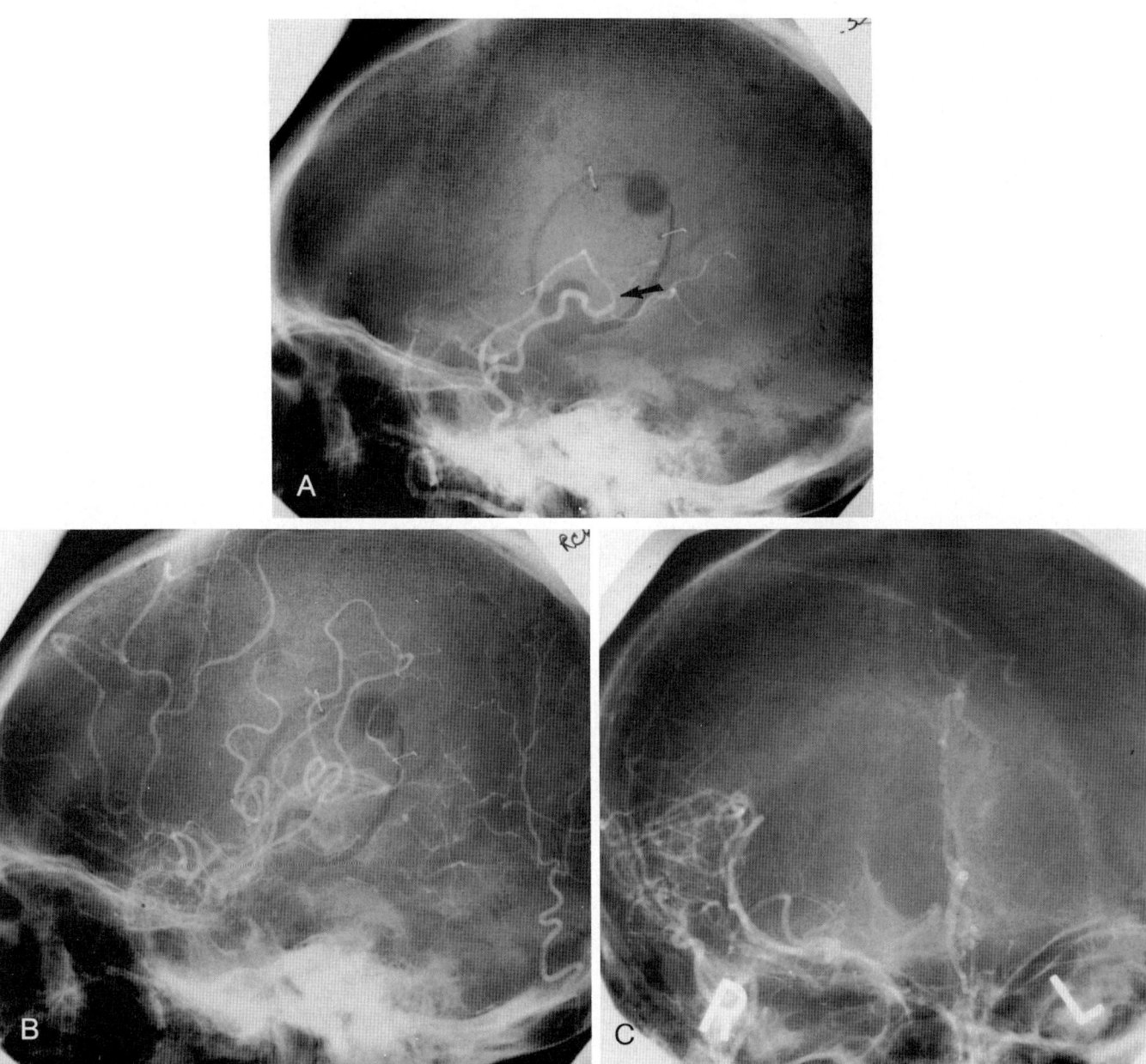

Figure 4.19 Bypass for multiple occlusions and dementia. Preoperative angiography showed left vertebral and bilateral carotid occlusions. Postoperative left carotid angiogram shows: A, patent bypass (arrow); B, widespread filling of left MCA branches; and C, some contralateral ACA filling from graft. Spells ceased after surgery and mentation improved.

perficial temporal artery-middle cerebral bypass (Fig. 4.20). Cerebral angiography confirmed continued patency of the stenotic vessel and good filling of the bypass graft into the middle cerebral circulation. The patient was treated with aspirin and persantin but the episodes persisted. Approximately 1 year later, the patient suffered a moderate right cerebral hemisphere stroke which cleared to a mild deficit. Cerebral angiography at that time disclosed occlusion of the internal carotid artery with newly enhanced filling of the middle cerebral territory via the graft. An appropriate cerebral infarction was demonstrated on CT scan. This case has persuaded us that should TIAs persist after bypass graft and anti-platelet therapy, strong consideration of coumadin therapy should be entertained.

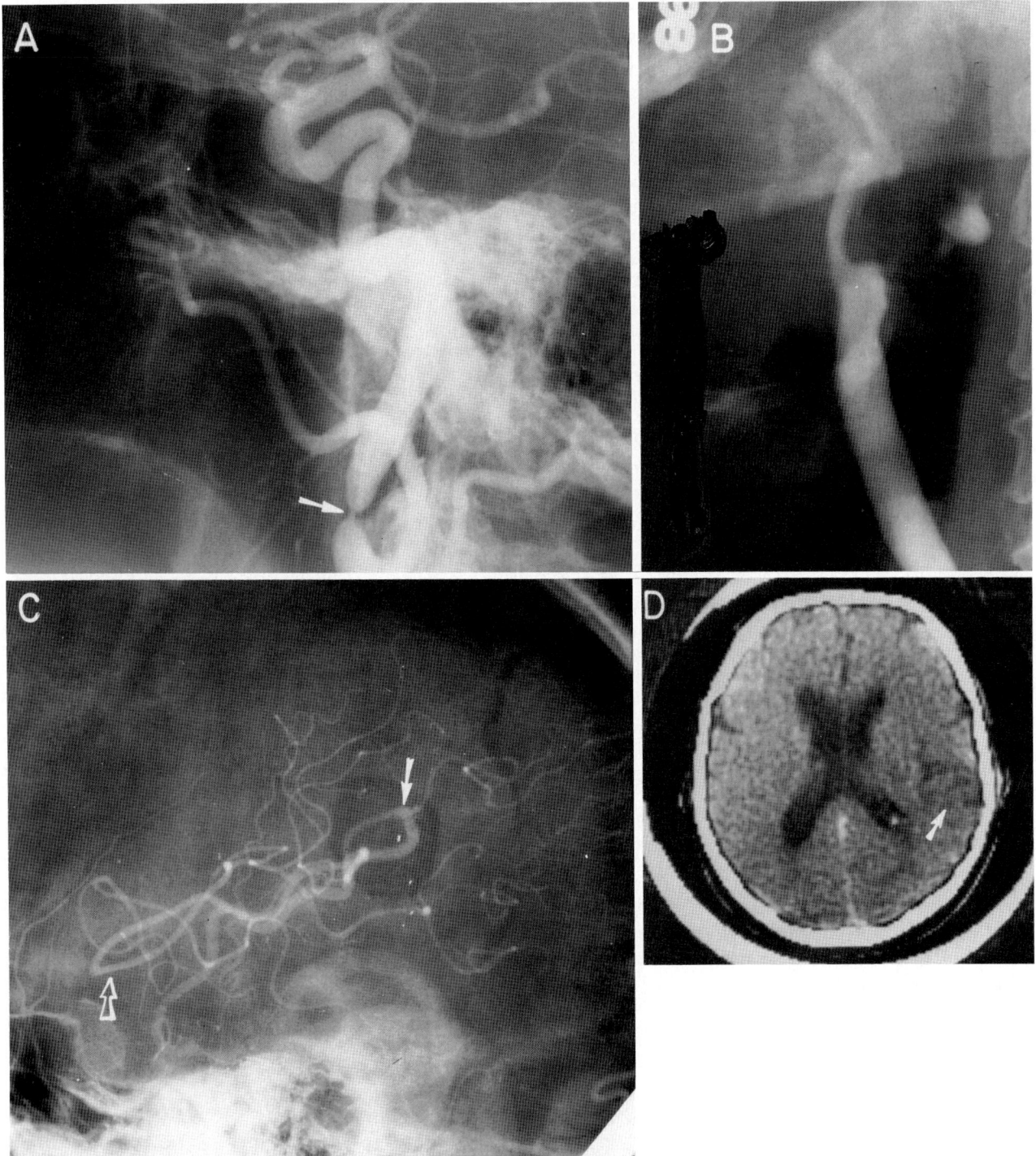

Figure 4.20 ICA occlusion after bypass. *A,* right high cervical ICA stenosis (*arrow*) caused TIAs. *B,* despite STA-MCA bypass, TIAs progressed to RICA occlusion with sudden left hemiparesis. *C,* a patent bypass (*closed arrow*) gave substantial MCA filling (*open arrow*). *D,* a small right parietal infarct persisted (*arrow*). The patient recovered virtually completely.

ALTERNATIVE PROCEDURES
Long Grafts from Cervical Arteries to MCA

A number of authors have recommended interposition of a free graft between an artery in the neck (subclavian or common carotid) and an intracranial artery (ICA or MCA) to provide immediate high flow revascularization. Initial results with saphenous vein grafts between common carotid artery and intracranial carotid artery were reported to be disappointing with high morbidity and low patency (23, 39). More recent experience with interposition of grafts between the common carotid or the subclavian artery and a cortical branch of MCA have been more promising with low complication rates and good postoperative patency rates, but the procedure remains in the developmental stage (20, 30, 34, 35).

For the graft, polytetrafluoroethylene, saphenous vein, or radial artery have been used. For cervical carotid-angular MCA branch saphenous grafting, three teams of surgeons work simultaneously, one to prepare the cervical carotid, one to prepare the angular artery, and a third to harvest the saphenous vein. The proximal graft is completed under loupes using a side-biting Satinsky clamp on the common carotid artery to avoid cross-clamping this vessel. The saphenous vein is routed subcutaneously behind the ear to the cranial wound (Fig. 4.21). Microsurgical end-to-side anastomosis is then carried out, with the donor vessel bevelled back toward MCA origin. To compensate for the very wide donor graft, a long cortical arteriotomy is performed. The techniques used in STA-MCA anastomosis apply to this operation. Early technical problems with this procedure reportedly have been overcome by using a 2-mm vein, avoiding hydrostatic dilation and use of the retroauricular tunnel (30).

Occipital-MCA Anastomosis

When the STA is inadequate, the occipital artery may sometimes be used (32). The angiogram shows whether this vessel is adequate; in some cases the artery is small or bifurcates early into small distal branches. Palpation and Doppler probe permit marking of the artery's course. Direct cutdown on the occipital artery provides the best exposure. Careful sharp dissection is needed to free the vessel from surrounding dense adhesions. Exposure and preparation of the MCA branch and anastomosis are completed as in STA-MCA bypass.

Other Procedures

When STA and occipital artery are inadequate, a short segment of forearm vein can be interposed between one of these arteries and an MCA branch (38). The vein should be 3–4 mm in diameter to avoid major discrepancy with the MCA. For both anastomoses, a marked bevel (60° or more) and long arteriotomy (7–9 mm) can maximize the ostium size.

Ordinarily, the middle meningeal artery is too

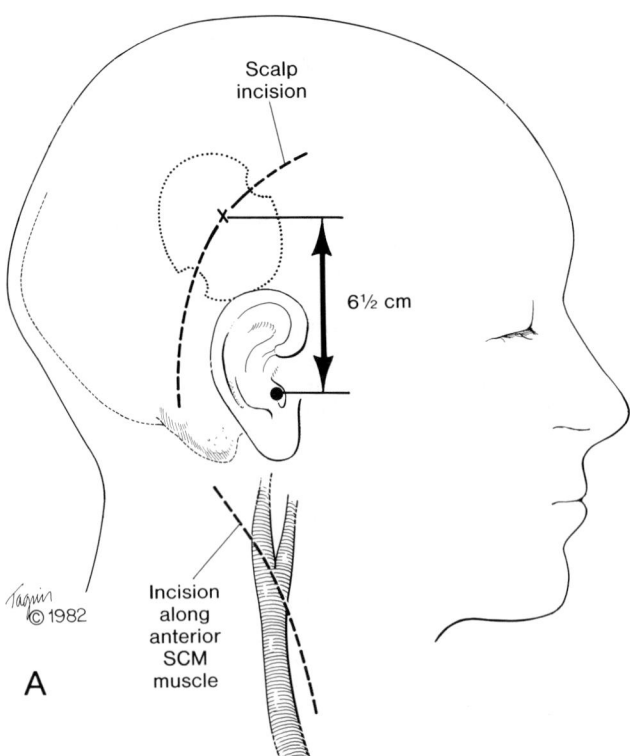

Figure 4.21 Common carotid artery to middle cerebral artery long vein graft. *A*, outline of incisions used for the neck and cranial exposures. *B* and *C*, details of the distal and proximal anastomosis. *D*, final position of the vein graft.

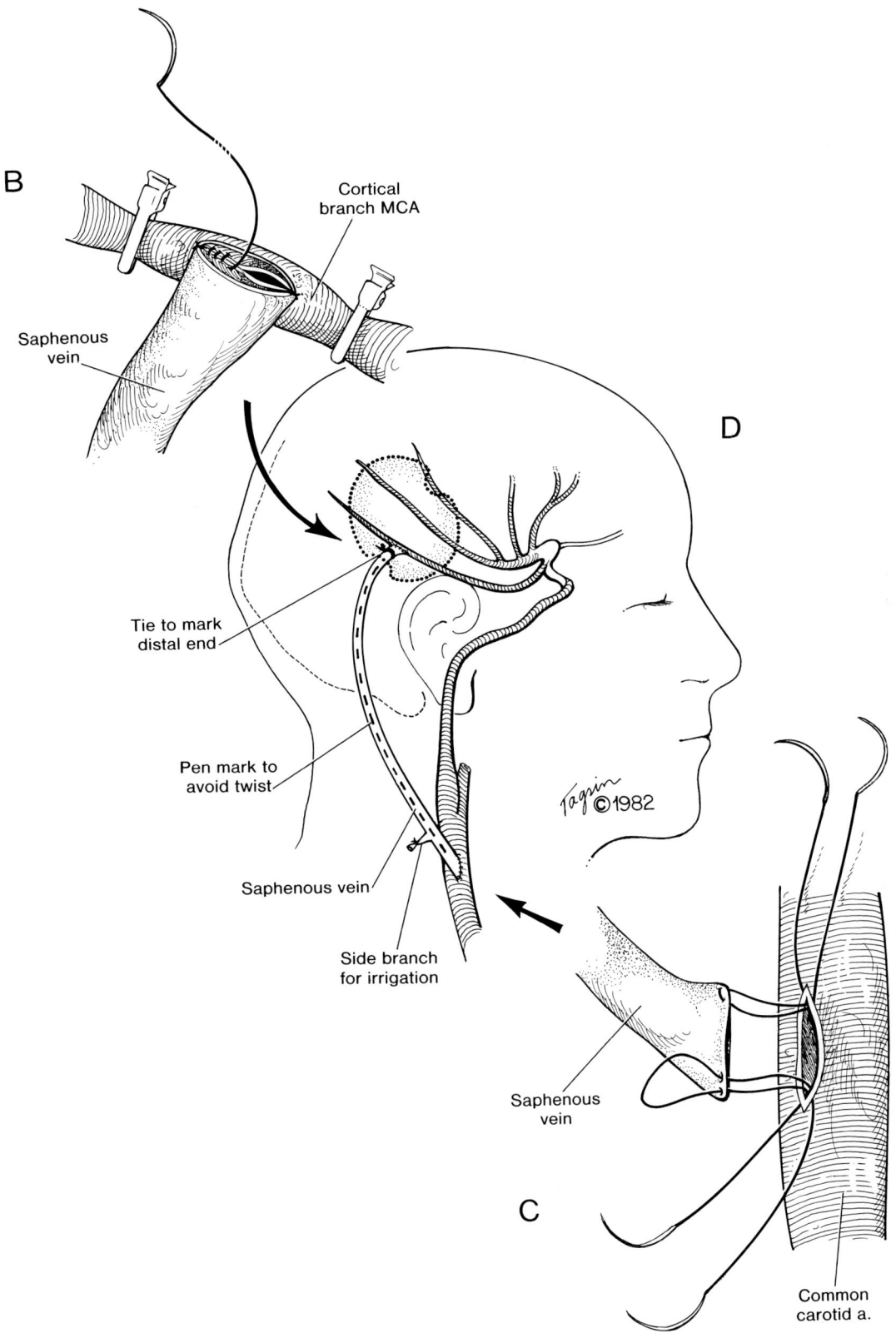

Figure 4.21 (*B* to *D*)

small to be useful for revascularization. Occasionally, the artery may be large enough for grafting, when it is enlarged due to the presence of a meningioma (25).

When no suitable recipient vessel is available, the STA may be ligated and laid on the cortex (3). Microanastomoses may develop later on. Several authors have recommended placement of vascularized omental grafts directly on the brain to add vascular supply (14, 16, 42).

REFERENCES

1. Amine AR, Moody RA, Meeks W: Bilateral temporal-middle cerebral artery anastomosis for moyamoya syndrome. Surg Neurol 8:3–6, 1977.
2. Ammerman BJ, Smith DR: Giant fusiform middle cerebral aneurysm: successful treatment utilizing microvascular bypass. Surg Neurol 7:255–257, 1977.
3. Ausman JI, Moore J, Chou SN: Spontaneous cerebral revascularization in a patient with STA-MCA anastomosis. J Neurosurg 44:84–87, 1976.
4. Barnett HJM, Peerless SJ, McCormick CW: In answer to the question: "As compared to what?" A progress report on the EC/IC bypass study. Stroke 11:137–140, 1980.
5. Chater N, Popp J: Microsurgical vascular bypass for occlusive cerebrovascular disease: review of 100 cases. Surg Neurol 6:115–118, 1976.
6. Chater N, Mani J, Tonnemacher K: Superficial temporal artery bypass for cerebrovascular occlusive disease. Cal Med 119:9–13, 1973.
7. Crowell RM: Emergency STA-MCA bypass for acute focal cerebral ischemia, in Schmidek P et al (eds): *Microneurosurgical Anastomoses for Cerebral Ischemia*. Berlin, Springer-Verlag, 1977.
8. Crowell RM: Direct brain revascularization, in Schmidek H, Sweet WH (eds): *Current Techniques of Operative Neurosurgery*. New York, Grune & Stratton, 1978.
9. Crowell RM, Olsson Y: Effect of extracranial-intracranial vascular bypass graft on experimental acute stroke in dogs. J Neurosurg 38:26–31, 1973.
10. Donaghy RMP, Yasargil MG: *Microvascular Surgery*. Stuttgart, Georg Thieme Verlag, 1967.
11. Ferguson GG, Peerless SJ: *Extracranial-Intracranial Arterial Bypass in the Treatment of Dementia and Multiple Extracranial Arterial Occlusion.* Presented at the Twenty-sixth Annual Meeting of the Congress of Neurological Surgeons, New Orleans, October 28, 1976.
12. Furlan AJ, Little JR, Dohn DF: Arterial occlusion following anastomosis of the superficial temporal artery to middle cerebral artery. Stroke 11:91–95, 1980.
13. Gelber BR, Sundt TM Jr: Treatment of intracavernous and giant carotid aneurysms by combined internal carotid ligation and extra- to intracranial bypass. J Neurosurg 52:1–10, 1980.
14. Goldsmith HS, Duckett S, Chen WF: Prevention of cerebral infarction in the monkey by omental transposition to the brain. Stroke 9:224–229, 1978.
15. Grubb RL, Ratcheson RA, Raichle ME, Klieboth AB, Gado MH: Regional cerebral blood flow and oxygen utilization in superficial temporal-middle cerebral artery anastomosis patients. J Neurosurg 50:733–741, 1979.
16. Henschen C. Operative revascularisation des zirkulatorisch geschädigten gehirns durch auflage gestielter muskellapen encephalo-myo-synangiose, Langenbecks Arch Klin Chir 264:392–401, 1950.
17. Heros RC, Nelson PB: Intracerebral hemorrhage after microsurgical cerebral revascularization. Neurosurgery 6:371–375, 1980.
18. Holbach K-H, Wassmann HW, Hoheluchter KL: Reversibility of the chronic post-stroke state. Stroke 7:296–300, 1976.
19. Holbach K-H, Wassmann HW, Hoheluchter KL, Jain KK: Differentiation between reversible and irreversible post-stroke changes in brain tissue: Its relevance for cerebrovascular surgery. Surg Neurol 7:325–331, 1977.
20. Iwabuchi T, Kudo T, Hatanaka M, Oda N, Maeda S: Vein graft bypass in treatment of giant aneurysm. Surg Neurol 12:463–466, 1979.
21. Karasawa J, Kikuchi H, Furuse S, Kawamura J, Sakaki T: Treatment of moyamoya disease with STA-MCA anastomosis. J Neurosurg 49:679–688, 1978.
22. Kearns TP, Siekert RG, Sundt TM Jr: The ocular aspects of bypass surgery of the carotid artery. Mayo Clin Proc 54:3–11, 1979.
23. Lougheed WM, Marshall BM, Hunter M, Michel ER, Sandwith-Smyth H: Common carotid to intracranial internal carotid bypass venous graft. J Neurosurg 34:114–118, 1971.
24. McDowell FH: The Extracranial/Intracranial Bypass Study. Stroke 8:545, 1977.
25. Miller CF II, Spetzler RF, Kopaniky DJ: Middle meningeal to middle cerebral arterial bypass for cerebral revascularization. Case report. J Neurosurg 50:802–804, 1979.
26. Reichman OH: Complications of cerebral revascularization. Clin Neurosurg 23:318–335, 1976.
27. Reichman OH, Davis DO, Roberts TS, et al: Anastomosis between STA and cortical branch of MCA for the treatment of occlusive cerebrovascular disease, in Marei FT (ed): *Reconstructive Surgery of Brain Arteries*. Budapest, Akademiai Kiado, 1974.
28. Robertson J: Personal communication, 1975.
29. Samson DS, Boone S: Extracranial-intracranial (EC-IC) arterial bypass: past performance and current concepts. Neurosurgery 3:79–86, 1978.
30. Samson DS, Gerwertz BL, Beyer CW Jr, Hodosh RM: Saphenous vein interposition grafts in the microsurgical treatment of cerebral ischemia. Arch Surg 116:1578–1582, 1981.
31. Schmiedek P, Gratzl O, Spetzler R, Steinhoff H, Enzenbach R, Brendel W, Marguth F: Selection of patients for extra-intracranial arterial bypass surgery based on rCBF measurements. J Neurosurg 44:303–312, 1976.
32. Spetzler RF, Chater N: Occipital artery-middle cerebral artery anastomosis for cerebral artery occlusive disease. Surg Neurol 2:235–238, 1974.
33. Spetzler RF, Shuster H, Roski RA: Elective extracranial-intracranial arterial bypass in the treatment of inoperable giant internal carotid artery aneurysms. J Neurosurg 53:22–27, 1980.
34. Spetzler RF, Rhodes RS, Roski RA, Likavec MJ: Subclavian to middle cerebral artery saphenous vein bypass graft. J Neurosurg 53:465–469, 1980.
35. Story JL, Brown WE Jr, Eidelberg E, Arom KV, Stewart JR: Cerebral revascularization: common carotid to distal middle cerebral artery bypass. Neurosurgery 2:131–135, 1978.
36. Sundt TM Jr, Siekart RG, Piepgras DG, Sharbrough FW, Houser OW: Bypass surgery for vascular disease of the carotid system. Mayo Clin Proc 51:677–692, 1976.
37. Sundt TM, Piepgras DG: Surgical approach to giant intracranial aneurysms: Operative experience with 80 cases. J Neurosurg 51:731–742, 1979.
38. Tew JM Jr: Reconstructive vascular surgery for prevention of stroke. Clin Neurosurg 22:264–280, 1975.
39. Woringer E, Kunlin J: Anastomose entre la carotide primitive et la carotide intra-cranienne on la Sylvienne par greffon selon la technique de la suture suspendue. Neurochirurgie 9:181–188, 1963.
40. Yasargil MG: *Microsurgery Applied to Neurosurgery*. Stuttgart, Georg Thieme Verlag, 1968.
41. Yasargil MG, Krayenbuhl HA, Jacobson JH: Microneurosurgical arterial reconstruction. Surgery 67:221–233, 1970.
42. Yonekawa Y, Yasargil MG: Brain vascularization by transplanted omentum: A possible treatment of cerebral ischemia. Neurosurgery 1:256–259, 1977.

Chapter 5 ATHEROSCLEROSIS OF THE VERTEBROBASILAR CIRCULATION: EVALUATION, MANAGEMENT, AND OPERATIVE PROCEDURES

CLINICAL SYNDROMES
Vertebrobasilar Ischemia

Symptoms of vertebrobasilar insufficiency and infarction are usually due to atherosclerotic occlusive disease within the intracranial vertebral artery, the basilar artery, or its branches (Fig. 5.1). Most patients with stenosis or occlusion at the origin of a vertebral artery do not have symptoms. When transient symptoms of vertebrobasilar ischemia are associated with stenosis of the extracranial vertebral artery, the patients usually do not go on to have infarction (9). This is probably due to the extensive collateral circulation that develops into the distal extracranial vertebral artery.

Extracranial stenosis or occlusion of one vertebral artery is somewhat more likely to be symptomatic if the other vertebral artery is also severely stenotic or occluded due to atheroma or is congenitally hypoplastic or absent (Fig. 5.2). Rarely, compression of the vertebral artery by an osteophyte associated with cervical spondylosis may cause symptoms (4). Vertebrobasilar ischemia symptoms secondary to carotid occlusive disease are discussed on p. 22.

The clinical picture is diverse. Dizziness, diplopia, dysarthria, and weakness or numbness in part or all of one or both sides of the body are the most common symptoms. Other manifestations include headache, staggering, veering to one side, blurred vision, partial or complete blindness, ptosis, dysphagia, confusion, syncope, and memory lapse.

Non-invasive vascular studies are of little help. Doppler imaging can at times demonstrate proximal vertebral stenosis or occlusion, but this does not give the necessary information about the intracranial circulation. The CT scan may provide information as to where infarction has occurred, but is of little value in the patient with transient ischemic symptoms. Angiography is required to adequately study these patients and must visualize the full extent of the innominate, subclavian and extracranial vertebral and carotid arteries, as well as the intracranial circulation.

Most patients with vertebrobasilar ischemia respond to anticoagulation with heparin and then coumadin. The rare patient who continues to have symptoms and has a precarious circulation should be evaluated for surgery. Several surgical procedures have been used to improve vertebrobasilar circulation. We believe that further experience will probably confirm useful roles for vertebral artery transposition in some patients with vertebral artery stenosis or occlusion and occipital artery-posterior inferior cerebellar ar-

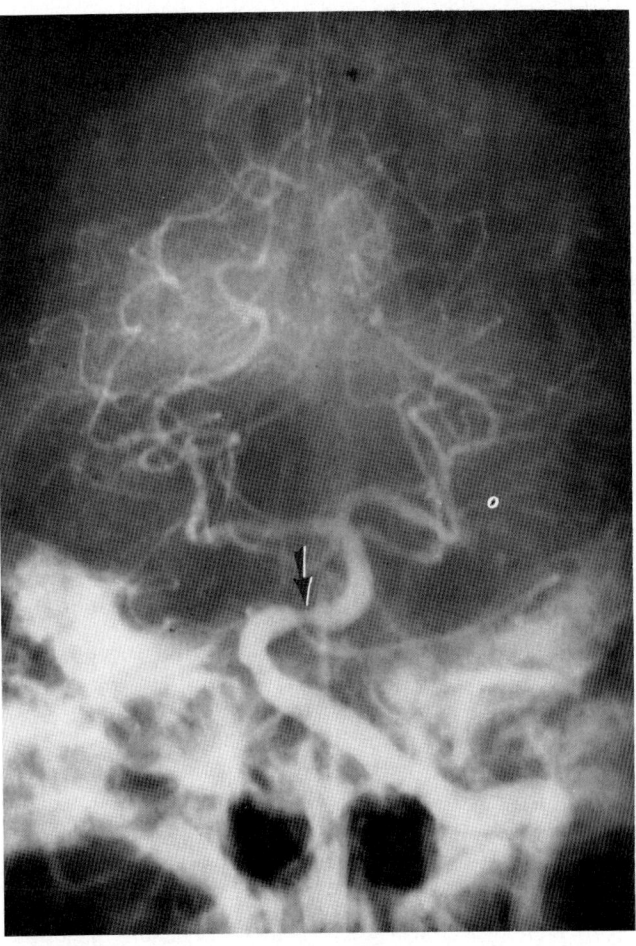

Figure 5.1 Basilar artery stenosis. Vertebral angiogram showing stenosis in the proximal basilar artery (*arrow*). The patient presented with TIAs. This is a common site for atherosclerosis to occur. At the present time anticoagulation is the best treatment.

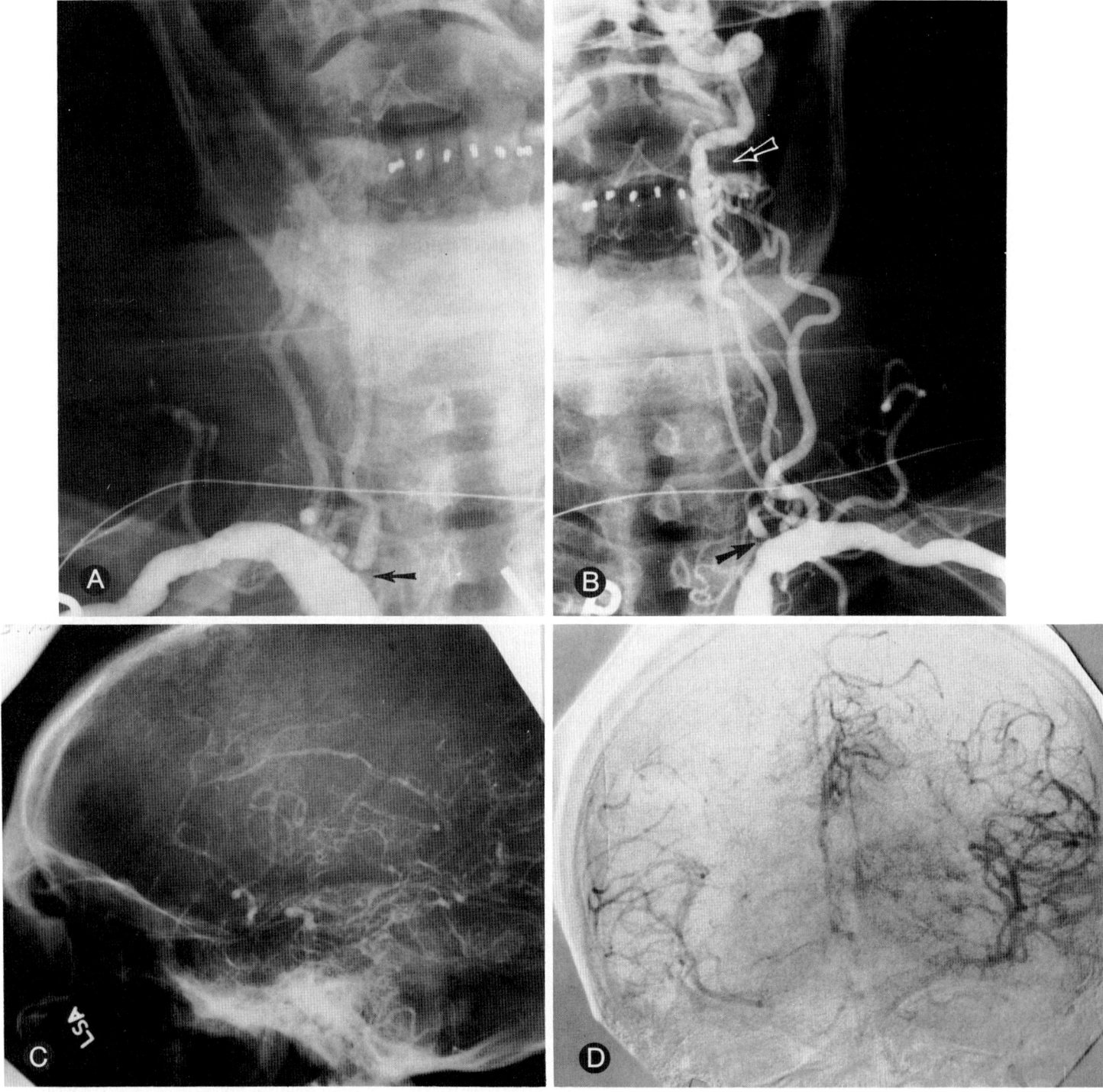

Figure 5.2 Vertebral artery stenosis. *A*, right subclavian angiogram showing severe stenosis (*arrow*) at the origin of the vertebral artery. The carotid artery is occluded. *B*, left subclavian angiogram showing severe stenosis (*closed arrow*) at the origin of the vertebral artery with narrowing of the proximal lumen, indicating reduced pressure. Note that the normal caliber of the distal vertebral artery is restored by collateral circulation (*open arrow*). *C* and *D*, intracranial views show that the entire circulation depends on the marginal flow in the vertebral arteries. Unilateral stenosis at the origin of the vertebral artery is usually asymptomatic. However, when other arterial supply to the brain is occluded, the stenosis may be significant. Complete angiography in this patient confirmed bilateral carotid occlusion. Ischemic episodes ceased and mentation improved after bypass right STA-MCA graft.

tery (PICA) bypass for some patients with distal vertebral artery pathology.

Subclavian Steal

A subclavian steal occurs when blood flows retrograde down the vertebral artery and into the distal subclavian artery. In most patients, the cause is atherosclerosis with stenosis or occlusion of the subclavian or innominate artery proximal to the origin of the vertebral artery. Other causes, though rare, are trauma, embolization, congenital vascular anomalies, or surgical interruption of the subclavian artery.

In many patients, the subclavian steal is asymptomatic, being found at the time of angiography for another problem. When it is symptomatic, most patients complain of vertebrobasilar neurological symptoms and a small number have symptoms of brachial ischemia. Production of neurological symptoms by exercising the affected arm has been frequent in some series but rare in others (6).

On examination there is usually a bruit over the subclavian artery. The brachial blood pressure is significantly lower on the affected side. Non-invasive studies indicate the degree of flow reduction in the upper extremity. Angiography requires study of both subclavian arteries and the carotid circulation. Late films are needed to see the retrograde flow down the vertebral artery and into the subclavian artery (Fig. 5.3A and B).

Most patients do not require treatment, because there are few if any symptoms, but in some a surgical procedure is indicated. The operations that have been used include: bypass graft from ipsilateral common carotid artery to subclavian artery distal to the site of the obstruction, vertebral artery transposition, vertebral artery ligation, subclavian thromboendarterectomy, and axilloaxillary bypass graft. When surgery was first done for subclavian artery stenosis or occlusion, a transthoracic approach for either endarterectomy or bypass graft from the aorta was done (27). However, because of significant morbidity and mortality from these procedures, other techniques were developed. Axilloaxillary grafts have been prone to thrombosis. The preferred operation has been bypass graft from the common carotid artery to the subclavian artery distal to the stenosis (27). However, some surgeons favor subclavian endarterectomy if it can be done through a supraclavicular approach (28). Vertebral artery transposition has been proposed when vertebrobasilar ischemia is more prominent than the brachial ischemic symptoms (8). Bohmfalk et al. reviewed the literature and found that vertebral ligation relieved or improved the neurological symptoms in patients with subclavian steal and did not adversely affect the arm (6). They concluded that vertebral-to-common carotid artery transposition would have the advantage of establishing a more sure antegrade flow in the vertebral artery than the carotid-to-subclavian bypass.

Vertebral Artery Stenosis or Occlusion Due to Neck Movement or Manipulation

Occlusive disease in the vertebral artery may be associated with symptoms of dizziness or syncope when turning the head into a certain position. Angiography usually reveals absence, occlusion, or hypoplasia of one vertebral artery and stenosis or occlusion of the other vertebral artery at the C1–C2 level when the head is turned. The vertebral artery is relatively fixed in the transverse foramen between C1 and C2 and between the exit from the foramen at C1 and the atlanto-occipital membrane (18). Since much of the rotation and tilting of the head occurs at C1–C2, the remaining patent vertebral artery may be temporarily occluded with these movements (21). Most patients avoid the positions causing symptoms and no treatment is needed. On rare occasion a fusion may be necessary.

A more common problem often caused by head and neck manipulation therapy is injury to the vertebral artery, where it is fixed at C1–C2 (18, 20, 21). Injury to the intima serves as a focus for thrombus formation, which is a source of embolus. Transient ischemic symptoms or stroke may occur either immediately or several days later. Angiography usually shows narrowing or occlusion of the vertebral artery at the C1–C2 level. There may also be an associated pseudoaneurysm.

When vertebrobasilar ischemic symptoms or a mild stroke are due to this cause, anticoagulation with heparin followed by coumadin is indicated. Occasionally, surgical treatment with a bypass graft may be needed.

OPERATIVE PROCEDURES AND RESULTS

Cervical Exposure of the Subclavian and Vertebral Arteries

The supraclavicular exposure can be used for most right vertebral and subclavian operations, some left vertebral and subclavian operations, and transpositions of the vertebral artery. Many operations on the left subclavian artery, on the left vertebral artery when it originates proximally, and on the innominate artery require a median sternotomy or transthoracic approach.

A supraclavicular incision is made centered over the clavicular head of the sternocleidomastoid muscle (Fig. 5.4). The platysma is incised and the clavicular head of the sternocleidomastoid muscle is divided. The scalene fat pad is entered and the omohyoid muscle is divided or retracted superiorly. This exposes the anterior scalene muscle, phrenic nerve, and internal jugular vein (Fig. 5.5). The phrenic nerve is mobilized and retracted with a soft rubber tape. The anterior scalene muscle is divided, bringing into view the subclavian artery and brachial plexus.

The subclavian artery is mobilized proximal and distal to the origin of the vertebral artery (Fig. 5.6).

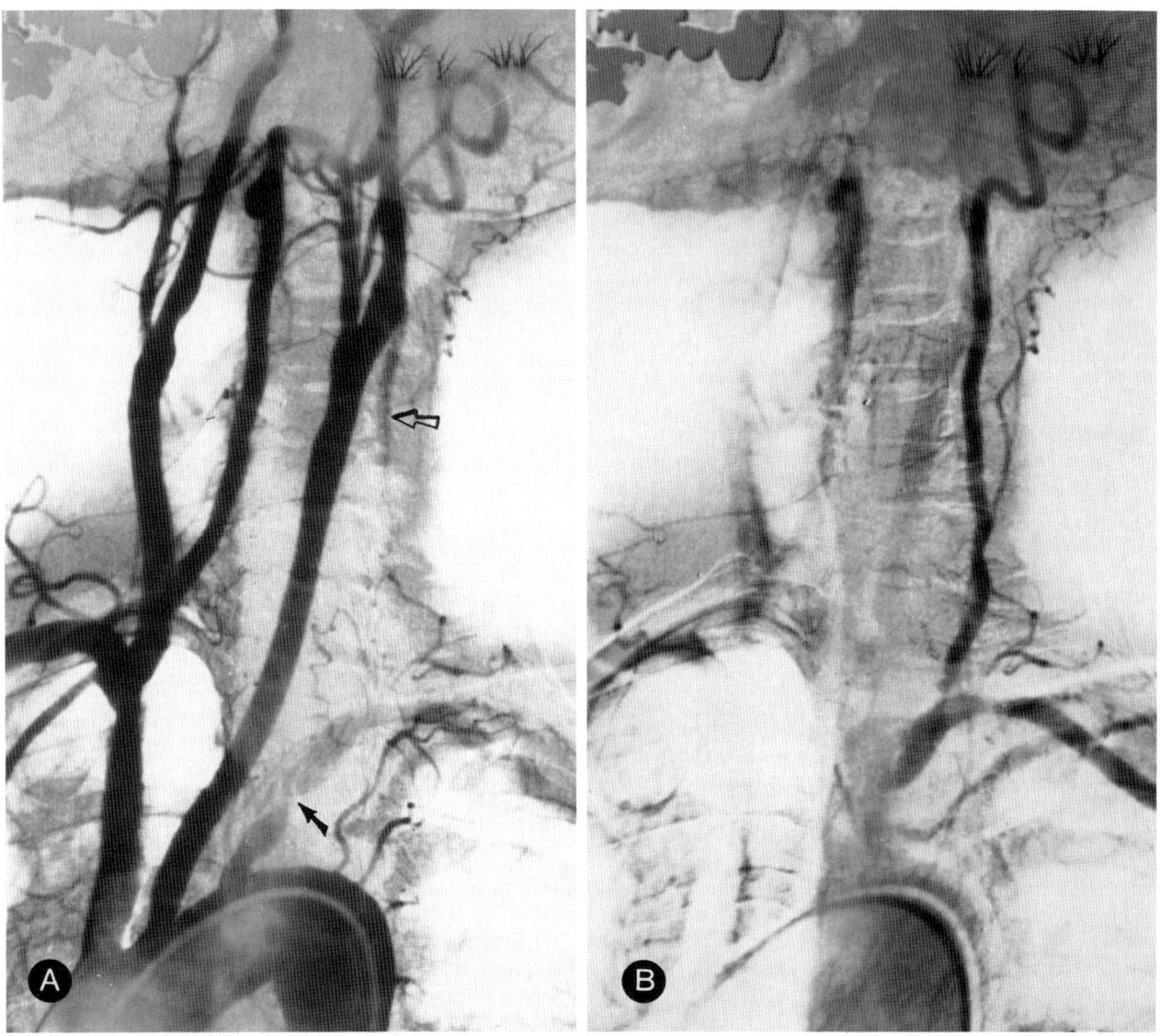

Figure 5.3 Subclavian steal. *A*, arch angiogram. This film shows severe stenosis in the proximal left subclavian artery (*closed arrow*), no antegrade filling of the vertebral artery, and beginning retrograde flow down the vertebral artery (*open arrow*). *B*, later film showing retrograde flow down the vertebral artery and denser opacification of the distal subclavian artery.

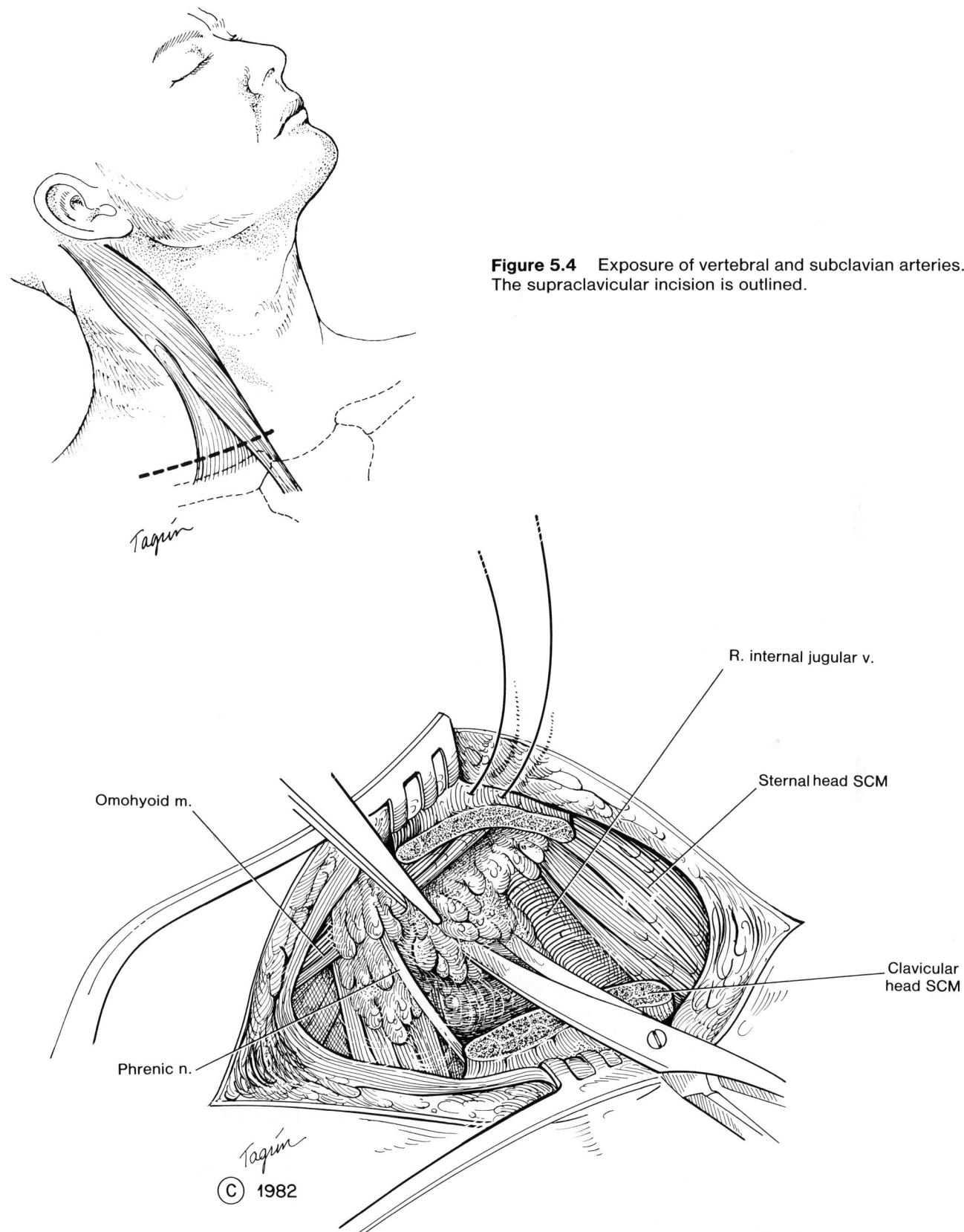

Figure 5.4 Exposure of vertebral and subclavian arteries. The supraclavicular incision is outlined.

Figure 5.5 Exposure of vertebral and subclavian arteries. The clavicular head of the sternocleidomastoid muscle has been divided. Adipose tissue and lymph nodes are being dissected to expose the internal jugular vein, anterior scalene muscle, and phrenic nerve.

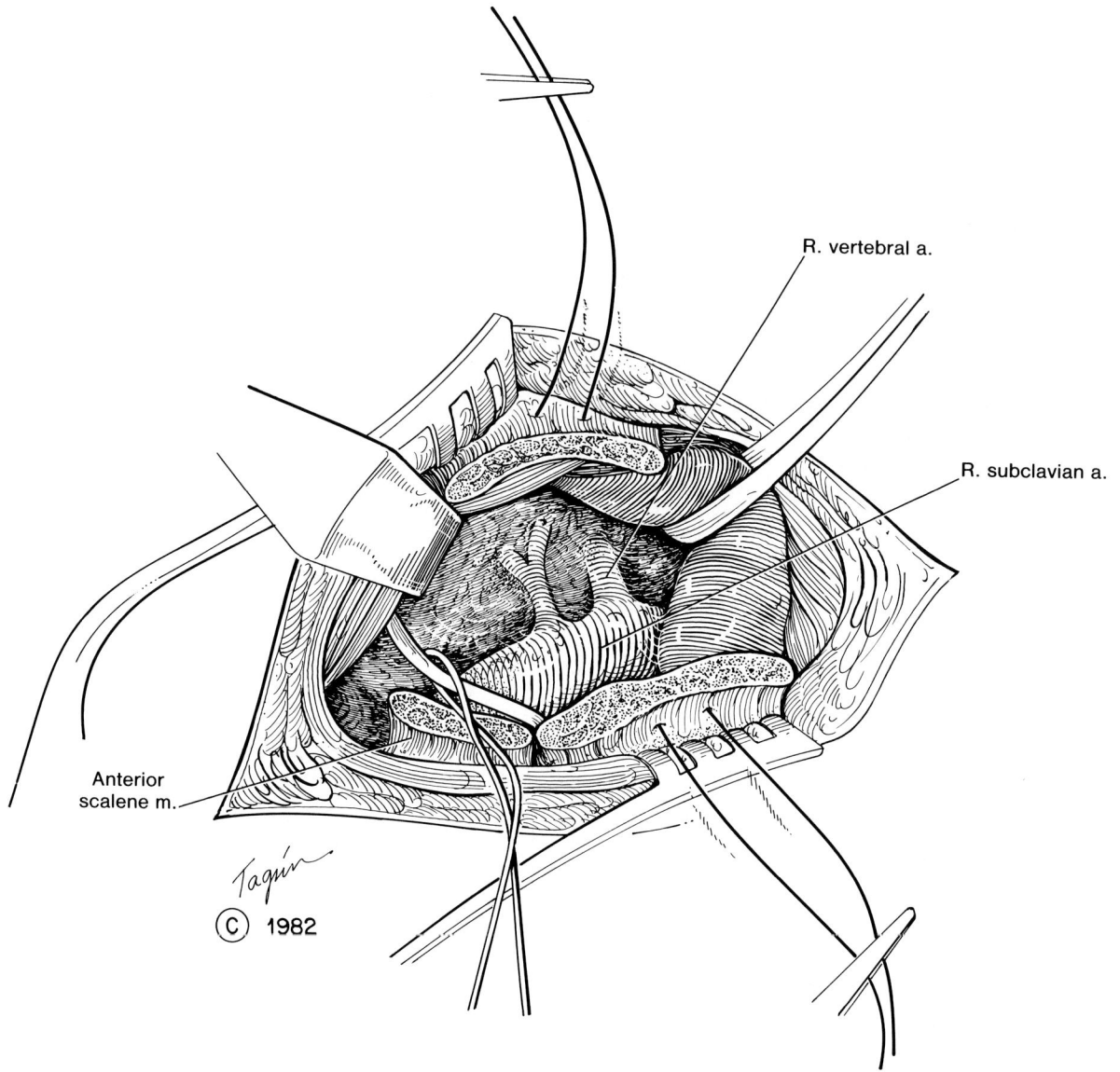

Figure 5.6 Exposure of vertebral and subclavian arteries. The anterior scalene muscle has been divided and the arteries brought into view.

On the left side, the thoracic duct is identified and spared. If it is injured, it should be ligated. The vertebral veins may need to be divided. Appropriate tapes are placed as indicated for proximal and distal control of the subclavian artery and around the vertebral artery. Separate control of the thyrocervical trunk and internal mammary artery may be necessary.

Vertebral Artery Endarterectomy

Vertebral endarterectomy is considered for atherosclerotic occlusive disease which involves the origin of the vertebral artery. The technique of the operation has been described (29). The vertebral artery is a much more fragile vessel than the carotid artery and extra care must be used with surgery on this vessel.

Direct incision into the proximal vertebral artery for endarterectomy is usually not indicated. The preferred approach is to perform the endarterectomy via a trans-subclavian artery incision. We have not seen a patient where this operation was indicated, but the exposure is illustrated (Fig. 5.7).

In a report from one center, 36 patients had vertebral endarterectomy (19, 28). Twenty were done on the right side by a supraclavicular cervical approach and two also required a median sternotomy. Only six of the 14 on the left side could be done by the cervical approach because of the low level of the vertebral artery origin. In the other eight, a transthoracic approach was used. If the patient was a poor risk for a thoracotomy and the origin of the left vertebral artery could not be reached by the cervical approach, the

Atherosclerosis of Vertebrobasilar Circulation

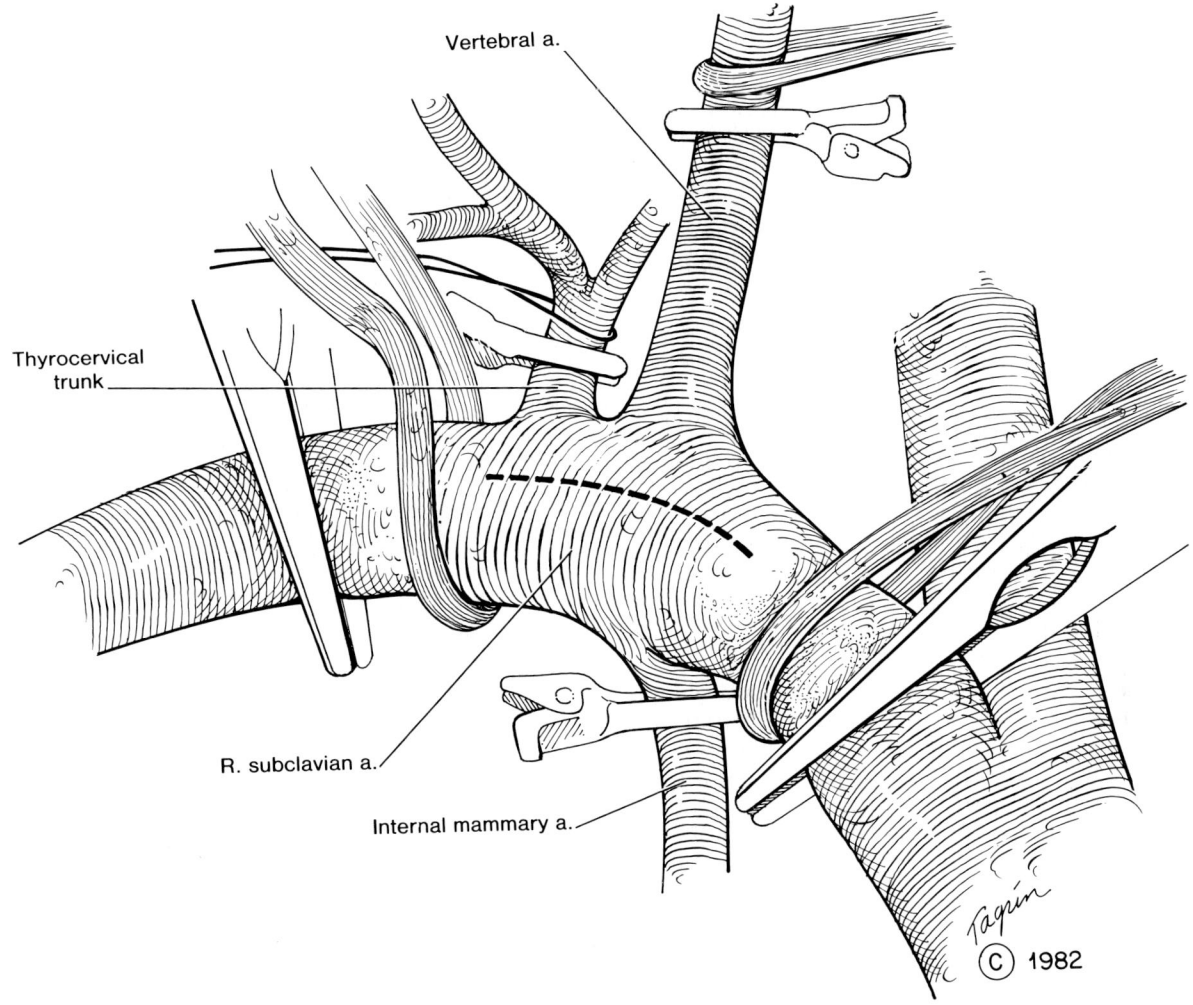

Figure 5.7 Vertebral endarterectomy. The placement of tapes and clamps is shown and the incision outlined.

vertebral artery was reimplanted into the subclavian or common carotid artery. In the last 26 operations no new neurological deficits occurred. Complications included occlusion of one vertebral artery with no symptoms, a lymphocele, and a myocardial infarction. In another report, 58 patients who had some type of unilateral vertebral reconstruction for brain stem symptoms (syncope was the most common) or combined cerebral and brain stem symptoms after any flow-obstructing lesion in the carotid artery had been corrected, had an average stroke rate over a 14-year period of only 1% per year (12).

A recent report has described intradural endarterectomy of the vertebral artery in the segment from entrance to the dura to its disappearance under the brain stem (1). The patient had TIAs that were refractory to anticoagulation. There was a satisfactory postoperative course and angiographic documentation of an open artery.

Percutaneous transluminal angioplasty has been attempted in five patients with stenosis at the origin of the vertebral artery (16). In four patients the procedure was successful with no complications and relief of symptoms.

Subclavian and Innominate Artery Endarterectomy

The approach for subclavian endarterectomy is described in Figures 5.4–5.6. In one report, 29 patients with right subclavian stenosis were all done through a cervical incision, while this could be done in only 14 of 43 patients where the stenosis was on the left, the others requiring a left thoracotomy (28). In another report, 13 of 14 patients who had subclavian endarterectomy for either neurological or arm symptoms remained free of symptoms over an average period of 53 months (11).

In a report of 33 patients with cerebral symptoms related to innominate stenosis, the surgical approach was through a median sternotomy (28). In 28 patients, an endarterectomy was done, while five required a bypass graft from the side of the aorta. All patients were reported to have been relieved of their symptoms.

The treatment of innominate artery stenosis by intraoperative transluminal angioplasty has been reported in one patient with a good result (14). In another report, two patients with subclavian steal syndrome due to left subclavian stenosis were treated with percutaneous transluminal angioplasty with relief of symptoms (15). The procedure was done using systemic heparinization, and then daily aspirin was given.

Vertebral Artery Transposition

The technique for the transposition of the vertebral to the common carotid artery has been outlined by Bohmfalk et al. The method is also described by Galbraith and McDowell and Wylie and Ehrenfeld (6, 10, 29), and has been amplified by Fein (8). The procedure should not be used when there is significant common carotid artery atheroma (6, 8). A few patients have been reported where the vertebral artery is transposed to another site on the subclavian artery (5, 28). An external carotid artery to mid-cervical vertebral artery end-to-side anastomosis and external carotid artery to distal cervical vertebral artery end-to-end anastomosis have also been reported (17).

The operative exposure combines features of the carotid and subclavian artery approaches which have been described. A parasternocleidomastoid incision is made which curves laterally across the insertion of the sternocleidomastoid muscle in the supraclavicular region. The platysma is incised. The sternomastoid fascia is opened and dissection along the border of the muscle exposes the carotid artery as described in Chapter 2, "Carotid Endarterectomy." Two tapes are placed around the proximal common carotid artery, the carotid bifurcation is exposed and tapes are placed around the external and internal carotid arteries.

The medial two-thirds of the sternocleidomastoid muscle is divided near its attachment to the clavicle and sternum (Figs. 5.5 and 5.6). The scalene fat pad is entered and the anterior scalene muscle, phrenic nerve, and internal jugular vein are identified. The phrenic nerve is mobilized and retracted. The anterior scalene muscle is divided near its origin from the first rib bringing into view the subclavian artery and brachial plexus. If the operation is being done on the right side, the vertebral origin is found by dissecting along the superior surface of the subclavian artery. On the left side the dissection is carried behind the subclavian vein along the subclavian artery medially. Care is taken to protect the thoracic duct which inserts on the lateral aspects of the junction between the left internal jugular and subclavian veins. If it is injured, it should be ligated. The vertebral artery is then followed from its origin to the transverse process at C6. An electromagnetic flowmeter may be used to record vertebral artery flow and direction (7, 8). The patient is heparinized and blood pressure elevated as indicated. If the operation is being done for subclavian steal, the brachial blood pressures are checked with temporary occlusion of the vertebral artery.

The proximal vertebral artery is then suture-ligated and a temporary Heifitz aneurysm clip used to occlude the distal portion of the vertebral artery (Fig. 5.8). The common carotid artery is temporarily occluded while monitoring the EEG. An oval arteriotomy is done in the lateral wall of the common carotid artery. A partial occluding clamp may then be placed to isolate the segment with the arteriotomy and reestablish some blood flow, or a temporary shunt can be placed if the need is indicated by EEG changes. Under magnification, an end-to-side anastomosis is done with a running 5-0 or 6-0 Prolene suture. The internal carotid artery is then temporarily occluded, the clamps are removed and blood flow is allowed up the external carotid artery, and then full circulation is reestablished.

In a recent report, this operation was associated with five excellent and one good result in patients with vertebral stenosis and two excellent results with subclavian steal (8). The only neurological complication was a persistent Horner's syndrome in one patient.

Carotid-Subclavian Artery Graft

This procedure is best done through a supraclavicular approach (Fig. 5.4). The subclavian artery is exposed as described. In order to expose the common carotid artery, the posterior border of the sternomastoid muscle is divided and the carotid sheath opened. Tapes are placed on the common carotid artery. An 8-mm knitted Dacron graft is used for the bypass graft. The graft is preclotted and the patient is given 7000 units of intravenous heparin. Blood pressure is elevated and the EEG monitored. Two clamps are placed on the common carotid artery and an arteriotomy is made. The Dacron graft is bevelled and sutured end-to-side to the common carotid artery (Fig. 5.9). Flow is then allowed into the graft which is clamped in its proximal portion and carotid artery blood flow is restored. The distal end of the graft is then brought to the side of the subclavian artery and an end-to-side anastomosis is done. Clamps are removed and flow restored. The incision is then closed in layers. The possibility of a steal from the carotid artery has been raised but not demonstrated. In some cases, symptoms have not been relieved and studies have shown that antegrade flow has not been reestablished in the vertebral artery (6).

In a series of 57 carotid-subclavian bypass operations, there was no mortality or new neurological problems (27). Two patients had to have further surgery because of an infected graft and one had a thoracic duct fistula that closed spontaneously. Follow-up from 3 months to 16 years revealed no new neurological or arm symptoms. In another report of

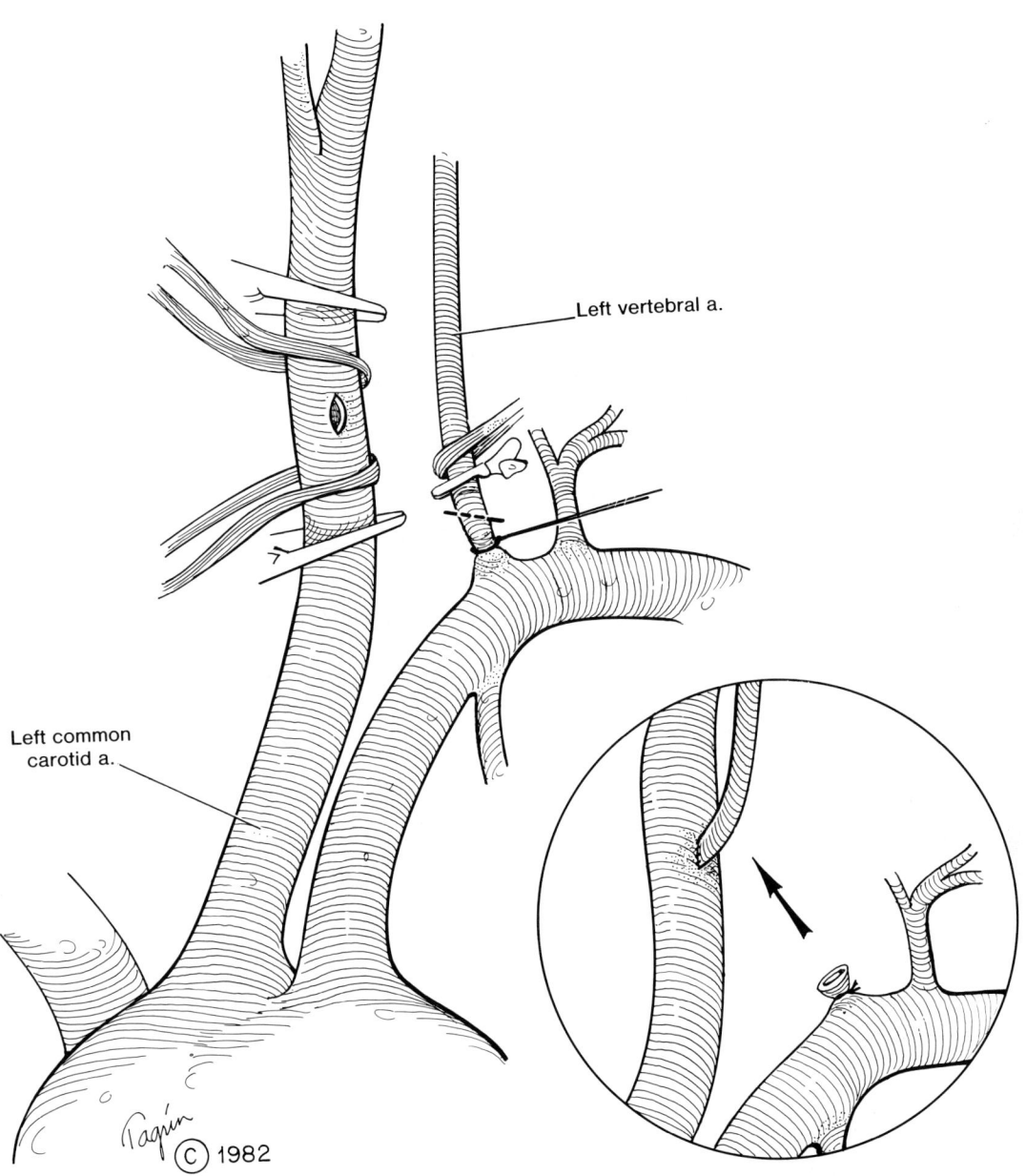

Figure 5.8 Vertebral artery transposition. The illustration shows a left side exposure. See text for details of operation.

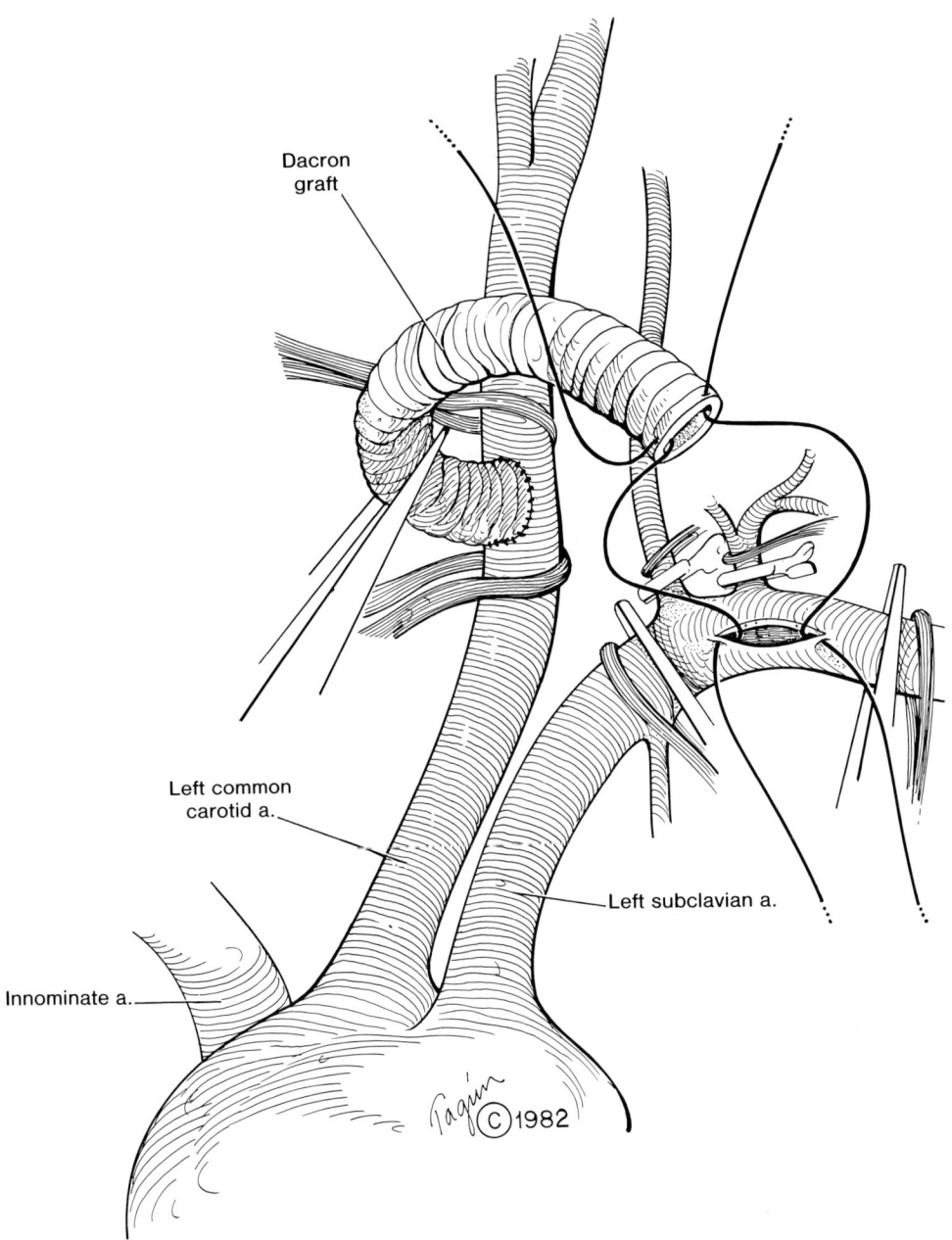

Figure 5.9 Carotid-subclavian artery graft. A Dacron graft is being used. An end-to-side anastomosis has been done on the common carotid artery. The anastomosis to the subclavian artery has been started.

20 patients, a Dacron graft was found to be superior to an autogenous saphenous vein graft (11).

Occipital Artery-Posterior Inferior Cerebellar Artery (Occipital-PICA) Bypass

The technical feasibility and relative safety of occipital to PICA bypass have been established (2, 13, 22–24). Impressive angiographic filling of the vertebrobasilar circulation has been demonstrated following this operation. However, the clinical indications for this procedure are not yet defined.

General anesthesia is required with strict attention to maintenance of normal blood pressure throughout the procedure. The lateral position seems to provide adequate exposure and avoid the danger of cerebral ischemia inherent in the sitting position. A modified hockey-stick incision, rising high in the midline above the inion, provides adequate length for the occipital artery and access to the caudal PICA loop (Fig. 5.10). To avoid scalp edge necrosis, no clamps are placed on the flap edge. The occipital artery, which is invested in dense fascia, must be freed up by meticulous sharp microdissection. A suboccipital craniectomy, with removal of the posterior rim of the foramen magnum and a hemilaminectomy of C1, allows exposure of the cerebellar tonsils. The caudal loop of PICA, which is localized angiographically, is dissected free of arachnoid and supported by a sling of rubber dam stitched to extracranial soft tissues.

The anastomosis is completed much like an STA-MCA bypass graft. The tip of the occipital artery is cleared of adventitia and bevelled. A clip is placed on the caudal loop of PICA, an oval window is excised, and a small stent is inserted. Anastomosis is done with interrupted 10-0 monofilament nylon sutures. The occipital artery is bevelled back toward the PICA origin in order to promote vertebrobasilar perfusion. During closure of the wound, one must be careful to avoid graft compression.

In a report of 22 patients, it was noted that the primary problem with the operative procedure was marginal neurological status prior to operation leading to respiratory complications from preoperative impairment of the cranial nerves (22). Only two patients had a permanent increase in neurological deficits (unilateral hearing loss and homonymous hemianopia). The same general complications noted with STA-MCA grafts were also encountered with this procedure.

Bypass Procedures for Basilar Artery Occlusive Disease

For basilar artery occlusive disease, direct revascularization may offer effective protection against stroke when TIAs continue in spite of anticoagulation. In order to enhance brain blood flow distal to the occlusive process, anastomosis must be to either the superior cerebellar artery or the posterior cerebral artery.

Superficial temporal to proximal superior cerebellar artery anastomosis has been reported (3, 25). Sundt et al. have been concerned about the volume of flow achieved in this anastomosis (25). For occlusive disease in the proximal posterior cerebral or distal basilar artery, they have used a side-to-side anastomosis of the posterior cerebral and superior cerebellar arteries.

The large caliber of the posterior cerebral artery in many patients makes this an attractive vessel for anastomosis. Use of a saphenous vein graft between the external carotid and proximal posterior cerebral artery has been done (26). For this procedure, the patient is positioned supine with the head turned level to the floor. A saphenous vein graft is harvested in the usual fashion. At the same time, the carotid bifurcation is exposed and a low temporal craniotomy is performed. The vein graft should be reversed to eliminate valvular obstruction. The saphenous vein is anastomosed to either the external carotid artery or end-to-side to the common carotid artery using a Satinsky clamp to partially occlude the artery. After appropriate tunneling, the saphenous vein segment is introduced without kinking, and routed from the carotid location to the posterior cerebral artery at the level of the tentorium. Significant temporal retraction may be required for this maneuver. Anastomosis of the saphenous vein in end-to-side fashion to the posterior cerebral artery is performed microsurgically after appropriate trimming of the vessel. The precise role and indications for this procedure have yet to be established.

Removal of Foreign Body from Vertebral Artery

One patient was seen because the end of a guide wire, used during angiography, had broken off and lodged in the vertebral artery at the C2–3 level just before the first turn in the artery (Fig. 5.11). Angiogram showed the artery to be open. The patient had syncopal attacks.

An incision was made paralleling the mid-portion of the sternocleidomastoid muscle. The posterior border of the sternocleidomastoid muscle was retracted medially and the nerve roots of the upper brachial plexus identified. The paravertebral muscles were separated from the anterior aspect of the transverse processes of C3 and C4, the level having been identified by x-ray. The anterior portions of the transverse processes of C3 and a portion of C4 were removed. Using the air drill with a diamond burr, bone was also removed from the medial and lateral aspects of the vertebral artery canal. Bleeding from epidural veins was controlled with bipolar coagulation. Tapes were placed around the vertebral artery at the superior and inferior margins of the exposure. Blood pressure was maintained above 150 mmHg. A small arteriotomy was made in the artery and the foreign body removed. A single suture closed the opening. The postoperative course was uncomplicated.

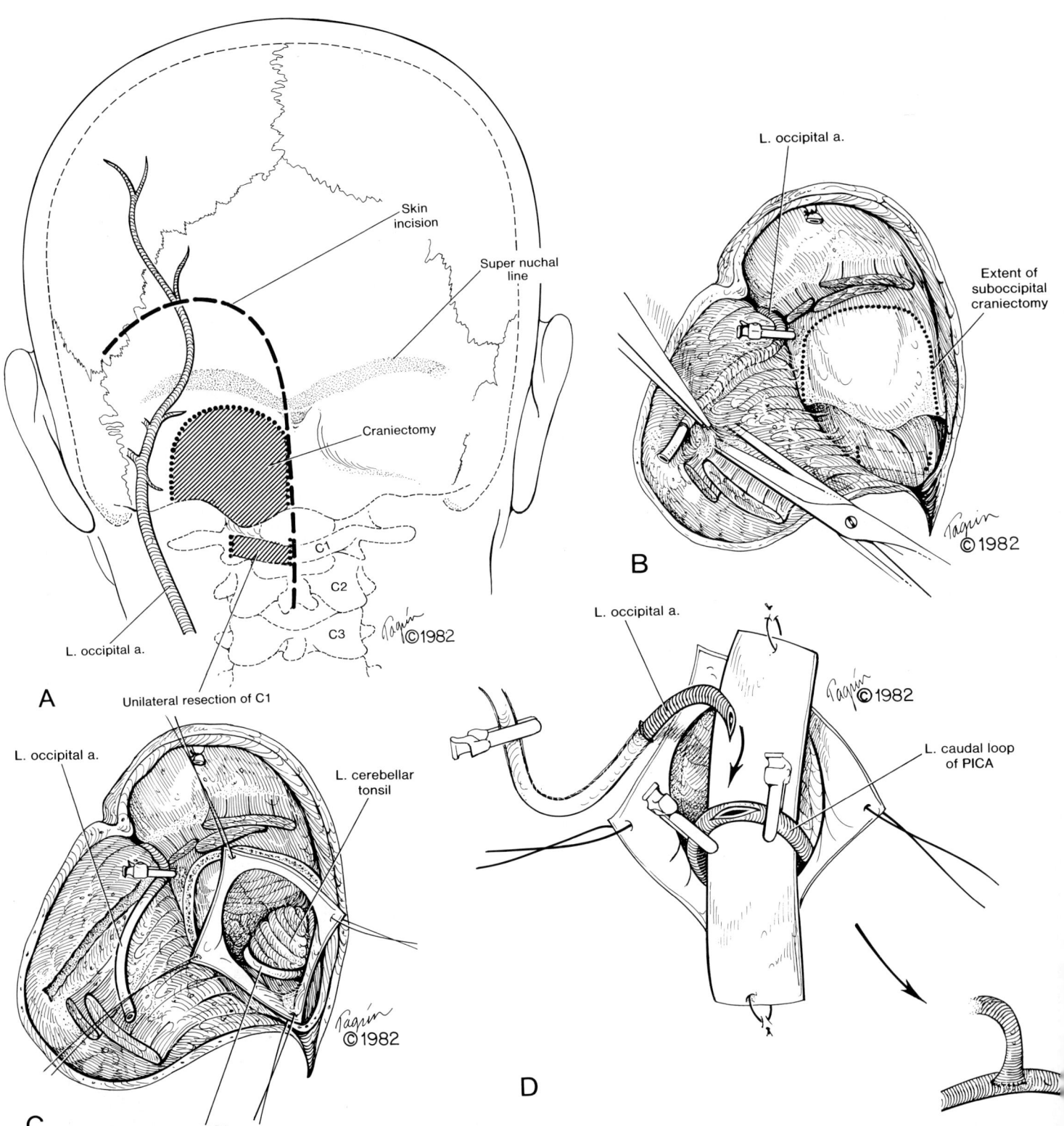

Figure 5.10 Occipital artery-PICA bypass. *A*, initial exposure. Hockey stick incision is carried well above the superior nuchal line to assure adequate length for the occipital artery segment. The bony removal includes the posterior rim of foramen magnum and hemilaminectomy of C1. *B*, preparation of occipital artery. The vessel is followed from the skin edge proximally through the muscle layers to the mastoid. Relatively little adventitia remains attached to the vessel. *C*, exposure of PICA. After craniectomy and C1 hemilaminectomy, the dura is opened in a cruciate fashion to expose the cerebellar tonsil and caudal loop of PICA. The vessel may be followed laterally to the area of maximum diameter. *D*, Anastomosis. PICA is gently lifted off the tonsil with a rubber dam which is sutured to dura. The occipital artery is freed of adventitia distally and a fish-mouthed bevelled ostium is prepared. After clipping the PICA with Kleinert-Kees clips, an arteriotomy is performed. End-to-side anastomosis is carried out with interrupted 10-0 monofilament nylon sutures.

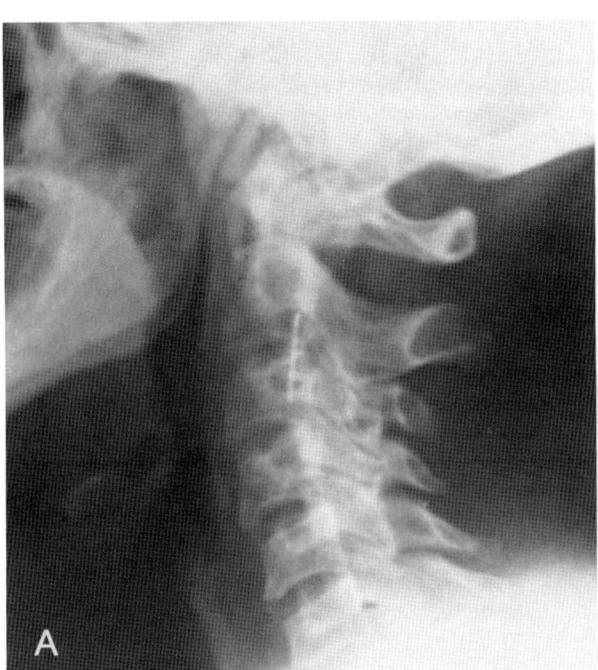
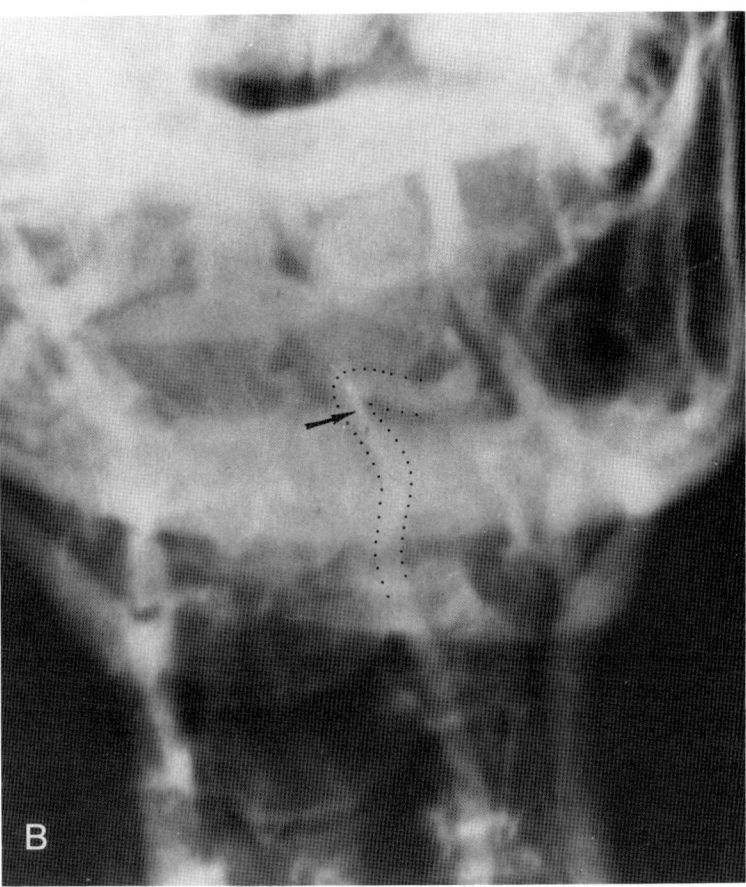

Figure 5.11 Foreign body in vertebral artery. A, lateral x-ray of neck showing the end of a guide wire at C2–3. B, A–P arch angiogram showing the wire (*arrow*) to be lodged at the first turn in the vertebral artery (*outlined with dots*).

REFERENCES

1. Allen GJ, Cohen RJ, Preziosi TJ: Microsurgical endarterectomy of the intracranial vertebral artery for vertebrobasilar transient ischemic attacks. Neurosurgery 8:56–59, 1981.
2. Ausman JI, Lee MC, Klassen AC, Seljeskog EL, Chou SN: Stroke: What's new? Cerebral revascularization. Minn Med 59:223–227, 1976.
3. Ausman JI, Dias FG, de los Reyes RA, Pak H, Patel S, Boulos R: Superficial temporal to proximal superior cerebellar artery anastomosis for basilar artery stenosis. Neurosurgery 9:56–59, 1981.
4. Bakay L, Leslie EV: Surgical treatment of vertebral artery insufficiency caused by cervical spondylosis. J Neurosurg 23:596–602, 1965.
5. Bergnen R̂, Bauer RB: Vertebral artery reconstruction. A successful technique in selected patients. Ann Surg 193:441–447, 1981.
6. Bohmfalk GL, Story JL, Brown WE Jr, Marlin AE: Subclavian steal syndrome. Part 1. Proximal vertebral to common carotid artery transposition in three patients and historical review. J Neurosurg 51:628–640, 1979.
7. Bohmfalk GL, Story JL, Brown WE Jr, Marlin AE: Subclavian steal syndrome. Part 2. Intraoperative vertebral artery blood flow measurement. J Neurosurg 51:641–643, 1979.
8. Fein JM: Vertebral artery transposition for vertebral basilar insufficiency. Presented at the 1981 meeting of the American Association of Neurological Surgeons.
9. Fisher CM: Occlusion of the vertebral arteries. Arch Neurol 22:13–19, 1970.
10. Galbraith JG, McDowell HA Jr: Stroke and occlusive cerebrovascular disease. Review and surgical results in 265 cases. J Med Assoc Ala 38:1107–1111, 1969.
11. Gerety RL, Andrus CH, May AG, Rob CG, Green R, DeWesse JA: Surgical treatment of occlusive subclavian artery disease. Circulation 64:228–230, 1981.
12. Imparato A, Riles T, Kim GE, Mintzer R: Vertebral artery reconstruction. Stroke 12:125, 1981.
13. Khodadad G, Singh RS, Olinger CP: Possible prevention of brain stem stroke by microvascular anastomosis in the vertebrobasilar system. Stroke 8:316–321, 1977.
14. Lowman BG, Queral LA, Holbrook WA, Estes JT, Bayly B: The treatment of innominate artery stenosis by intraoperative transluminal angioplasty. Surgery 89:565–568, 1981.
15. Moore T, Russell MT, Parent A, Parker L, Smith R: Nonsurgical treatment of "subclavian steal syndrome" with percutaneous transluminal angioplasty. Neurosurgery 9:466, 1981.
16. Motarjeme A, Keifer JW, Zuska AJ: Percutaneous transluminal angioplasty of the vertebral arteries. Radiology 139:715–717, 1981.
17. Pritz MB, Chandler WF, Kindt GW: Vertebral artery disease: Radiological evaluation, medical management and microsurgical treatment. Neurosurgery 9:524–530, 1981.
18. Robertson JT: Neck manipulation as a cause of stroke. Stroke 1:1, 1981.
19. Roon AJ, Ehrenfeld WK, Cooke PB, Wylie EJ: Vertebral artery

reconstruction. Am J Surg 138:29–36, 1979.
20. Schellhas KP, Latchaw RE, Wendling LR, Gold LHA: Vertebrobasilar injuries following cervical manipulation. JAMA 244:1450–1453, 1980.
21. Sherman DG, Hart RG, Easton JD: Abrupt change in head position and cerebral infarction. Stroke 12:2–6, 1981.
22. Sundt TM Jr, Piepgras DG: By-pass surgery for vertebral artery occlusive disease: Technique and complications. Clin Neurosurg 26:346–352, 1979.
23. Sundt TM Jr, Piepgras DG: Occipital to posterior inferior cerebellar artery By-pass surgery. J Neurosurg 48:916–928, 1978.
24. Sundt TM Jr, Whisnant JP, Piepgras DG, Campbell JK, Holman CB: Intracranial bypass grafts for vertebral-basilar ischemia. Mayo Clin Proc 53:12–18, 1978.
25. Sundt TM Jr, Campbell JK, Houser OW: Transposition and anastomosis between the posterior cerebral and superior cerebellar arteries. J Neurosurg 55:967–970, 1981.
26. Sundt TM Jr, Houser OW, Piepgras DG: Interposition saphenous vein grafts between the external carotid and proximal posterior cerebral artery for advanced occlusive disease and large aneurysms. J Neurosurg (to be published).
27. Thompson BW, Read RC, Campbell GS: Operative correction of obstructed subclavian or innominate arteries. South Med J 71:1366–1369, 1978.
28. Wylie EJ, Effeney DJ: Surgery of the aortic arch branches and vertebral arteries. Surg Clin N Am 59:669–680, 1979.
29. Wylie EJ, Ehrenfeld WK: *Extracranial Occlusive Cerebrovascular Disease: Diagnosis and Management.* Philadelphia, WB Saunders, 1970.

Chapter 6 FIBROMUSCULAR DYSPLASIA OF THE INTERNAL CAROTID ARTERY

PATHOGENESIS

Fibromuscular dysplasia (FMD) was first described in the renal artery. In the head and neck, the most common area of involvement is one or both distal extracranial internal carotid arteries. Other arteries that can be affected include the common carotid, external carotid, vertebral, and large intracranial arteries. The etiology is unknown. Several reports have suggested the possibility of a hormonal influence because of a marked female preponderance, but this has not been proven.

Three types of pathological change have been described (3). The most common change primarily involves the media. There are multiple small saccular dilations due to areas of destruction and fragmentation of the media alternating with rings of fibrous and muscular hyperplasia. This type predominately affects females. The second type, occurring in a small percentage of cases, is associated with an increase in the fibrous elements of the intima producing concentric narrowing of the lumen. This type affects both sexes. The third type of pathological finding is a periadventitial fibroplasia which is quite rare.

CLINICAL PRESENTATION

The diagnosis of FMD is not usually made until angiography is done. In two reported series, the incidence of FMD was 0.6% in 13,955 and 0.53% in 6,100 cerebral angiograms (3, 10). The symptoms that led to angiography in several series of patients found to have FMD are summarized in Table 6.1. It is apparent that many of these patients had symptoms related to problems other than FMD. Several of the patients with TIAs and infarction had significant atherosclerosis which probably accounted for the symptoms. In the majority of patients, FMD is an incidental finding. Probably only a small number of these patients had focal cerebral ischemia due to reduced flow or emboli related to FMD in the internal carotid artery. On rare occasion, an acute stroke may be associated with development of a thrombus in an area of FMD in the internal carotid artery (1). A few patients will have a bruit that is disturbing enough to warrent angiography. Other symptoms that may relate to FMD include headache, facial pain, dizziness, tinnitus, seizure, or syncope (10, 11, 14).

The age at the time of diagnosis and sex incidence are summarized from nine reports in Table 6.2. The vast majority of patients were women with symptoms occurring in the fourth, fifth, and sixth decades.

The natural history of the disease has not been fully defined, but most patients seem to have a benign course (3, 14). The results in Table 6.3 suggest that FMD is often an incidental finding with a low incidence of subsequent cerebral ischemia (3). In fact, two of the three patients had ischemic events in the territory of an artery other than the one involved with FMD. Seven of the 13 patients with focal cerebral ischemia were treated. Five had atherosclerosis that may have been the cause of the symptoms.

In another series of 17 patients, one was operated but 16 were followed for 1–9 years (average, 3.8) (13). Fourteen showed no evidence of progression of FMD, while two patients with significant atherosclerotic disease had strokes. Four had received aspirin, three anticoagulants, and the others no specific therapy.

ANGIOGRAPHY

The typical angiographic finding is an area of alternating zones of widening and narrowing of the arterial lumen (Fig. 6.1, A and B). This has been described as a "string of beads" appearance. It was seen in 80% of the angiograms in two series of 25 patients (9, 12) and in 31 of 32 patients in another series (10). The next most common finding is a tubular stenosis. Other angiographic findings include a diverticulum, a web at the carotid bifurcation, and dissection (9, 10, 12, 15). In the patient with the typical angiographic findings, the area of involvement begins at the level of the first to third cervical vertebrae and extends distally for one or more centimeters (9, 10, 11). Rarely is the first 2.0–3.0 cm of the internal carotid artery involved. Intracranial involvement is also rare. None was reported in a series of 82 patients (3), four in a series of 25 patients (9), and in one of 17 patients the intracavernous portion of the internal carotid was involved (14). In one series, the incidence of bilateral internal carotid involvement was 37% (3), 86% in another series (10), and 44% in the summary of the 109 cases reported up to 1974 (6).

FMD has been associated with spontaneous dissection, intracranial aneurysm, carotid cavernous fistula, embolism, and reduced flow in the artery distal to the pathology (3). In the 109 cases reported up to

Table 6.1
Symptoms that Led to Angiography in Patients Found to Have FMD

Reference	No. of Patients	Focal TIA	Ischemia or Infarction	SAH	Signs of Mass Lesion	Asymptomatic Bruit Alone	Nonfocal Neurological Symptoms	Other
3	79	6	7	10	29	8	3	16
10	32	9	9	5	0	2	4	3
14	17	7	2	0	0	0	8	0
9	25	8	6	9	0	0	2	0
11	15	1	2	3	1	3	4	1

Table 6.2
Age and Sex Distribution from Reports of Patients with FMD

Reference	No. of Patients	Sex		Age Range (yr)
		M	F	
3	82	8	74	18–76 (mean, 58)
14	17	0	17	34–74 (mean, 58)
9	25	5	20	4–71 (avg., 45)
10	32	0	32	34–70 (avg., 57)
12	25	6	19	30–70 (avg., 58)
11	15	0	15	21–79 (avg., 51)
5	20	2	18	30–79 (avg., 52)
2	18	0	18	40–83 (mean, 60)
4	86	3	83	27–83 (mean, 58)

Table 6.3
Subsequent Cerebral Ischemic Events in Patients with FMD[a]

Reason for Angiogram	No. of Patients with FMD	Average Follow-up (mo)	Subsequent Cerebral Ischemic Events
Intracranial mass lesion	29	50	3
Aneurysm	10	52	0
Other non-ischemic disorders	27	80	0
Focal cerebral ischemia	13	75	0

[a] From Corrin et al. (3).

1974, 23 had aneurysms, and a high incidence of associated aneurysm has also been a finding in other series (Table 6.1) (6). Associated atherosclerosis has been seen in several patients.

A small number of patients have had repeat angiograms. In one report, two of six patients showed progression of the lesion (10). In one of these patients, recurrent embolic infarctions led to repeat angiography 2 years later which showed enlargement of the septum at the carotid bifurcation with an associated thrombus. Recurrent symptoms stopped after the septum was excised. In the second patient, angiography was done 4 years later for evaluation of diffuse headache and revealed progression of bilateral FMD. Dilatation resulted in relief of the headaches. In the other four patients, angiograms 1.5–7 years after the initial study showed no change. Other reports described 12 patients with follow-up angiography ranging from 2 months to 6 years (10, 14). Progression of the lesion was seen in three.

TREATMENT

Since FMD is often an incidental angiographic finding and there is a low incidence of subsequent cerebral ischemia events, many patients do not require any treatment. When there are neurological symptoms, medical therapy with anticoagulation or antiplatelet drugs is recommended. In the rare case where this treatment is not effective or there is evidence of a significant hemodynamic or progressive lesion, surgery may be indicated.

The preferred surgical treatment for most cases has been the use of graduated internal dilation (2, 11, 12, 15). The exposure for this operation is the same as that utilized for a carotid endarterectomy. The principal of treatment is to dilate the stenotic segment (12). Common duct dilators (Bakes) are used. After the exposure is completed, appropriate tapes are placed and the patient is heparinized. The common and external carotid arteries are clamped and the internal carotid artery is controlled with a tourniquet. A small transverse arteriotomy is made in the distal common carotid artery. The dilators are passed into the internal carotid artery beginning with 3.0 mm or smaller and progressing to 5.0 mm in 0.5-mm increments. The wall of the internal carotid artery may be thin, so care is taken as the dilator encounters resistance at the intraluminal septae. As the dilator is passed through the septum, a distinct give is felt. This procedure is continued until the base of the skull is reached. When the dilatation is complete, the arteriotomy is closed with a continuous 5-0 Prolene suture. Heparin is not reversed, and antiplatelet therapy is started in the immediate postoperative period.

This procedure has been associated with a very low risk. In a series of 19 patients treated by dilatation and followed for 2–12 years (mean, 7.3 years), there was no operative morbidity or mortality and only two late recurrences of mild symptoms (12). In another report of 66 patients who had 97 arteries dilated, there were two postoperative strokes, but both recovered within a month (4). Other reports also record good results with dilatation (2, 5, 10, 11).

Patients with symptomatic FMD have done well following excision of a septum, resection of the area

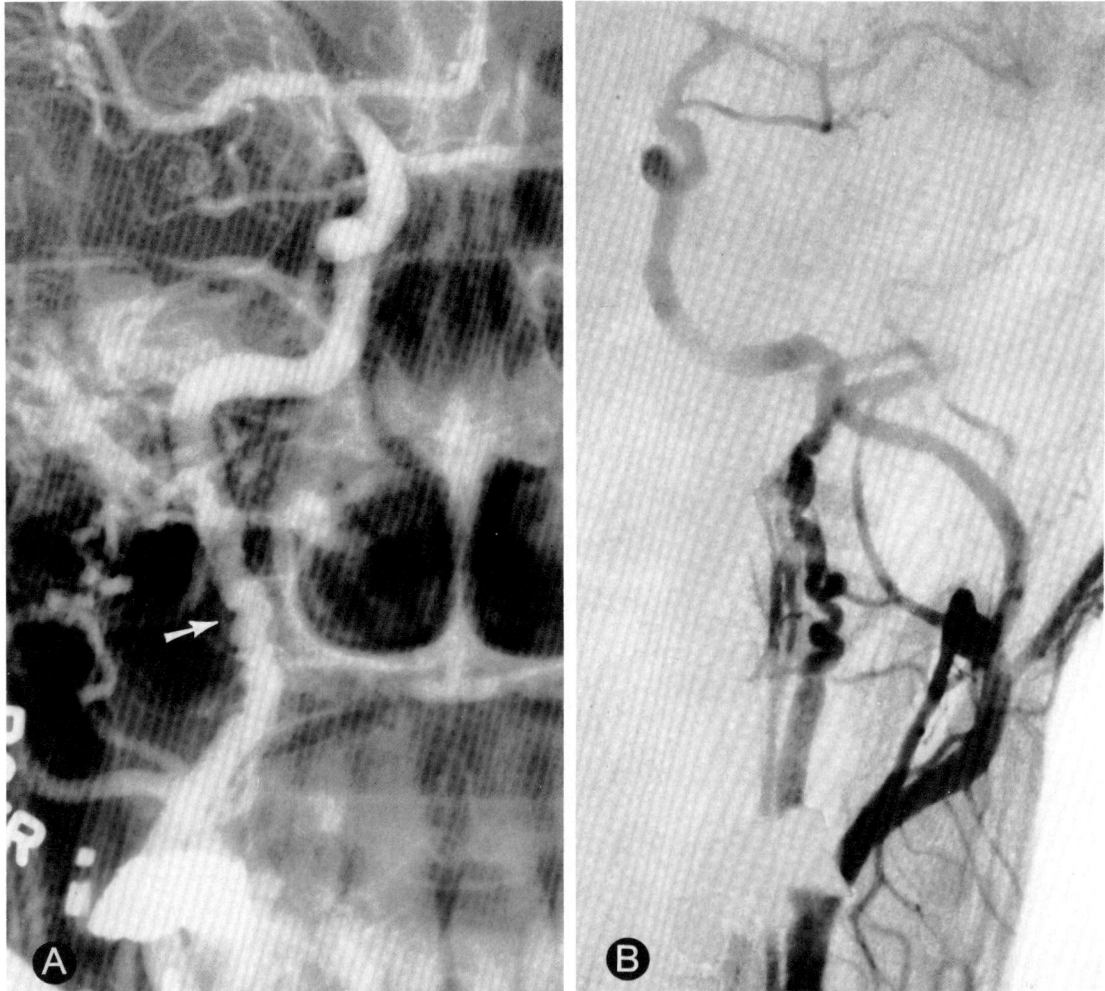

Figure 6.1 Typical angiographic appearances of fibromuscular dysplasia in the distal aspect of the extracranial internal carotid artery. A, note the "corregated" or "string of beads" appearance (arrow). B, subtraction study in another patient showing tortuosity, as well as segmental constrictions.

of pathology, endarterectomy for atherosclerosis, and combined dilatation and endarterectomy (4, 5, 10). An occasional patient has been treated with an extracranial to intracranial bypass graft (3, 13, 14). In one patient a saphenous vein graft was placed from the carotid bifurcation to the distal extracranial internal carotid artery (16). When a web is present at the carotid bifurcation, endarterectomy is an effective treatment (15).

The dilatation of FMD of the internal carotid artery by percutaneous transluminal angioplasty using a balloon dilating catheter has been described in three patients (8). Systemic heparin was not used but the patients were placed on aspirin. A catheter has also been placed in the common carotid artery at operation and the artery dilated under fluoroscopic control (7). The authors believe this is safer than the percutaneous method should an intimal flap develop or arterial perforation occur. Further experience will be needed to establish the role of this method of treatment.

REFERENCES

1. Balaji MR, DeWeese JA: Fibromuscular dysplasia of the internal carotid artery: Its occurence with acute stroke and its surgical reversal. Arch Surg 115:984–986, 1980.
2. Collins GJ, Rich NM, Clagett GP, Spebar MJ, Salander JM: Fibromuscular dysplasia of the internal carotid arteries. Ann Surg 194:89–96, 1981.
3. Corrin LS, Sandok BA, Houser OW: Cerebral ischemic events in patients with carotid artery fibromuscular dysplasia. Arch Neurol 38:616–618, 1981.
4. Effeney DJ, Ehrenfield WK, Stoney RJ, Wylie EJ: Why operate on carotid fibromuscular dysplasia? Arch Surg 115:1261–1267, 1980.
5. Ehrenfeld WK, Wylie EJ: Fibromuscular dysplasia of the internal carotid artery. Arch Surg 109:676–681, 1974.
6. Frens DB, Petajan JH, Auderson R, Deblanc HJ: Fibromuscular dysplasia of the posterior cerebral artery; Report of a case and review of the literature. Stroke 5:161–166, 1974.
7. Garrido E, Montoya J: Transluminal dilatation of internal

carotid artery in fibromuscular dysplasia. A preliminary report. Surg Neurol 16:469-471, 1981.
8. Hasso AN, Bird CR, Zinke DE, Thompson JR: Fibromuscular dysplasia of the internal carotid artery. Percutaneous transluminal angioplasty. Am J Neurorad 2:175-180, 1981.
9. Osborn AG, Anderson RE: Angiographic spectrum of cervical and intracranial fibromuscular dysplasia. Stroke 8:617-626, 1977.
10. So EL, Toole JF, Dalal P, Moody DM: Cephalic fibromuscular dysplasia in 32 patients. Arch Neurol 38:619-622, 1981.
11. Stanley JC, Fry WJ, Seeger JF, Hoffman GL, Gabrielsen TO: Extracranial internal carotid and vertebral artery fibrodysplasia. Arch Surg 109:215-222, 1974.
12. Starr DS, Lawrie GM, Morris GC Jr: Fibromsucular disease of carotid arteries: Long term results of graduated internal dilatation. Stroke 12:196-199, 1981.
13. Sundt TM Jr, Siekert RG, Piepgras DG, Sharbough FW, Houser OW: Bypass surgery for vascular disease of the carotid system. Mayo Clin Proc 51:677-692, 1976.
14. Wells RP, Smith RR: Fibromuscular dysplasia of the internal carotid artery. A long term follow-up. Neurosurgery (in press).
15. Wirth FP, Miller WA, Russell AP: Atypical fibromuscular hyperplasia. J Neurosurg 54:685-689, 1981.
16. Young PH, Smith KR Jr, Crafts DC, Barner HB: Traumatic occlusion in fibromuscular dysplasia of the carotid artery. Surg Neurol 16:432-437, 1981.

Chapter 7 DISSECTION OF INTERNAL CAROTID, VERTEBRAL, AND INTRACRANIAL ARTERIES

Dissection in the wall of the carotid, vertebral, or intracranial artery causing narrowing or occlusion of the arterial lumen or acting as a source of emboli is an established cause of cerebral ischemia (1–40). The dissection develops when blood penetrates an intimal defect and strips the intima from the media. The etiology of the dissection is either spontaneous or traumatic. The term spontaneous indicates that no obvious precipitating injury was recognized, although pathology may be found in the arterial wall in some cases. Traumatic causes include non-penetrating injury to the head and neck, direct injury to the vessel, and angiography.

SPONTANEOUS DISSECTION: INTERNAL CAROTID ARTERY

Pathogenesis

Dissection of the internal carotid artery begins at two sites of predilection: just distal to the origin and between C2 and the base of the skull. The possible relationship of congenital defects in the wall of the artery, of cystic medial necrosis, and of fibromuscular hyperplasia to the cause of the dissection has been discussed (13, 16, 32).

In seven of the first 11 reported cases, the involved internal carotid artery as well as the opposite carotid and aorta were said to show cystic medial necrosis (13). However, this was not found in the detailed pathological study of a specimen we removed at surgery (30). In that case, the wall of the artery showed no underlying intrinsic disease, but the muscle and elastic tissue had an irregular disorganized arrangement rather than the usual laminar pattern. In another report, examination of four arteries removed at operation showed dissection occurring in the outer layers of the media, decrease in the smooth muscle cells and elastic tissue, and degeneration and fragmentation of the internal elastic membrane (12). Fibromuscular dysplasia has been associated with six reported cases of dissection (9, 12, 13, 32).

In spontaneous dissection, even when obvious external trauma is not a factor, it is possible that other factors relate to the onset. In three cases, symptoms began during a period of heavy coughing (13). Minor falls may be significant as noted in the report of a patient who, while skiing, developed acute dissection of both internal carotid arteries, of the right vertebral artery at the level of the second vertebra, and of the left vertebral artery at the sixth cervical vertebra (32). The relationship of head rotation to injury of the internal carotid artery is discussed in the section on traumatic dissections.

It is likely that intracranial emboli from the area of the carotid dissection may be a primary cause of symptoms in many cases. This has been demonstrated in cases of both spontaneous and traumatic dissection (3, 14, 32).

Clinical Manifestations

The average age of patients with dissection is the mid 40's, considerably younger than patients with stroke due to atherosclerosis (13, 16, 26). Approximately two-thirds of the patients are male. Hypertension is present in only a small number.

A history of headache and unilateral head or facial pain followed by TIAs or neurological deficit is highly suggestive of the diagnosis, and the findings of oculo-sympathetic palsy (miosis and ptosis) adds further support to this impression (11, 13, 16, 26). The period of evolution of symptoms leading to the diagnosis is relatively short, ranging from a few hours to 10 days (13, 28).

In a report of 16 patients where the diagnosis of

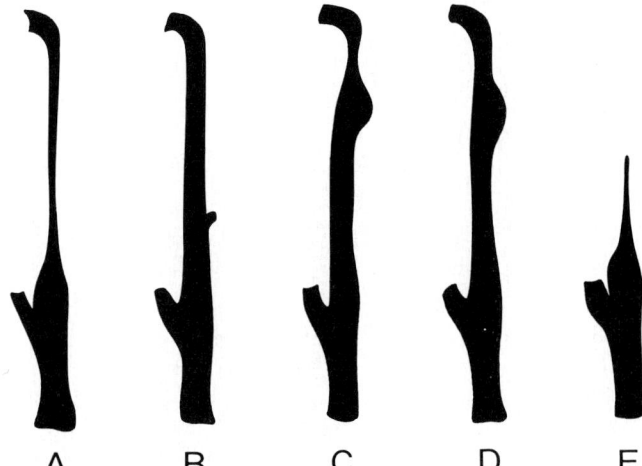

Figure 7.1 Angiographic profiles seen with internal carotid dissection. *A*, characteristic "string sign." The extracranial internal carotid artery is narrowed from above the bifurcation to the base of the skull. *B*, proximal internal carotid pouch. This may be evidence of a previous dissection that has healed. *C*, distal extracranial internal carotid pouch with narrowing of the adjacent lumen—another characteristic finding. *D*, distal extracranial pouch alone. This may occur acutely but can also remain indefinitely after the dissection heals. *E*, complete occlusion. There is no characteristic feature.

carotid dissection was definite or highly likely, 11 had transient ischemic attacks, 10 headache or facial pain, and eight noted a subjective bruit (13). At the time of the initial examination, only three of the 16 patients were hemiplegic or aphasic; four had a slight hemiparesis or monoparesis; six had a normal neurological examination except for oculo-sympathetic palsy; and three had an entirely normal examination. Subsequently, five patients were reported who had angiographic changes suggestive of internal carotid dissection, in whom the initial clinical manifestations were unilateral head and face pain associated with ipsilateral oculo-sympathetic paresis (28). The pain was described as constant and non-throbbing, but fluctuating in intensity. In some patients there was scalp tenderness.

Unilateral head pain is presumably due to the direct effect of the arterial dissection on pain receptors within the wall of the artery (28). Oculo-sympathetic palsy is due to involvement of sympathetic fibers that accompany the internal carotid artery.

In the early reports of spontaneous dissection, a

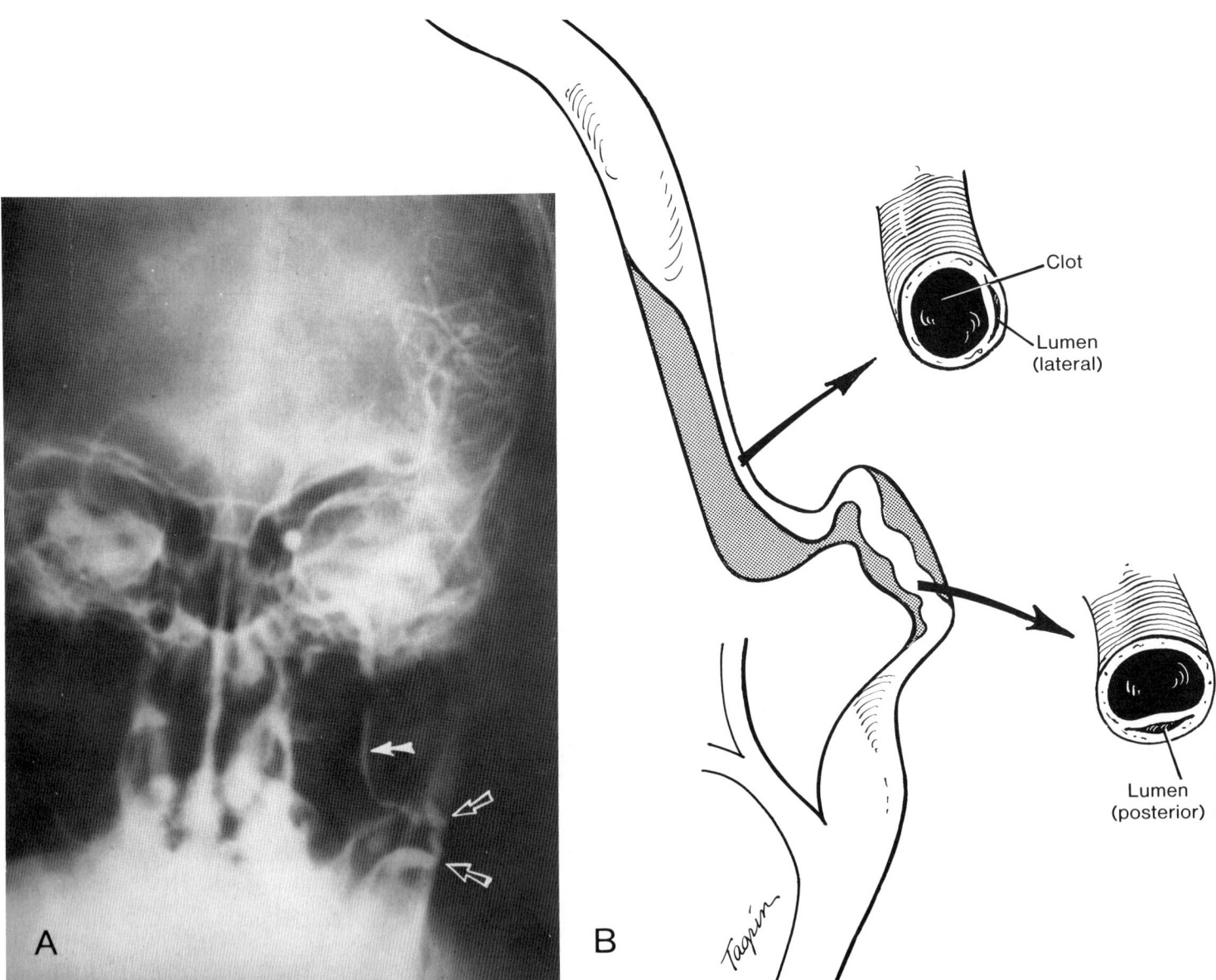

Figure 7.2 Typical angiographic finding (string sign), pathology, and surgical treatment. This 41-year-old man was well until 2 days before admission when he suddenly felt weak and noted transient blurring of vision in the left eye. He was well until the next day when he developed a right hemiparesis which improved. On the morning of admission, he awakened with a right hemiplegia and aphasia. *A*, this AP angiogram led to the original designation of the "string sign" (30). The long area of narrowing in the internal carotid artery (*solid arrow*) is highly suggestive of the diagnosis. In this patient there was also an abnormally narrowed and kinked segment in the proximal internal carotid artery (*open arrows*). *B*, the nature of the pathology found at operation is shown. The internal carotid artery was dilated and had a bluish color throughout its length.

high incidence of severe neurological deficits was noted (30). However, with increased recognition of the problem, it has been found that many cases will have a benign clinical course (13, 14). Several patients in the series reported by Fisher et al. made a good recovery and had no recurrent symptoms, even though no specific therapy was given (13). In another report of five patients where the only neurological finding was an oculo-sympathetic palsy, one had a major stroke and the other four remained well without specific treatment (28). In a report of six patients who had follow-up angiograms, the carotid artery had become nearly normal in five and one showed a complete occlusion. Resolution of the problem on follow-up angiography has also been confirmed by others (14, 26). However, development of complete occlusion may be associated with a serious neurological deficit (3).

Angiographic Findings

The diagnosis is usually established by angiography except where complete occlusion has occurred.

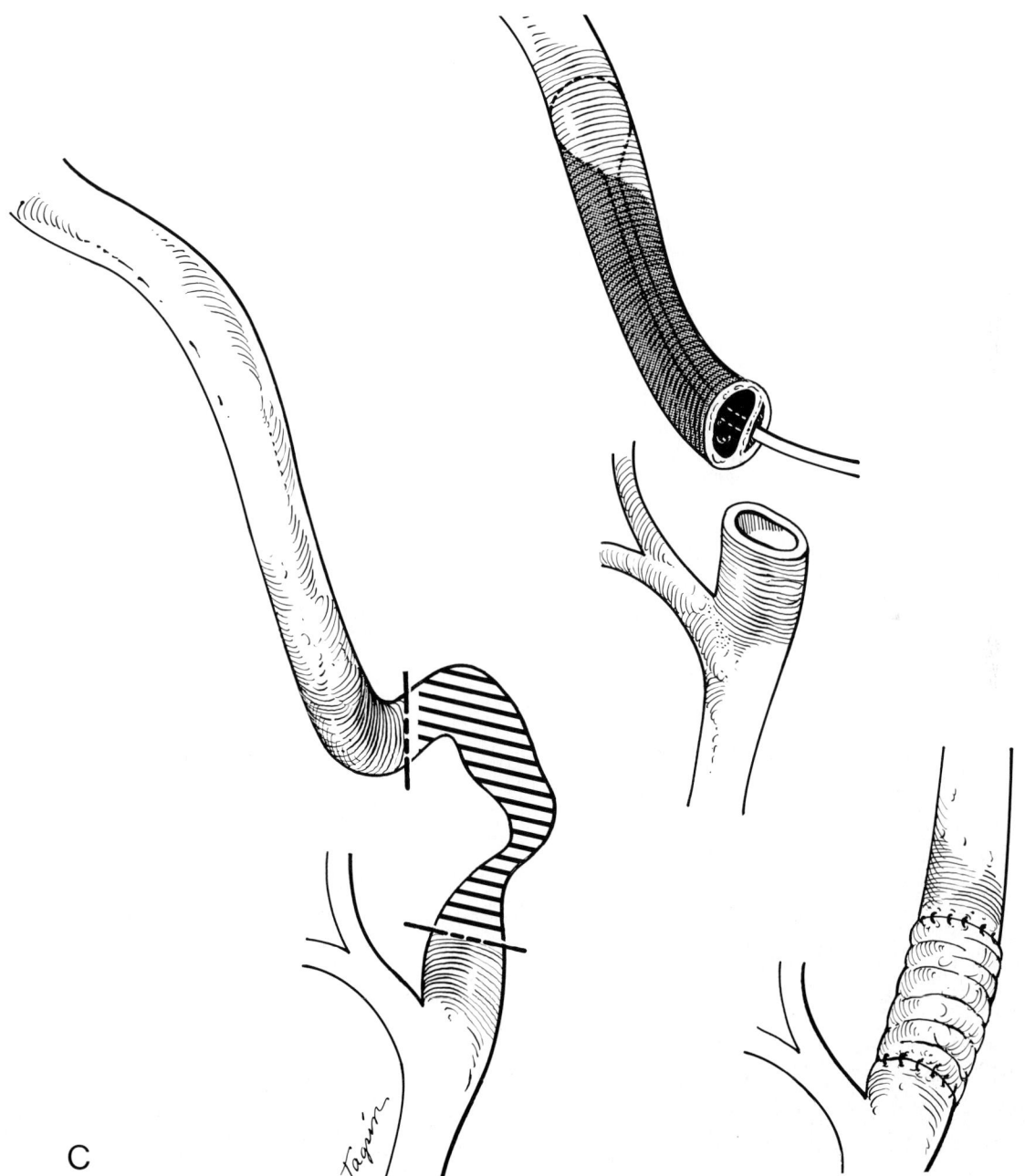

Figure 7.2 *C*, diagram of operative procedure performed. The proximal part of the dissection and the narrowed kinked segment were resected. A Fogarty catheter was inserted, inflated, and retracted, removing the dissection clot and elevated intima. A Dacron graft was sewn into place. (From Ojemann RG, Fisher CM, Rich JC: Spontaneous dissecting aneurysm of the internal carotid artery. Stroke 3:434–440, 1972, by permission of the American Heart Association, Inc.)

The angiographic profiles seen with carotid dissection are illustrated in Figure 7.1. Characteristic findings include: 1) the "string sign," a long, irregular narrowing beginning above the carotid bifurcation in the neck and extending throughout much of the extracranial course of the internal carotid artery (Figs. 7.2A and 7.3, A and B); 2) a distal internal carotid pouch occurring between C2 and the base of the skull (Fig. 7.4, A and B); 3) a proximal internal carotid pouch (1, 12, 13, 15, 30). Long areas of dissections may be combined with short dissection pouches (Fig. 7.5 A to D). Occasionally, a double lumen has been reported but we have not seen this. When a complete occlusion occurs there is no characteristic feature.

In our report of a single case of spontaneous carotid dissection, it was noted that the long stenotic segment of the cervical internal carotid artery (the "string sign") might be a reliable indication of carotid dissection (Fig. 7.1A) (30). Subsequently, 22 cases of dissection of the cervico-cerebral arteries were reported, and in 16 patients, angiography demonstrated a long narrow column of contrast material (13). In another report, 11 of 19 patients showed this finding (12). The "string sign" is the result of the dissecting hemorrhage compressing the natural lumen. It differs markedly from the short stenotic lesion of atherosclerosis and rarely occurs with other types of occlusive cerebrovascular disease such as atheroma, fibromuscular dyspasia, arteritis, moyamoya disease, and vasospasm (13). These long dissections usually extend to the base of the skull without entering the petrous canal, but there are exceptions (Fig. 7.3). In one case, the dissection involved only the petrous portion of the artery (15).

Another distinctive angiographic finding in carotid dissection is a localized aneurysmal sac or out-pouching on the cervical portion of the internal carotid artery between C2 and the base of the skull (Fig. 7.2, A and B). The case reported by Hardin et al. (18) was proved at surgery and that of Bostrom and Liliequest (4) at autopsy. Similar pouches in the distal internal carotid artery have been described frequently in trau-

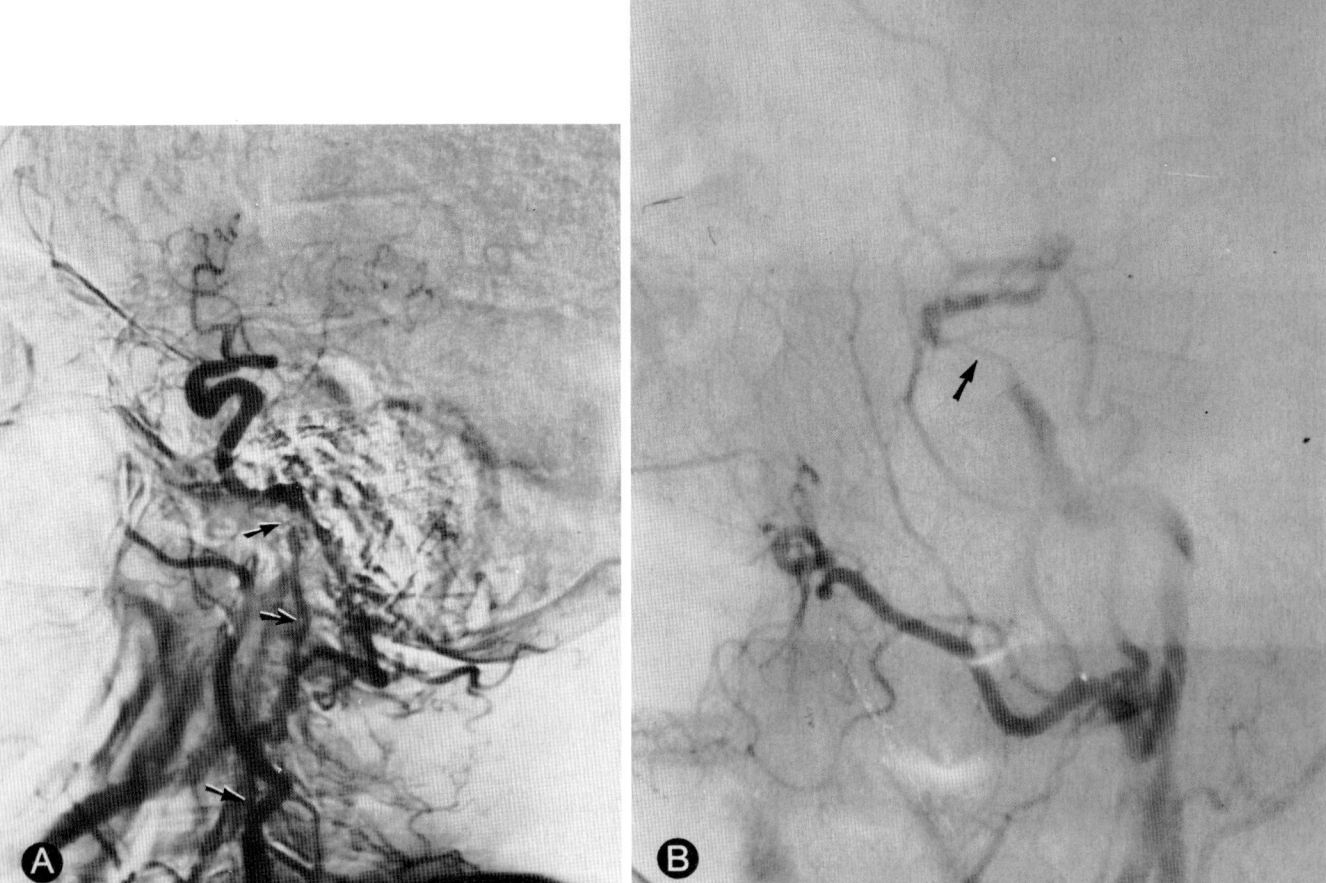

Figure 7.3 Other examples of the "string sign." A, the internal carotid artery (*arrows*) is narrowed from its origin to the base of the skull where it abruptly widens to a normal lumen. B, localized "string sign" in the petrous portion of the internal carotid artery (*arrow*). A presumptive diagnosis of dissection was made since this artery subsequently developed a normal caliber.

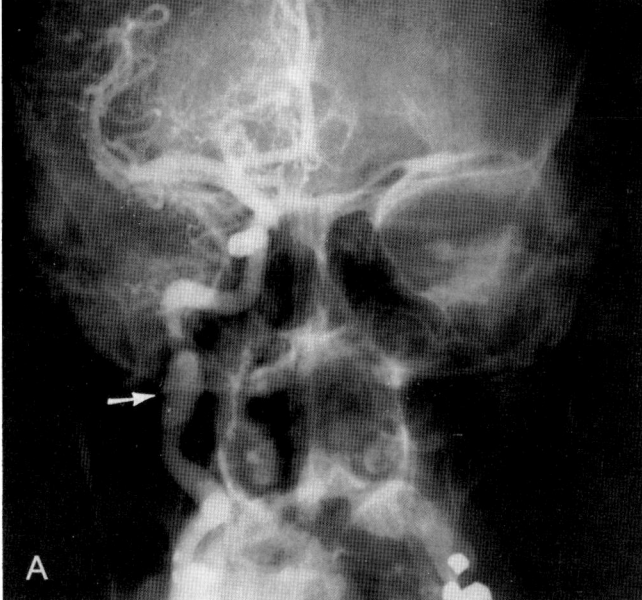
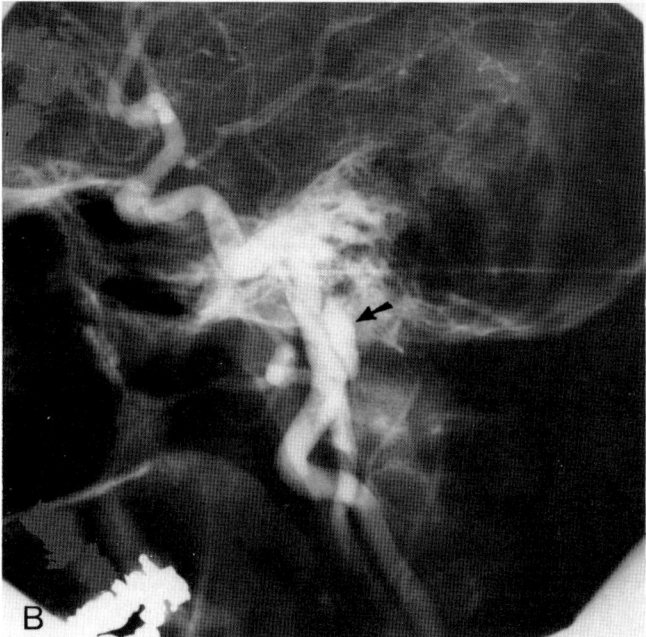

Figure 7.4 Typical angiographic finding (distal internal carotid pouch. *A* and *B*, left carotid angiogram showing a sac protruding posteriorly (*closed arrows*) from the internal carotid artery between C1 and the base of the skull. The lumen of the internal carotid artery is slightly narrowed. Comment: A 46-year-old woman had an acute upper respiratory infection with a severe cough. She developed a superficial pain on the left side of the head with superimposed jabs of severe pain. The scalp was sensitive. At the same time, a pulsating sound was noted in the left ear. A deep left neck pain developed. She noted that the left eye was half closed due to a drooping of the upper lid. A left miosis was found. Angiography 1 year later showed the sac to be about the same size, but the arterial lumen no longer narrowed. The bruit disappeared after 5 months. The head pain persisted intermittently. The neck pain subsided after

matic carotid dissection, and it is possible that this finding means the lesion was, in fact, traumatic in origin (36, 37).

Fisher et al. in their case 7 describe another angiographic finding in a patient who had serial angiograms (13). When first studied because of recent transient TIAs, there was a typical carotid "string sign" 7 cm long. The patient was treated with anticoagulation. Eight days later another angiogram revealed that the residual lumen had widened slightly. A third anigogram 7 months later showed full restoration of the lumen. At the site of the proximal end of the previous narrowing, there was an oval-shaped sac or pouch measuring 10 × 4 mm. The occasional finding of a small sac of this type on the proximal internal carotid artery probably represents a healed dissection.

In some cases, the internal carotid artery has become totally occluded. In these patients, the occlusion usually begins 2 cm or more distal to the origin of the internal carotid artery with a gradual taper of the vessel proximal to the occlusion. There is usually no evidence of atheroma in the cases studied at operation or autopsy. However, this type of carotid occlusion is not distinctive since intracranial occlusion of the distal internal carotid artery from any cause may be associated with retrograde thrombus extending into the neck and giving the same angiographic picture.

Treatment

The initial treatment of most patients with internal carotid dissection should be anticoagulation to prevent embolization. Satisfactory recovery of several patients treated with heparin and then coumadin has been reported (10, 11, 13, 14, 26, 27). One patient was treated with 5 months of continuous intravenous heparin using an implantable infusion device (8). The ideal duration of heparinization has not been established. Probably heparin should be used for at least 2 weeks. Thereafter, coumadin seems to be effective in preventing recurrent symptoms. Coumadin should be used for at least 3 months. Angiography has documented the resolution of the lesion in several cases. Even if the angiogram still shows some narrowing of the lumen, treatment probably does not need to be continued beyond this point.

If symptoms progress or recur in spite of medical treatment, surgical therapy should be considered. In addition, the patient who has an acute progressing or fluctuating neurological deficit and evidence of diminished flow probably is a candidate for direct carotid surgery. At operation, the diameter of the internal carotid artery is enlarged and the vessel has a bluish appearance. This finding is characteristic for a dissection.

---

2 months but then recurred 8 months later. No symptoms have returned over a period of 28 months.

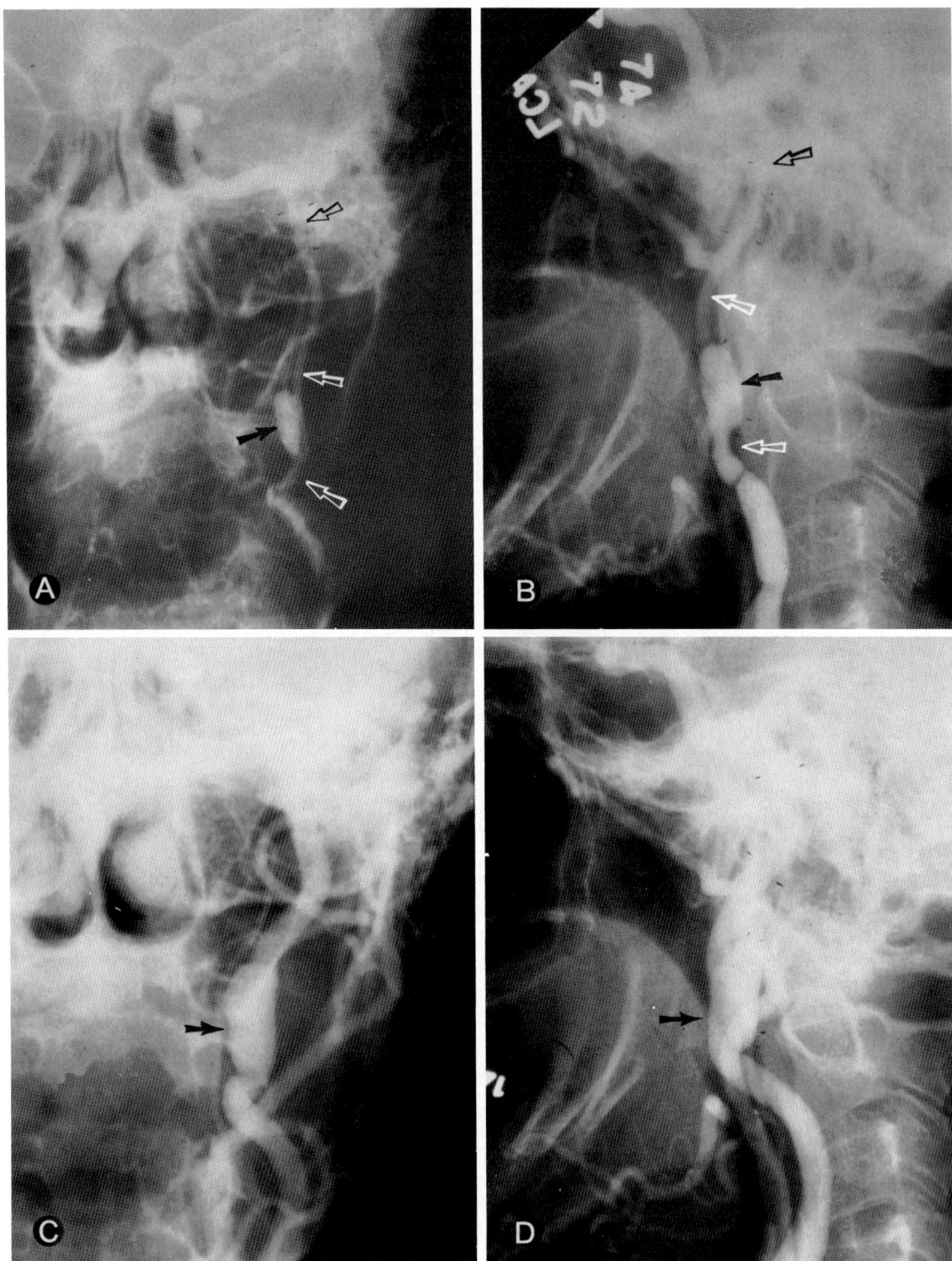

Figure 7.5 Typical angiographic finding (distal internal carotid pouch and narrowed artery). *A* and *B*, AP and lateral carotid angiograms showing narrowing of the internal carotid artery (*open arrows*) and an aneurysmal sac (*closed arrows*) in the proximal part of the dissection. This study was done eight days after starting heparin. On the original angiogram, the dissection was seen but not the sac. *C* and *D*, 7 months later the lumen has returned to normal size. The localized pouch persists (*closed arrows*). Comment: This 45-year-old man had a SAH 6 years before admission. Angiography showed three aneurysms on the right side and two on the left. A right common carotid ligation had been done. One week before admission while ill with the flu, he developed headache above the left eye and side of the head and pain on the side of the nose. Intermittent shining scintillations in the left visual field were noted. From the onset of the headache it was noted that the left upper lid drooped slightly and the left pupil was smaller. He could feel a pulsation deep in the left ear. On the day of admission there was a 15-minute episode of numbness of the right fingers, slurred speech, and sagging of the face. Left oculo-sympathetic palsy was the only abnormal neurological finding on examination.

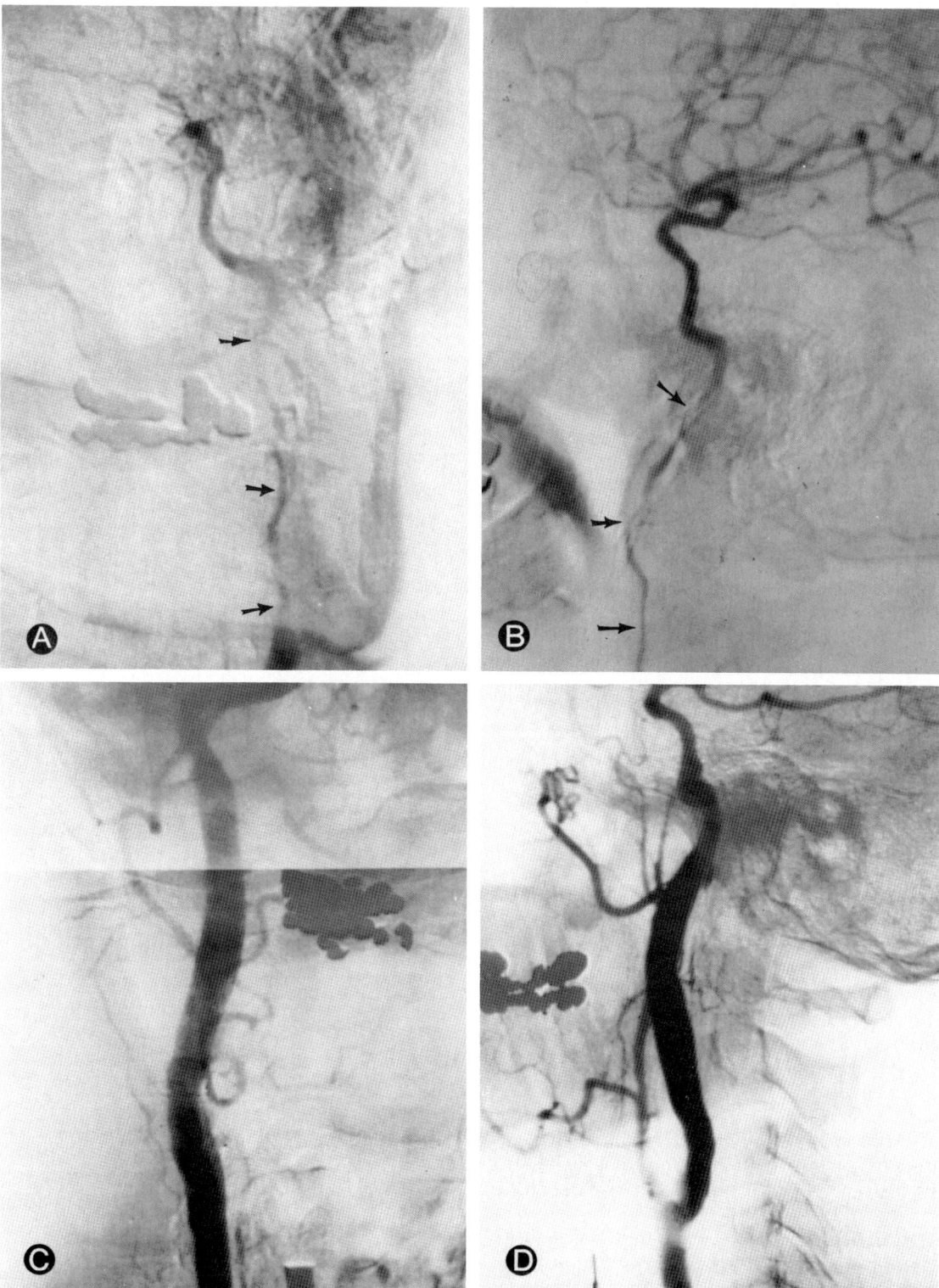

Figure 7.6 Acute neurological syndrome with dissection of internal carotid artery: surgical treatment. This 45-year-old woman presented with a fluctuating neurological deficit. Transient neurological disability occurred in spite of heparin. Surgery was performed immediately. Full recovery occurred. *A* and *B*, AP and lateral carotid angiogram showing "string sign" in internal carotid artery (*closed arrows*). At operation the internal carotid artery was enlarged and the wall had a typical bluish appearance. An arteriotomy was made in the proximal internal carotid artery and a Fogarty catheter inserted in the true lumen. The dissected intima and the clot were removed. There were no further neurological symptoms after the operation. *C* and *D*, postoperative angiogram showing restoration of an enlarged widely patent internal carotid artery lumen.

Surgical treatments which have been used for this problem include endarterectomy, resection and insertion of a graft, use of a balloon catheter, carotid ligation, and STA-MCA bypass graft. In three cases, the dissected area was resected and a vein graft inserted (12). Osteotomy of the mandible has been used to aid this exposure but this is probably not necessary (18, 39). Removal of the dissected intima and subintimal thrombus has also been done by arteriotomy and primary closure without a patch (6, 33). Postoperative angiography was reported to show good restoration of flow.

The use of a balloon catheter to remove the dissected intima has been described in one case (Fig. 7.2C) (30). A second case who presented with a fluctuating neurological deficit was treated in a similar manner (Figs. 7.6, A to D). In two other cases this technique was reported (12). In one, the postoperative angiogram was normal, but in the other, a ragged appearance on the intraoperative angiogram and high stump pressure led to internal carotid artery ligation. In another patient from the same report, the carotid artery was ligated when the dissection could not be removed. No complications were noted.

Bypass surgery, with anastomosis of the superficial temporal artery to a middle cerebral artery branch, has been used in a few patients with severely compromised cerebral circulation (28), with encouraging results. It was noted on follow-up angiography 3 to 6 months later that all these patients showed complete or partial resolution of the angiographic abnormality.

SPONTANEOUS DISSECTION: INTRACRANIAL ARTERIES

Pathogenesis

Dissection has been reported to involve all major intracranial arteries. This problem has been summarized in 1971 (22, 34), in 1977 (40), and in 1979 (1).

The middle cerebral artery has been the most frequently reported site of intracranial involvement (22, 34, 40). The internal carotid and basilar arteries are also common sites, and there are reports of involvement of the vertebral, posterior cerebral, and anterior cerebral arteries (1).

Examination of the wall of the artery shows the dissection with associated thrombus to be either circumferential or eccentric. It is usually between the intima and media, but may be located within either of these layers (1, 19, 40).

Discussion of the pathogenesis includes consideration of trauma, congenital medical defects, atherosclerotic changes in the wall, fibromuscular dysplasia, arteritis, infection, and homocystinuria (1, 15, 19, 21, 40). Cystic medial necrosis has rarely been found (1). The possible association with migraine has been raised (1, 34). Usually, a definite cause cannot be conclusively demonstrated. In the pathological examination of a case of middle cerebral dissection, there was splitting, fraying, disintegration, and irregular thickening of the elastic lamina, but similar, although less severe changes were seen in two other patients without dissection (7). In the detailed pathological examination of a case of middle cerebral dissection, no specific cause could be found (19).

Trauma as a possible cause of dissection of intracranial vessels is discussed in the next section. As with internal carotid dissection, the possible relationship with minor trauma is uncertain.

Clinical Manifestations, Diagnosis and Treatment

The onset of symptoms is most common in young adults (1, 22, 34). The age of reported patients has ranged from 6 months to 69 years (1). The majority of cases were between 15 and 35 (22). Recent reports of spontaneous middle cerebral dissection have included a number of patients under 20 years of age (7, 13, 19, 21). No sex predominance has been noted.

Unusually frequent and severe headache is a prominent symptom (35). A detailed analysis of reports of intracranial dissection containing sufficient data revealed that 19 of 20 cases had headache, often severe, with localization to the side of the involved artery in supratentorial dissections (40).

The onset of neurological symptoms is variable, but an acute severe neurological deficit due to infarction often develops (11, 22, 40). In 12 patients with intracranial dissection, six presented with sudden loss of consciousness, three with stroke, and three with subarachnoid hemorrhage (11). One patient with a dissection of the basilar artery had symptoms from compression of the pyramidal tracts and chronic subarachnoid hemorrhage before developing severe infarction (1). In another patient, an intracerebral hematoma followed rupture of the vessel and three other reports of such cases have been noted (22).

Angiography usually shows either a narrowed or occluded artery (1). The unusual segmental narrowing ("string sign") has been seen in the vertebral, middle, and posterior cerebral arteries (13, 19, 22) (Fig. 7.7). A double lumen has been demonstrated (20).

Most patients with intracranial dissection have not survived (17). In a recent report of the management of 11 patients, three with hemisphere ischemia and carotid stenosis underwent STA-MCA bypass, and five presenting with SAH had a direct surgical procedure (11), but treatment was complicated by recurrent SAH in one patient, stroke in four, and death in three.

TRAUMATIC DISSECTION

Pathogenesis

Dissection of the internal carotid artery and its branches can occur following non-penetrating injury to the head and neck, direct injury to the artery, and carotid angiography (23, 36, 37). Non-penetrating in-

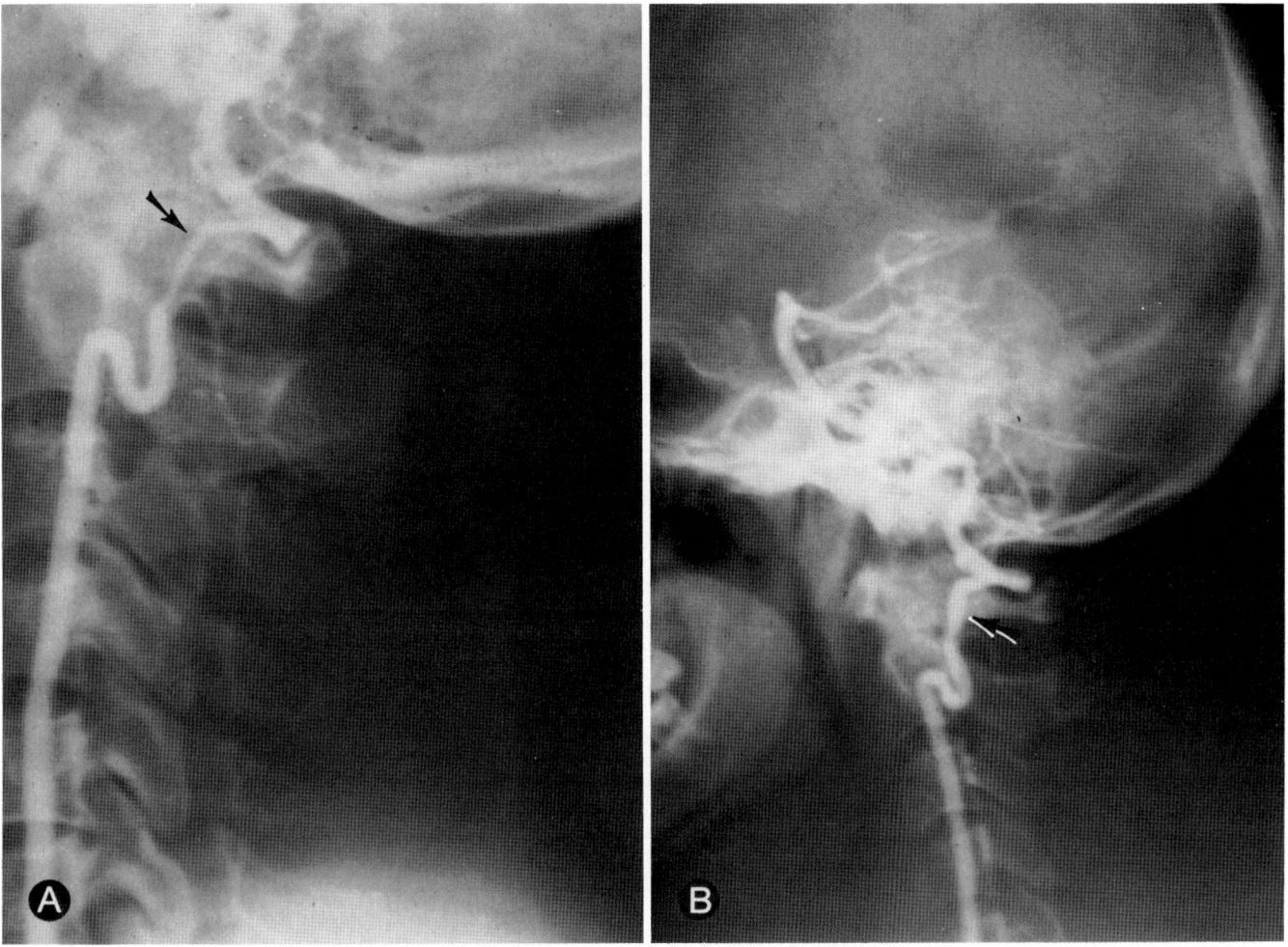

Figure 7.7 Dissection of the vertebral artery. *A,* lateral vertebral angiogram shows dissection at the C1 level. *B,* lateral vertebral angiogram taken 3 weeks later. A normal lumen is restored. No specific treatment had been given. Comment: This 35-year-old man was vigorously spanking his son when he felt something snap on the right side of the upper neck posteriorly. He immediately felt weak and lost his equilibrium. There was dysarthria, burning of the eyes, headache extending from the back of the head forward to behind the eye, numbness of both upper extremities and the right leg, dysphagia, and incoordination of the right extremities. He was unable to sit because of the balance problem. Examination showed a right lateral medullary syndrome. The signs and symptoms cleared over 2 weeks.

jury to the head and neck may cause an intimal tear in the cervical carotid vessels. The tear may lead to the development of a localized dissection or aneurysmal out-pouching (7, 10, 18). Thrombus may be the source of cerebral emboli and occlusion of the artery may develop (7). The most likely mechanism for production of this tear is the sudden severe stretch of the internal carotid artery over the upper cervical spine when the neck is hyperextended and laterally flexed to the opposite side (7, 10, 18). It may also be caused by a direct blow to the artery (2).

The cases of intracranial dissection where trauma has been suggested have followed closed head injury without fracture (19). Surgical trauma to the internal carotid artery during tonsillectomy and to the middle cerebral artery after ligation of an aneurysm have also been reported as causes of dissection (36, 37).

Clinical Manifestations, Diagnosis and Treatment

Traumatic dissection can produce the same picture as spontaneous dissection. The patient may present with a head injury with the initial diagnosis of cerebral concussion or contusion.

The interval between the trauma and onset of symptoms is variable. In the majority of patients with internal carotid artery dissection, symptoms occur within 24 hours of the trauma (2). However, long, symptom-free intervals may occur. In a report of six cases, three developed rapid deterioration in neurological status within 3 hours, one had the onset of symptoms in 8 days, another developed a TIA 2 weeks after an accident, and the last patient was well until 1 year after recovery from a serious head injury when he developed a stroke due to an embolus from the area of dissection and aneurysmal formation (36).

Symptoms in patients with intracranial dissection may be acute or delayed (1). In a review of the reported cases of post-traumatic middle cerebral occlusion, including those where dissection had been demonstrated at autopsy, the interval between trauma and onset of symptoms varied from a few hours to several days (20).

When a patient with a history of trauma develops neurological symptoms and the CT scan does not clarify the causes, angiography is needed to help establish a diagnosis. It is also imperative that adequate views of both the head and neck be obtained.

When non-pentrating trauma to the head and neck cause arterial injury, the most common angiographic finding is internal carotid occlusion 1 to 3 cm above the bifurcation (37). However, in some patients an intimal tear leads to development of a dissection. In a report of six patients, the angiographic abnormality between C2 and the base of the skull consisted of a localized narrowing of the vessel and/or an aneurysmal out-pouching (36). Another important finding present in four of the six patients was evidence of intracranial emboli.

The natural history of the illness is unknown. However, the results of a recent report suggest that the problem may be, like spontaneous dissection, a more benign process than originally thought (36). All six patients in that report were treated medically and had an uncomplicated course. Anticoagulation was used when emboli were demonstrated, and there was no complication from this therapy. Follow-up angiograms were done in four of the six patients and showed that none of the dissections progressed to complete occlusion; one had disappeared, in three, the ipsilateral false aneurysm had enlarged, and in three, an aneurysmal out-pouching in the opposite, asymptomatic, internal carotid artery was seen which had not been demonstrated on the initial angiographic study. These aneurysmal sacs may remain unchanged for several years or they may spontaneously thrombose (36, 37). In both circumstances, the patient has usually remained asymptomatic.

REFERENCES

1. Alexander CB, Burger PC, Goree JA: Dissecting aneurysms of the basilar artery in two patients. Stroke 10:294–298, 1979.
2. Bergquist BJ, Boone SC, Whaley RA: Traumatic dissection of the internal carotid artery treated by ECIC anastomosis. Stroke 12:73–76, 1981.
3. Bladin PF: Dissecting aneurysm of carotid and vertebral arteries. Vasc Surg 8:203–223, 1974.
4. Bostrom K, Liliequist B: Primary dissecting aneurysm of the extracranial part of the internal carotid and vertebral arteries. Neurology 17:179–186, 1967.
5. Brown OL, Armitage JL: Spontaneous dissecting aneurysms of the cervical internal carotid artery: two case reports and a survey of the literature. Am J Roentgenol 118:648–653, 1973.
6. Burklund CW: Spontaneous dissecting aneurysm of the cervical carotid artery: a report of surgical treatment in two patients. Johns Hopkins Med J 126:154–159, 1970.
7. Chang V, Rewcastle NB, Harwood-Nash DCF, Norman MD: Bilateral dissecting aneurysms of the intracranial internal carotid arteries in an 8-year-old boy. Neurology 25:573–579, 1975.
8. Chapleau CE, Robertson JT: Spontaneous cervical carotid artery dissection: Outpatient treatment with continuous heparin infusion using a totally implantable infusion device. Neurosurgery 8:83–87, 1981.
9. Collins GJ, Rich NM, Clagett GP, Speban MJ, Salander JM: Fibromuscular dysplasia of the internal carotid artery. Ann Surg 194:89–96, 1981.
10. Dagi TF, Beal MF, Brem S, Welch J, Ojemann RG, Poletti CE: Internal carotid artery dissection after pregnancy (to be published).
11. Durward QJ, Peerless SJ, Barnett HJM, Fox AJ, Friedman A, Drake CG: *Spontaneous Cerebrovascular Dissection, Presented at the 1981 Meeting of the Society of University Neurosurgeons.*
12. Ehrenfeld WK, Wylie EJ: Spontaneous dissection of the internal carotid artery. Arch Surg 111:1294–1301, 1976.
13. Fisher CM, Ojemann RG, Roberson GH: Spontaneous dissection of cervico-cerebral arteries. Can J Neurol Sci 5:9–19, 1978.
14. Friedman WA, Day AL, Quisling RG, Sypert GW, Rhoton AL Jr: Cervical carotid dissecting aneurysms. Neurosurgery 7:207–214, 1980.
15. Giedke H, Kriebel J, Sindermann F: Dissecting aneurysm of the petrous portion of the internal carotid artery. Case report and review of previous cases. Neuroradiology 10:121–124, 1975.
16. Greiner AL: Spontaneous dissecting aneurysms of the cervical internal carotid artery. Stroke 7:6, 1976.
17. Grosman H, Fornasier VL, Bonder D, Livingston KE, Platts ME: Dissecting aneurysm of the cerebral arteries. J Neurosurg 53:693–697, 1980.
18. Hardin CA, Snodgrass RG: Dissecting aneurysm of internal carotid artery treated by fenestration and graft. Surgery 55:207–209, 1964.
19. Hochberg FH, Bean CS, Fisher CM, Roberson GH: Stroke in a 16-year-old girl secondary to terminal carotid dissection. Neurology 25:725–729, 1975.
20. Hollin SA, Sukoff MH, Silverstein A, Gross SW: Post-traumatic middle cerebral artery occlusion. J Neurosurg 25:526–535, 1966.
21. Johnson AC, Graves VB, Pfaff JP Jr: Dissecting aneurysm of intracranial arteries. Surg. Neurol 7:49–51, 1977.
22. Kunze S, Schiefer W: Angiographic demonstration of a dissecting aneurysm of the middle cerebral artery. Neuroradiology 2:201–206, 1971.
23. Lai MD, Hoffman HB, Adamkiewicz JJ: Dissecting aneurysm of internal carotid artery after non-penetrating neck injury. Case report. Acta Radiol 5:290–295, 1966.
24. Liliequist B: The roentgenologic appearance of spontaneous dissecting aneurysm of the cervical internal carotid artery: report of a case. Vasc Surg 2:223–226, 1968.
25. Lloyd J, Bahnson HT: Bilateral dissecting aneurysms of the internal carotid arteries. Am J. Surg 122:549–551, 1971.
26. Luken MG, Ascherl GF Jr, Correll JW, Hilal SK: Spontaneous dissecting aneurysms of the extracranial internal carotid artery. Clin Neurosurg 26:353–375, 1979.
27. McNeill DH Jr, Dreisbach J, Marsden RJ: Spontaneous dissection of the internal carotid artery. Arch Neurol 37:54–55, 1980.
28. Mokri B, Sundt TM Jr, Houser OW: Spontaneous internal carotid dissection, hemicrania and Horner's syndrome. Arch Neurol 36:677–680, 1979.
29. New PFJ, Momose KJ: Traumatic dissection of the internal carotid artery of the atlantoxial level, secondary to non-penetrating injury. Radiology 93:41–49, 1969.

30. Ojemann RG, Fisher CM, Rich JC: Spontaneous dissecting aneurysm of the internal carotid artery. Stroke 3:434–440, 1972.
31. Pilz P, Hartjes HJ: Fibromuscular dysplasia and multiple dissecting aneurysms of intracranial arteries. A further cause of moyamoya syndrome. Stroke 7:393–398, 1976.
32. Ringel SP, Harrison SH, Norenberg MD, Austin JH: Fibromuscular dysplasia: Multiple "spontaneous" dissecting aneurysms of the major cervical arteries. Ann Neurol 1:301–304, 1977.
33. Roome NS Jr, Aberfeld DC: Spontaneous dissecting aneurysm of the internal carotid artery. Arch Neurol 34:251–252, 1977.
34. Sato O, Bascom JF, Logothetis J: Intracranial dissecting aneurysm. Case report. J Neurosurg 35:483–487, 1971.
35. Scott GE, Neubuerger KT, Denst J: Dissecting aneurysms of intracranial arteries. Neurology 10:22–27, 1960.
36. Stringer WL, Kelly DL: Traumatic dissection of the extracranial internal carotid artery. Neurosurgery 6:123–130, 1980.
37. Sullivan HG, Vines FS, Becker DP: Sequelae of indirect internal carotid injury. Radiology 109:91–98, 1973.
38. Thapedia IM, Ashenhurst EM, Rozdilsky B: Spontaneous dissecting aneurysm of the internal carotid artery in the neck: report of a case and review of the literature. Arch Neurol 23:549–554, 1970.
39. Wylie EF, Ehrenfeld WK: *Extracranial Occlusive Cerebrovascular Disease*. Philadelphia, WB Saunders, 1970, pp 48 and 192.
40. Yonas H, Agamanolis D, Takaoka Y, White RJ: Dissecting intracranial aneurysms. Surg Neurol 8:407–415, 1977.

Chapter 8 EMBOLISM

In most patients with embolism to the intracranial circulation, the embolic material consists of a fragment which has broken away from a thrombus within the heart (1, 2). The most common type of heart disease to be associated with embolism is chronic atrial fibrillation due to atherosclerosis, rheumatic heart disease, or other less common diseases. The source of the embolus is a thrombus deposited within the atrial appendage. The second most frequent source of cerebral emboli is a mural thrombus deposited on the damaged endocardium overlying an area of myocardial infarction. Emboli can also arise from atrial thrombosis associated with severe mitral stenosis without atrial fibrillation. The problem can also develop as a complication of cardiac surgery.

Usually, the embolus from the heart is small enough so that it does not block a major extracranial artery but becomes arrested at an intracranial bifurcation. On occasion, however, the internal carotid or vertebral artery may be blocked. If the embolus does not promptly break up or collateral circulation is inadequate, ischemic infarction occurs. A hemorrhagic infarction usually means an embolic cause, but non-hemorrhagic infarction can also occur. Any region of the brain may be affected, but the territory of the middle cerebral artery is most frequently involved.

Emboli from a thrombus that has formed on an ulcerated or stenotic atheromatous plaque of the aorta or carotid artery can cause cerebral symptoms as noted in Chapter 1. However, in most patients these fragments are not large enough to occlude major arteries and, therefore, do not have surgical implications.

Of all strokes, those due to cerebral embolism develop most rapidly, with the full clinical picture developing in several seconds to a minute. Usually there are no warning episodes. When a large embolus blocks the internal carotid artery or the stem of the middle cerebral artery, a severe neurological deficit is usually produced.

When the embolus enters the vertebral artery, it most often goes into one of the posterior cerebral arteries causing a homonymous hemianopia. In one report, 22% of cerebellar infarctions were reported to be due to emboli (4).

The diagnosis is usually based on the history. In the circumstance where embolic occlusion of the internal carotid artery or middle cerebral artery is suspected, emergency angiography may be indicated.

The problems in evaluating and treating these patients are difficult. Since the occlusion is sudden, there is little or no chance for collateral circulation to develop to help protect the brain. Therefore, diagnosis must be made and treatment started promptly. In some patients, the embolus will break up and spontaneous recovery follow. The patient with embolus is at risk for recurrent embolism. Therefore, anticoagulant therapy must be considered. The advisability of

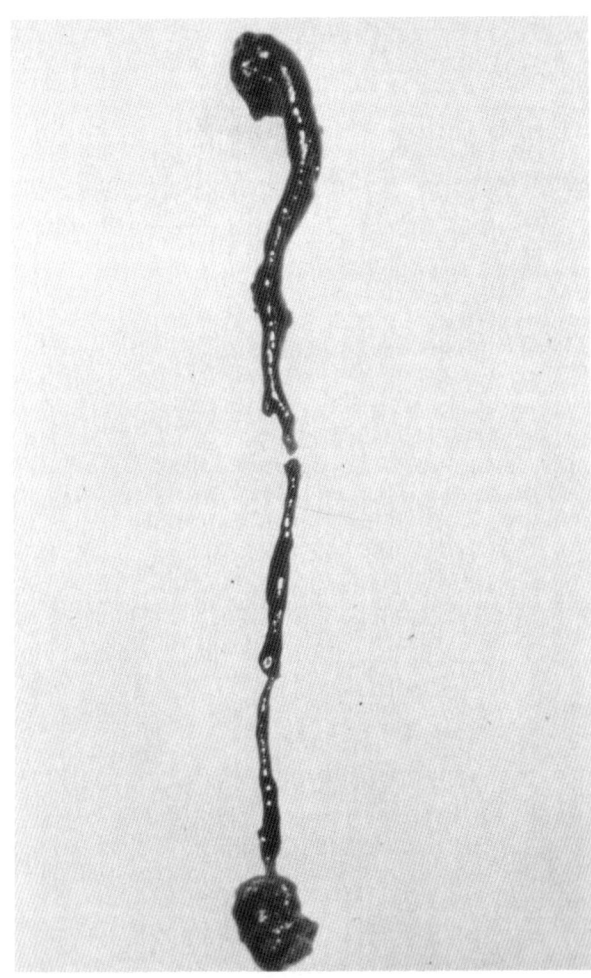

Figure 8.1 Occlusion of common carotid bifurcation by embolus from the heart. This 41-year-old man with a history of a myocardial infarction had the sudden onset of hemiplegia. Examination also disclosed an absent superficial temporal pulse. Immediate operation removed an organized thrombus at the carotid bifurcation (at bottom of picture) and a fresh thrombus in the internal carotid artery. Good back flow followed. The patient recovered with a moderate residual neurological deficit.

delaying anticoagulation for several days to avoid the risk of hemorrhage into an area of infarction has been discussed (1). If the CT scan does not show hemorrhage into the infarct, heparin may be started and then followed in several days by coumadin. This question must also be evaluated when a surgical procedure is being planned which may preclude the use of anticoagulants for several days.

CAROTID ARTERY EMBOLUS

The clinical features are the same as those described previously for carotid occlusive disease. Usually the onset of the stroke is sudden, without warning, and with the almost immediate development of severe hemiplegia. When the embolus is large enough to block the internal carotid artery, it will usually lodge at the common carotid artery bifurcation and obstruct both the external and internal carotid arteries (Fig. 8.1). Therefore, loss of superficial temporal pulse in the clinical setting described should make the physician suspicious of an embolus. This is particularly true if there is a history of heart disease or atrial fibrillation.

If the superficial temporal pulse is gone, immediate exploration without any other tests should be considered. Angiography, with digital subtraction if available, should be done in other patients where the diagnosis is suspected. At the same time, intravascular volume and blood pressure are increased to promote maximum collateral circulation. The guidelines for surgical treatment are similar to those described for treating acute carotid occlusion when a thrombus forms on an atheromatous plaque (Chapter 1). The surgical exposure is the same as outlined for carotid endarterectomy (Chapter 2).

MIDDLE CEREBRAL ARTERY EMBOLUS

Most intracranial emboli lodge in distal arterial branches, but occasionally the proximal middle cerebral artery may be occluded by an embolus. The technical feasibility of middle cerebral embolectomy has been clearly established and satisfactory patency rates may be obtained. Unfortunately, the process of cerebral infarction in most cases proceeds to irreversibility before the surgeon can restore blood flow. Early diagnosis and effective drug therapy to prolong

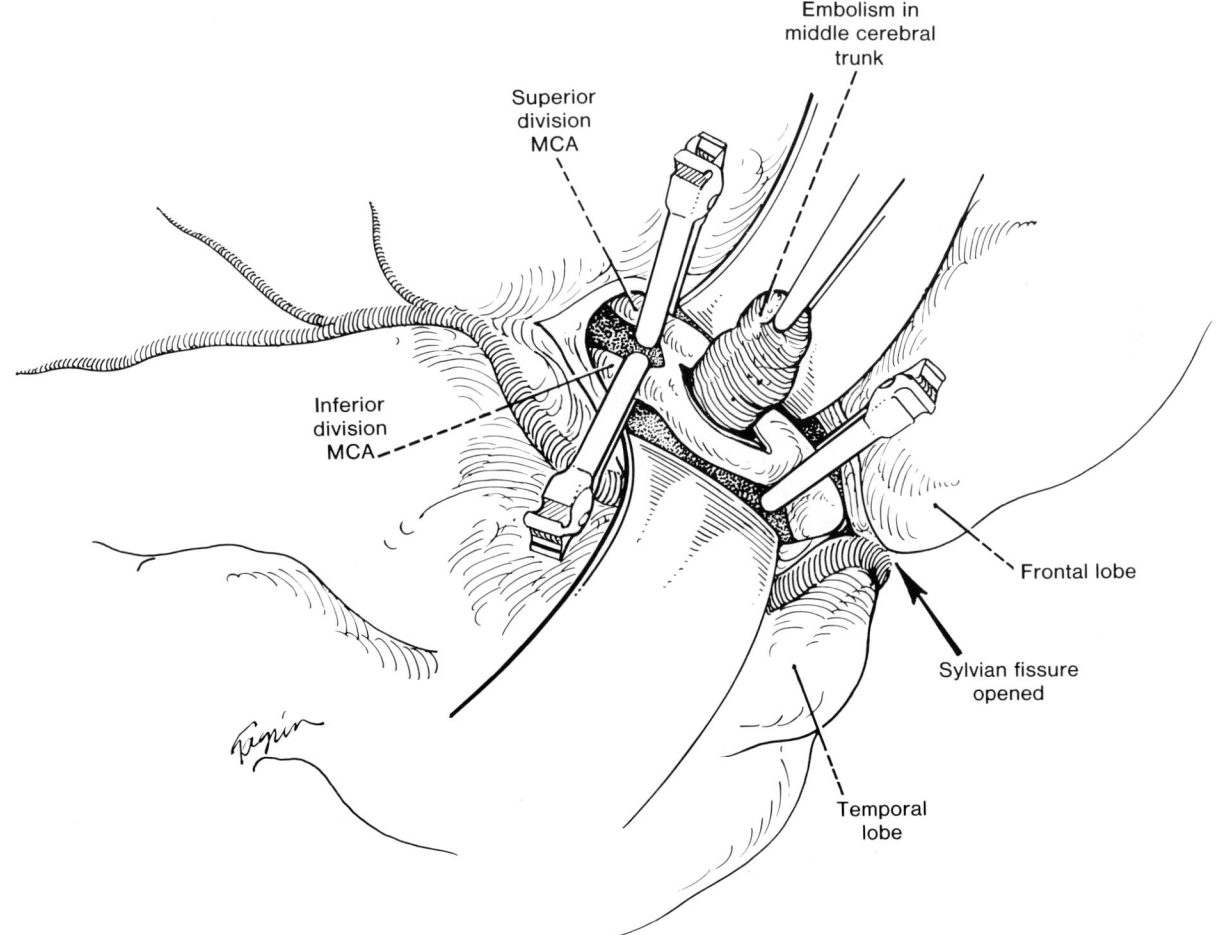

Figure 8.2 Middle cerebral artery embolectomy. Exposure of right middle cerebral artery in the Sylvian fissure and removal of an embolus from the M1 segment.

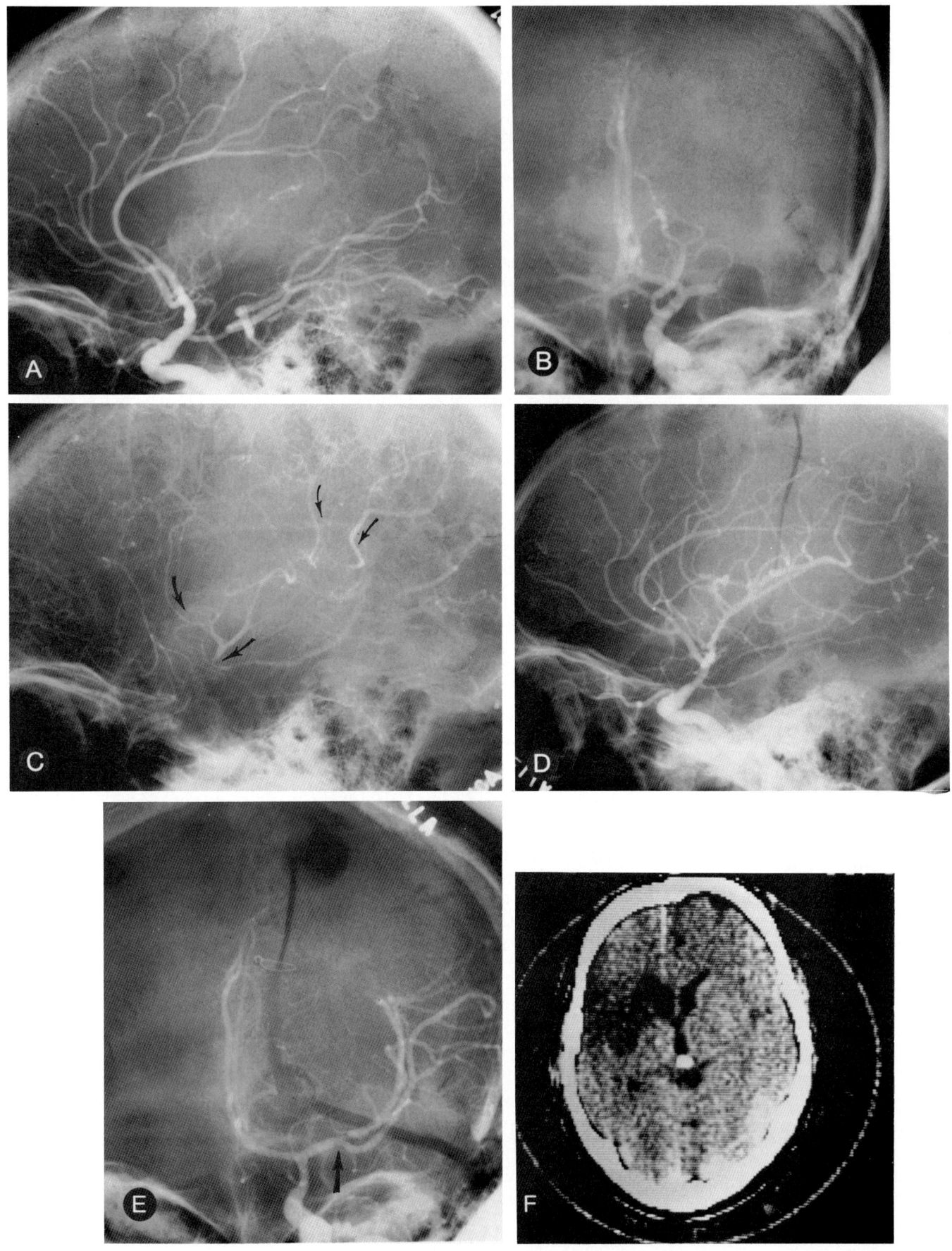

the period of reversibility will be needed to make this procedure widely useful.

At the present time, only an occasional patient will be a candidate for this procedure. The most common presentation is a young patient, already in the hospital for evaluation of a cardiac problem, with sudden onset of a hemiplegia which is promptly diagnosed. Immediate treatment with intravenous pentobarbital, modest hypertension, and adequate intravascular volume and hematocrit may retard the infarction process. Immediate intubation may be needed to protect the airway and maintain normal arterial blood gases. Emergency angiography is necessary to localize the MCA obstruction. Surgery can be proposed reasonably only where the obstruction is localized to the M1 segment and proximal MCA divisions with good distal collateral filling of the MCA territory.

A frontotemporal craniotomy should be performed rapidly. If the cortex shows marked pallor, swelling, and petechiae, irreversible infarction has occurred and embolectomy will not be helpful. If the brain appears less damaged, the MCA trunk is exposed by splitting the Sylvian fissure. In case this proves difficult, one may rapidly approach the MCA bifurcation through a corticectomy in the superior temporal gyrus (see Chapter 16 for details of this approach). Careful inspection of the MCA and its bifurcation serves to identify the site of the embolus, which will appear dark purple. Care should be taken not to dislodge the embolus at this stage. Heifetz clips are placed proximal and distal to the occlusion. An arteriotomy is made directly over the embolus (Fig. 8.2). Ordinarily, this can be very short, about half the breadth of the M1 segment, to facilitate closure. When the embolus is lodged at the MCA bifurcation, three short arteriotomies may be best, one over the M1 segment, and two in the proximal MCA divisions. Arteriotomies are best performed with a broken razor blade, or #11 knife blade. The embolus is removed with forceps or a fine sucker. In most cases, no effort should be made to remove MCA atheroma, should it be encountered. The lumen is irrigated with heparinized saline. Back flow is checked by briefly opening the clips. Arteriotomies are closed with running 7-0 monofilament nylon. A patch graft is generally not necessary. A Silastic tubing for a stent may be helpful for the M1 trunk closure. We have occasionally used tissue adhesive to assure watertight closure. In case of brain swelling, the bone flap may be left out, and barbiturate coma may be maintained for 24–72 hours. Blood pressure should be maintained in the high normal range. Postoperative angiography and CT can document impact of therapy.

In the three embolectomy cases from our series, angiography confirmed patency in two (Fig. 8.3). Revascularization was completed within 8 hours after onset in each patient. Neurological improvement, beyond that expected from recuperation after cerebral infarction, was documented in two cases. In the patient without neurological improvement postoperatively, there had been marked brain swelling, pallor, and petechiae at surgery. In one case, where neurological improvement was noted early after surgery, a massive pulmonary embolus 1 week later took the patient's life.

In 1976, the results in 35 cases of intracranial arteriotomy for embolus or thrombosis, reported in the English literature, were summarized (3). In 18 of 37 operated vessels, postoperative angiography demonstrated patency. There was no definite evidence to indicate any difference in the outcome between those with open or occluded arteries. It was concluded that the best surgical candidate is a young person, in good general medical condition, in whom the occlusion has occurred within a few hours of surgery.

REFERENCES

1. Adams RD, Victor M: *Principles of Neurology*. New York, McGraw-Hill, 1977, pp 530–534.
2. Fisher CM, Dalal PM, Adams RD: Cerebrovascular Disease and Stroke Syndrome, in Harrison TR (ed): *Principles of Internal Medicine*. McGraw-Hill, New York, 1962.
3. Garrido E, Stein BM: Middle cerebral artery embolectomy. J Neurosurg 44:517–521, 1976.
4. Sypert GW, Alvord EC Jr: Cerebellar infarction. A clinicopathological study. Arch Neurol 32:357–363, 1975.

Figure 8.3 Middle cerebral artery embolectomy. Four days after coronary artery bypass and infarctectomy, a 42-year-old man suffered sudden aphasia and right hemiplegia. A and B, immediate left carotid angiography documented MCA stem occlusion. C, good retrograde filling of distal MCA branches back to the bifurcation (arrows). Embolectomy restored flow about 7 hours after onset of deficit. D and E, postoperative angiography documented patency. Arrow indicates where embolus was removed at MCA bifurcation. There is some narrowing at that point. F, CT shows the infarction. The patient recovered to a mild right hemiparesis with normal language.

Chapter 9 CEREBRAL AND CEREBELLAR INFARCTION

Irreversible damage to brain tissue due to lack of blood is called infarction or ischemic necrosis. Brain infarcts vary greatly in size and in the amount of congestion and hemorrhage within the area. Some infarcts are pale and devoid of blood and others show varying degrees of extravasation of blood from small vessels in the infarcted area. The latter are usually associated with embolism (see Chapter 8).

The CT scan defines the extent of the infarction. Details regarding the use of this test in patients with infarction are presented in Chapter 1.

Most patients with infarction will be alert with a neurological deficit related to the area of infarction. Treatment is directed to the cause of the infarction. Occasionally, symptoms due to swelling and edema will develop but this usually responds to medical treatment. In a few patients, surgery may be required to provide decompression because the swollen infarcted brain tissue does not respond to medical therapy.

CEREBRAL INFARCTION

When acute massive ischemic cerebral infarction with progressive signs of brain stem compression fails to respond to medical therapy, treatment with hemicraniectomy and opening of the dura may be indicated. A dural graft is sewn in place or Gelfoam placed over the opening to protect the brain. We have done this operation in two patients with relief of pressure and eventual partial recovery of function.

In one report, three patients with acute massive multilobular ischemic infarction with uncal herniation, who were unresponsive to medical therapy, were treated with hemicraniectomy and opening of the dura (9). All three survived, although a severe fixed neurological deficit persisted in two. The factors that influenced undertaking this surgery were the relatively young age of the patients, involvement of the non-dominant hemisphere, lack of systemic illness, and a positive attitude of the family.

CEREBELLAR INFARCTION
Etiology

The swollen infarcted cerebellar hemisphere may also cause brain stem compression leading to the need for neurosurgical treatment, often on an urgent basis. In the majority of patients, the infarction is in the posteroinferior half of the cerebellar hemisphere in the region supplied by the ipsilateral vertebral and posterior inferior cerebellar arteries (6, 12). Occasionally an infarct is found in the territory of the superior cerebellar artery (7, 10, 12).

Atherosclerotic occlusion with associated thrombosis is the most common cause of arterial occlusions. Embolism was implicated as the cause in 22% of the patients in one report (12). The problem has also been seen with traumatic occlusion of the vertebral artery, including neck manipulation (5).

Clinical Presentation and Diagnosis

The onset is usually sudden. The acute symptoms are rotatory dizziness, nausea and vomiting, and inability to stand or walk unaided (1, 5, 8, 11). Initially these symptoms may mimic a benign labyrinthine disorder (2).

In the early stages, examination may reveal nystagmus, usually horizontal and rapid in the direction of gaze, truncal ataxia, dysarthria, and stiff neck. Hypertension is present in about half the patients. As the problem progresses, drowsiness and confusion are noted. Ocular abnormalities are common with findings of an abducens nerve paresis or a gaze palsy, either paresis of ipsilateral gaze or deviation of the eyes to the opposite side. Bilateral extensor plantar responses are often noted. Occasionally there may be a peripheral facial palsy. Of note is the absence of significant hemiparesis. At least half of these patients stabilize and improve. However, progression to decerebrate posturing with stupor or coma and other evidence of severe brain stem compression can occur, often fairly rapidly.

Any patient suspected of having a posterior fossa mass lesion should have an immediate CT scan. The clinical features may not separate cerebellar hemorrhage and infarction. Emergency CT scanning locates the lesion, establishes the pathology, and documents the degree of hydrocephalus (Fig. 9.1). It must be remembered that the low density lesion in the cerebellum may not develop for some hours to a few days and, therefore, the initial CT scan may be inconclusive and serial scans may be helpful. In some cases, contrast enhancement will show the lesion.

In a report of 21 cases of cerebellar infarction documented by CT scan, six had progressive deterioration of consciousness, signs of brain stem compression, and the appearance of hydrocephalus on the CT scan (11). In 15 the course was uncomplicated and gradual improvement occurred. In another re-

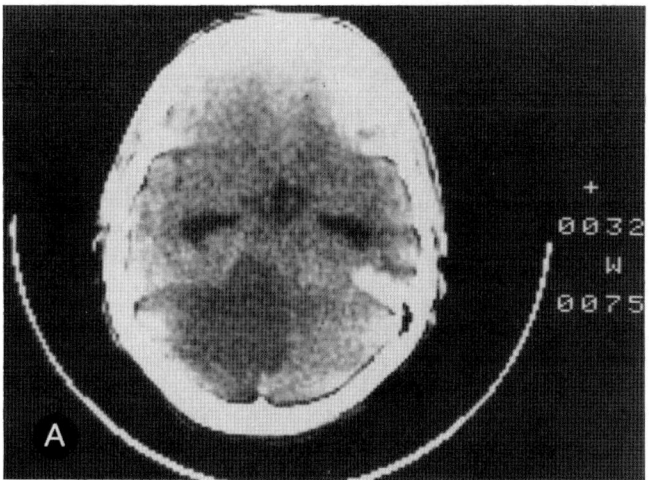

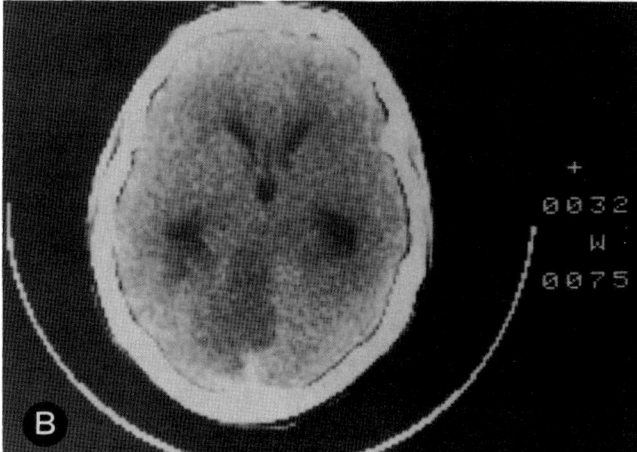

Figure 9.1 CT scan of cerebellar infarction. A, large infarct of the cerebellum causing brain stem compression. Note that the low density seems to be sharply demarcated and involves most of the cerebellar hemisphere. B, the infarct extends superiorly and there is evidence of hydrocephalus (confirmed on higher scans) with enlarged temporal horns and a dilated third ventricle. Comment: The patient developed increasing signs of brain stem compression which did not respond to medical treatment. Full recovery followed resection of the lateral cerebellum.

port, about half of the patients improved spontaneously (3).

Treatment

If the patient is alert and the neurological status is stable or improving, medical treatment with steroids and/or mannitol is given. If there is a decreasing level of consciousness in spite of medical treatment or there are signs of brain stem compression when the patient is first evaluated, immediate surgical treatment for removal of the infarcted cerebellar tissue is usually indicated. In one report, the presence of hydrocephalus was used as an important factor in deciding about surgery (10).

The operation has usually been done in the prone position, using a midline incision and performing a craniectomy that includes removal of the midline bone and posterior rim of the foramen magnum, as well as bone over the involved cerebellar hemisphere. The dural opening exposes the cerebellar hemisphere and extends across the midline and over the cerebellar tonsils. The resection includes at least the lateral half or more of the cerebellar hemisphere. To give a full decompression, the dura is closed using a graft of pericranial tissue from the occipital region. A satisfactory alternative approach is the lateral "park bench" position. The sitting position should not be used to avoid the risk of hypotension.

In a review summarizing the reports of 55 patients who developed signs of brain stem compression due to cerebellar infarction, it was found that 5 of 18 treated surgically and 31 of 37 not treated surgically died (2). In other reports it was concluded that medical treatment of large cerebellar infarcts was associated with an 80% mortality rate, while with surgery this figure dropped to 40% (4); and in 51 patients who had rapid worsening of signs of brain stem compression, it was found that 28 of 37 (76%) who were operated survived, while only 1 of 14 (7%) non-operated patients lived (11). It was concluded that to be effective, surgical treatment must be initiated as soon as possible after consciousness begins to deteriorate.

REFERENCES

1. Duncan GW, Parker SW, Fisher CM: Acute cerebellar infarction in the PICA territory. Arch Neurol 32:364–368, 1975.
2. Feely MP: Cerebellar infarction. Neurosurgery 4:7–11, 1979.
3. George B, Cophignon J, George C, Lougnon J: Surgical aspects of cerebellar infarction. Based upon a series of 79 cases. Neurochirurgie 24:83–88, 1978.
4. Greenberg J, Skubick D, Shenkin H: Acute hydrocephalus in cerebellar infarct and hemorrhage. Neurology 29:409–413, 1979.
5. Heros RC: Cerebellar infarction resulting from traumatic occlusion of a vertebral artery. Case report. J Neurosurg 51:111–113, 1979.
6. Heros RC: Cerebellar hemorrhage and infarction. Current concepts of cerebrovascular disease. 16:17–22, 1981.
7. Ho SU, Kim KS, Berenberg RA, Ho HT: Cerebellar infarction: A clinical and CT study. Surg Neurol 16:350–352, 1981.
8. Lehrich JR, Winkler GF, Ojemann RG: Cerebellar infarction with brain stem compression. Diagnosis and surgical treatment. Arch Neurol 22:490–498, 1970.
9. Rengachary SS, Batnitzky S, Morantz RA, Arjunan K, Jeffries B: Hemicraniectomy for acute massive cerebral infarction. Neurosurgery 8:321–328, 1981.
10. Sayama I, Sakotani AY, Yasui N, Ito Z, Kobayashi T, Nakajimak K: Cerebellar infarction: Early predication to the operative indication of posterior fossa decompression. Brain and Nerve (Tokyo) 33:801–810, 1981.
11. Scotti G, Spinnler H, Sterzi R, Vallar G: Cerebellar softening. Ann Neurol 8:133–140, 1980.
12. Sypert GW, Alvord EC Jr: Cerebellar infarction. A clinicopathological study. Arch Neurol 32:357–363, 1975.

Section 2: INTRACRANIAL ANEURYSMS, ARTERIOVENOUS MALFORMATIONS, AND BRAIN HEMORRHAGE

Chapter 10: INTRACRANIAL ANEURYSMS AND SUBARACHNOID HEMORRHAGE: INCIDENCE, PATHOLOGY, CLINICAL FEATURES, AND MEDICAL MANAGEMENT

Ruptured intracranial aneurysm, the most common cause of subarachnoid hemorrhage, often leads to serious neurological disability or death (19, 35, 53, 69, 74). Medical and technical advances have improved the surgical treatment for patients with intracranial aneurysms (19, 14, 40, 57, 69, 70, 84). CT scanning provides immediate atraumatic diagnosis of intracranial hemorrhage and hydrocephalus (17). Amicar decreases the rate of early recurrent hemorrhage (45, 48, 50). Delay of surgery for 1–2 weeks allows resolution of cerebral swelling and is associated with good operative results (19, 25, 54). Microsurgery minimizes the degree of brain retraction, and provides good illumination and precise visualization to spare tiny but critical perforating arteries (40). Modern neuroanesthesia facilitates surgery by "defusing the bomb" with deep hypotension and relaxing the brain with hyperventilation and diuresis (1).

Results gained with microsurgical direct operation (14, 19, 40, 57, 69, 70) are superior to results from bed rest (51) or indirect procedures (35, 76). Only rarely do special circumstances, e.g., certain giant aneurysms, require internal carotid occlusion (18, 46, 67), with or without cerebral revascularization with a bypass graft (see Chapter 20). For most patients who reach the operating room, a good to excellent outcome can be expected. We recommend operation for ruptured aneurysms in patients up to age 70 who achieve grade 3 status or better and in some older patients who are grade 1 or 2 (4). In addition, surgery may be indicated for unruptured aneurysms 7 mm or larger in diameter, since these lesions probably bleed with significant frequency (52, 78, 83) (see Chapter 19).

Vasospasm, particularly in the preoperative period, continues to cause disability and death (3, 9, 12, 22, 30, 37, 49, 56, 81, 85). There is evidence that a CT scan done early after SAH can accurately predict which patients may suffer serious symptomatic vasospasm (22, 75). It may be that such patients warrant vigorous prophylactic management with drugs (81), special management of fluid and blood volume, early surgery, or a combination of therapies. Reports of early surgery from Japan have been equivocal (72, 73), and a large cooperative study to evaluate this approach is underway.

PREVALENCE

Cerebral aneurysm and subarachnoid hemorrhage are common problems. It has been estimated that 400,000 Americans harbor unruptured cerebral aneurysms (59). The incidence of subarachnoid hemorrhage is estimated at 26,000 annually in the U.S., and about 80% of these hemorrhages are attributable to intracranial aneurysm (19, 39, 74). A serious concern is the fact that only about one-half of these patients reach the hospital and less than one-quarter have surgery (19). A large percentage of the remainder go unoperated to death or major disability. Only diagnosis prior to SAH can help these patients (59). Hopefully the development of digital subtraction angiography and high resolution CT scan will help identify more aneurysms before they rupture (42).

The prevalence of aneurysm in the population is correlated with age; the peak incidence is in the sixth decade of life, while aneurysms are rare in childhood and adolescence. A slight tendency toward female preponderance is characteristic. When subarachnoid hemorrhage occurs in pregnancy, the incidences of aneurysms and arteriovenous malformations are about the same (58).

Familial intracranial aneurysms are rare. Review of the literature revealed reports of 47 families in whom more than one member had a proven aneurysm (31). It was concluded that elective investigation of the asymptomatic members of these families should be considered.

ETIOLOGY

No clear etiology has been established for idiopathic intracranial aneurysm. The occasional occurrence of cerebral aneurysm with congenital disorders, such as coarctation of the aorta and polycystic kidney disease, has lent some credence to the concept of a developmental mechanism. The familial occurrence of aneurysms also gives support to a developmental etiology. However, the very low prevalence of cerebral aneurysm in infancy and childhood indicates that the lesions themselves are not congenital; at best, a predisposition toward later aneurysm formation might be present at birth. Some reports indicate a degenerative or inflammatory mechanism (66, 71). Evidence includes the finding of abundant destruction of elastica in aneurysmal walls (11) and liposome-like granules in close association with the disintegrating elastica (13).

Occasionally, aneurysms may be caused by trauma (7, 26), infection (8), or tumor (16). Traumatic aneurysms caused by head injury are an infrequent cause of subarachnoid hemorrhage. Bacterial aneurysms usually arise as a sequel to bacterial endocarditis and typically occur in distal branches of the cerebral arterial tree (see Chapter 21). Atrial myxoma is occasionally associated with multiple intracranial aneurysms, which result from tumor emboli that invade and destroy the arterial wall.

PATHOLOGY

Intracranial aneurysms arise at specific sites in the cerebral circulation (13). Approximately 85% occur in the anterior circulation. Most aneurysms of the anterior circulation are located on the anterior communicating, the internal carotid, and the middle cerebral arteries. Except for aneurysms in the region of the genu of the pericallosal artery, aneurysms arising on the distal branches of these vessels are almost always bacterial in origin. Aneurysms in the posterior circulation are most common at the apex of the basilar artery and at the origin of the posterior-inferior cerebellar artery. The reported incidence of multiple intracranial aneurysms ranges from 12–31%, and of bilateral aneurysms, particularly in mirror locations, 9–19% (82). In patients with aneurysms, 1.1% are reported to have intracranial arteriovenous malformations (55). The majority of aneurysms in this situation are on the major feeding artery or proximal portion of the feeding artery system (82). For these reasons, complete angiography should be performed in every patient known to harbor a single lesion.

Gross examination of aneurysms indicates origin from bifurcations of major proximal intracranial arteries (Fig. 10.1 A and B) (13, 71). Most of these lesions have a definable neck for surgical clipping. Aneurysms may be classified according to size: small lesions are less than 15 mm in diameter; large lesions 15–25 mm, and giant lesions above 25 mm. In giant aneurysms, thickening, thrombosis, and calcification of the wall are often seen.

Histopathologic examination reveals thinning of the arterial wall with absence of internal elastic lamina (Fig. 10.1C). The location of this attenuation corresponds to medial defects which appear at branch points in normal arteries. Cerebral arteries are particularly vulnerable to the mechanical effects of pulse pressure, as they have little external elastic lamina and no extrinsic tissue support.

PATHOPHYSIOLOGY

A summary of pathophysiologic features and complications of subarachnoid hemorrhage is presented in Fig. 10.2 and Table 10.1. Growth of aneurysms has been documented by serial angiography (2, 62). Because of the propensity of aneurysms to enlarge, and the fact that larger aneurysms are more inclined to rupture (82), small aneurysms (less than 7 mm) should be followed with angiographic examination at 1-year intervals. The water hammer effect of the pulse causes ballooning of the normal gap in internal elastic lamina found at an arterial bifurcation. Proliferation of adventitia thickens the neck of the aneurysm, while the fundus expands in response to transmural pulsatile forces.

Aneurysmal rupture may lead to minor or catastrophic intracranial hemorrhage (Fig. 10.1A) (43, 74). The pressure of the pulse finally pierces a tiny hole in the aneurysm fundus. Bleeding is probably very brief in most instances, leading to headache, nausea, vomiting, and (less frequently) loss of consciousness. In some cases, massive hemorrhage quickly fills the basal cisterns and ventricular system, leading to coma and death. More commonly, bleeding is stopped by tissue pressure and the formation of fibrin-platelet plug at the site of rupture (21).

Increased intracranial pressure is a common sequel of acute subarachnoid bleeding from intracranial aneurysms. Hayashi et al. showed that impaired consciousness in patients with acute subarachnoid hemorrhage is usually related to increased intracranial pressure rather than cerebral vasospasm (32). Raised intracranial pressure may act to retard recurrent subarachnoid hemorrhage. Subsequently, communicating hydrocepahlus with normal or increased ICP may develop, particularly when bleeding is severe in the basal cisterns.

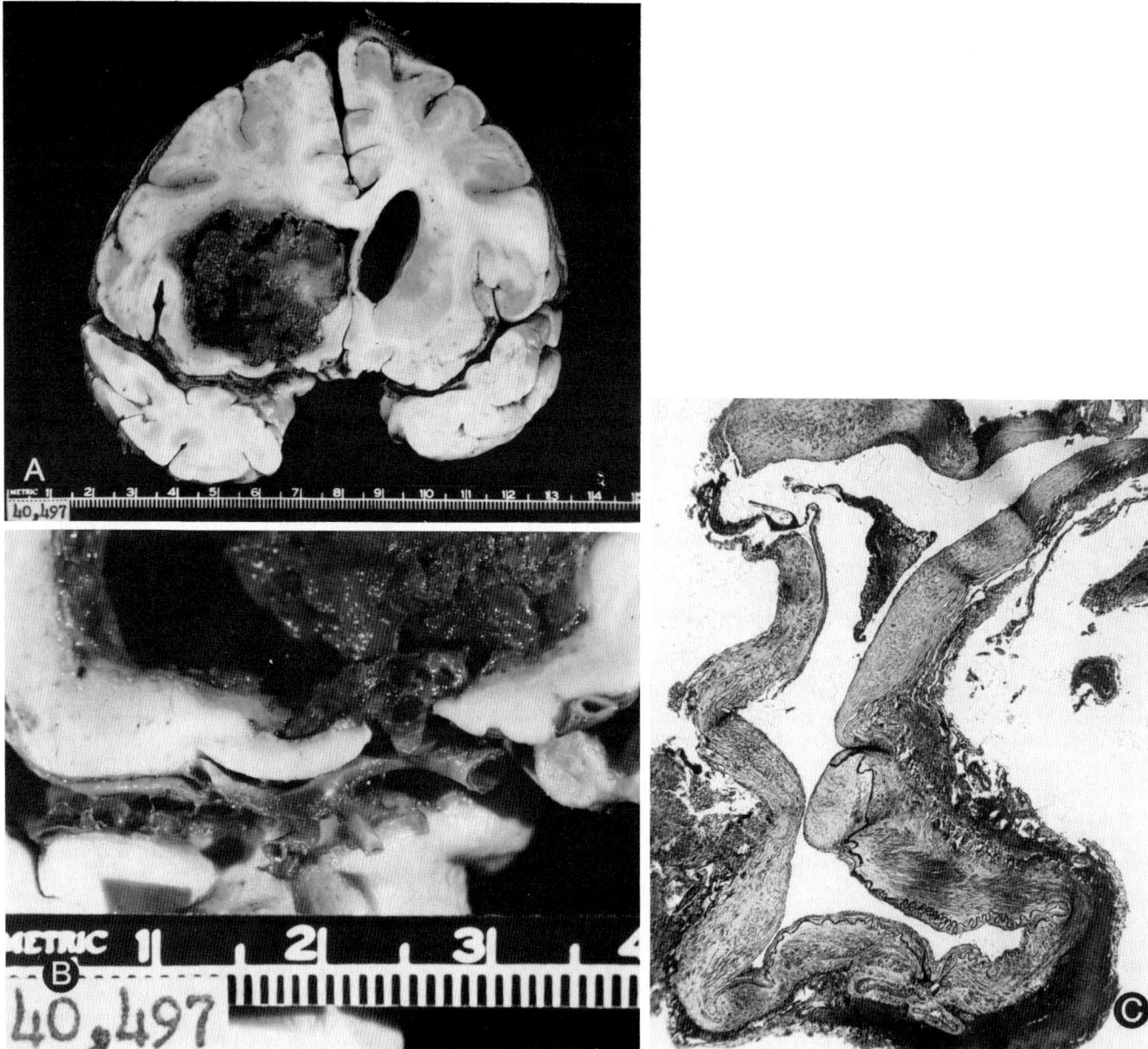

Figure 10.1 Ruptured internal carotid artery bifurcation aneurysm. *A*, intracerebral hemorrhage. Patient expired from intracranial mass effect with shift of midline structures. *B*, closer view shows aneurysm projecting superiorly into the hematoma. There is a well-defined neck. *C*, microscopic section of aneurysm shows the parent artery (*bottom*) with thick muscular walls and elastic laminae. The aneurysm (*above*) has absent elastica and rupture point at upper left.

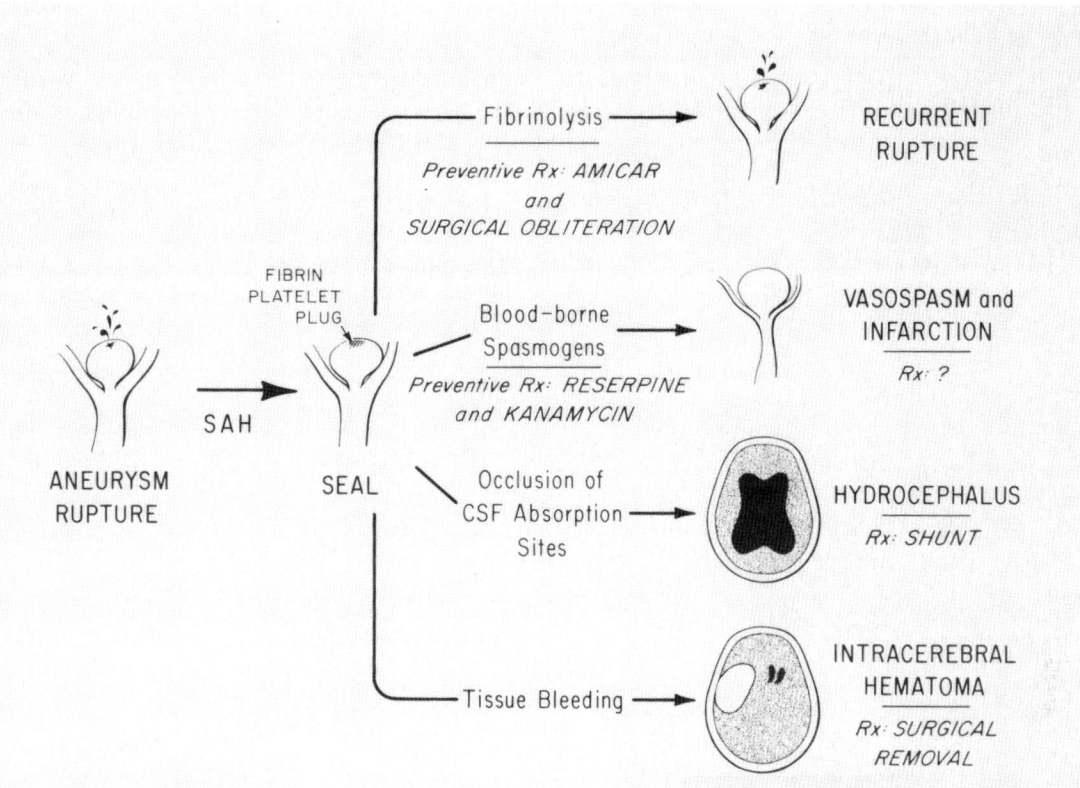

Figure 10.2 Complications of aneurysmal subarachnoid bleeding.

Hypothalamic irritation by subarachnoid bleeding may lead to a variety of systemic abnormalities (36, 79). Electrolyte imbalance is common and may be due to contraction of intravascular volume or inappropriate secretion of antidiuretic hormone (44, 49). Cardiac abnormalities are sometimes observed, including cardiac arrhythmias (15). In some patients, electrocardiographic changes may suggest myocardial infarction. More commonly, electrocardiographic changes are transient and unaccompanied by cardiac enzyme abnormalities. Q waves, elevated ST segments, and ST- and T-wave changes are commonly observed. Hormonal abnormalities have been observed, including abnormal levels of hydroxycorticosteroids, abnormal dexamethasone suppression test, and disturbance of the normal circadian secretion of steroid hormones (15).

Neurological complications are common following subarachnoid hemorrhage (Fig. 10.2) (Table 10.1). These include deficits due to intracerebral hematoma, ischemia, hydrocephalus and recurrent subarachnoid hemorrhage. Seizures may occur. Vision may be impaired secondary to subhyaloid hemorrhage, and rarely vitreous hemorrhage.

Cerebrovascular vasospasm with cerebral infarction is a poorly understood and frequent complication of subarachnoid hemorrhage (Figs. 10.3 and 10.4) (24, 33, 37, 81). Vasospasm is defined as radiographically measurable constriction of cerebral arteries after aneurysm bleeding. This arterial constriction may lead to cerebral ischemia and infarction with attendant delayed ischemic deficit.

Two general mechanisms seem important in the evolution of cerebral vasospasm: In one, vasoconstrictive substances are released by activated platelets, cerebral tissue, or red blood cells (9, 12, 30, 56). Serotonin, prostaglandins, and thromboxanes are among the substances thought to be important. Additionally, the decomposing products of hemolyzing blood, including protein and hemoglobin catabolites, may possibly be vasoactive agents. In the second mechanism hypothalamic dysfunction may result in the generalized discharge of catecholamines which in turn constrict cerebral arteries, particularly those irritated by subarachnoid blood and unable to deactivate circulating catecholamines (80). If regional cerebral blood flow is not reduced below a critical threshold, constriction of the large conducting vessels may produce no symptoms at all. If the constriction is severe and blood flow falls below the critical threshold, there may be symptomatic cerebral ischemia and perhaps infarction (Figs. 10.3 and 10.4).

Subarachnoid hemorrhage also causes other cerebrovascular sequelae. In a study using O^{15}, cerebral blood flow and cerebral oxygen utilization were significantly decreased, whether or not vasospasm was

Table 10.1
Complications of Subarachnoid Hemorrhage

Complications	Clinical Features	Diagnostic Tests	Therapy
Increased intracranial pressure	Headache, decreased alertness	CT, ventricular puncture, subarachnoid bolt	Steroids, mannitol, hyperventilation
Intracerebral hematoma	Immediate focal deficit	CT	Steroids, mannitol, consider evacuation
Vasospasm and infarction	Delayed focal deficit	CT, angiography, cerebral blood flow	Volume replacement, blood pressure maintenance (? drugs)
Seizures	Focal motor seizures	CT, EEG	Anticonvulsants
Hydrocephalus	Decreased alertness, increased deficit	CT	Ventricular drainage or ventriculoperitoneal shunt
Recurrent subarachnoid hemorrhage	Recurrent headache or deterioration	CT or lumbar puncture	Aneurysm obliteration
Hypothalamic disturbance: SIADH, cerebral salt wasting	Neurologic deterioration	Serum and urine electrolytes, blood volume	Fluid restriction (IV saline in some cases)
Cardiac abnormalities	Arrhythmia, myocardial infarct	EKG, cardiac enzymes	Therapy of arrhythmia; therapy of myocardial infarction
Hypertension	Increased blood pressure		Antihypertensive medication
Vitreous hemorrhage	Blindness	Fundoscopy	Observation; sometimes vitrectomy

present (29, 30). In patients with severe narrowing of cerebral arteries, there was marked depression of cerebral blood flow and cerebral oxygen utilization, and a significant increase in cerebral blood volume.

CLINICAL PRESENTATION

Premonitory symptoms may precede rupture in as many as 60% of the cases (38). Localized periorbital pain with diplopia and/or ptosis indicates compression of the third nerve, generally by an internal carotid-posterior communicating artery aneurysm. This presentation is of sufficient diagnostic accuracy as to warrant emergency angiography and surgical intervention, if indicated (38). Headache with poor localization, nausea, back pain, lethargy, and photophobia may also be associated with intracranial aneurysm, but these symptoms are not specific or diagnostic.

Giant cerebral aneurysms may present as mass lesions. These lesions, arising most frequently from the middle cerebral and internal carotid arteries, may give rise to slow and progressive hemiparesis and dysphasia (see Chapter 20). Careful CT evaluation with and without contrast material may lead to the correct diagnosis (Fig. 10.5) (18).

Ischemic deficit is unusual in the absence of vasospasm. Occasionally, embolization from an aneurysmal sack partially filled with clot may cause TIAs or symptomatic infarction (5).

Subarachnoid hemorrhage is the most frequent presentation of intracranial aneurysm (43, 59). Some episodes of subarachnoid bleeding are of a minor nature, with little or no resultant neurological dysfunction. The headache of subarachnoid hemorrhage is described as excruciating, usually of sudden onset, sometimes associated with brief loss of consciousness, nausea and vomiting, neck pain, back pain, photophobia, and generalized malaise. If the patient reports "the worst headache of my life," SAH must be suspected. In many instances, the ictus of subarachnoid hemorrhage is related to physical effort, and a history of subarachnoid bleeding in relation to intercourse is not uncommon. In some cases, "seizure" is the presenting complaint. These symptoms may be accompanied by immediate transient neurological deficits, including hemiparesis, aphasia, or third-nerve palsy.

Immediate neurological deficits persist in many patients. The generalized insult from bleeding may be expressed as acute confusion, fever, or hyperten-

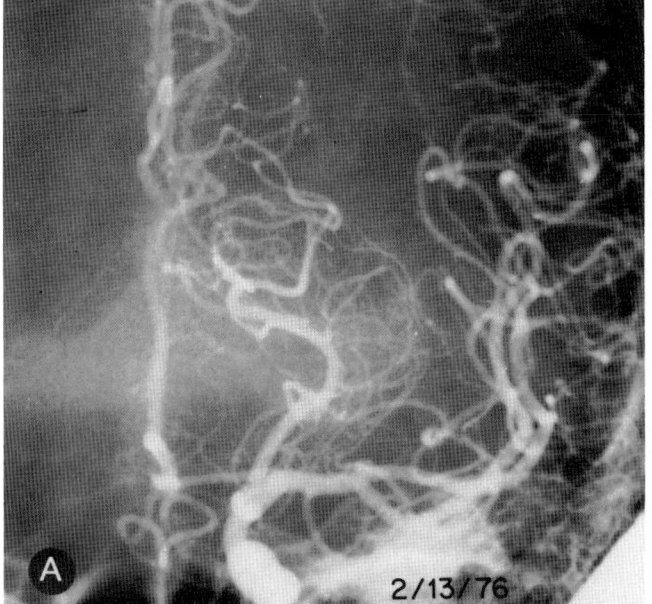
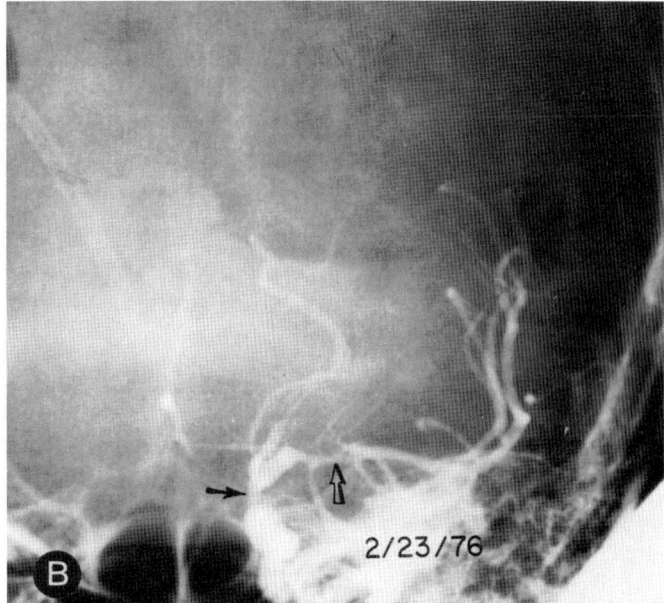
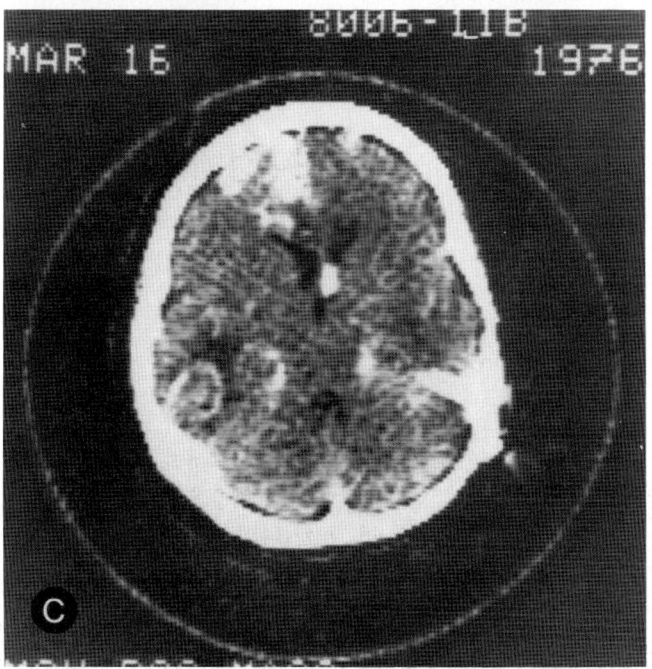

Figure 10.3 Delayed cerebral vasopsasm and infarction after SAH (no source identified). *A*, AP left carotid angiogram 1 day after SAH is normal with fetal left posterior cerebral artery. *B*, angiogram 11 days after SAH shows marked narrowing of ICA (*closed arrow*), MCA (*open arrow*), P1 segment of PCA, and anterior cerebral artery which barely fills. *C*, CT with contrast 29 days after SAH shows marked left frontal enhancement consistent with infarction. Shunt catheter tip in right lateral ventricle with resolution of hydrocephalus.

sion. Pre-retinal hemorrhage, a distinctive fingerprint of subarachnoid bleeding, is frequently present. A Babinski sign, hemiparesis, or dysphasia may point to contralateral middle cerebral or internal carotid territory disease. A sixth-nerve palsy or other lower cranial nerve dysfunction may suggest posterior fossa pathology, although an isolated sixth-nerve palsy may simply reflect increased intracranial pressure. Acute confusion, memory disturbance, and personality change may result from an anterior communicating aneurysm.

The classification offered by Botterell (10), and modified by Hunt (34) has proved useful to many clinicians (Tables 10.2 and 10.3). In general, patients in grades 1 and 2 are managed medically for about 10 days; operation is then indicated to prevent recurrent hemorrhage. Patients in grades 3 and 4 are allowed 2 to 3 weeks to stabilize before surgery. Patients showing a progressive neurological deficit may need operation for removal of life-threatening hematomas or for placement of a shunt for hydrocephalus.

Delayed complications of subarachnoid hemorrhage are frequent and protean (Table 10.1) (Fig. 10.2) (14). The three common causes of delayed neurological deficit are vasospasm, hydrocephalus, and recurrent subarachnoid hemorrhage. Symptomatic vaso-

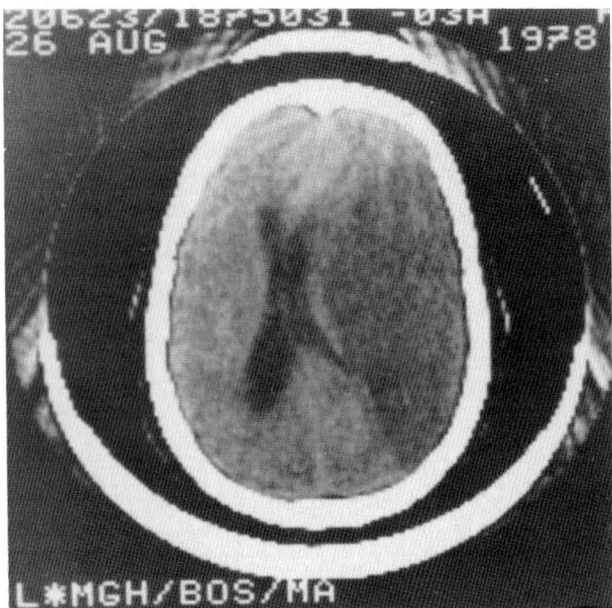

Figure 10.4 CT depicts cerebral infarction due to vasospasm. The entire MCA territory shows low density change from infarction. MCA aneurysm ruptured 2 weeks prior to this scan.

Table 10.2
Assessment of Patients with SAH (Botterell (10))

Grade 1	Conscious ± signs of subarachnoid blood
Grade 2	Drowsy without significant deficit
Grade 3	Drowsy with a neurological deficit
Grade 4	Deteriorating with major neurological deficit
Grade 5	Moribund with extensor rigidity and failing vital signs

Table 10.3
Assessment of Patients with SAH (Hunt and Hess (34))

Grade I	Asymptomatic, or minimal headache and slight nuchal rigidity.
Grade II	Moderate to severe headache, nuchal rigidity, no neurological deficit other than cranial nerve palsy.
Grade III	Drowsiness, confusion, or mild focal deficit.
Grade IV	Stupor, moderate to severe hemiparesis, possibly early decerebrate rigidity and vegetative disturbances.
Grade V	Deep coma, decerebrate rigidity, moribund appearance.

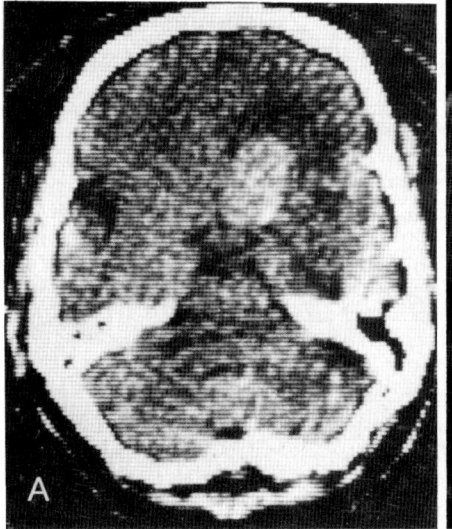 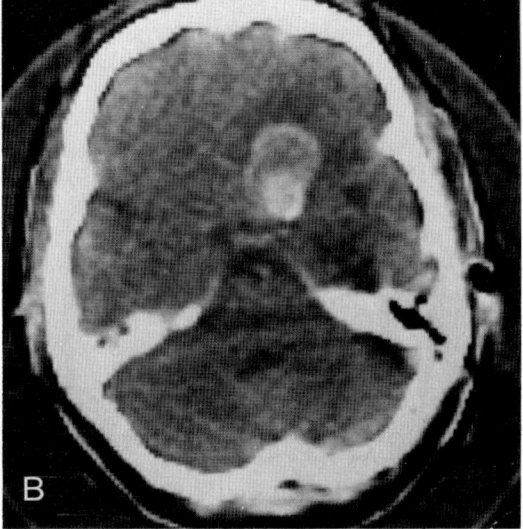

Figure 10.5 CT demonstration of giant carotid-ophthalmic aneurysm. Before (A) and after (B) contrast enhancement. Dense zone is residual lumen. Mixed density zone is mural thrombus. Frontal low density is edema (findings confirmed at surgery).

spasm rarely develops before the third day. Hydrocephalus generally decreases the level of alertness and may exacerbate focal neurological deficit. Subarachnoid hemorrhage may recur with or without obvious headache. CT scanning and lumbar puncture can identify recurrent subarachnoid hemorrhage or hydrocephalus.

The problem of rebleeding has been reviewed by Jane et al. (35, 82). Recurrent hemorrhage is most likely early after SAH with the rebleeding incidence curve falling to a plateau at about 6 weeks. Thereafter, anterior and posterior communicating aneurysms rebleed at a rate of 3–4% per year for at least 20 years and two-thirds of the patients who rebleed die. Factors associated with rebleeding include poor clinical grade on admission, hypertension, older age, aneurysm pointing upward, short broad aneurysms, and aneurysm enlargement on serial angiograms.

The clinical syndrome of delayed ischemic deficit, occurring in 20-36% (57), is marked by neurological deterioration occurring from 4 to 16 days after initial hemorrhage, with peak incidence on day 8 after SAH (24). Minor symptoms of drowsiness are commonly followed by hemiparesis or hemiplegia, aphasia, or other focal neurological abnormalities. In the most severe cases, increased intracranial pressure and death may occur. When the problem is less severe, gradual recovery may begin within a few days and in some cases be quite complete.

It has been clearly demonstrated that severe vasospasm is the cause of delayed neurological symptoms. In 50 patients with subarachnoid hemorrhage, 31 had severe arterial constriction and 25 developed delayed ischemic deficits (24). Cerebral symptoms were not present unless major cerebral arteries were narrowed to less than 1 mm in diameter.

Diagnosis of cerebral vasospasm cannot rest on clinical criteria alone. Headache and neurological deterioration, including focal neurological signs, may stem from inappropriate secretion of antidiuretic hormone, dehydration, drug intoxication, rebleeding, or hydrocephalus. Definitive diagnosis of vasospasm rests on angiographic demonstration of severely constricted arteries.

MEDICAL EVALUATION

When admitted, every patient with SAH should have an electrocardiogram, bleeding studies (prothrombin time, partial thromboplastin time, and platelet count), serum electrolytes, and serum osmolarity. Noninvasive vascular evaluations of the lower extremities (plethysmography) may be used to screen for deep vein thrombosis, which may occur in patients treated with epsilon animocaproic acid. In patients where there are EKG abnormalities or where induced hypotension is planned during surgery, cardiac consultation is indicated.

Computed Tomography

Computed tomography (CT) has revolutionized the investigation of subarachnoid hemorrhage (17, 61). CT may establish the diagnosis by showing blood in the basal cisterns, interhemispheric fissure, ventricles or adjacent brain tissue (Fig. 10.6). In patients with suspected SAH, especially those with significant neurological deficit, CT should be performed as the initial diagnostic study. This test should be done before lumbar puncture is considered to avoid the risk of transtentorial herniation.

CT scanning permits accurate diagnosis of the etiology of subarachnoid hemorrhage in many patients. The location, form, and distribution of hemorrhage, together with direct enhancement of the aneurysm itself, may establish the diagnosis of intracranial aneurysm. Cerebral arteriovenous malformations may be demonstrated in unenhanced and, more

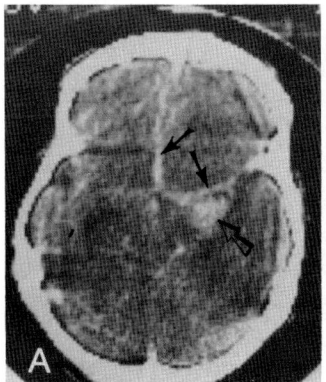 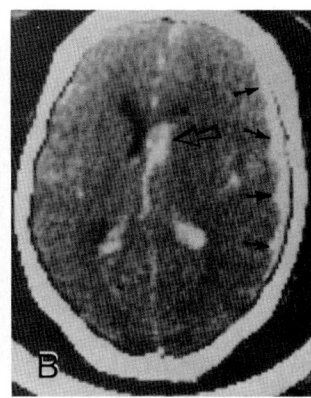

Figure 10.6 CT depicts aneurysmal hemorrhage. *A, closed arrows* show subarachnoid blood. *Open arrow* shows intracerebral clot. *B, closed arrows* indicate subdural hematoma. *Open arrow* shows intraventricular hematoma.

commonly, in enhanced CT scans. The appearance of giant intracranial aneurysms, with enhanced residual lumen and unenhanced high density mural thrombus, is particularly distinctive in CT depiction (Fig. 10.5) (41). In some patients with multiple cerebral aneurysms or arteriovenous malformation, CT may specify which of the various lesions has actually bled.

Computed tomography is also useful for the diagnosis of complications of subarachnoid hemorrhage, including recurrent SAH, hydrocephalus, and cerebral infarction (Figs. 10.3C, 10.4, and 10.7C). To permit the rapid accurate diagnosis of these adverse developments, CT scanning should be performed promptly after any deterioration and compared to the CT done on admission.

CT can help predict vasospasm (23, 75). Fisher and colleagues found a high incidence of severe vasospasm in cases with CT demonstration of globular clots or thick layers of subarachnoid blood (23 of 24 cases) (23). All of the patients with severe vasospasm showed signs of ischemia in the cerebral territories corresponding to the vasospastic arteries. Thus, the presence of extensive subarachnoid hematoma seemed a reliable prognostic index to later development of symptomatic vasospasm and in the absence of thick subarachnoid clot, vasospasm usually failed to develop.

These findings have important implications for therapy. Because patients in jeopardy from vasospasm may be identified, preventive measures can be considered for these high risk patients and initiated early after hemorrhage. Early operation might be used to remove the offending clot and obliterate the aneurysm in order to permit the use of induced hypertension if ischemia develops.

For patients without SAH where intracranial aneurysm is suspected, CT may also be useful. Thin sections (2 mm) with contrast enhancement may reveal an aneurysm on or near the circle of Willis (82). In the future, ultrahigh resolution and reconstruction techniques may be helpful, but at the present time only angiography can establish the diagnosis.

Lumbar Puncture

In cases of suspected subarachnoid bleeding lumbar puncture should be used only when CT is not available or where CT is negative because it occasionally precipitates aneurysm rupture or transtentorial herniation. To make certain that bloody CSF is not the result of a traumatic tap, a CSF sample should be centrifuged to detect xanthochromic supernatant. Occasionally, repeat lumbar puncture is required to document subarachnoid bleeding, as cisternal blood may take several hours to migrate to the lumbar subarachnoid space.

Angiography

Angiography should demonstrate the aneurysmal sac and neck and their relation to parent arteries (Fig. 10.7 (2, 3, 19). Satisfactory visualization will often require oblique and base views. To exclude an arterial loop, the aneurysm should be demonstrated in two projections. To assure visualization of the anterior communicating artery complex, compression of one carotid artery may be used during injection of the contralateral carotid artery. To exclude multiple lesions, 4-vessel angiography is recommended. Subtraction techniques are often useful to delineate vascular anatomy near the base of the skull. Stereoscopic views contribute to a three-dimensional appreciation of cerebral aneurysms.

Careful inspection of the initial CT scan may diagnose the cause of SAH. If not, angiography can be done shortly after admission if the patient is grade one or two. However, some surgeons wait until a day or two before operation before performing this study in order to determine the degree of vasospasm and to avoid doing two studies.

Suspected vasospasm is also an indication for angiography. Since angiography may exacerbate spasm, the study is terminated once arterial narrowing has been documented. We have found it helpful to grade spasm according to the diameter of the residual arterial lumen: 0 = no narrowing, + = slight narrowing, ++ = about 1 mm in diameter, +++ = lumen about 0.5 mm with indistinct outline, and ++++ = lumen less than 0.5 mm, flow is delayed, and often collateral flow crosses borderzone anastomoses. These figures apply to proximal ACA and MCA; for supraclinoid ICA, they are about 1 mm greater (24).

The technique of digital intravenous subtraction angiography (DSA) will likely find a role in the evaluation of some aneurysm patients (42). Already, some giant lesions have been imaged with this method. If resolution improves, DSA may supplant standard angiography for some patients being evaluated for aneurysm who have not had a subarachnoid hemorrhage.

Table 10.4
Medical Therapy for Aneurysmal SAH

1) Bed rest in a quiet, darkened room.
2) Fluid administration aimed to maintain normal circulating volume and central venous pressure.
3) Elastic stockings or pneumatic compression boots.
4) Epsilon aminocaproic acid (30 gm per day intravenously via continuous infusion).
5) Anticonvulsants (diphenylhydantoin, 300 mg/day).
6) Stool softeners (Colace, 100 mg TID).
7) For agitation, phenobarbital (15–30 mg IM or PO Q3H).
8) For hypertension, hydralazine (5–20 mg IM Q3h), to bring the systolic pressure below 150 mm Hg without causing drowsiness. In some cases propranolol is used, and occasionally resistant hypertension requires intravenous nitroprusside for control.
9) Methylprednisolone (16–80 mg PO or IV Q6h), to reduce cerebral swelling in symptomatic patients.
10) Cimetidine is given (300 mg PO or IV Q8h), along with antacid by mouth or gastric tube every 3 hours.
11) Codeine for headache (30–60 mg PO or IM Q3-4h).
12) Kanamycin, 1 gm TID, and reserpine, 0.2 mg SC TID may be considered to reduce the chance of postoperative vasospasm. These drugs are given only to grade 1 and 2 patients without other contraindications.

MEDICAL MANAGEMENT

Several reports have outlined medical treatment for patients with subarachnoid hemorrhage (25, 54). Our program is summarized in Table 10.4. "Aneurysm precautions" usually include a quiet room, limited visitors, and complete bed rest (51). Fluid administration is designed to maintain a normal blood volume. Stool softeners are given to avoid straining. Sedatives are administered to avoid upset and consequent hypertension. Anticonvulsants are prescribed to prevent seizures. Corticosteroid therapy is begun in patients with neurological deficit, increased intracranial pressure, or intractable headache.

Since fibrinolysins in cerebrospinal fluid lyse the clot sealing the aneurysm leak, antifibrinolytic therapy is a logical approach to prevent recurrent bleeding. Several studies indicate that the incidence of rebleeding is substantially diminished in patients who receive the antifibrinolytic agent epsilon aminocaproic acid (EACA) (27, 45, 47, 48, 50). The recommended dose of EACA is 30–36 gm/day, administered intravenously until surgery or for three weeks if surgery is not performed. Some authors have recommended oral therapy (63). The use of antifibrinolytic therapy, however, carries a small risk of thrombotic or ischemic complications, and some authorities recommend caution in its use (65). To prevent deep vein thrombosis in the lower extremities, intermittent pneumatic calf compression may be useful.

Antihypertensive therapy is used in many centers to prevent recurrent bleeding. However, lowering the

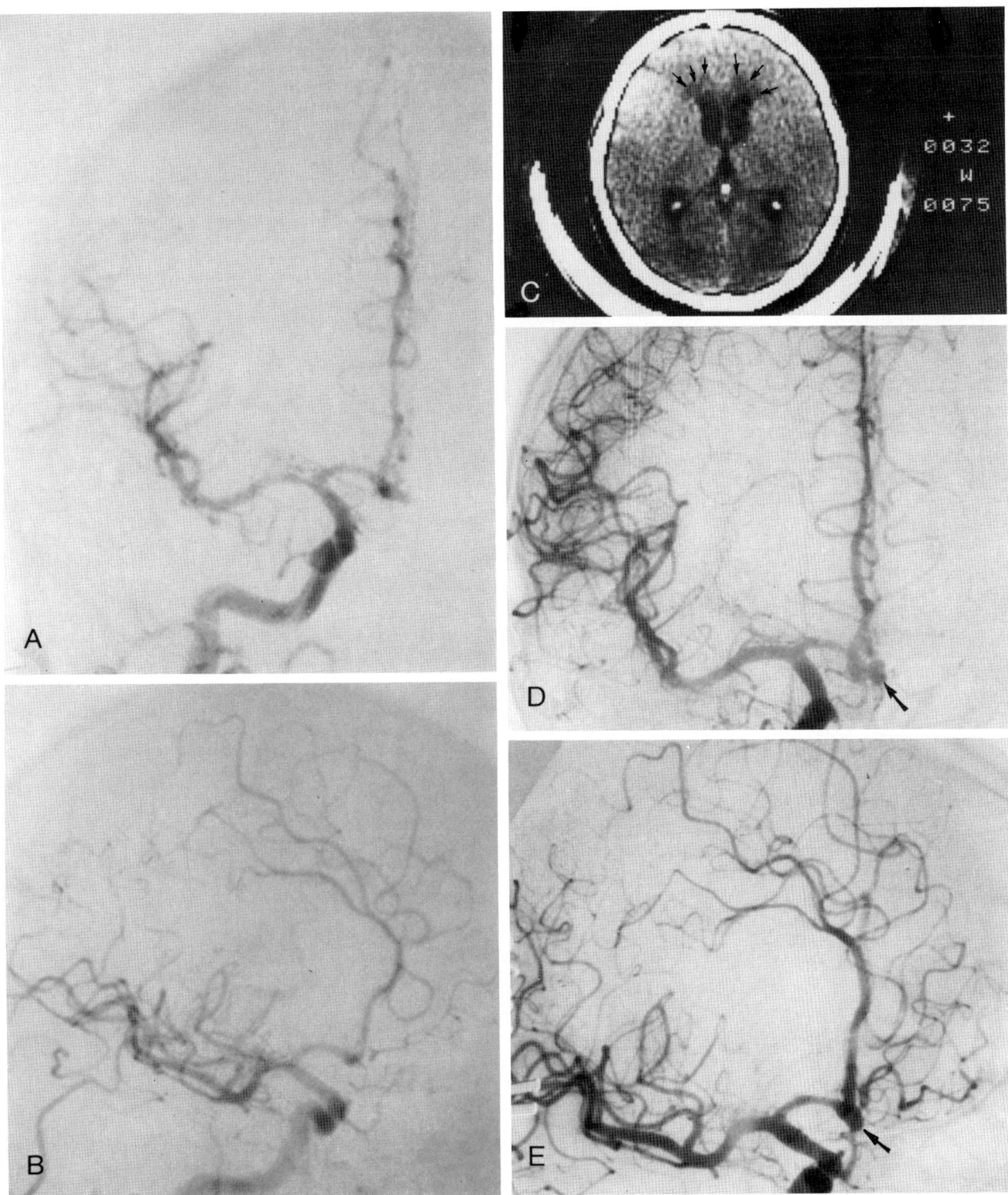

Figure 10.7 Repeat angiography discloses anterior communicating aneurysm. A and B, right carotid angiogram performed 2 days after SAH shows no definite aneurysm or spasm even with an oblique view to show the anterior communicating complex. Left carotid angiogram was normal. C, CT scan 1 week after SAH shows low density anterior to ventricles (*arrows*) suggesting infarction due to anterior cerebral spasm. D and E, repeat right carotid angiogram 3 weeks after SAH shows anterior communicating aneurysm (*arrow*).

blood pressure to hypotensive levels may exacerbate ischemia in patients with ruptured aneurysms. We administer antihypertensive medication (hydralazine, propranolol) only to achieve normal blood pressure. Occasionally, marked hypertension can be controlled only with intravenous agents, such as trimethaphan camsylate or nitroprusside (60).

Should a patient deteriorate, metabolic studies and CT are rechecked. Electrolyte imbalance may require correction. CT may reveal evidence of recurrent hemorrhage, hydrocephalus, cerebral edema or infarction. If a clear explanation of deterioration is not found, and the clinical picture suggests recurrent hemorrhage, lumbar puncture may be indicated; if the clinical picture suggests vasospasm, angiography is performed.

Management of increased intracranial pressure may be guided by neurological symptoms and signs, CT scanning, and at times monitoring with a Richmond bolt or ventriculostomy. In deteriorating patients (grades 3-5), mannitol and hyperventilation may be beneficial. Progressive hydrocephalus requires ventriculoperitoneal shunting for relief of symptoms.

Cerebrovascular vasospasm remains a difficult problem in management. A large number of experimental and clinical therapies have been used in the treatment of vasospasm (64, 68, 81). Reserpine and Kanamycin reduce blood serotonin, an agent known to cause vasoconstriction. Prophylactic administration of these agents has been reported to diminish the incidence of delayed ischemia deficits, particularly after operation (84, 85).

Volume expansion and moderate hypertension appear to be beneficial for angiographically proven, symptomatic vasospasm (20, 28). For these patients, a program of therapy is begun, with monitoring of radial arterial pressure and central venous pressure. The intravascular volume is increased with colloid or packed cells to achieve a central venous pressure of 10-12 cm of water and a hematocrit of 35-40%. A pressor is given to increase the systolic blood pressure to about 30 mm Hg above basal levels with a maximum of 160 mm Hg. Phenylephrine or Dopamine may be used for this purpose.

If the initial angiographic study is normal, medical therapy is continued until about 2-3 weeks after SAH. The study is then repeated (6, 77). On occasion, a lesion may be seen, presumably because a thrombus has lyzed, spasm has improved, or compression from edema or clot has subsided (Fig. 10.7). If the second study is negative, EACA is stopped and the patient gradually ambulated. Such patients are readmitted for angiogram 3 months later. If this study is negative, the prognosis is good.

REFERENCES

1. Aitken RR, Drake CG: A technique of anesthesia with induced hypotension for surgical correction of intracranial aneurysms. Clin Neurosurg 21:107-114, 1974.
2. Allcock JM, Canham PB: Angiographic study of the growth of intracranial aneurysms. J Neurosurg 45:617-621, 1976.
3. Allcock JM, Drake CG: Ruptured intracranial aneurysms—the role of arterial spasm. J Neurosurg 22:21-29, 1965.
4. Amacher AL, Ferguson GG, Drake CG, Girvin JP, Barr HWK: How old people tolerate intracranial surgery for aneurysm. Neurosurgery 1:242-244, 1977.
5. Antunes JL, Correll JW: Cerebral emboli from intracranial aneurysms. Surg Neurol 6:7-10, 1976.
6. Forster DMC, Steiner L, Hakanson S, Bergvall U: The value of repeat pan-angiography in cases of unexplained subarachnoid hemorrhage. J Neurosurg 48:712-716, 1978.
7. Benoit BG, Wortzman G: Traumatic cerebral aneurysms: clinical features and natural history. J Neurol Neurosurg Psychiat 36:127-138, 1973.
8. Bingham WF: Treatment of mycotic intracranial aneurysms. J Neurosurg 46:428-437, 1977.
9. Blaso WP, Mistry G, duBoulay GH, Forster DMC, Boullin, DJ: The Relationship of Vasoactive Substances in CSF of Subarachnoid Hemorrhage Patients to Cerebral Vasospasm and Prognosis, in Wilkins RH (ed): Cerebral Arterial Spasm, Baltimore, Williams & Wilkins, 1979, pp 144-157.
10. Botterell EH, Lougheed WM, Scott JW, Vandewater SL; Hypothermia, and interruption of carotid, or carotid and vertebral circulation, in the surgical management of intracranial aneurysms. J Neurosurg 13:1-42, 1956.
11. Cajander S, Hassler O: Enzymatic destruction of the elastic lamella at the mouth of cerebral berry aneurysm? An ultrastructural study with special regard to the elastic tissue. Acta Neurol Scand 53:171-181, 1976.
12. Clower BR, Haining JL, Smith, RR: Pathophysiological Changes in the Cerebral Artery after Subarachnoid Hemorrhage, in Wilkins RH (ed): Cerebral Arterial Spasm, Baltimore, Williams & Wilkins, 1979, pp 124-131.
13. Crompton MR: The pathology of subarachnoid hemorrhage. J R Coll Physicians Lond 7:235-237, 1973.
14. Crowell RM, Zervas NT: Management of intracranial aneurysm. Med Clin N Am 63:695-713, 1979.
15. Cruickshank JM, Neil-Dwyer G, Stott AW: Possible role of catecholamines, corticosteroids, and potassium in production of electrocardiographic abnormalities associated with subarachnoid hemorrhage. Br Heart J 36:697-706, 1974.
16. Damasio H, Seabra-Gomes R, da Silva JP, Damasio AR, Antunes JL: Multiple cerebral aneurysms and cardiac myxoma. Arch Neurol 32:269-270, 1975.
17. Davis KR, New PFJ, Ojemann RG, Crowell RM, Morawetz RB, Roberson GH: Computed tomographic evaluation of hemorrhage secondary to intracranial aneurysm. Am J Roentgen 127:143-153, 1976.
18. Drake CG: Giant intracranial aneurysms: Experience with surgical treatment in 174 patients, Clin Neurosurg, 25:12-95, 1979.
19. Drake CG: Management of cerebral aneurysm. Stroke 12:273-283, 1981.
20. Farhat SM, Schneider RC: Observations on the effect of systemic blood pressure on intracranial circulation in patients with cerebrovascular insufficiency. J Neurosurg 27:441-445, 1967.
21. Fisher CM, Ojemann RG: Basal rupture of saccular aneurysm. A pathological case report. J Neurosurg 48:642-644, 1978.
22. Fisher CM, Kistler JP, Davis JM: The Correlation of Cerebral Vasospasm and the Amount of Subarachnoid Blood Detected by Computerized Cranial Tomography after Aneurysm Rupture, in Williams RH (ed): Cerebral Arterial Spasm, Baltimore, Williams & Wilkins, 1979, pp 397-408.
23. Fisher CM, Kistler JP, Davis JM: Relation of cerebral vasospasm to subarachnoid hemorrhage visualized by computerized tomographic scanning. Neurosurgery 6:1-4, 1980.
24. Fisher CM, Roberson GH, Ojemann RG: Cerebral vasospasm with ruptured saccular aneurysm—the clinical manifestations. Neurosurgery 1:245-248, 1977.
25. Flamm ES: Parasurgical treatment of aneurysms. Clin Neurosurg 24:240-247, 1977.

26. Fleischer AS, Patton JM, Tindall GT: Cerebral aneurysms of traumatic origin. Surg Neurol 4:233–239, 1975.
27. Fodstad H, Liliequist B, Schannong M, Thulin CA: Tranexamic acid in the preoperative management of ruptured intracranial aneurysms. Surg Neurol 10:9–15, 1978.
28. Gianotta SL, McGillicuddy JE, Kindt GW: Diagnosis and treatment of postoperative cerebral vasospasm. Surg Neurol 8:286–290, 1977.
29. Grubb RL, Raichle ME, Eichling JO, Gado MH: Effects of subarachnoid hemorrhage on cerebral blood volume, blood flow, and oxygen utilization in humans. J Neurosurg 46:446–453, 1977.
30. Grubb L, Jr: Cerebral Hemodynamics and Metabolism in Subarachnoid Hemorrhage and Vasospasm, in Wilkins RH (ed): *Cerebral Arterial Spasm*, Baltimore, Williams & Wilkins, 1979, pp 341–349.
31. Hashimoto I: Familial intracranial aneurysms and cerebral vascular anomalies. J Neurosurg 46:419–427, 1977.
32. Hayashi M, Marukawa S, Fujii H, Kitano T, Kobayaski H, Yamamoto S: Intracranial hypertension in patients with ruptured intracranial aneurysm. J Neurosurg 46:584–590, 1977.
33. Heros RC, Zervas NT, Negoro M: Cerebral vasospasm. Surg Neurol 5:354–362, 1976.
34. Hunt WE, Hess RM: Surgical risk as related to time of intervention in the repair of intracranial aneurysms. J Neurosurg 28:14–20, 1968.
35. Jane JA, Winn HR, Richardson AE: The natural history of intracranial aneurysms: rebleeding rates during the acute and long-term period and implication for surgical management. Clin Neurosurg 24:176–184, 1976.
36. Jenkins JS, Buckell M, Carter AB, Westlake S: Hypothalmic-pituitary-adrenal function after subarachnoid hemorrhage. Br Med J 20:707–709, 1969.
37. Kassell NF, Peerless SJ, Drake CG: Cerebral Vasospasm: Acute Proliferative Vasculopathy? I. Hypothesis. in Wilkins RH (ed): *Cerebral Arterial Spasm*, Baltimore, Williams & Wilkins, 1979, pp 85–87.
38. King RB, Saba MI: Forewarnings of major subarachnoid hemorrhage due to congenital berry aneurysm. N Y St J Med 74:638–639, 1974.
39. Kurtzke JF: *Epidemiology of Cerebrovascular Disease*. Joint Council CVD, Survey Report, Rochester, Minnesota, Whiting Press, 1980.
40. Krayenbuhl HA, Yasargil MG, Flamm ES, Tew JM Jr: Microsurgical treatment of intracranial saccular aneurysms. J Neurosurg 37:678–686, 1972.
41. Lavyne MH, Kleefield J, Davis KR, Ojemann RG, Crowell RM: Giant intracranial aneurysms of the anterior circulation: clinical characteristics and diagnosis by computed tomography. Neurosurgery 3:356–363, 1978.
42. Little JR, Furlan AJ, Modic MT, Bryerton B, Weinstein MA: Intravenous digital subtraction angiography: Application to cerebrovascular surgery. Neurosurgery 9:129–136, 1981.
43. McCormick WF: The natural history of intracranial saccular aneurysms. Weekly Update. Nuerol Neurosurg 1:1–8, 1978.
44. Maroon JC, Nelson PB: Hypovolemia in patients with subarachnoid hemorrhage therapeutic implications. Neurosurgery 4:223–226, 1979.
45. Maurice-Williams RS: Prolonged antifibrinolysis: an effective non-surgical treatment for ruptured intracranial aneurysms? Br Med J 1:945–947, 1978.
46. Miller JD, Jawad K, Jennett B: Safety of carotid ligation and its role in the management of intracranial aneurysms. J Neurol Neurosurg Psychiat 40:64–72, 1977.
47. Mullen S, Dawley J: Antifibrinolytic therapy for intracranial aneurysms. J Neurosurg 28:21–23, 1968.
48. Mullen S, Hanlon K, Brown F: Management of 136 consecutive supratentorial berry aneurysms. J Neurosurg 49:794–804, 1978.
49. Nelson PB, Seif SM, Maroon JC, Robinson AG: Hyponatremia in Patients with Subarachnoid Hemorrhage: A Study of Vasopressin and Blood Volume, in Wilkins RH (ed): *Cerebral Arterial Spasm*, Baltimore, Williams & Wilkins, 1979, pp 654–658.
50. Nibbelink DW, Torner JC, Henderson WG: Intracranial aneurysms and subarachnoid hemorrhage. A cooperative study. Anti-fibrinolytic therapy in recent onset subarachnoid hemorrhage. Stroke 6:622–629, 1975.
51. Nibbelink DW, Torner JC, Henderson WG: Intracranial aneurysms and subarachnoid hemorrhage—report on a randomized treatment study. IV-A. Regulated bed rest. Stroke 8:202–221, 1977.
52. Ojemann RG: Management of the unruptured intracranial aneurysm. N Engl J Med 304:725–726, 1981.
53. Pakarinen S: Incidence, aetiology, and prognosis of primary subarachnoid hemorrhage. Acta Neurol Scand 43:1–127, 1967.
54. Peerless SJ: Pre- and postoperative management of cerebral aneurysms, Clin Neurosurg 26:209–231, 1979.
55. Perret G, Nishioka H: Report on the cooperative study of intracranial aneurysms and subarachnoid hemorrhage. Section VI arteriovenous malformations. J Neurosurg 25:467–490, 1966.
56. Pitts LH, MacPherson P, Wyper DJ, Jennett B, Blair I, Cooke MBD: Effects of Vasospasm on Cerebral Blood Flow after Subarachnoid Hemorrhage, in Wilkins RH (ed): *Cerebral Arterial Spasm*. Baltimore, Williams & Wilkins, 1979, pp 333–337.
57. Post KD, Flamm ES, Goodgold A, Ransohoff J: Ruptured intracranial aneurysms. Case morbidity and mortality. J Neurosurg 46:290–295, 1977.
58. Robinson JL, Hall CS, Sedzimir CB: Arteriovenous malformations, aneurysms and pregnancy. J Neurosurg 41:63–70, 1974.
59. Sahs AL, Nibbelink DW, Torner JC (eds): *Aneurysmal Subarachnoid Hemorrhage*, Baltimore, Urban & Schwarzenberg, 1981.
60. Samson DS, Hodash RM, Reid WR, Beyer CW, Clark WK: Risk of intracranial aneurysm surgery in the good grade patient: early versus late operation. Neurosurgery 5:422–426, 1979.
61. Scotti G, Ethier R, Melancon D, Terbrugge K, Tchang S: Computed tomography in the evaluation of intracranial aneurysms and subarachnoid hemorrhage. Radiology 123:85–90, 1977.
62. Sekhar LN, Heros RC: Origin, growth and rupture of saccular aneurysms: a review. Neurosurgery 8:248–260, 1981.
63. Sengupta RP, So SC, Villarejo-Ortega FJ: Use of epsilon aminocaproic acid (EACA) in the preoperative management of ruptured intracranial aneurysms. J Neurosurg 44:479–484, 1976.
64. Simeone FA, Vinall PE: Current concepts in the management of cerebral vasospasm, in Nelson E, Price TR (eds): *Cerebral Vascular Diseases. Proceedings of the Eleventh Princeton Conference*. New York, Raven Press, 1978.
65. Sonntag VKH, Stein BM: Arteriopathic complications during treatment of subarachnoid hemorrhage with epsilon-aminocaproic acid. J Neurosurg 40:480–485, 1974.
66. Stehbens WE: Ultrastructure of aneurysms. Arch Neurol 32:798–807, 1975.
67. Sundt T: Surgical technic for giant intracranial aneurysms, in Ransohoff J (ed): *Modern Technics in Surgery: Neurosurgery*. Mount Kisco, New York, Futura, 1981, pp 1–40.
68. Sundt TM Jr: Management of ischemic complications after subarachnoid hemorrhage. J Neurosurg 43:418–425, 1975.
69. Sundt TM, Jr, Whisnant JP: Subarachnoid hemorrhage from intracranial aneurysms. Surgical management and natural history of disease. N Engl J Med 299:116–122, 1978.
70. Suzuki J (ed): *Cerebral Aneurysms. Experiences with 1000 Directly Operated Cases*. Tokyo, Neuron, 1979.
71. Suzuki J, Ohara H: Clinicopathological study of cerebral aneurysms. Origin, rupture, repair, and growth. J Neurosurg 48:505–514, 1978.
72. Suzuki J, Yoshimoto T, Onuma T: Early operations for ruptured intracranial aneurysms—study of 31 cases operated on within the first four days after ruptured aneurysm. Neurol Med Chr 18:82–89, 1978.
73. Suzuki J, Onuma T, Yoshimoto T: Results of early operations on cerebral aneurysms. Surg Neurol 11:407–412, 1979.
74. Sypert GW: Intracranial aneurysms: Natural history and surgical management. Compr Ther 4:64–73, 1978.
75. Takemae T, Mizukami M, Kin H, Kawase T, Araki G: Computed tomography of ruptured intracranial aneurysm in acute stage—relationship between vasospasm and high density on CT scan. No To Shinkei 30:861–866, 1978.

76. Tindall GT: The treatment of anterior communicating aneurysms by proximal anterior cerebral artery ligation. Clin Neurosurg 21:134–150, 1974.
77. West HH, Mani RL, Eisenberg RL, Tuerk K, Stucker TB: Normal cerebral arteriography in patients with spontaneous subarachnoid hemorrhage. Neurology 27:592–594, 1977.
78. Wiebers DO, Whisnant JP, O'Fallon WM: The natural history of unruptured intracranial aneurysms. N Engl J Med 304:696–698, 1981.
79. Wilkins RH: Hypothalmic dysfunction and intracranial arterial spasm. Surg Neurol 4:472–480, 1975.
80. Wilkins RH: The role of intracranial artery spasm in the timing of operations for aneurysm. Clin Neurosurg 24:185–207, 1977.
81. Wilkins RH: Attempted Prevention or Treatment of Intracranial Arterial Spasm: A Survey, in Wilkins RH (ed): *Cerebral Arterial Spasm*. Baltimore, Williams & Wilkins, 1979, pp 542–555.
82. Wilkins RH: Update-subarachnoid hemorrhage and saccular intracranial aneurysm. Surg Neurol 15:92–101, 1981.
83. Winn HR, Richardson AE, Jane JA: The long-term prognosis in untreated cerebral aneurysms: I. The incidence of late hemorrhage in cerebral aneurysm: a 10-year evaluation of 364 patients. Ann Neurol 1:358–370, 1977.
84. Zervas NT, Candia M, Candia G, Kido D, Pessin MS, Rosoff CB, Bacon V: Reduced incidence of cerebral ischemia following rupture of intracranial aneurysm. Surg Neurol 11:339–344, 1979.
85. Zervas NT, Kistler JP, Ploetz J: Effect of Reserpine and Kanamycin on Postoperative Delayed Ischemic Deficits in Patients with Subarachnoid Hemorrhage after Aneurysm Rupture, in Wilkins RH (ed): *Cerebral Arterial Spasm*. Baltimore, Williams & Wilkins, 1979, pp 514–517.

Chapter 11 INTRACRANIAL ANEURYSMS: GENERAL ASPECTS OF SURGICAL TREATMENT

Management of the patient with ruptured intracranial aneurysm is concerned with recovery from the initial bleed and the prevention of recurrent hemorrhage (20). Treatment of most of the complications of subarachnoid hemorrhage (SAH) and the immediate prevention of recurrent hemorrhage is best accomplished with medical therapy. For the long term, the most effective means for prevention of recurrent hemorrhage is surgical obliteration of the aneurysmal sac.

For most patients, the ideal procedure is direct operation to eliminate the aneurysm and to preserve all normal vasculature, including tiny perforating arteries. Modern tactics to preserve intact circulation and minimize brain damage include: 1) microsurgical dissection and obliteration, 2) controlled exposure with self-retaining brain retractors, 3) a slack brain to promote exposure, and 4) a slack aneurysm to reduce the chance of intraoperative rupture (4, 9, 27).

Good judgment is crucial in selecting the proper procedure for the individual case. At times it may be wiser to settle for a partial clipping, e.g., when a dogear of firm aneurysmal wall remains unclipped, in order to spare a critical branch vessel. In some cases, the condition of the patient or location of the aneurysm will indicate an indirect operation, with ligation of the principal feeding artery or no surgery at all.

TIMING

Controversy exists regarding the timing of operation. Delaying surgery 10–14 days permits resolution of edema, and good results have been obtained (12, 21, 26). With this approach, some patients deteriorate from spasm while awaiting surgery. Early surgery within 1–2 days after SAH may allow removal of subarachnoid clot to reduce the chance of vasospasm (11, 12, 21, 25). Surgical risk may be greater, but overall management risk may be diminished. Preliminary results of early microsurgical treatment have been equivocal.

At present, we favor delayed surgery for most patients. The timing of operation is determined primarily by clinical condition, judged by the Botterell classification (Table 10.2) (2, 10, 13). For patients in good condition without significant deficit (grade 1–2), angiography is performed 8–12 days after SAH, and surgery is performed the following day if there is no significant spasm. Since patients with anterior communicating aneurysms appear more sensitive to the effects of surgery, surgery may be deferred a bit longer, from 10–14 days after SAH. If there is significant vasospasm, we defer operation another week, and then proceed with surgery, regardless of residual spasm, if the patient remains grade 1–2 (Figs. 11.1 and 11.2). Vasospasm in the first 2 weeks after SAH may be exacerbated by surgery with clinical deterioration. Vasospasm after 2 weeks apparently does not carry this ominous significance.

For patients with substantial neurological deficits (grade 3–4), operation is deferred 2–3 weeks; but may be done sooner if the deficits improve significantly. For patients with very severe deficits (grade 4–5), surgery is deferred until improvement indicates the likelihood of a useful functional outcome. Younger age of the patient and positive attitude of the family tend to favor operation in this group. In moribund patients, operation is usually not indicated.

A major predictor of symptomatic vasospasm is the CT scan done within 48 hours after SAH. When there is thick clot in the basal cisterns, the likelihood of eventual symptomatic spasm is high (see Chapter 10). In a few of these high risk patients, we have performed immediate surgery (within 48 hours of SAH) for removal of clot and aneurysm clipping. Clot extraction has not been easy. After clipping of the lesion, postoperative vasospasm can be treated with hypertension and hypervolemia. Limited results thus far are encouraging for this approach.

ANESTHESIA

Premedication

The night before surgery, steroids are begun if not already included in the regimen. In addition, propranolol (Inderal) is given. This agent appears to improve the stability of blood pressure control intraoperatively. Four units of packed red blood cells are requested. Premedication often includes diazepam (Valium) 10 mg intramuscularly or a neurolept agent (Innovar, 0.5 cc IM).

Preparation

An intravenous line, preferably a large bore plastic cannula, is established in the induction room. In many patients receiving ϵ-amino caproic acid, suitable veins are hard to identify, and rather than cause agitation by repeated venipuncture efforts, it is better to place a small gauge needle intravenously, and then establish two large bore IV routes after the patient is anesthetized. If necessary, the external jugular vein or a leg vein may be used. If no intravenous line can be easily established, a mask induction of anesthesia may be necessary. Prophylactic antibiotics are given after a good IV is in place.

A catheter is introduced into the radial artery for continuous monitoring of arterial pressure. The pressure transducer is fixed at the level of the external auditory meatus. Such monitoring is particularly important during induction, when wide swings of arterial pressure may occur. Pressor and antihypertensive agents are available for infusion; phenylephrine hydrochloride (10 mg in 250 cc 5% dextrose and water) and sodium nitroprusside (50 mg in 250 cc 5% dextrose in water shielded with tinfoil) serve well for these needs.

Induction

Once all preparations are complete, a slow induction is carried out over 10 minutes or more prior to intubation. One common technique of anesthesia is described in detail. After initial preoxygenation, sodium pentobarbital is given by increments (50–150 mg per increment up to 1 gm total). Once the patient is deeply drowsy, Halothane is administered by mask (0.5–1.5%). Prior to intubation, a muscle relaxant is given. A twitch monitor is applied to the ulnar nerve to assess the completeness of neuromuscular blockade. An additional increment of pentobarbital is given just prior to intubation. Ideally, at this point, the blood pressure is in the range of 100 mm Hg systolic. Laryngoscopy is carried out, and the vocal cords are sprayed with a local anesthetic solution. The blood pressure response to laryngoscopy is noted; if a substantial increase in blood pressure has occurred, an additional increment of pentobarbital is administered, or the concentration of Halothane increased, or both are done. Finally, with the patient stable and well anesthetized, laryngoscopy is done with gentle endotracheal intubation. The cuff of the endotracheal tube is inflated and checked for leaks. Controlled ventilation is preferred, with arterial PCO_2 maintained in the range of 30 torr, as demonstrated by frequently sampled arterial blood gases. The arterial blood gases likewise provide a frequent check on the adequacy of oxygenation. Prior to the application of the 3-point Mayfield headrest, more pentobarbital is given to prevent hypertension.

Reduction of Brain Tension

Most patients receive 100 gm of Mannitol (1 gm/kg IV) while the bone flap is being turned; in many cases, this is preceded by furosemide (20 mg IV). This usually gives excellent relaxation of the brain. For smaller patients, 50 gm Mannitol may suffice. Solu-medrol (80 mg IV) is continued every 4 hours.

For most cases, intraoperative aspiration of cerebrospinal fluid (CSF) is helpful to reduce brain tension. In many patients, this can be accomplished by gradual removal of CSF from the basal cisterns during the initial exposure. Where this method is ineffective, especially with obliteration of cisterns by blood, direct ventricular puncture may be used to drain CSF. In some patients it may be anticipated that a lumbar subarachnoid spinal catheter for drainage of CSF may be helpful. We often use spinal drainage for anterior communicating, distal anterior cerebral and basilar aneurysms. After the induction of anesthesia, a catheter (22-gauge polyethylene tubing from Portex) is introduced via a Touhy needle. Only a small amount of fluid is allowed to escape at the time of introduction. The catheter is placed in such a fashion that upon request, further fluid may be removed by the anesthesiologist after dural incision.

Controlled Hypotension

Frequent communication between the neuroanesthesiologist and the neurosurgeon is crucial for pharmacologic control of blood pressure during surgery. Controlled hypotension is used to slacken the aneurysm in order to aid dissection and decrease the likelihood of intraoperative rupture (1). In most patients, the systolic blood pressure is maintained at about 100 mm Hg (mean 75 mm Hg) during the initial exposure. Once the aneurysm is in view, the blood pressure is further dropped to about 80 mm Hg systolic (mean 60 mm Hg). During critical dissection of the neck of the aneurysm, deep hypotension may be required with systolic blood pressure about 60 mm Hg (mean about 40 mm Hg). Occasionally, a particularly difficult portion of an aneurysm may justify a burst of very deep hypotension for 2–3 minutes at a mean of 20–25 mm Hg. Most patients tolerate this type of deep hypotension without postoperative sequelae. In normal brain, autoregulation maintains local cerebral blood flow to mean arterial blood pressures of 40–45 mm Hg. In patients with subarachnoid hemorrhage, however, autoregulation may be lost in some zones. Moreover, in some elderly patients with a history of hypertension and ischemic heart disease, prolonged and deep hypotension may not be well tolerated by the brain, heart, and kidneys. In such cases, levels of controlled hypotension may be moderated. If vasospasm is suspected clinically or documented by angiography, it may be wise to avoid the use of hypotension and to maintain the systolic blood pressure over 100 mm Hg.

Several techniques for controlled hypotension are available. In many cases, moderate hypotension may be achieved simply by increasing the concentration of inspired Halothane. In most patients, an additional agent such as sodium nitroprusside will be required to further diminish the blood pressure. Trimethaphan

Intracranial Aneurysms: General Aspects of Surgical Treatment

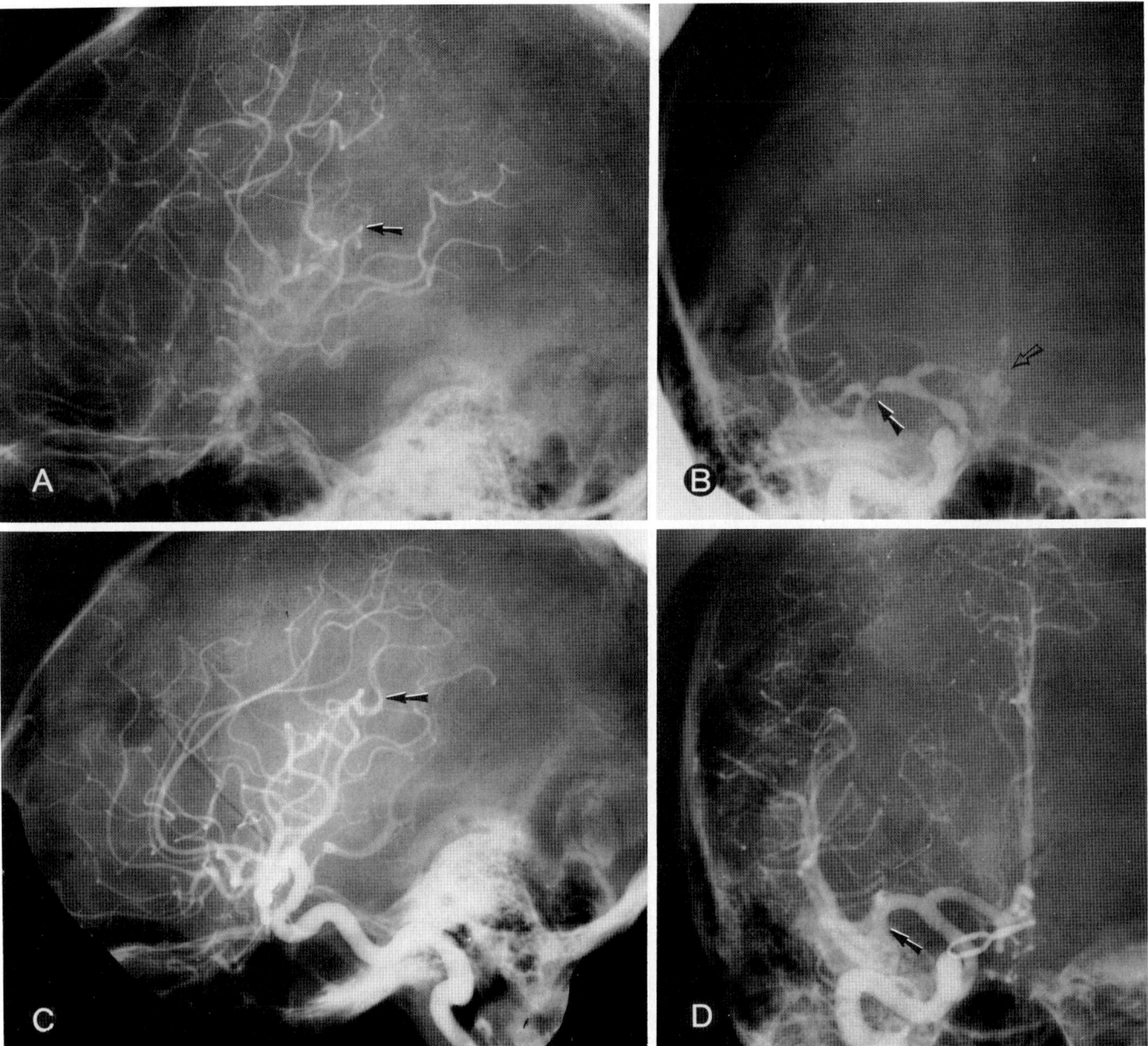

Figure 11.1 Timing of surgery. *A* and *B*, right carotid angiogram 4 days after SAH shows anterior communicating aneurysm (*open arrow*) and vasospasm with slow flow in MCA branches (*closed arrows*). Patient had left hemiplegia, (grade 3). *C* and *D*, postoperative right carotid angiogram performed 5 weeks after SAH and 2 weeks after surgery shows aneurysm obliterated, spasm lysed (*arrow*). Surgery was performed 3 weeks after SAH, without repeat angiogram, in alert left hemiplegic patient (grade 3). Beginning shortly after surgery, hemiplegia improved slowly to mild paresis.

camsylate (Arfonad) or trinitroglycerine may also be used for this purpose. Propranolol, given preoperatively and then intraoperatively in doses as high as 1–2 mg intravenously, may be used for more prolonged, stable hypotensive effect. Once the aneurysm is obliterated, cerebral perfusion is maximized by volume expansion with colloid and packed cells to keep hematocrit at 35–40%. Blood pressure is elevated to about 140 mm Hg systolic, using a pressor as needed.

SURGICAL TECHNIQUE

Every aspect of surgery for intracranial aneurysm is designed to minimize brain injury during obliteration of the lesion. Neuroanesthetic techniques discussed in the preceeding section reduce brain tension to allow for safer exposure and slacken the aneurysm for safer dissection. Surgical techniques aim for safe exposure and dissection through application of microsurgical principles. Two centimeters of retraction

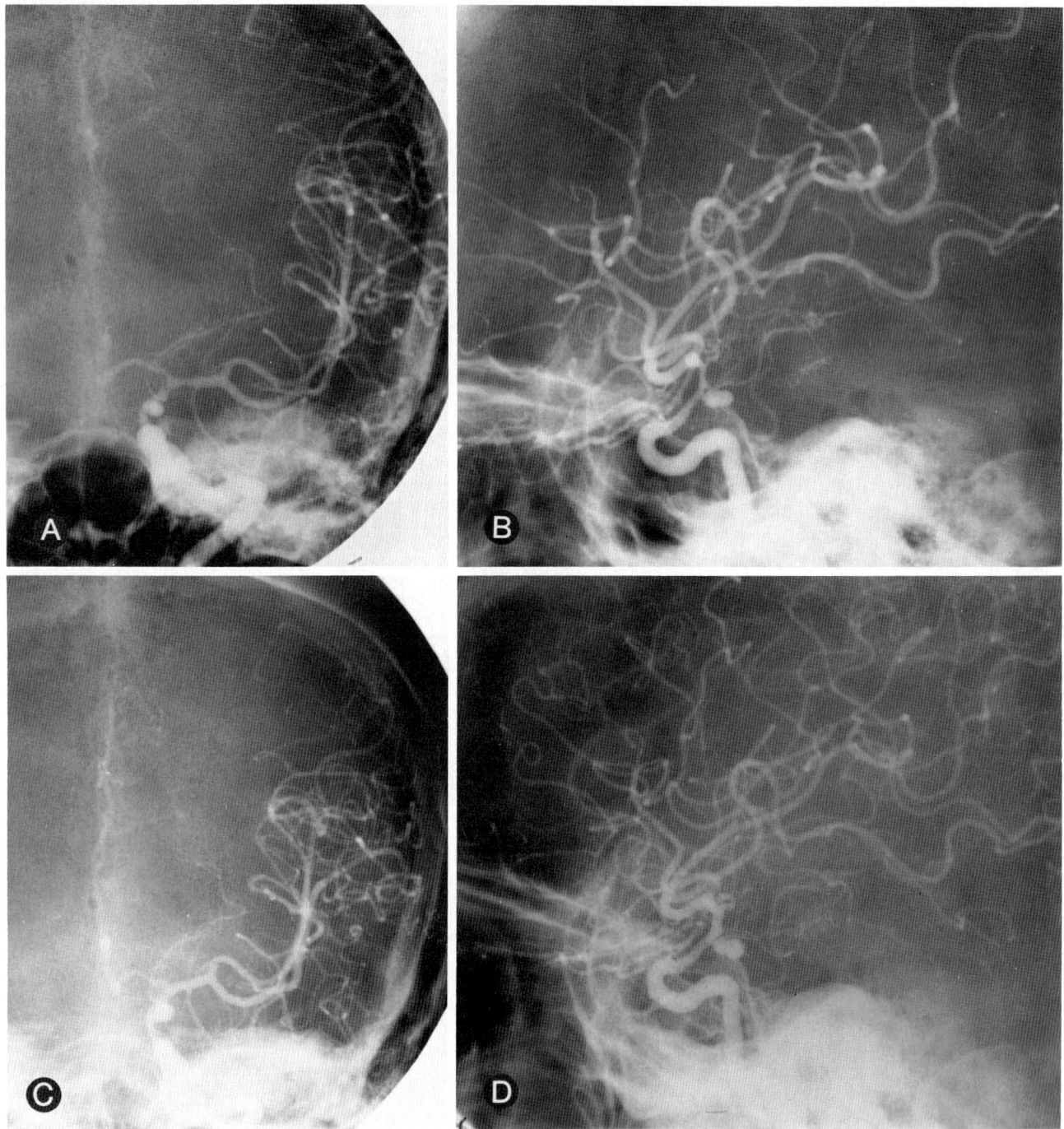

Figure 11.2 Preoperative cerebral vasospasm. *A* and *B*, left carotid angiogram 4 days after SAH when patient developed right hemiparesis and dysphasia. There is an aneurysm at the internal carotid-posterior communicating artery junction and spasm of the internal carotid and anterior cerebral arteries. *C* and *D*, left carotid angiogram 14 days after SAH. The spasm is resolving after treatment with hypervolemia and induced hypertension (systolic BP, 170 mm Hg). Aneurysm is unchanged in size. Deficits are mild. Surgery was done the next day. *E* and *F*, postoperative angiogram shows aneurysm clipped and spasm fully resolved at 24 days after SAH. The anterior choroidal artery is preserved.

usually provides adequate exposure. With microsurgical visualization and instrumentation, the neurosurgeon can see and dissect the plane between the aneurysm and surrounding structures. These factors have led to improved results in aneurysm surgery.

Operating Room Layout

Though many layouts may be used, we have found the one shown in Fig. 11.3 useful. The operating table is positioned in the center of the room. The surgeon

Intracranial Aneurysms: General Aspects of Surgical Treatment

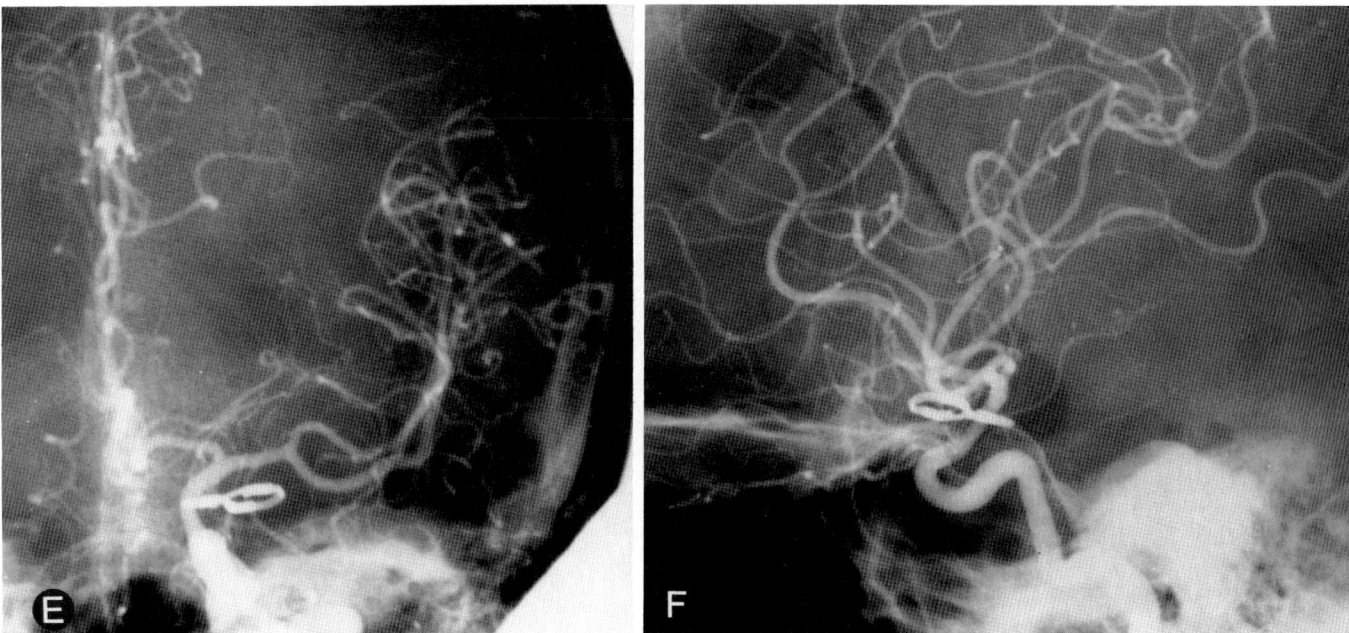

Figure 11.2 (*E* and *F*)

stands or sits at the head. For a right-handed surgeon, the scrub nurse stands to his right to facilitate passing instruments. The neuroanesthetist sits at the patient's left side, with extension tubes from patient to anesthesia machine as needed, particularly when the head is turned to the right. The assistant usually stands to the surgeon's left. During microsurgery, a floor-mounted Zeiss (OpMi 1) microscope stands just to the left of the rostral end of the operating table. The television monitor for microsurgery is attached to the ceiling for viewing by the scrub nurse, neuroanesthetist, and other observers. An overbed table, or attached Mayo stand, brought up to the patient's shoulder, conveniently holds the instruments. The surgeon generally sits on a soft stool, with a covered narrow Mayo stand supporting his right arm, and the microscope up-down pedal to his right.

Instrumentation

The development of microsurgery has revolutionized the surgery of intracranial aneurysms (4, 16). The use of the Zeiss operating microscope, as developed by Yasargil, provides dramatic magnification and brilliant illumination of tiny arterial anatomy, with reduced requirements for retraction. The floor-mounted OpMi 1 remains our choice for its simplicity, flexibility, and ease of servicing. For most aneurysms, we prefer a 275- or 300-mm objective, variable-angle binoculars, and high-eye point 12.5X eyepieces. For the "park bench" position, straight binoculars are convenient. The sitting position requires straight binoculars and the 250-mm lens. If the surgeon is right-handed, the stereoscopic binocular observer tube is placed on the left. A Telstil adaptor is placed on the right side of the microscope to provide a place for video monitoring and intermittent photography.

Microsurgical instrumentation has kept pace with the development of the surgical microscope. The Greenberg self-retaining retractor provides steady, minimally traumatic brain retraction. Its primary post is attached horizontally to the left side of the Mayfield headrest, and secondary parts and retractor arms take a low profile to avoid inadvertent bumps. Bipolar coagulating forceps permit precise hemostasis, gentle dissection with spreading motions, and shrinkage of the aneurysmal neck. A variety of microsurgical dissectors aid blunt dissection of arteries and aneurysms. The fine curved Rhoton dissectors (#6–8) and a straight flat microdissector are particularly helpful. Fine microscissors and arachnoid knives may be used for sharp dissection of adhesions to the sac.

For aneurysm surgery, three suctions should be available. Two of these are #16 suctions set to low vacuum on the controlled suction unit. The third suction is a #1 sucker at full vacuum placed to the left, to be used if the aneurysm should rupture.

Positioning

For surgery, the patient is generally positioned horizontally. This posture minimizes cardiovascular stress and promotes cerebral perfusion, especially during induced hypotension. For most anterior circulation lesions, a supine position is best. The operating table may be flexed slightly to elevate the head. A supine position with the head turned is chosen for the subtemporal approach to basilar aneurysms. A

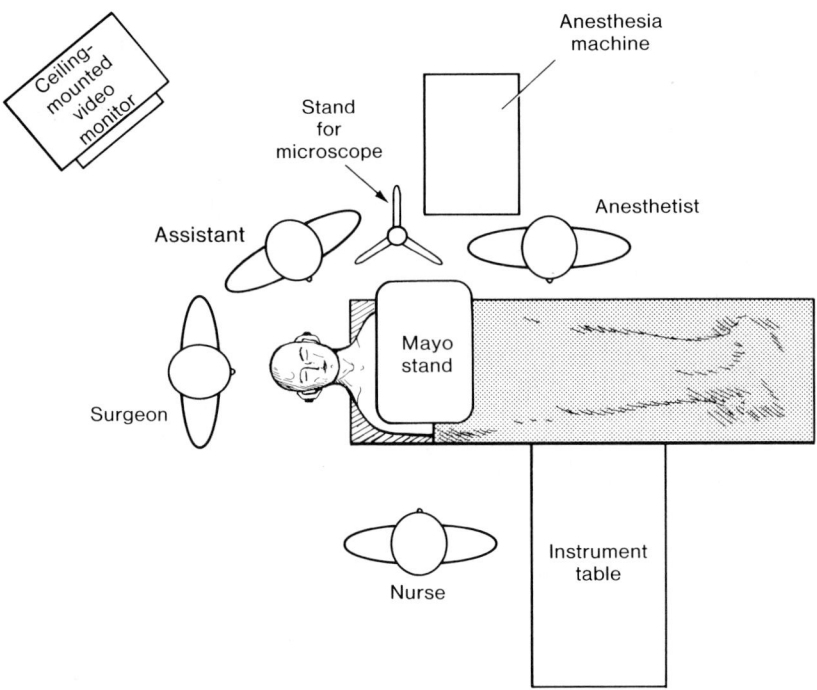

Figure 11.3 Operating room layout for most aneurysm operations performed by a right-handed surgeon.

lateral position with the head turned may be chosen for a suboccipital approach to a vertebral aneurysm. Here the knees and hips are flexed and a roll is placed under the dependent axilla, usually the left.

Occasionally, the sitting position may be warranted for vertebral artery aneurysms. In some instances, the advantages of exposure may outweigh the disadvantages of cardiovascular stress and impaired cerebral perfusion.

Several general principles govern head position. The head is held above heart level to avoid venous engorgement. A space of two finger breadths is maintained between the jaw and the clavicle to avoid jugular compression. The vertex is tilted about 15° toward the floor so the brain falls away from the base. The three-point Mayfield headrest provides solid fixation.

Turning of the head depends on the specific aneurysm site (Fig. 11.4). Generally, the head is turned to give the surgeon a vertical view into the field (except for posterior fossa lesions). For azygos and pericallosal artery aneurysms, the head is straight (0° turn) and flexed about 20°. For internal carotid artery (ICA) aneurysms, a 45° turn gives good access. For anterior communicating artery aneurysms and middle cerebral artery (MCA) aneurysms approached through the Sylvian fissure, a 60–70° turn gives good exposure—less turning forces the surgeon to tilt his own head uncomfortably. For MCA aneurysms, approached via superior temporal gyrus, a 90° turn may be used with a roll under the shoulder. The same head position is used for the subtemporal approach to basilar tip aneurysms. If head position is not ideal, modification by changing the headrest can be achieved intraoperatively.

Cranial Approaches

The flap is determined by the lesion site (Fig. 11.5). In general, smaller flaps are needed for microsurgical exposure. Headlight and 2.5X loupes improve macrosurgical vision for turning the flap.

A pterional flap provides versatile exposure of the anterior circle of Willis (27). Exposure is excellent for aneurysms of the internal carotid and anterior communicating arteries (Fig. 11.5). In some cases, basilar bifurcation aneurysms and medial MCA lesions can be approached via this route. The key to this exposure is access to the floor of the anterior fossa. This access is assured by accurate placement of the key burr hole, a low craniotome cut anteriorly, and extensive removal of the lateral sphenoid ridge (see Chapter 12).

A full frontotemporal flap provides good exposure for middle cerebral aneurysms (8) (Fig. 11.5). Access to the ICA and proximal MCA is achieved with the pterional flap. Additional temporal exposure is helpful for distal MCA lesions, particularly when a superior temporal gyrus corticectomy is utilized. This flap can also serve to expose an ICA lesion through the Sylvian fissure and a basilar tip aneurysm under the temporal lobe.

A coronal flap and interhemispheric approach provide exposure for clipping azygos and pericallosal aneurysms (17) (Fig. 11.5). Though the non-dominant right side is preferable if there is a choice, reference to the angiogram will indicate which side has the less

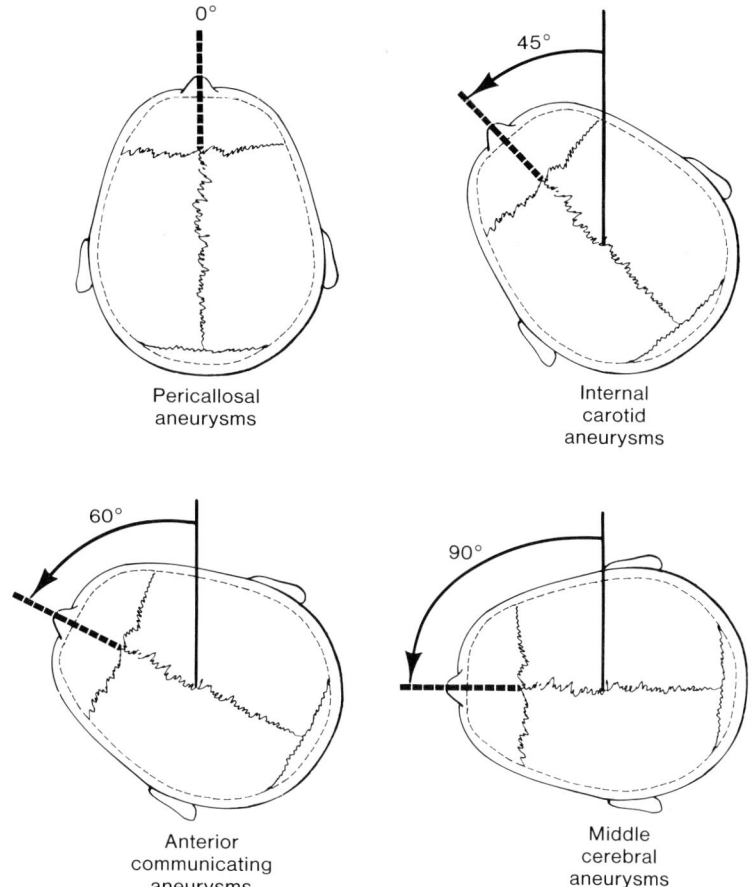

Figure 11.4 Positioning the head. For most anterior circulation aneurysms, turning of the head depends on the aneurysm site. For *pericallosal* (A$_2$CA) lesions, the head is straight ahead and flexed 0° to the floor. For *internal carotid* (ICA) aneurysms, the head is turned 45° away from the lesion. For *anterior communicating* aneurysms, the head is rotated 60° away from the side of the approach. For *middle cerebral* aneurysms (MCA), the head is horizontal.

formidable veins crossing the field. Care is needed to avoid injury to posterior frontal bridging veins and to superior sagittal sinus, since occlusion of these structures can lead to hemiplegia. The surgeon avoids injury to the motor cortex by positioning the flap just anterior to the coronal suture. Since the anterior burr holes are in front of the hairline, they are filled with methylmethacrylate at the conclusion of the procedure.

A small temporal bone flap, turned via a straight ("tic") incision, provides nice subtemporal access to a basilar tip aneurysm (19) (Fig. 11.5). The bony exposure should extend down to the zygoma and floor of middle fossa.

A hockey-stick incision (Fig. 11.5) permits unilateral suboccipital craniectomy with removal of the foramen magnum and the arch of C$_1$ for exposure of vertebral artery aneurysms (19). The key is a lateral exposure to the sigmoid sinus. This facilitates a view into the cerebellopontine angle with minimal cerebellar retraction.

A combined subtemporal-suboccipital approach is occasionally useful for exposure of the basilar trunk (14) (Fig. 11.5). Angiography should demonstrate a contralateral patent transverse sinus if the ipsilateral lateral sinus is to be sacrificed to widely divide the tentorium.

The precise site of the lesion will determine the details of operative approach. The soft-tissue exposure and craniotomy must provide adequate access to the aneurysm with minimum brain retraction. Removal of bone to the base of the skull is usually needed, for example, rongeuring away of lateral sphenoid ridge in a pterional craniotomy. The dural incision is fashioned to provide optimum access and still protect the brain. For these maneuvers, headlight and loupes provide good visualization and mobility.

Retraction

The brain is slowly elevated with a hand-held retractor. Depending on the location of the aneurysm, CSF is aspirated by opening the basal cisterns or by a spinal catheter until the brain is slack enough to insert a self-retaining retractor.

We prefer the Greenberg retractor for its stability and controllability. For craniotomies, the primary bar

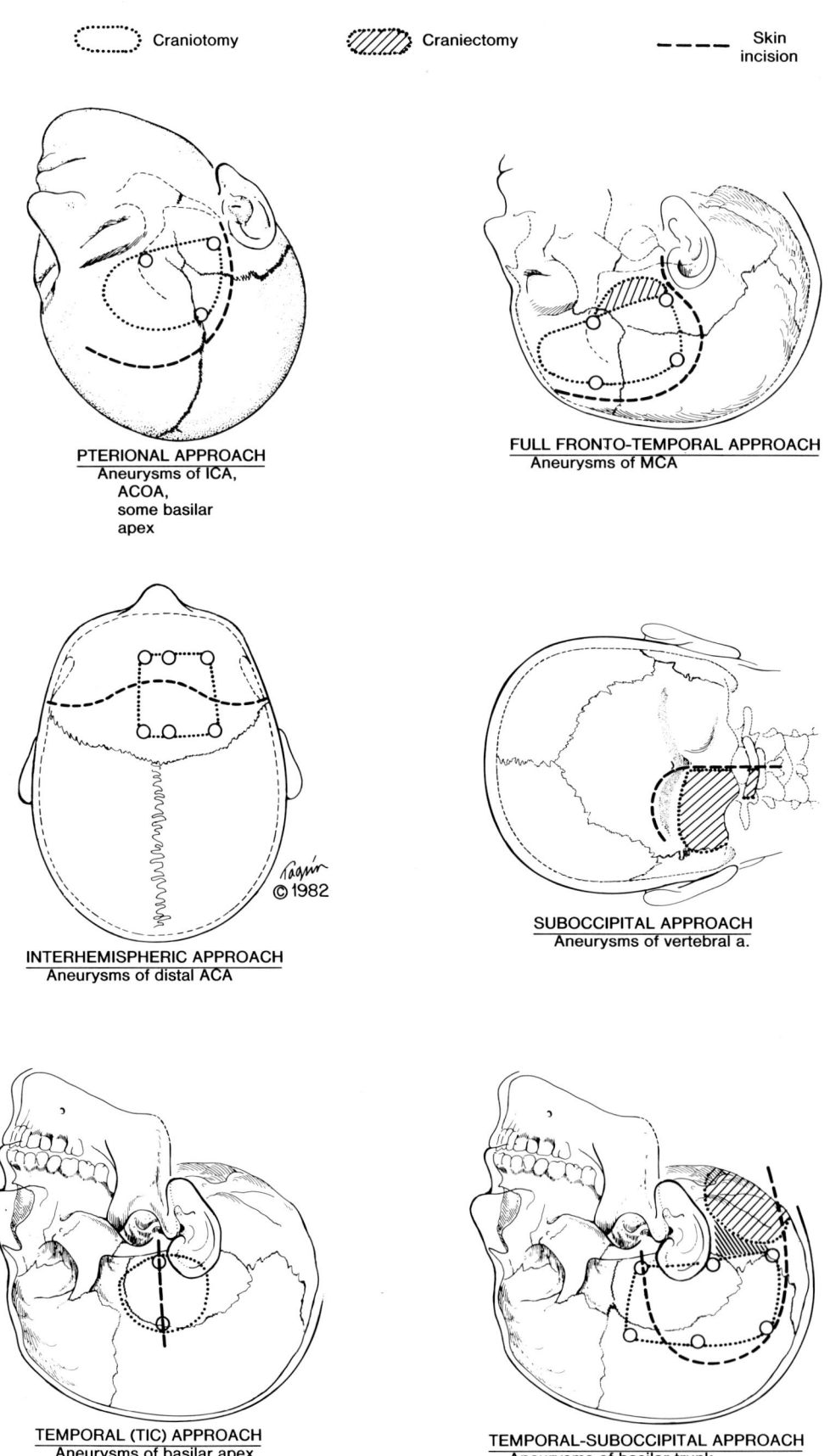

Figure 11.5 Cranial approaches for aneurysm surgery.

is attached horizontally to the Mayfield headrest to the surgeon's left. A secondary bar is fixed vertically to the primary bar. Another secondary bar is attached obliquely about an inch from the vertex. Long retractor arms can then be placed on this oblique secondary. Retractor arms are contoured in low-profile to avoid being bumped. Each retractor arm (usually 2 or 3) holds a thin or medium width Teflon-coated brain retractor blade. The retractor blades rest on rubber dam or Telfa pledgets protecting the brain and distributing the retraction pressure. For small alterations in retraction, tension is maintained in the retractor arm. For larger changes in position, the retractor arm is loosened, then retightened. For a subfrontal approach to the circle of Willis, the brain is retracted from the base but also lifted gently off the optic nerve. Ordinarily, the cleft of retraction need be no more than 1–2 cm for microsurgery, and as a result, retraction injury may be minimized.

Deep Exposure

Once brain retractors are placed, visual mobility is no longer at a premium, and the microscope is wheeled into the field for magnified visualization of the small, relatively fixed field. Sometimes retractor manipulation and arachnoid dissection will suffice for a beautiful exposure of the aneurysm. But often a small corticectomy in silent brain serves to diminish the pressure of retraction and its attendant injury. The gyrus rectus corticectomy is well-known and recommended for almost all anterior communicating artery aneurysms. For some ICA aneurysms, particularly those at the bifurcation, deeper exposure can be obtained by opening the medial Sylvian fissure. When this proves difficult, a 1-cm medial frontal corticectomy, with sparing of perforant arteries, can safely give the needed exposure. For laterally placed middle cerebral aneurysms, a superior temporal gyrus corticectomy gives the required view with a minimum of retraction.

Microsurgical Dissection

The aneurysm is approached under 10–16X magnification. Moderate hypotension is employed in the early stages, and deep hypotension may be used to complete the job if the sac is thin-walled. On parent arteries, blunt dissection is often used. A #16 sucker with low vacuum in the left hand can provide counter traction for a Rhoton #6 or other fine dissector in the right hand. The side of the dissector is less likely to perforate than the tip. A microcottonoid in the field can be used for retraction and to protect aneurysm and brain. Near the aneurysm, sharp dissection is preferred when the lesion's margins can be clearly visualized. Delicate tissue attachments are coagulated and cut with microscissors. After dissecting the parent vessels, the surgeon frees the neck. A broad path must be prepared for each blade of the clip lest the neck be torn during clipping. Mobilization of the dome may be needed to adequately prepare the neck and to facilitate sparing adherent critical vessels. When the dome is to be mobilized, it is wise to leave a layer of brain or arachnoid attached.

Aneurysm Clips

A host of different surgical clips may be used effectively (Fig. 11.6). For many lesions, we have used the Heifetz clip. This clip is held rigidly in the clip applying forceps for precision of application, and its jaws open broadly to accept even large necks. Its disadvantage is the breadth of its blade, which may be too wide for safe insertion in a narrow aperture. In this respect, the Yasargil clip, with its millimeter wide blade, is superior. This clip, which we have also found very useful, has two drawbacks: the limited opening of its jaws, which precludes clipping of larger lesions, and its tendency to stick in the clip applying forceps during release. This latter problem may be overcome by opening the jaws of the clip applying forceps wider than usual by separating the handles with the third and fourth fingers inserted therein.

The Drake clip, with its proximal aperture, is best for basilar tip aneurysms, since the aperture may conveniently encircle the P_1 segment and its perforating vessels. The aperature on Drake clip may also be used to encircle other structures (19): the A-1 or A-2 branch when clipping anterior communicating aneurysms, another clip blade when more than one clip is necessary for a complex lesion, or a middle cerebral divisions when clipping a middle cerebral bifurcation aneurysm. Drake clips are available in clip lengths from 6–24 mm. In clipping basilar bifurcation aneurysms, the correct length must be used to avoid vascular occlusion. Occasionally, it is necessary to trim the blade to an appropriate length and file its rough tip. Because of its strength, the clip is helpful for large or even giant aneurysms. It should be borne in mind, however, that an atheromonous aneurysmal neck may foil even such a strong clip. In such instance, preparation with bipolar cauterization or ligature, or even crushing with a hemostat, may set the stage for clipping.

The Sugita clip is also strong, and its bayonet-formed shank allows excellent visualization of the tips of the clip during application. The offset of its shank from its blades makes this a very handy clip for parallel application alongside a previously applied clip, avoiding the problem of the hubs of two clips interfering with each other. When a two-clip solution is entertained, another clip to consider is the triangular-formed clip in the Heifetz-Weck series which can sometimes nicely eliminate a pesky dog-ear. The Sundt-Kees clip is sometimes used for a posteromedially directed internal carotid artery aneurysm (24). The variety with a cutout window may be used for preservation of the anterior choroidal artery. The McFadden clip, with its ideal metallurgy, is similar in many respects to the Yasargil clip. The Vari-angle clip is occasionally used for an especially awkward angle of application. The right angle clip applier

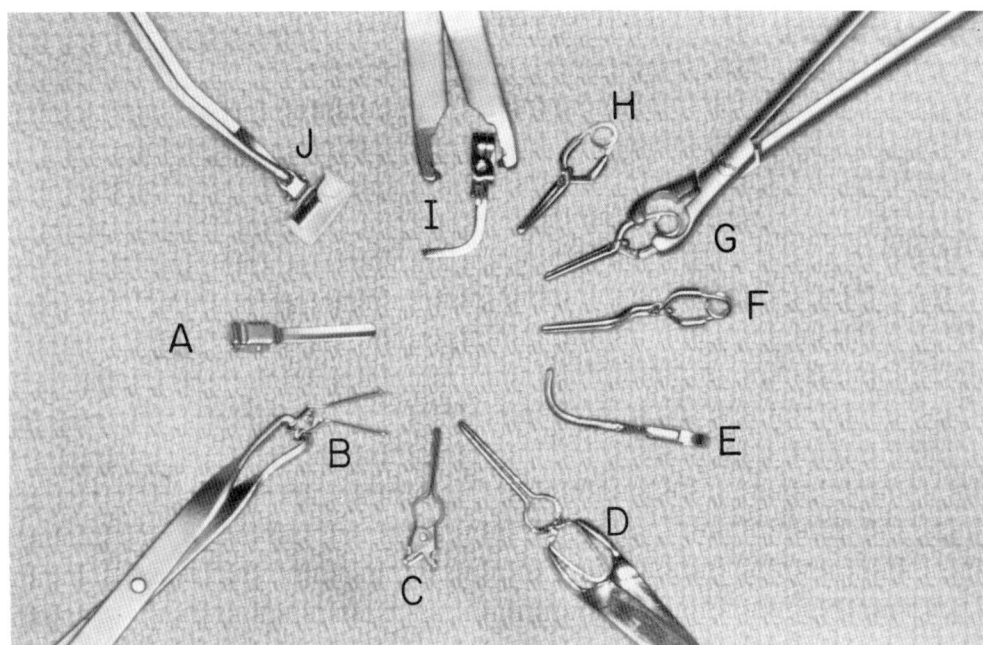

Figure 11.6 Aneurysm clips. *A*, 12-mm straight Heifetz clip is one of the most useful all around clip with blades that open quite widely. *B*, "angled on the flat" Heifetz clip is useful for proximal ICA aneurysm to avoid hitting the base of the skull. *C*, Drake-Heifetz clip can be cut cleanly with wire cutters and filed smooth for intermediate blade length. *D*, Drake-Kees clip can encircle vessels (or nerves) to avoid injury; also comes in lengths up to 24 mm to occlude giant aneurysms. *E*, large right-angle curved Yasargil clip snugs in nicely to a carina as for pericallosal aneurysms. *F*, Sugita clip's bayonet form contours to some aneurysms and also can be applied side by side to another clip without hubs interfering. *G*, straight Yasargil clip has very narrow blades which are useful for carotid-ophthalmic aneurysms. *H*, shallow curved Yasargil clip is nice for many small or cauterized lesions. *I*, right-angle McFadden Variangle clip has ideal (tantalum) metallurgy and can be slipped beneath ICA on posteromedial pointing lesions. *J*, Sundt-Kees clip-graft (here with window) is good for some ICA trunk aneurysms which point posteromedially, and can also be used to repair torn vessels.

designed by Sundt, for use with Mayfield type clips, is also useful for awkward angles of application. In some situations, applications of a Heifetz clip using a slender hemostat will provide a right angle application.

Obliteration of the Aneurysm

The surgeon is well advised to approach the aneurysm with a broad array of techniques for dealing with the problem. For the great majority of aneurysms clipping or ligature is the most effective. Occasionally, an aneurysm will defy safe clipping and reinforcement must be used, either with tissue adhesive or muslin. Insertion of thrombogenic wire has been recommended for some giant aneurysms.

Precise application of the clip is required. The clip is advanced gently, with axial rotational tiny wiggling to reduce drag until the tips are just beyond the opposite side of the neck. Generally, it is possible to visualize one of the two blades as it advances. If significant resistance is encountered, one should stop and remove the clip. Usually dissection, with freeing of arachnoid attachments, will take care of the problem. In some cases, with a paper-thin aneurysmal neck, a brief deepening of hypotension may be needed just at the time of clip application.

After clip application, one must check the adequacy of clipping and condition of circulation. Clip tips must be visualized beyond the opposite edge of the lesion, and the entire aneurysm should be obliterated. Satisfactory clipping of the lesion should be proved by aspiration of the aneurysm with a 25-gauge spinal needle. If bleeding from the aneurysm persists after the needle perforation, further obliteration will be needed. Finally, the surgeon should satisfy himself that as retractors are removed, the clip will not produce dangerous torque on the aneurysmal neck or compression of adjacent neural or vascular structures.

Bipolar cauterization of the neck of the aneurysm may be helpful in some cases (27) (Fig. 11.7). This technique, initiated by Yasargil, may narrow the neck for easier clipping. In addition, it may thicken the neck, eradicating dangerous thin spots in this critical area. When undertaking this manuever the bipolar cautery should be set low, with prior testing of its electrocautery effect and the blades of the forceps should pass completely across the neck of the lesion, to reduce the danger of rupture. As current is turned on, the surgeon alternately applies very gentle pressure and release. Ideally, a slow coagulation with whitening and thickening of the neck is produced without charring or popping. During this time, continuous irrigation of the area of coagulation should be done. In some cases, the coagulation may completely obliterate the neck.

For some aneurysms a ligature may be helpful, particularly in lesions with a wide neck, making it difficult to define a clear area for a clip (Fig. 11.8). A variety of ligature passers are available. If space is limited, a ligature may be placed deep to the aneurysm with fine forceps. The surgeon then reflects the lesion to the opposite side searching for the ligature beyond the aneurysm neck and retrieving it gently with a forceps. After the ligature is placed about the neck, a surgeon's knot is fashioned and gently pulled taut. In some cases, the neck may be obliterated totally by these maneuvers. In other cases, the ligature narrows the neck for subsequent clipping.

Under the microscope, an aneurysm rarely defies clipping and ligation. When it does, reinforcement may be the safest technique. The usual approach is the application of muscle or acrylic. Recently, tissue adhesives have been utilized, but delayed reaction may be a problem (Fig. 11.9).

Following completion of the obliteration of the aneurysm, Surgicel is applied to the edges of any corticectomy. At this point, the neuroanesthetist gradually raises the blood pressure to the normal level for that patient. The surgeon carefully checks to make certain that hemostasis at the aneurysm site is adequate.

Intraoperative Rupture

Deliberate action is necessary in the event of aneurysmal rupture at any point during the dissection. The surgeon must proceed in an orderly fashion with temporary hemostasis, precise visualization of the source of hemorrhage and its relation to critical structures, and then accurate hemostasis. Small areas of hemorrhage can be controlled with suction and a cottonoid. Very careful direction of the suction tip to the precise point of bleeding should be attempted to clear the field entirely of bleeding. Then precise coagulation with the bipolar cautery or application of a bit of Surgicel or muscle with compression for a few minutes may seal a minor leak. If hemostasis can be obtained in this way, it is best to direct the dissection to another corner and return to the hemorrhage area at a later time.

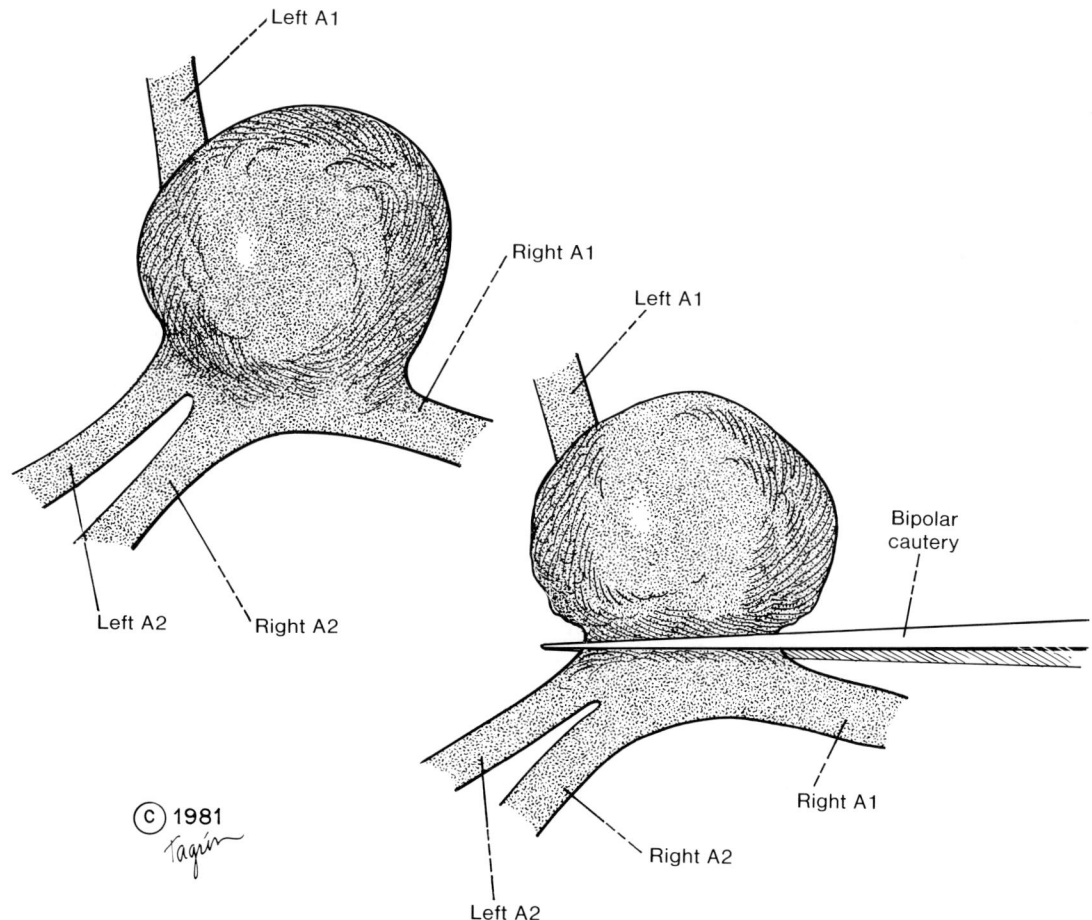

Figure 11.7 Bipolar cauterization of neck of aneurysm. This technique will both shrink the neck of the aneurysm and toughen the wall.

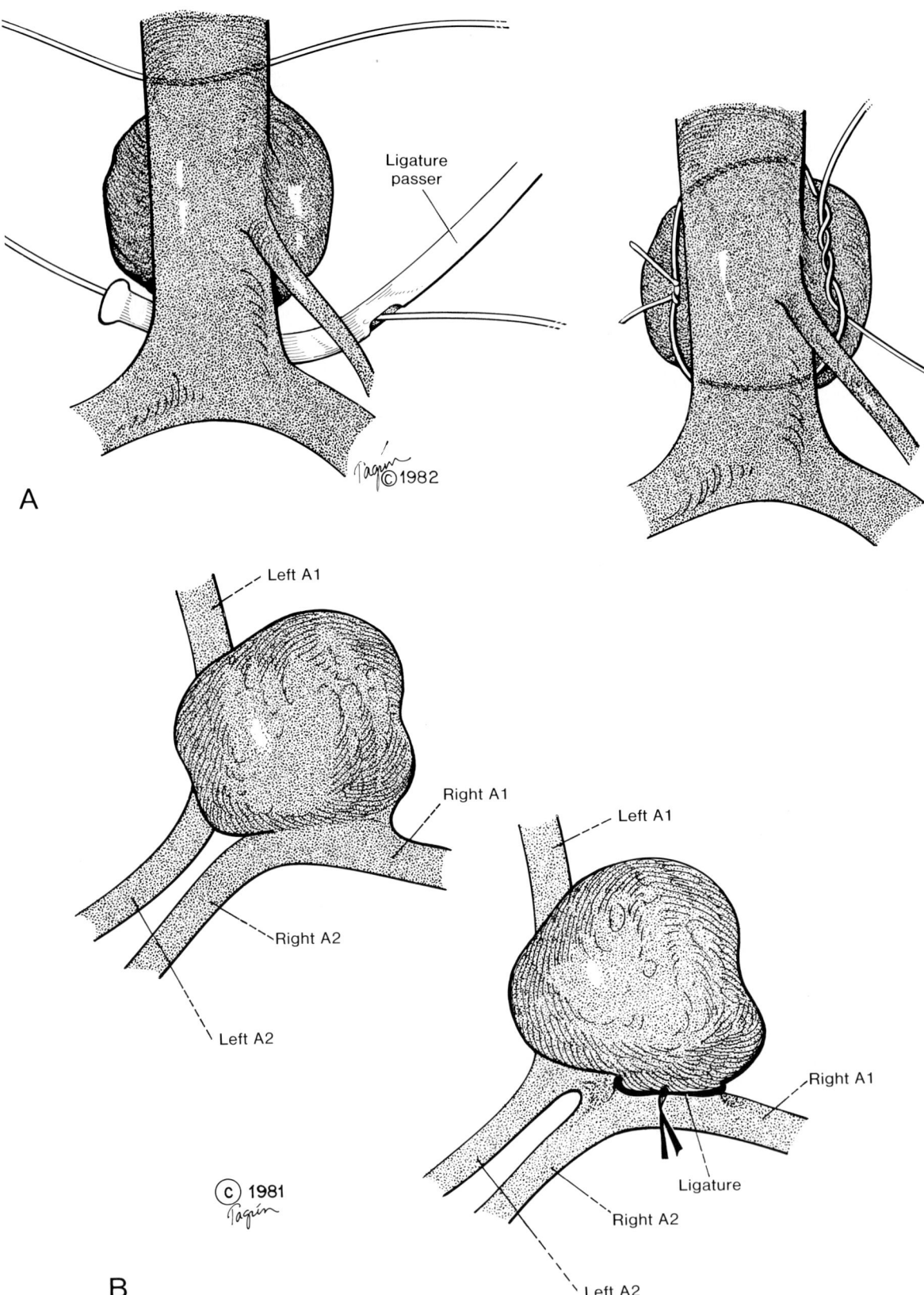

Figure 11.8 Use of a ligature to help occlude an aneurysm. This technique can be used to help prepare the lesion for clipping when there is a broad base. *A*, technique of using two ties when it is difficult to get around the aneurysm. *B*, narrowing of base of anterior communicating aneurysm with a single tie.

Intracranial Aneurysms: General Aspects of Surgical Treatment

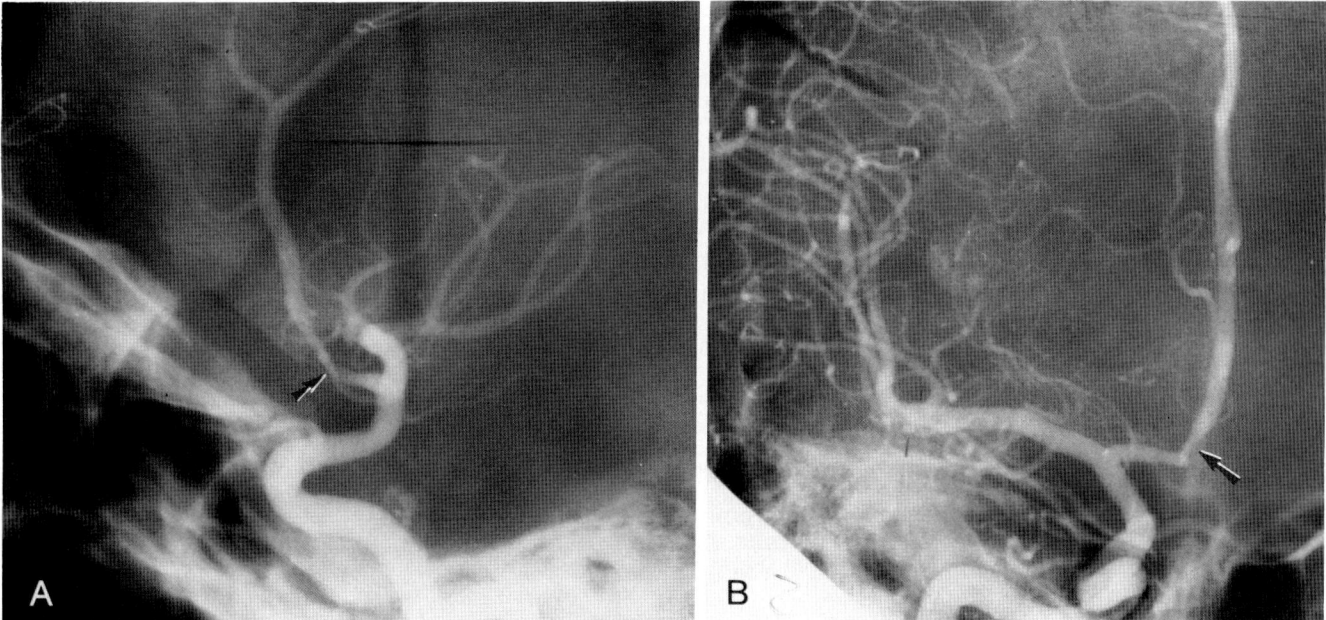

Figure 11.9 Postoperative arterial narrowing after application of tissue adhesive. A and B, right carotid angiogram 6 months after application of tissue adhesive to anterior communicating aneurysm. No aneurysm seen, arterial narrowing present (*arrow*). Patient showed delayed deterioration in memory and affect.

Brisk bleeding requires the use of the large or multiple suction. If this occurs tell the anesthesiologist to give blood and alter the technique to keep the blood pressure up because blood loss can be rapid and maximum collateral circulation may be required if temporary arterial occlusion is needed. Application of a temporary clip to the dome may be helpful. If a tear at the neck of an aneurysm cannot be controlled with a clip, repair with either an interrupted suture technique (10-0 nylon) or tissue adhesive may be used.

Closure

Irrigation is carried out with saline. All visible clots around accessible arteries are removed. Papaverine is applied to these vessels. When the brain is slack, substantial saline may be added to fill the dead space. The dura is closed and Surgicel is placed in the epidural space for hemostasis. The bone flap is wired in place with #28-gauge stainless steel wire sutures, and the dura is apposed to the bone flap with a central suture. The operative area is irrigated with bacitracin solution. The muscle, fascia, galea, and skin are closed with appropriate sutures.

Indirect Surgery

For some lesions, particularly giant aneurysms, direct attack may be too risky (see Chapter 20) (3, 24). A safe treatment may be ligation of a proximal parent artery, either in the neck or in the head (18). Occlusion of the internal carotid artery with a gradually occluding clamp diminishes pressure and often results in thrombosis of internal carotid aneurysms. A snare ligature can be used to occlude the middle cerebral or basilar arteries to thrombose aneurysms of these vessels (3). To prevent ischemic infarction, several methods for revascularization of the brain can be used prior to arterial occlusion (22) (see Chapter 4).

POSTOPERATIVE MANAGEMENT

Guidelines for postoperative care have been presented (6, 11, 20). At the conclusion of the procedure, the patient is treated prophylactically against vasospasm. The central venous pressure is brought to 10 cm of water with colloid if there is no cardiac contraindication. The hematocrit is maintained at 35–40% by the transfusion of packed cells if necessary. The blood pressure is maintained in the range of 110–140 mm Hg systolic with volume and pressors as required. Medications include steroids, an antacid, and diphenyl hydantoin. Elastic stockings or pneumatic compression boots are used until the patient is ambulatory.

If the patient awakens with a new deficit or develops later neurological deterioration, a CT scan is performed looking for intracranial hematoma, hydrocephalus, or cerebral edema. Rarely, infection may be disclosed (Fig. 11.10, A to C). Appropriate treatment is instituted if these conditions are found. If the CT scan fails to disclose an adequate explanation for the deterioration, an angiogram is performed. If significant vasospasm (grade 3+ or 4+) is seen (Fig. 11.11, A to D), additional medical treatment is indicated (7). The systolic blood pressure is increased to 160–170 mm Hg; using dopamine or neosynephrine (7, 15).

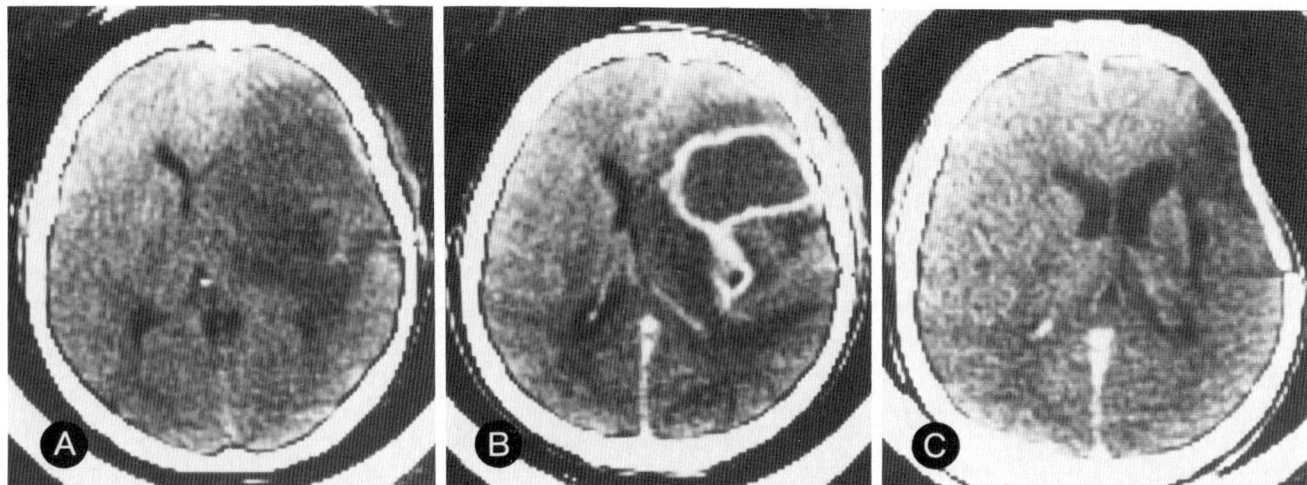

Figure 11.10 Obliteration of MCA aneurysm and successful treatment of postoperative brain abscess. *A* and *B*, CT scan (plain and enhanced) 2 weeks after surgery shows brain abscess in site of hematoma removal. Patient had delayed onset of increasing left hemiparesis and was drowsy. *C*, enhanced CT 3 months after original surgery shows encephalomalocia and no mass effect. Treatment by aspiration of abscess contents, removal of bone flap, and antibiotics. Complete recovery.

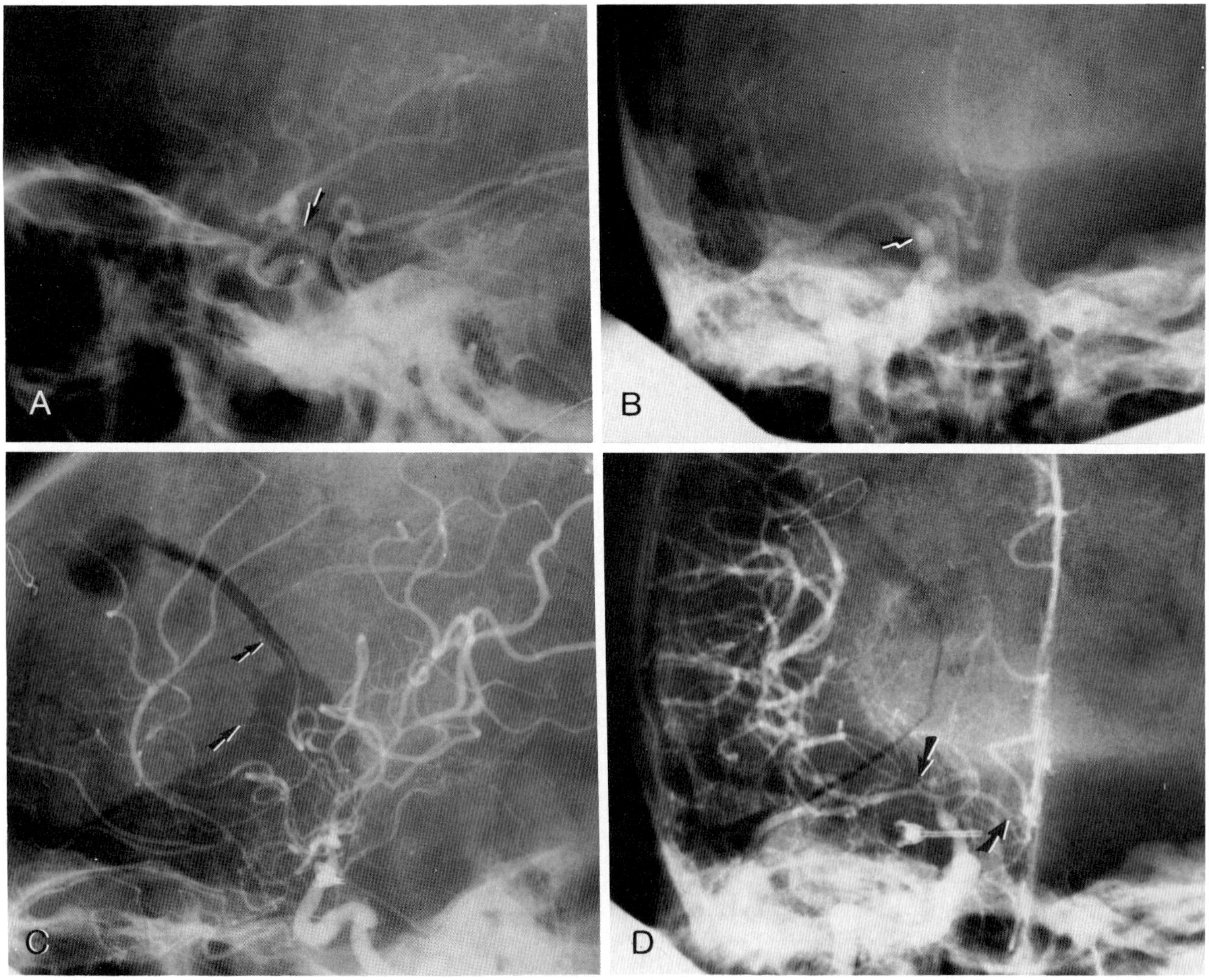

Figure 11.11 (*A* to *D*)

Intracranial Aneurysms: General Aspects of Surgical Treatment

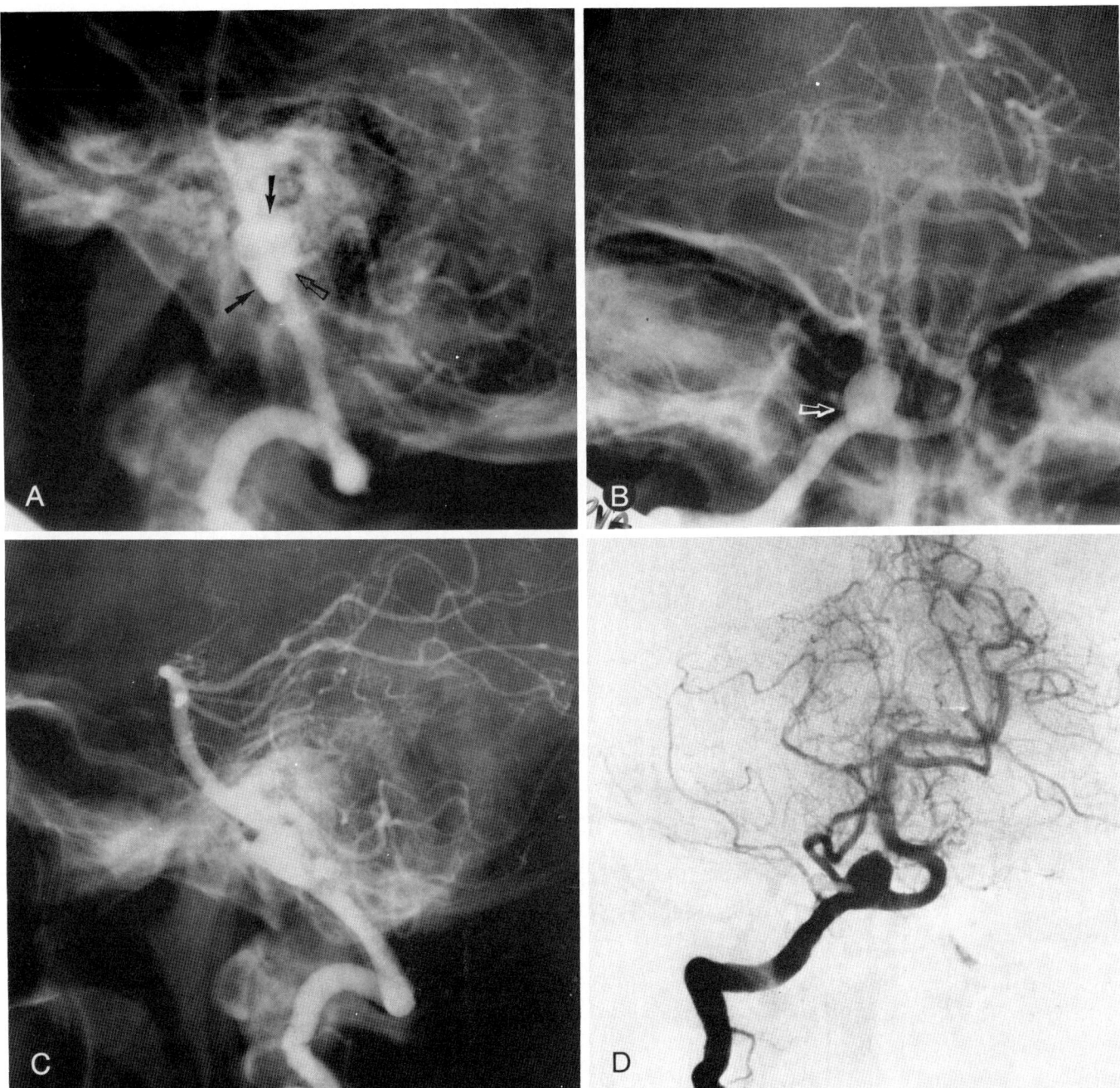

Figure 11.12 "Slipped clip." *A* and *B*, preoperative right vertebral angiogram shows large aneurysm (*closed arrows*) arising from vertebral artery at origin of posterior inferior cerebellar artery (*open arrows*). At surgery, Heifetz clip was applied up to the hilt. *C* and *D*, postoperative angiogram shows clip only a few millimeters across aneurysm neck. Patient refused reoperation.

Figure 11.11 Postoperative cerebral vasospasm. *A* and *B*, right carotid angiogram shows aneurysm (*arrow*) of internal carotid-posterior communicating arteries and no spasm 8 days after SAH. *C* and *D*, postoperative right carotid angiogram performed 1 day after surgery and 9 days after SAH shows obliteration of aneurysm with intense spasm of internal carotid, anterior cerebral, and middle cerebral arteries, and delayed flow in MCA branches (*arrows*). Despite hypertensive therapy, marked left hemiparesis persisted. CT scan 2 weeks later showed right cerebral infarction.

In most patients, postoperative angiography is recommended to ascertain the adequacy of aneurysm obliteration and maintenance of normal vasculature (5). In the rare case of a "slipped clip," reoperation for replacement of the clip is usually indicated (Fig. 11.12, A to D).

REFERENCES

1. Aitken RR, Drake CG: A technique of anesthesia with induced hypotension for surgical correction of intracranial aneurysms. Clin Neurosurg 21:107–114, 1974.
2. Botterell EH, Lougheed WM, Scott JW, Vanderwater SL: Hypothermia, and interruption of carotid, or carotid and vertebral circulation, in the surgical management of intracranial aneurysms. J Neurosurg 13:1–42, 1956.
3. Drake CG: Giant intracranial aneurysms: Experience with surgical treatment in 174 patients. Clin Neurosurg 26:12–95, 1979.
4. Drake CG: Management of cerebral aneurysm. Stroke 12:273–283, 1981.
5. Drake CG, Allcock JM: Postoperative angiography and the "slipped" clip. J Neurosurg 39:683–689, 1973.
6. Flamm ES: Parasurgical treatment of aneurysms. Clin Neurosurg 24:240–247, 1976.
7. Giannotta SL, McGillicuddy JE, Kindt GW: Diagnosis and treatment of postoperative cerebral vasospasm. Surg Neurol 8:286–290, 1977.
8. Heros RC, Ojemann RG, Crowell RM: Superior temporal gyrus approach to middle cerebral aneurysms. Technique and results. Neurosurgery (in press).
9. Hollin SA, Decker RE: Effectiveness of microsurgery for intracranial aneurysms. Postoperative angiographic study of 50 cases. J Neurosurg 39:690–693, 1973.
10. Hunt WE, Hess RM: Surgical risk as related to time of intervention in the repair of intracranial aneurysms. J Neurosurg 28:14–20, 1968.
11. Hunt WE, Kosnik EJ: Timing and perioperative care in intracranial aneurysm surgery. Clin Neurosurg 21:79–89, 1974.
12. Hunt WE, Miller CA: The results of early operation for aneurysm. Clin Neurosurg 24:208–215, 1976.
13. Jenkins JS, Buckell M, Carter AB, Westlake S: Hypothalamic-pituitary-adrenal function after subarachnoid hemorrhage. Br Med J 4:707–709, 1969.
14. Kasdon DL, Stein BM: Combined supratentorial and infratentorial exposure for low-lying basilar aneurysms. Neurosurgery 4:422–426, 1979.
15. Kosnik EJ, Hunt WE: Postoperative hypertension in the management of patients with intracranial arterial aneurysms. J Neurosurg 45:148–154, 1976.
16. Krayenbuhl HA, Yasargil MG, Flamm ES, Tew JM, Jr: Microsurgical treatment of intracranial saccular aneurysms. J Neurosurg 37:678–686, 1972.
17. Lougheed WM, Marshall BM: Management of aneurysms of the anterior circulation by intracranial procedures, in Youmans JR (ed): *Neurological Surgery.* Philadelphia, WB Saunders, 1973, pp 731–767.
18. Miller JD, Jawad K, Jennett B: Safety of carotid ligation and its role in the management of intracranial aneurysms. J Neurol Neurosurg Psychiat 40:64–72, 1977.
19. Nelson PB, Seif SM, Maroon JC, Robinson AG: Hyponatremia in patients with subarachnoid hemorrhage: a study of vasopressin and blood volume, in Wilkins RH (ed): *Cerebral Arterial Spasm.* Baltimore, Williams & Wilkins, 1979, pp 654–658.
20. Peerless SJ: Pre- and postoperative management of cerebral aneurysms. Clin Neurosurg 26:209–231, 1979.
21. Samson DS, Hodosh RM, Reid WR, Beyer CW, Clark WK: Risk of intracranial aneurysm surgery in the good grade patient: Early versus late operation. Neurosurgery 5:422–426, 1979.
22. Spetzler RF, Shuster H, Roski RA: Elective extracranial-intracranial arterial bypass in the treatment of inoperable aneurysms of the giant internal carotid artery. J Neurosurg 53:22–27, 1980.
23. Sundt T: Surgical technic for giant intracranial aneurysms, in Ransohoff J (ed): *Modern Technics in Surgery, Neurosurgery.* Mount Kisco, New York, Futura, 1981, vol 24, pp 1–40.
24. Sundt TM, Jr, Murphey F: Clip grafts for aneurysm and small vessel surgery. Part 3: Clinical experience in intracranial internal carotid artery aneurysms. J Neurosurg 31:59–71, 1969.
25. Suzuki J, Yoshimoto T, Onuma T: Early operations for ruptured intracranial aneurysms: Study of 31 cases operated on within the first four days after ruptured aneurysm. Neurol Med Chr (Tokyo) 18:82–89, 1978.
26. Suzuki J, Onuma T, Yoshimoto T: Results of early operations on cerebral aneurysms. Surg Neurol 11:407–412, 1979.
27. Yasargil MG, Fox JL: The microsurgical approach to intracranial aneurysms. Surg Neurol 3:7–14, 1975.

Chapter 12 INTERNAL CAROTID ANEURYSMS

Aneurysms of the internal carotid artery are the most common intracranial aneurysms in clinical and autopsy series (3, 5, 10, 11, 12). The precise origin of these lesions is variable, often involving the posterior communicating or anterior choroidal arteries and sometimes arising at the bifurcation of the internal carotid artery. Those arising at the ophthalmic artery origin are discussed in Chapter 13. The operative technique in individual cases depends on the specific origin of the lesion. Sometimes the operative management of internal carotid artery aneurysms is relatively straightforward, but the larger lesions, particularly those at the bifurcation, may prove extremely difficult to handle (8, 9, 11, 12, 13).

PRESENTATION

Most patients with internal carotid artery aneurysms come to medical attention because of symptoms of subarachnoid hemorrhage. A substantial minority reach the hospital because of a third nerve palsy, which is usually but not always accompanied by pain in and behind the orbit. The oculomotor palsy may be incomplete, and pupillary sparing is rare. Though other conditions, including diabetes and the Tolosa-Hunt syndrome, can mimic this condition, the syndrome of painful ophthalmoplegia generally warns of an enlarging internal carotid artery aneurysm and is sufficiently characteristic to warrant urgent angiography. Rarely, a patient with internal carotid aneurysm will present with TIAs or seizure (1).

EVALUATION AND MANAGEMENT

In general, the program of evaluation and medical management does not differ from the standard regimen described in Chapter 10. A CT scan may demonstrate subarachnoid hematoma near the internal carotid artery or the aneurysm itself filled with contrast material. Subarachnoid hematoma in the interpeduncular cistern may be related to a posterior pointing internal carotid-posterior communicating artery aneurysm rather than a basilar bifurcation lesion.

Selective internal carotid artery angiography should show the neck of the aneurysm and its relation to ophthalmic, anterior choroidal, and posterior communicating arteries (Fig. 12.1). In some cases, special views including oblique or off lateral projections will be needed to provide this information. When the posterior cerebral artery is not visualized with internal carotid injection, one may assume this vessel is irrigated from the vertebrobasilar circulation. If the posterior cerebral artery does fill from the internal carotid artery injection, then evaluation of washout may suggest alternate filling from the posterior circulation. However, a direct vertebral angiographic study is preferable to establish this point (Fig. 12.1). This information is needed to decide if the posterior communicating artery may be sacrificed with clipping of the aneurysm. Careful inspection of the films will aid the surgeon in determining the relationship of the aneurysm to the cavernous sinus. When the lesion is at or below the anterior clinoid process, part or all of the aneurysm may lie within the cavernous sinus.

General aspects of surgical treatment are discussed in Chapter 11. We have generally chosen to operate these cases 8-10 days after subarachnoid hemorrhage. Since vasospasm appears to be more common with internal carotid aneurysms (7), it may be that operation in the first 24 hours after rupture to clip the aneurysm and evacuate the subarachnoid clot should be considered but this treatment approach needs further evaluation.

OPERATIVE TECHNIQUE

Positioning

The three-point Mayfield headrest is utilized to hold the head which is turned away from the side of the lesion at about 45° to the vertical (Fig. 12.2). The vertex is tilted 15° below the horizontal to permit the brain to fall away from the base of the skull and the head is held slightly above heart level. Additional pentobarbital (50-150 mg IV) is given just prior to this painful stimulation to avoid blood pressure elevation.

Incision and Scalp Flap

Pterional craniotomy is useful for most anterior circulation aneurysms and is therefore described here in some detail (12). In most patients, an incision just behind the hairline is preferred, proceeding from the widow's peak in curvilinear fashion to a point just above the zygoma in front of the tragus (Fig. 12.2). The superficial temporal artery is palpated and marked. The incision should lie posterior to the root of the superficial temporal artery in order to preserve this structure with the flap. Occasionally, in bald individuals or in cases where additional exposure is

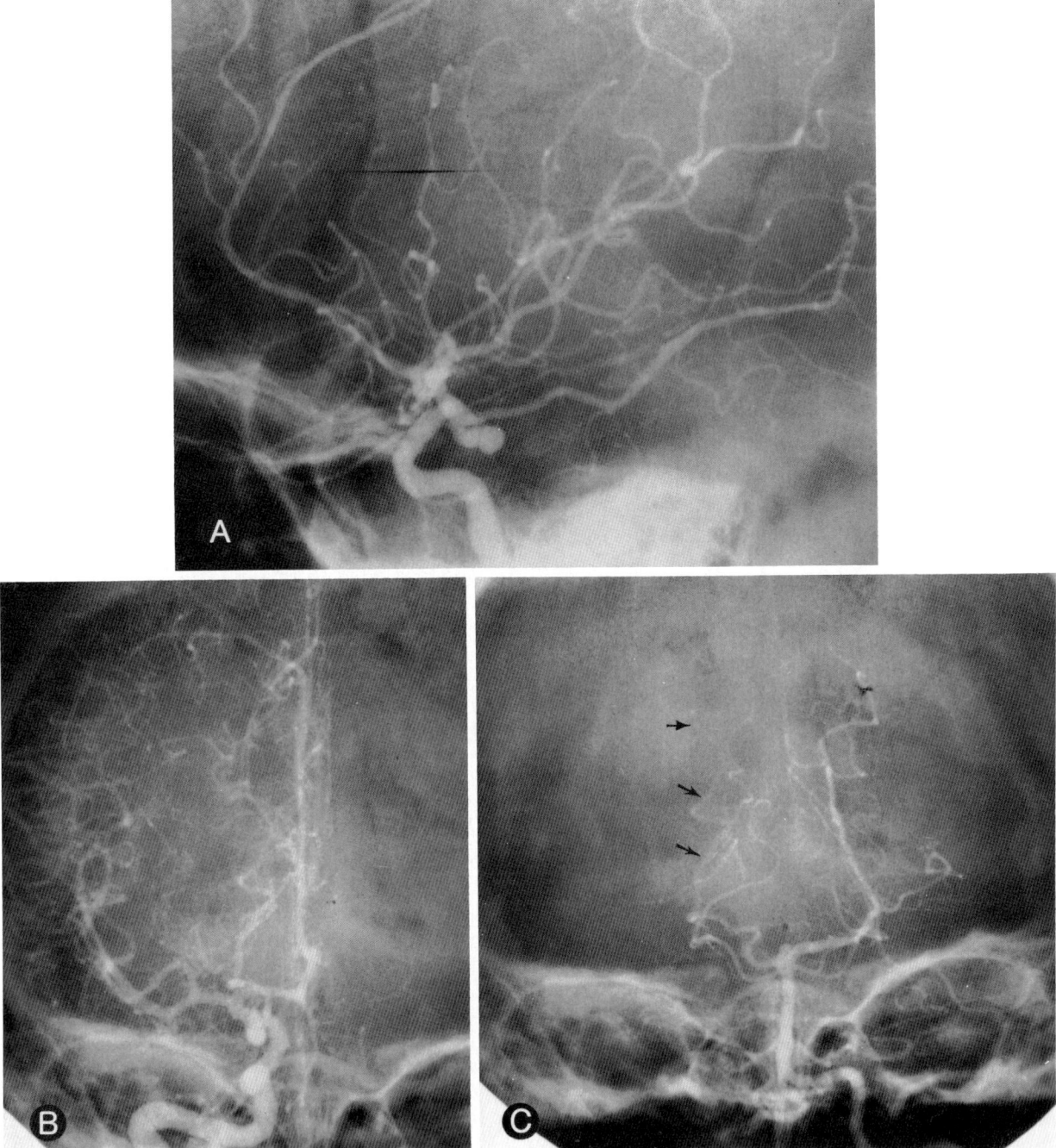

Figure 12.1 Internal carotid-posterior communicating aneurysm: importance of vertebral angiography. A and B, right carotid angiogram shows large internal carotid aneurysm at origin of fetal-type posterior cerebral artery. No washout from posterior circulation. C, AP vertebral angiogram however, shows filling of the right posterior cerebral artery (arrows) which is faint due to washout. There is a tiny aneurysm at the basilar apex.

desired for another aneurysm, an alternative incision may be planned, utilizing a wrinkle high in the forehead or a coronal incision extending across the midline. As the area is draped, the post for the Greenberg retractor is attached horizontally on the three-point headrest to the left of the patient's head.

Both surgeon and assistant utilize loupes and headlights during the initial phases of the procedure. Local anesthesia (Xylocaine 0.5% or Marcaine 1% without epinephrine) is injected along the incision except in the area of the superficial temporal artery. The incision is begun anteriorly and cuts down to but not

Internal Carotid Aneurysms

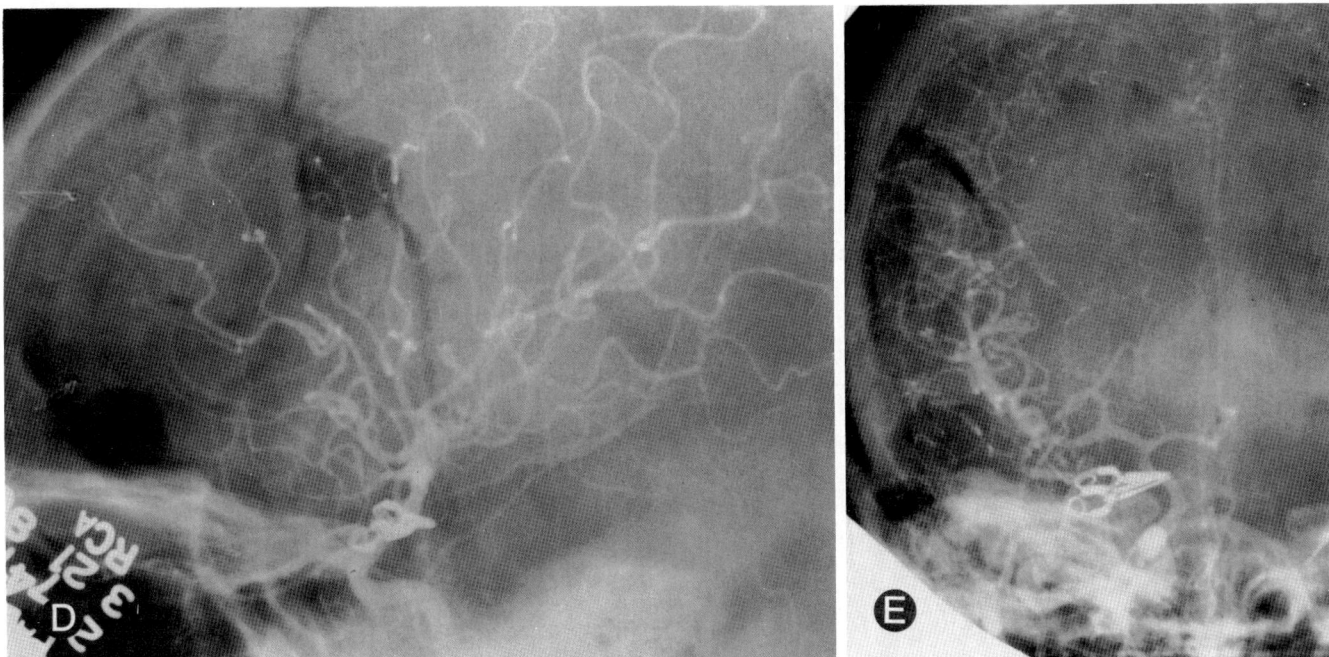

Figure 12.1 *D* and *E*, postoperative right carotid angiograms show 1) non-filling of aneurysm, and 2) non-filling of fetal posterior cerebral artery which required clipping to collapse aneurysm. Vertebral angiogram had demonstrated that this maneuver would likely be safe. The postoperative examination was normal.

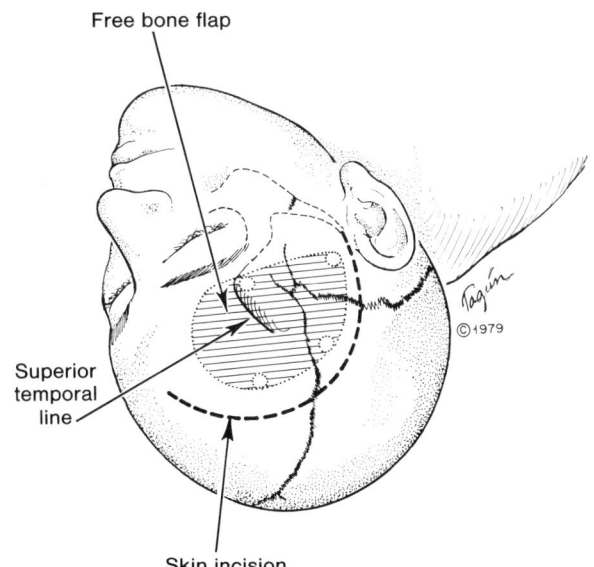

Figure 12.2 Pterional craniotomy. Head is turned 45°. Incision is behind hairline for low free bone flap. After removal of pterion and lateral sphenoid ridge, retractors are inserted to approach optic nerve and internal carotid artery.

through periosteum. A scissors is inserted in the plane between galea and periosteum and then the knife incises down to the scissors, thus preventing injury to the underlying temporalis muscle and superficial temporal artery. Care is taken to avoid injuring this artery, particularly near its root. The posterior branch of the superficial temporal artery is dissected free and divided between 3-0 silk ligatures, thus permitting the trunk and frontal branch of this vessel, which might be needed for later cerebral revascularization, to be reflected forward with the soft tissue flap. Hemostasis is obtained by the application of Dandy hemostats to the posterior margin and Köln clips to the anterior margin of the incision, taking particular care to avoid injury to the superficial temporal artery.

Next, the temporalis fascia is incised with a knife, and the temporalis muscle is opened with the cutting cautery. A branch of the deep temporal artery is usually encountered within the muscle, and this must be cauterized accurately to avoid annoying bleeding. The periosteum is swept off the skull to the edge of the orbit using a periosteal elevator. The muscle is reflected from the skull, with the cutting cautery until the zygomatic process of frontal bone is approached. The soft tissue flap is folded over a sponge to prevent ischemic compression, protected with a rubber dam and Bacitracin-soaked sponge, held in place with sutures sewn into the muscle and attached by rubber bands to the drapes. A final maneuver, which permits maximum visualization beneath muscle, is the application of Cushing retractors to the muscle along the zygomatic process of frontal bone, with tension applied to these retractors via rubber bands and Allis clamps attached to the drapes. This approach provides excellent exposure once the bone flap is removed. We have tried the Z-formed temporalis fascia opening suggested by Yasargil and found it no better

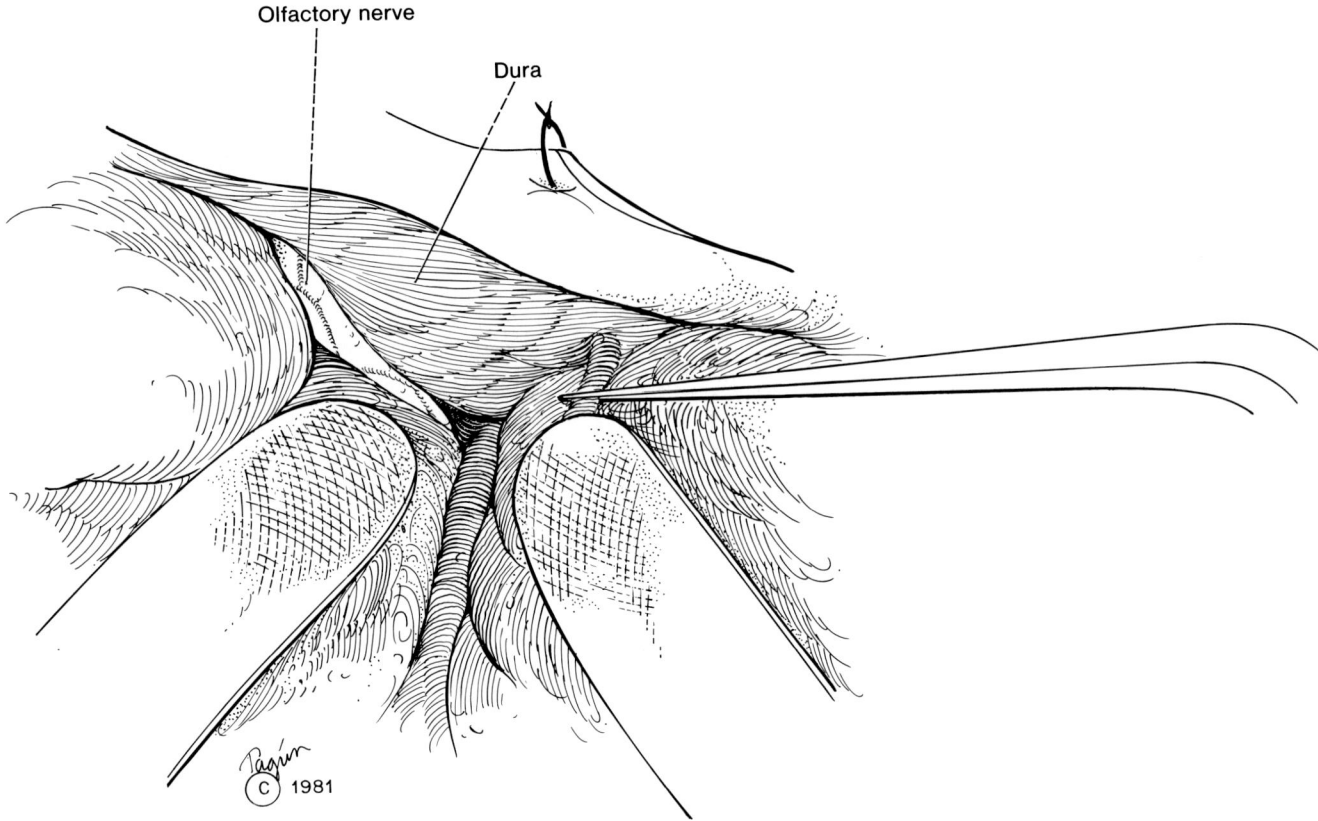

Figure 12.3 Approach to the internal carotid artery. If the lesion does not point laterally, temporal tip veins are divided to mobilize the temporal lobe.

for exposure and less satisfactory from the cosmetic standpoint (15).

Initial Exposure

A free pterional bone flap is turned with the power drill and craniotome (12) (Fig. 12.2). The critical burr hole is placed just behind the zygomatic process of frontal bone and below the end of the superior temporal line. Additional burr holes are placed in the frontal and temporal regions, the latter just at the superior temporal line. The unsightly depression of an inferomedial frontal burr hole can be eliminated by the use of a curved bony cut with the craniotome. Dura is separated from the inner table of the skull with a #3 Penfield dissector. The craniotome cut is made starting along the floor of the anterior fossa, proceeding medially about 3–4 cm, and then curving in an easy arch posteriorly to the high temporal burr hole. It is well to angle this saw curve slightly, beveling outward to provide nice seating for the bone flap when it is replaced. The lateral sphenoid ridge is preserved with the bone flap, which is finally broken off with prying by a periosteal elevator. The bone flap is carefully peeled off the dura, and the middle meningeal artery is identified, coagulated, and cut if necessary. Bony edges are waxed for hemostasis. Additional bone is rongeured from the lateral sphenoid ridge. Care is taken at this point to avoid injury to structures in the superior orbital fissure. Frequently, a small arterial branch to the dura in this region must be coagulated. These maneuvers effectively level the sphenoid ridge between frontal and temporal lobe, thus creating an unobstructed visual access to the anterior clinoid area. In some patients, the inner table of bone forming the floor of anterior fossa over the orbit will be characterized by mountainous irregularities impeding exposure. A high speed drill may be used to smooth the area. If a small opening into the orbit occurs, it is plugged with Gelfoam. If additional access is needed along the floor of the anterior fossa behind the supraorbital ridge, the inner table bone at the edge of the craniotomy just anterior to the key hole may also be removed with the rongeur without compromising the cosmetic appearance of the outer table. Occasionally a very prominent and lateral frontal sinus may be encountered with the saw cut or bone removal. If this occurs, the mucosa should be removed, the sinus packed with Bacitracin-soaked Gelfoam, and the bone opening covered with a flap of pericranium tissue dissected from the back of the scalp flap and sewn to the adjacent dura. A fine drill point is used to create holes for wires to hold the flap in place at the time of closure. Dural to pericranial sutures of 4-0 Neurolon are placed around the periphery of the bone opening

Internal Carotid Aneurysms

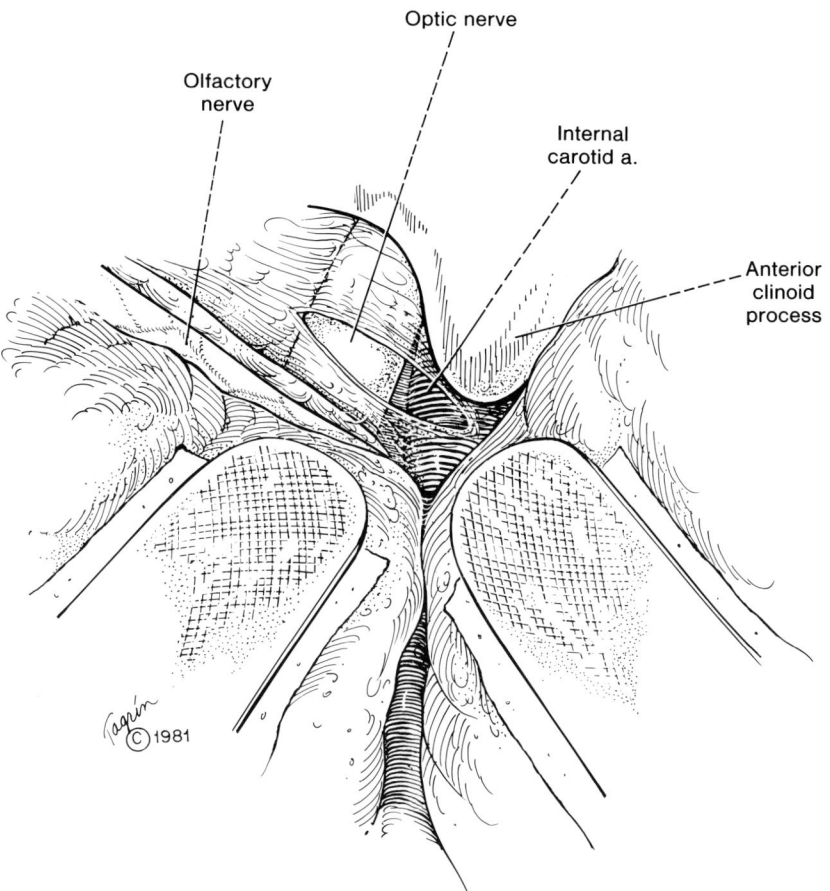

Figure 12.4 Opening arachnoid. Microscissors and a fine right-angled hook are used to open the arachnoid over optic nerve and ICA. This permits the frontal lobe to be elevated safely.

to achieve epidural hemostasis. Tiny strips of Surgicel are inserted in the epidural space as needed. Bacitracin-soaked sponges are placed over the skin edges and all exposed tissue except the dura.

During this phase, the surgeon can readily determine whether the brain is slack. If brain seems full, then measures must be taken to obtain adequate reduction in brain tension; the PCO_2 may need adjustment, additional dehydration may be required, or CSF drained. Occasionally, ventricular puncture will be needed to obtain a slack brain.

A linear dural incision is made approximately 1.0 cm above the inferior margin of the bony opening with inferior turning at the frontal and temporal corners. The inferior dural flap is tacked up flush with the bone edge and held with sutures under tension, being certain to avoid a buckle in the center of this flap which could interfere with intradural visualization.

The surface of the brain is inspected for evidence of subdural hematoma, subarachnoid hemorrhage, or evidence of cerebral infarction. A medium width, Teflon-coated, hand-held brain retractor is used to gently elevate the frontal lobe. A sucker on a cottonoid can be used to gradually remove CSF which may appear inferior to the frontal lobe. The retractor is slowly advanced just in front of the edge of the sphenoid wing. When the aneurysm arises from the supraclinoid internal carotid artery and points laterally, the temporal lobe is left undisturbed to avoid the threat of tearing an embedded aneurysm. Otherwise, the temporal lobe is carefully elevated and temporal tip bridging veins are divided (Fig. 12.3).

The olfactory tract, an important landmark, will come into view, and following this a few millimeters posteriorly will lead one to the region of the optic nerve (Fig. 12.3). Usually the arachnoid is thin and the optic nerve and carotid artery are visualized, but at times the arachnoid may be thickened, obscuring these structures. The arachnoid is opened using a fine right angle hook, microdissector and/or microscissors (Fig. 12.4). Time should then be spent allowing further CSF to drain. It is most important that the brain be so slack that only mild retraction is needed for adequate exposure.

A protective layer of Telfa or rubber dam, precut to the proper shape, is placed like a rug over the exposed frontal lobe down to the olfactory tract. At this point, the Greenberg self-retaining retractor blade bent to about 60°, is placed to elevate the frontal lobe. The retractor should take a low profile so as to give easy access to the subfrontal region.

Once the temporal tip is free, a covering of Telfa is placed, and the lobe is held posteriorly with a slender retractor blade fixed on the Greenberg apparatus. The two retractor blades should be separated by only several millimeters. Up to this point, the combination of loupes and headlight illumination has been used for maximum mobility with adequate visualization.

Microsurgical Dissection

The operating microscope is now positioned. We prefer a 300-mm objective, angled oculars, and 12.5X eyepieces. A small beam splitter is used with the stereoscopic observer tube on the left (in the case of a right-handed surgeon) and the color television camera on the right. Stools for the surgeon and assistants are positioned to allow the surgeons to work seated. A Mayo stand is placed next to the head on the surgeon's right to provide an armrest. The mean arterial pressure is lowered to approximately 70–80 mm Hg. Controlled suction is utilized with low vacuum pressure.

The surgeon must be particularly flexible in his surgical approach to these lesions. This requires a broad armamentarium, of clips, as well as ligature carriers, tissue adhesives, and special dissectors (see Chapter 11). All of these items should be readily at hand as the aneurysm is approached.

The frontal lobe is gently elevated with the retractor after the arachnoid between the optic nerve and frontal lobe has been incised with microscissors. This permits visualization of the optic nerve and the proximal internal carotid artery. The arachnoid over the internal carotid artery is opened, and dissection proceeds proximal to distal to obtain control of the artery on both sides of the lesion's neck (Fig. 12.4).

Retraction alone usually suffices to expose lesions of the proximal supraclinoid internal carotid artery. To expose aneurysms of the distal supraclinoid internal carotid artery, we use a small medial frontal corticectomy (see p. 166 and Fig. 12.13). A short cortical incision (about 1 cm) serves to expose the aneurysm and parent vessel without undue retraction. Small branch arteries in this area which may include lenticulostriate and Heubner's arteries, must be spared since they may supply important areas.

Manipulation of the aneurysm is avoided until the neck is isolated. Dissection with a Rhoton #6 dissector is helpful to free the internal carotid artery. Sharp dissection, with microscissors or a #11 knife blade, is preferred for arachnoid and for some adhesions to the aneurysm. In general, it is best to dissect the white, tough portions of the lesion before proceeding to the red, thin areas, which are more likely to rupture. Dangerous red areas and adherent small branches are best left for dissection after the aneurysm neck is fully prepared. Usually the aneurysm is left adherent to the third cranial nerve, since clipping can be accomplished without mobilization which could injure the nerve. Occasionally, the aneurysm must be dissected off the third nerve to permit safe obliteration. The specific anatomy dictates which clip will be selected. Some lesions will need bipolar coagulation of the neck to narrow and toughen it prior to clipping.

During the final preparation of the aneurysm, controlled hypotension may be essential to avoid rupture. Healthy patients will tolerate a mean arterial pressure of 40–50 mm Hg for the final dissection and clipping. Occasionally, a particularly thin walled aneurysm may require brief profound hypotension with mean arterial pressure 20–30 mm Hg for 2–3 minutes. Only such hypotension as is critically necessary should be used. In patients with evidence of coronary artery disease, occlusive cerebrovascular disease, or residual neurological signs due to vasospasm, it may not be wise to use hypotension.

ANEURYSMS OF THE INTERNAL CAROTID ARTERY TRUNK

This section will consider aneurysms arising from the internal carotid artery distal to the origin of the ophthalmic artery. Most of these lesions arise at or near the origin of the posterior communicating artery. They usually point posteriorly or posterolaterally (Fig. 12.5). After subarachnoid hematoma is removed from around the proximal internal carotid artery, dissection proceeds distally along the internal carotid artery on its medial aspect, away from the aneurysm. If angiography has not shown an important contribution from the posterior communicating artery to the posterior cerebral artery, then no special effort to identify the posterior communicating artery is needed. If the artery does indeed give potentially critical supply to the posterior cerebral artery, then a search for the posterior communicating artery will be required. Sometimes the vessel may be located by deflection of the internal carotid artery medially to reveal the posterior communicating artery wrapped around the inferior pole of the aneurysm. In other cases, retraction of the internal carotid artery laterally will show the posterior communicating artery draped across the medial aspect of the lesion (Fig. 12.6). The aneurysm is avoided as dissection proceeds distally beyond the neck.

The requirements for distal dissection, retraction, and exposure will be dictated by the need to identify the anterior choroidal artery. Ordinarily, this vessel is found by dissecting laterally on the internal carotid artery just distal to the aneurysm. The anterior choroidal artery, which may be in duplicate and is generally located on the distal surface of the neck of the lesion, sweeping posteriorly and superiorly. In exposing this region, significant temporal lobe retraction may be required. To maximize safety during this

Internal Carotid Aneurysms

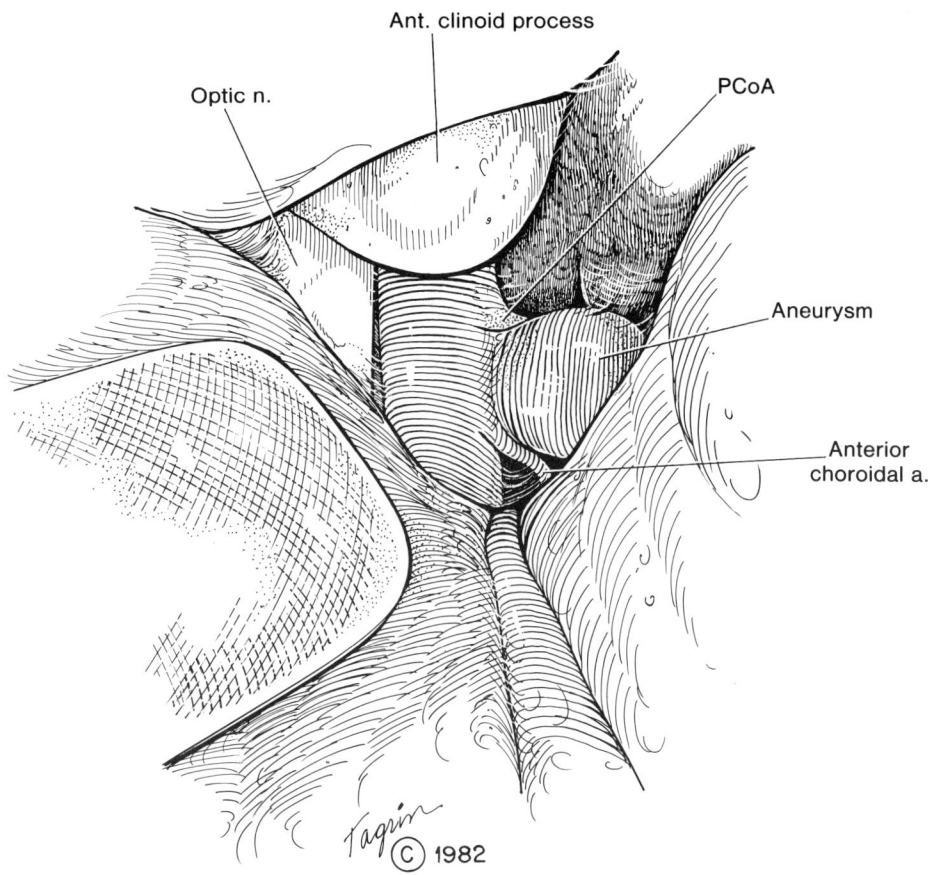

Figure 12.5 Posterior-lateral projection of ICA-PCoA aneurysm. Temporal lobe is not retracted. The dome is usually left adherent to the oculomotor nerve. Anterior choroidal artery must be spared.

exposure, the surgeon should carefully observe the relationship of the aneurysm to the temporal tip and the effects of temporal traction on the lesion. In some instances, it is necessary to free the dome of the aneurysm from the temporal lobe, leaving an area of protective arachnoid, in order to obtain satisfactory distal exposure.

If the posterior communicating artery does not provide critical arterial supply to the posterior cerebral artery, the origin of the artery may be included within the blades of the clip (Fig. 12.7). With the posterior communicating artery origin included in the clip, there may be back filling of the aneurysm from the distal artery. The surgeon can check this possibility after clipping by aspiration of the aneurysm with a 25-gauge spinal needle. If there is back filling, this may be eliminated by application of a clip to the posterior communicating artery just distal to the aneurysm. This clip should avoid perforators arising from the posterior communicating artery which can then be filled in retrograde fashion from the posterior circulation. When the posterior communicating artery provides important circulation to the posterior cerebral artery, the artery must be carefully dissected and preserved.

An alternative cause of persistent filling is inadequate obliteration of the neck which is most frequently the result of thick atherosclerosis in the neck of the lesion. A ligature or bipolar cauterization may prepare the neck for complete obliteration by clipping.

When there is a significant portion of the lesion directly posterior to the internal carotid artery, a curved clip can be applied flush with the internal carotid artery and give total obliteration (Fig. 12.8). A Sundt clip may also be used in this situation (Fig. 12.9). The 4-mm size is most frequently utilized with the cutout going around the anterior choroidal artery.

Sometimes a large aneurysm in this location may provide the surgeon with a difficult challenge, particularly when a fetal type posterior communicating artery must be preserved. In this situation, substantial dissection both medially and laterally may be required to prepare the lesion for obliteration. In order to obtain enough room to work, the surgeon may need to aspirate the lesion with a suction needle during the dissection of the neck and proximal dome. Careful inspection of the angiograms should warn the surgeon of this situation preoperatively. Rarely, a fusiform aneurysm of the internal carotid artery

164 Surgical Management of Cerebrovascular Disease

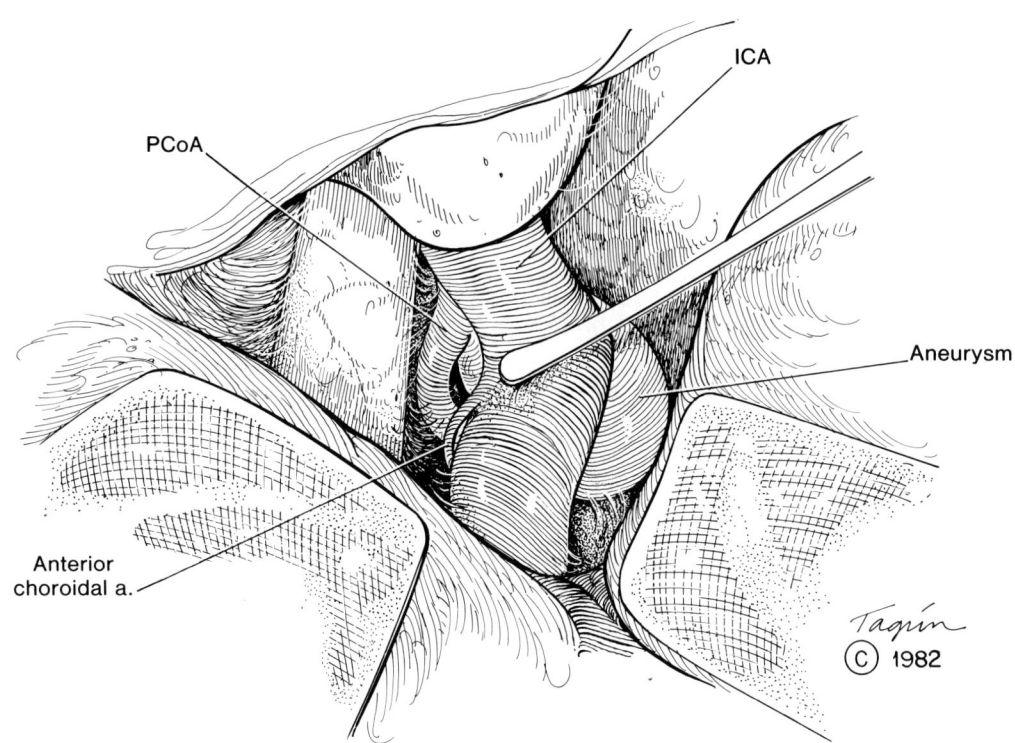

Figure 12.6 Posterior projection of ICA aneurysm. Deflection of ICA laterally may expose medial wall of aneurysm and its relation to ICA branches.

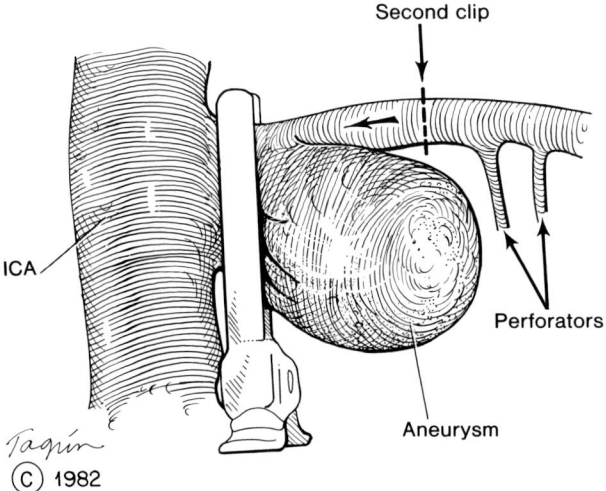

Figure 12.7 ICA-posterior communicating aneurysm. This lesion may back-fill from posterior communicating artery (PCoA) after clipping. A second clip to occlude PCoA must avoid important perforator branches. Preoperative angiography indicates whether the PCoA may be sacrificed safely.

Internal Carotid Aneurysms

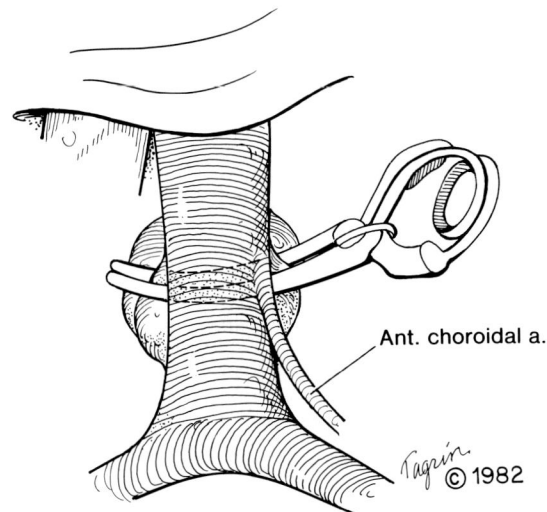

Figure 12.8 Posterior projection of ICA aneurysm. A markedly curved or right-angle clip may be effective.

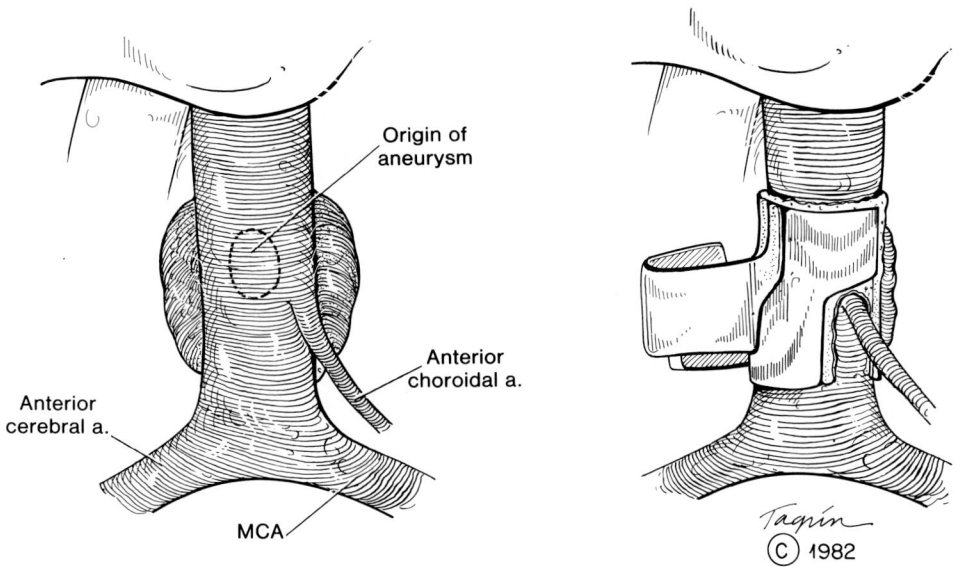

Figure 12.9 Posterior projection of ICA aneurysm. A Sundt clip-graft (with or without window) may be the answer.

may defy clipping and require reinforcement with tissue adhesive, muslin, or muscle.

Aneurysms of the proximal ICA may be exposed best by removal of the anterior clinoid process, as described for carotid-ophthalmic aneurysm (Chapter 13) (Fig. 12.10). Occasionally, such a lesion will be partially within the cavernous sinus, and opening the sinus will permit application of the deep blade of a clip (Fig. 12.11).

Occasionally, an aneurysm will rise at the anterior choroidal artery origin (Fig. 12.12). Preparation and obliteration of such aneurysms must preserve the anterior choroidal artery. Clipping of this artery will result in hemiplegia in one-third of the cases and temporary weakness in another one-third (2). Often bipolar cauterization may be used to prepare lesions in this area with adequate preservation of the anterior choroidal artery. Generally, a narrow clip with a curved blade, is convenient in this location. Sometimes a Sundt clip graft with a cutout for the branch artery offers the best solution.

Fifty-three aneurysms of the internal carotid trunk including lesions arising at the carinae of the posterior communicating artery and anterior choroidal artery were operated using microsurgical techniques (Table 12.1). Of these, 49 (92.5%) were judged to have good-excellent results. There were four poor results, all of which occurred in patients who were Grade 3 or 4 preoperatively. There were no deaths in this series of patients. These results are comparable to

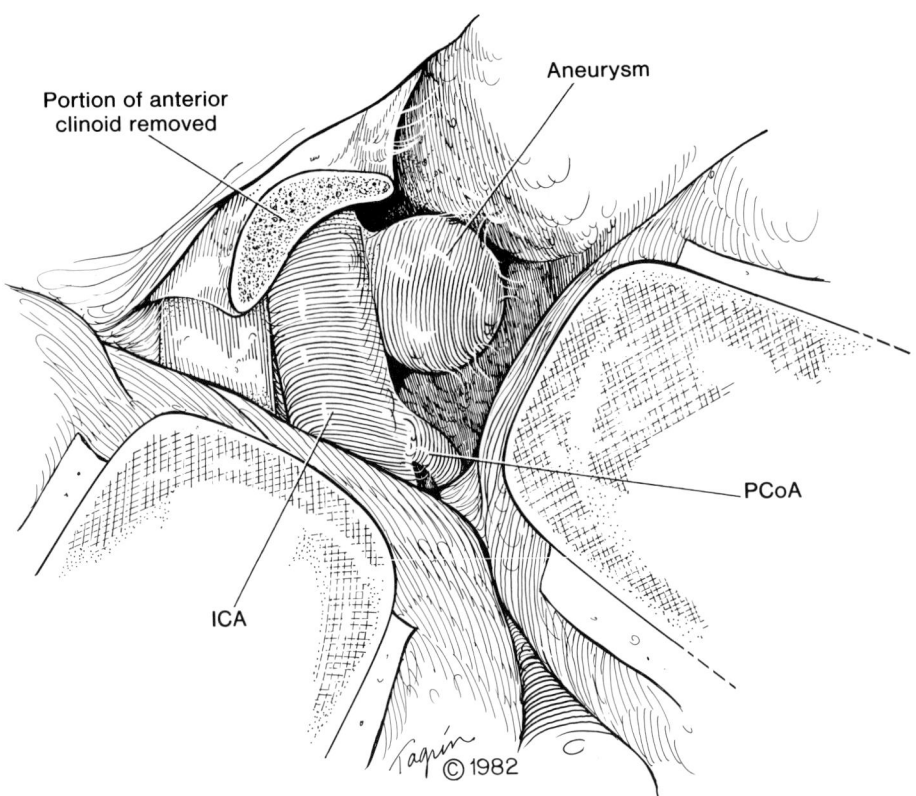

Figure 12.10 Proximal ICA aneurysm. Like a carotid ophthalmic lesion, this aneurysm may require removal of the anterior clinoid process for adequate exposure.

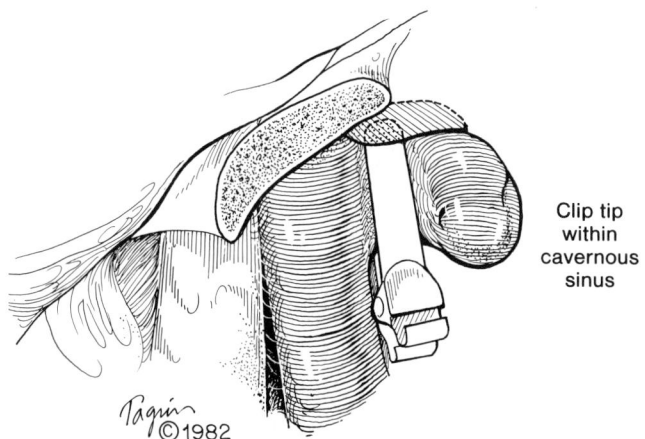

Figure 12.11 Proximal ICA aneurysm, partially within cavernous sinus. Similar to carotid-ophthalmic aneurysm. Anterior clinoid process may be removed for exposure. The cavernous sinus may be opened to permit clipping.

reports in the literature (4, 5, 6, 7, 10, 11, 14). For ICA trunk aneurysms, Yasargil and Smith record 81% good-excellent results with 7.4% mortality (14), and Hollin and Decker report 84% excellent results with 4.3% mortality (4). Poor results and deaths occurred in grade 4 and 5 patients in these two series.

ANEURYSMS OF THE INTERNAL CAROTID ARTERY BIFURCATION

These aneurysms are not uncommon and present a fundamentally different surgical problem from other proximally originating carotid artery aneurysms (13). Exposure is more difficult, typically requiring substantial retraction of frontal and temporal lobes. In some cases, the Sylvian fissure may be conveniently opened. With the fissure under tension, arachnoid is divided, either with a scissors or blunt hook, with the neighboring small arteries and veins being preserved. In many instances, a small frontal corticectomy will provide the needed exposure without further dangerous retraction (Fig. 12.13). In this instance, the proximal internal carotid artery is exposed as described on p. 161. The retractors are placed a few millimeters apart with an area of frontal lobe exposed just medial to the sylvian fissure. A small corticectomy approximately 1 cm in length is made along the Sylvian fissure. This corticectomy may sacrifice surface vessels on the lateral frontal lobe. Dissection is deepened by sucker removal of brain tissue directly overlying the distal internal carotid artery and its bifurcation. The final portions of pia-arachnoid overlying the distal carotid bifurcation and aneurysmal neck are carefully inspected to preserve small arteries which might represent important

Internal Carotid Aneurysms

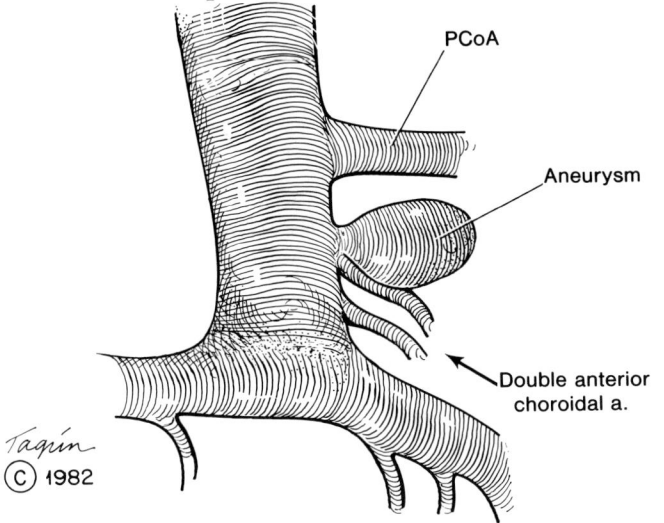

perforator vessels such as the lenticulostriate or Heubner arteries. Retractors are gently advanced into this opening with direct visualization of the effects of the traction on the vessels and the aneurysmal neck. In this fashion, the distal internal carotid and its bifurcation, together with the aneurysm neck, may be gently and safely exposed. Generally, it is not necessary to dissect and expose the entire dome of the bifurcation aneurysm. Instead, careful dissection with a Rhoton #6 instrument may separate the neck, both medially and laterally from myriad perforating arteries which may be adherent and must be preserved (Fig. 12.14). The most difficult portion of the

Figure 12.12 Internal carotid-anterior choroidal artery aneurysm. The anterior choroidal artery, which may be in duplicate, must be preserved even if a small corner of aneurysm must be left unclipped.

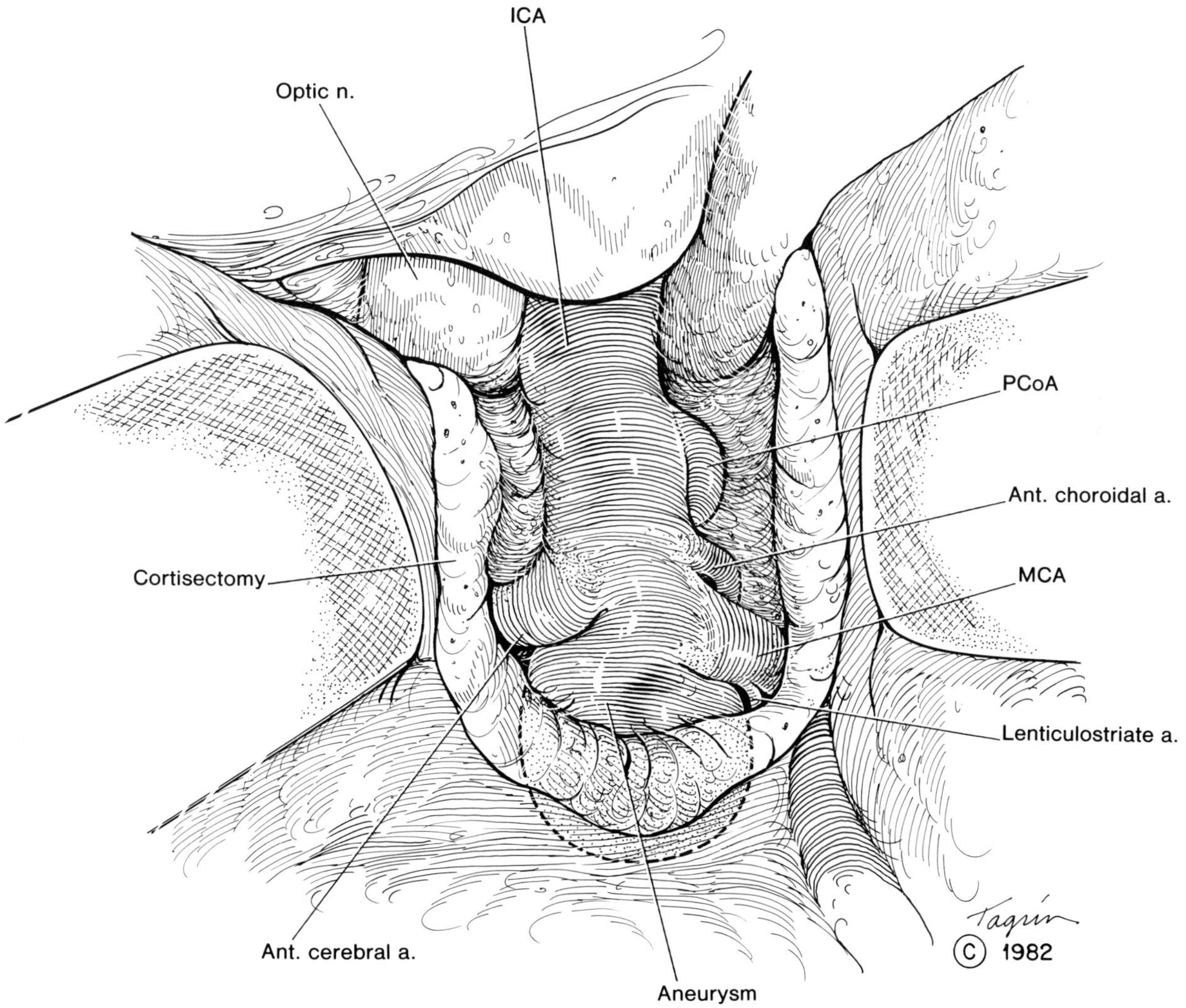

Figure 12.13 Internal carotid bifurcation aneurysm. Small medial frontal corticectomy (or opening Sylvian fissure) provides distal exposure of lesion with limited retraction.

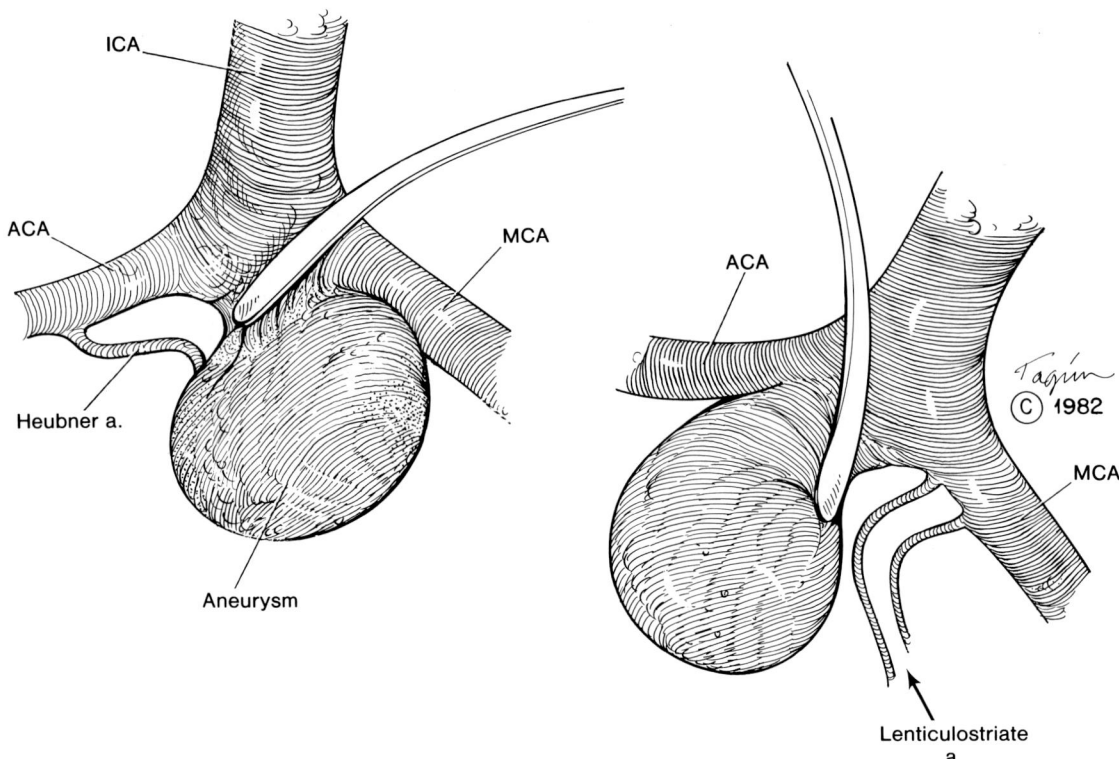

Figure 12.14 Internal carotid bifurcation aneurysm. Careful dissection of neck insures preservation of critical perforating branches from anterior and middle cerebral arteries.

dissection is freeing of the posterior medial neck of the lesion, which lies directly away from the surgeon's vision. Angling of the microscope to one side and then the other may be necessary for this dissection, which can be especially difficult if the lesion points posteromedially. In this situation, dissection inferior to the anterior cerebral artery and the middle cerebral artery may provide additional visualization. A larger corticectomy and more extensive mobilization of the aneurysmal dome may be required for safe preparation of the neck and adjacent small arteries. Occasionally, such a lesion may even extend to the area of the third nerve causing an oculomotor palsy (Fig. 12.15).

Obliteration of aneurysms of the internal carotid artery bifurcation can be accomplished with a variety of tactics, depending on the precise nature of the lesion. For many small lesions pointing in the axis of the internal carotid artery, a straight clip with narrow blades will do the job. Where there is a significant posteromedial segment, a curved clip may be required. When the aneurysm is directed posteromedially or posterolaterally, application of a right-angle clip may be the best solution. Such an application may proceed from the area distal to the bifurcation with the tips deep to the internal carotid artery pointing proximally along it. Occasionally, where the lesion is intimately adherent to the anterior cerebral A-1 segment, this vessel may be included in the clip, provided there is an adequate anterior communicating artery.

Eight aneurysms of the internal carotid bifurcation were operated in our series (Table 12.1). Of these, six were judged excellent or good results (75%). One poor result occurred in a grade 1 patient who developed spasm postoperatively with a moderate hemiparesis. This patient had not been on Reserpine-Kanamycin therapy prior to surgery. The other poor result was in a grade 3 patient who underwent uneventful clipping of the aneurysm 10 days after subarachnoid hemorrhage. Postoperatively, he remained obtunded with a mild hemiparesis, and developed massive pulmonary edema and disseminated intravascular coagulation which eventually proved fatal. Angiography showed obliteration of the aneurysm with good positioning of clip, preservation of normal vasculature, and only minimal spasm. Results from the literature are similar. Yasargil and Smith report 88% good-excellent results with 2.3% mortality (14).

Table 12.1
Results of Surgery for ICA Aneurysm

	Excellent	Good	Poor	Dead	Total
Trunk (PCoA, AChA)	44	5	4[a]	0	53
Bifurcation	4	2	1	1[a]	8
Total	48	7	5	1	61

[a] Grade 3-4 preoperatively.

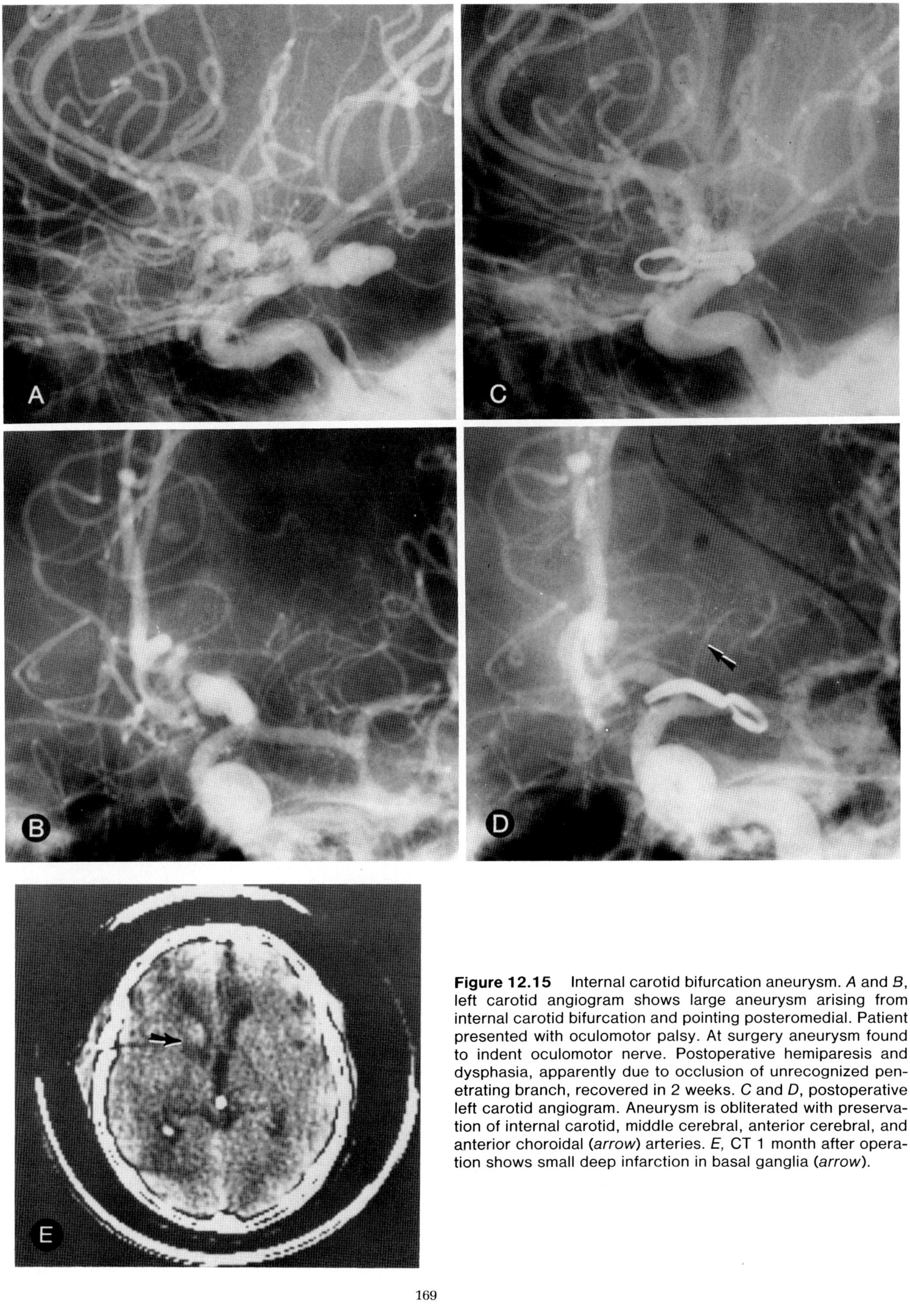

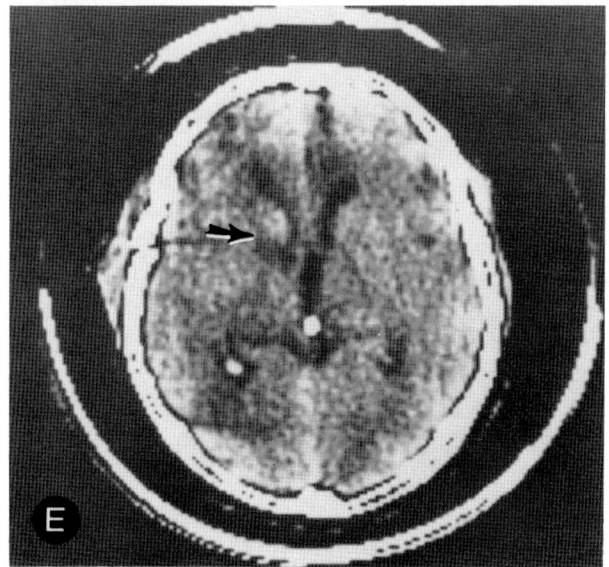

Figure 12.15 Internal carotid bifurcation aneurysm. *A* and *B*, left carotid angiogram shows large aneurysm arising from internal carotid bifurcation and pointing posteromedial. Patient presented with oculomotor palsy. At surgery aneurysm found to indent oculomotor nerve. Postoperative hemiparesis and dysphasia, apparently due to occlusion of unrecognized penetrating branch, recovered in 2 weeks. *C* and *D*, postoperative left carotid angiogram. Aneurysm is obliterated with preservation of internal carotid, middle cerebral, anterior cerebral, and anterior choroidal (*arrow*) arteries. *E*, CT 1 month after operation shows small deep infarction in basal ganglia (*arrow*).

REFERENCES

1. Antunes JL, Correll JW: Cerebral emboli from intracranial aneurysms. Surg Neurol 6:7-10, 1976.
2. Cooper IS: Surgical alleviation of Parkinsonism: Effects of occlusion of the anterior choroidal artery. J Am Geriatr Soc 11:691-717, 1954.
3. Crompton MR: The pathology of subarachnoid hemorrhage. J Roy Coll Physicians Lond 7:235-237, 1973.
4. Hollin SA, Decker RE: Microsurgical treatment of internal carotid artery aneurysm. J Neurosurg 47:142-149, 1977.
5. Krayenbuhl HA, Yasargil MG, Flamm ES, Tew JM Jr: Microsurgical treatment of intracranial saccular aneurysms. J Neurosurg 37:678-686, 1972.
6. Lougheed WM, Marshall BM: Management of aneurysms of the anterior circulation by intracranial procedures, in Youmans JR (ed): *Neurological Surgery*. Philadelphia, WB Saunders, 1973, pp 731-767.
7. Peerless SJ: Pre- and postoperative management of cerebral aneurysms. Clin Neurosurg 26:209-231, 1979.
8. Sengupta RP, Lassman LP, de Moraes AA, Garvan N: Treatment of internal carotid bifurcation aneurysms by direct surgery. J Neurosurg 43:343-351, 1975.
9. Sundt TM Jr, Murphey F: Clip grafts for aneurysm and small vessel surgery. Part 3: Clinical experience in intracranial internal carotid artery aneurysms. J Neurosurg 31:59-71, 1969.
10. Sundt TM Jr, Whisnant JP: Subarachnoid hemorrhage from intracranial aneurysms. Surgical management and natural history of disease. N Engl J Med 299:116-122, 1978.
11. Suzuki J (ed): *Cerebral Aneurysms: Experiences with 1000 Directly Operated Cases*. Tokyo, Neuron, 1979.
12. Yasargil MG, Fox JL: The microsurgical approach to intracranial aneurysms. Surg Neurol 3:7-14, 1975.
13. Yasargil MD, Boehm WG, Ho RE: Microsurgical treatment of cerebral aneurysms at the bifurcation of the internal carotid artery. Acta Neurochir (Wien) 41:61-72, 1978.
14. Yasargil MG, Smith RD: Management of aneurysms of anterior circulation by intracranial procedures, in Youmans JR (ed): *Neurological Surgery* (Second Edition). Philadelphia, WB Saunders (in press).

Chapter 13 CAROTID-OPHTHALMIC ANEURYSMS

PRESENTATION

Carotid-ophthalmic artery aneurysms usually present with subarachnoid hemorrhage (SAH) (6). Giant aneurysms may cause visual field abnormalities (3, 8). Rarely, a carotid-ophthalmic aneurysm may be associated with transient ischemic attacks in the territory of the internal carotid artery, presumably on an embolic basis. We have observed one case in which a giant ophthalmic aneurysm produced frontal cortical irritation with a presenting seizure disorder. There is a female preponderance for ophthalmic aneurysms and an unusual tendency for multiple aneurysms (3).

These lesions typically arise from the internal carotid artery just distal to the ophthalmic artery origin. Aneurysms of the ophthalmic artery itself are very rare. Carotid-ophthalmic aneurysms may point: 1) medially beneath the optic nerve, 2) laterally beneath the anterior clinoid process, 3) superomedially above the optic nerve, or 4) within the cavernous sinus.

EVALUATION

The overall program of evaluation and management is outlined in Chapters 10 and 11.

If a carotid-ophthalmic artery aneurysm is disclosed, special angiographic views must be obtained for complete characterization of the sac, its neck, and their relationship to internal carotid and ophthalmic arteries. Standard AP and lateral projections may require supplementary views, including base, oblique, or off lateral projections (Fig. 13.1). Subtraction is often helpful in visualizing the ophthalmic artery. In the event the aneurysm proves unapproachable and is best treated by an indirect procedure, views of the carotid bifurcation, external carotid and superficial temporal arteries, and collateral circulation to the carotid territory will be required.

OPERATIVE TECHNIQUE

The initial surgical approach is via a frontotemporal craniotomy described in detail in Chapter 12. The craniotomy in most instances is ipsilateral to the ophthalmic artery aneurysm. Occasionally, for a lesion which points medially or inferiorly from the internal carotid artery, contralateral craniotomy will provide the best visualization of the sac and neck (8). For bilateral ophthalmic artery aneurysms, careful selection of the most appropriate side for craniotomy may permit direct operation on both lesions from one side. The surgical approach differs from the standard pterional craniotomy in several respects, as the aneurysm is approached from beneath the frontal lobe.

Removal of Anterior Clinoid Process

The overlying dura is removed (Fig. 13.2) in order to expose the anterior clinoid process. The monopolar electrocautery, set at low current, is used with a coated Penfield #4 dissector to coagulate a semicircular path in the dura over the clinoid process. Great care must be exercised to avoid injury to the optic nerve which may lie under the dura, unprotected by bone in this area. Lateral coagulation must be terminated at the edge of the cavernous sinus. This coagulated area is incised with a #15 knife blade. The resulting flap of dura may be conveniently elevated with a fine angled microcurette and reflected posteriorly. This flap of dura lies over the internal carotid artery, thus protecting it during subsequent drilling.

The anterior clinoid process is removed with a high speed drill with angled hand-piece and diamond burr (Fig. 13.3). The surgeon can conveniently control this instrument with his right hand, resting his wrist firmly while the fine sucker is held in the field with the left hand. During controlled drilling, a fine stream of irrigation is directed onto the drill point using the combined suction irrigation system or a microirrigator is used by the assistant (12-cc syringe with a 22-gauge Medicut plastic catheter). The clinoid process may be isolated by drilling its medial and lateral bony supports. Usually, one drilling spot accurately placed on either side of the process will achieve this goal. Once underlying soft tissue is encountered, drilling is redirected slightly superiorly or inferiorly until each buttress, lateral and medial, is weakened. Then a 5-0 straight bone curette is used to gradually fracture and mobilize the resulting anterior clinoid fragment (Fig. 13.4). This is accomplished with utmost care and control to avoid abrupt movement of the fragment with possible injury to nearby structures. The 5-0 curette and microcurettes are used to dissect the fragment free from underlying soft tissues. If the bony exposure seems inadequate, additional drilling may be used to widen the field of view. If space permits a fine microantrostomy punch may be used for additional bony removal (Fig. 13.5). Note that paranasal sinus mucosa may in some cases extend into bone in this area. If mucosa is encountered, the overlying bony opening must be carefully waxed. If bleeding from soft tissue occurs, application of tiny amounts of Surgicel or Gelfoam may be used for hemostasis.

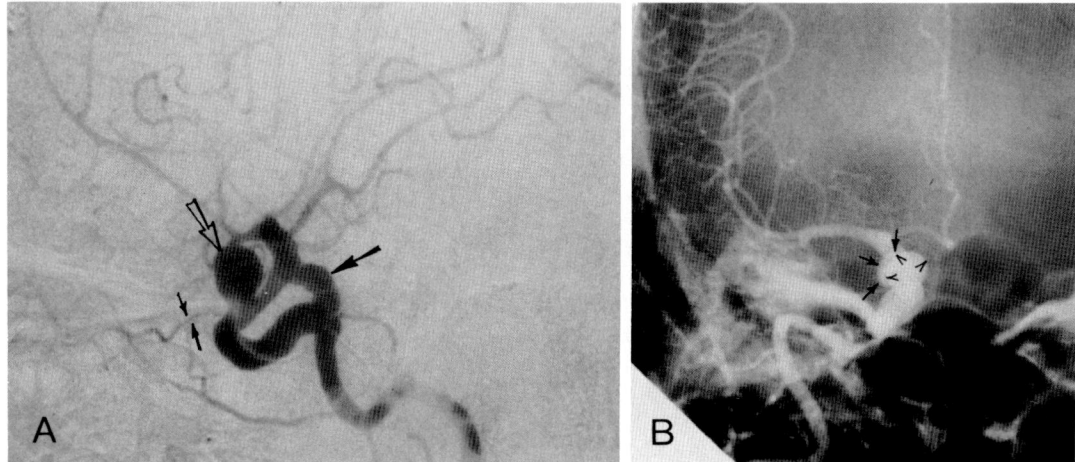

Figure 13.1 Clipping of carotid-ophthalmic and carotid-posterior communicating aneurysms. *A,* lateral right carotid angiogram shows ophthalmic aneurysm (*open arrow*), carotid-posterior communicating aneurysm (*large closed arrow*), and ophthalmic artery (*small arrows*). *B,* AP right carotid angiogram shows that the carotid-ophthalmic aneurysm (*arrowheads*) projects rostrally and carotid-posterior communicating aneurysm (*small arrows*) projects posteriorly. *C,* intraoperative illustration during right pterional craniotomy. Anterior clinoid process has been removed. Both aneurysms are dissected for clipping and the ophthalmic and anterior choroidal arteries are preserved.

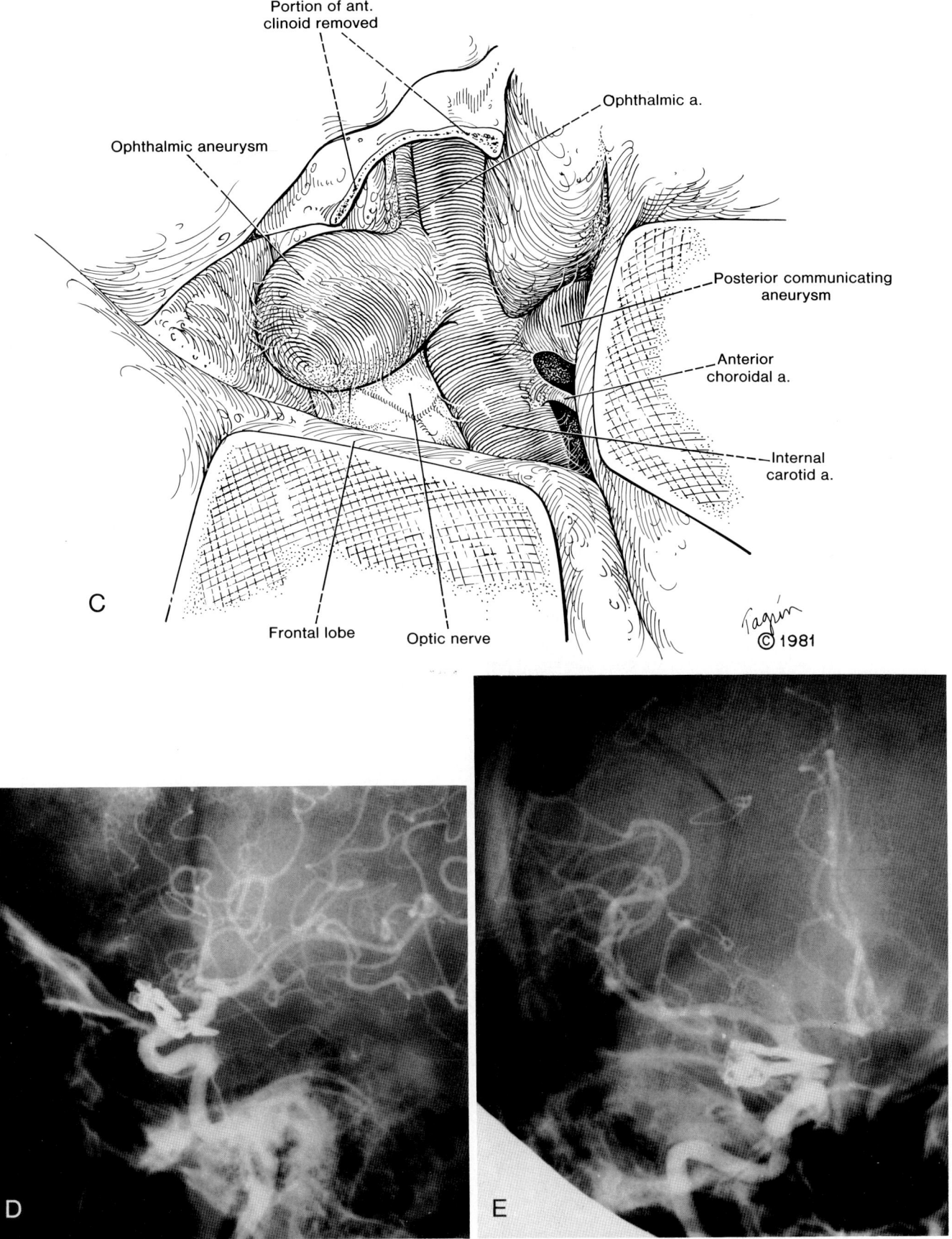

Figure 13.1 *D* and *E*, postoperative angiogram shows non-filling of aneurysms and preservation of anterior choroidal artery and ophthalmic artery.

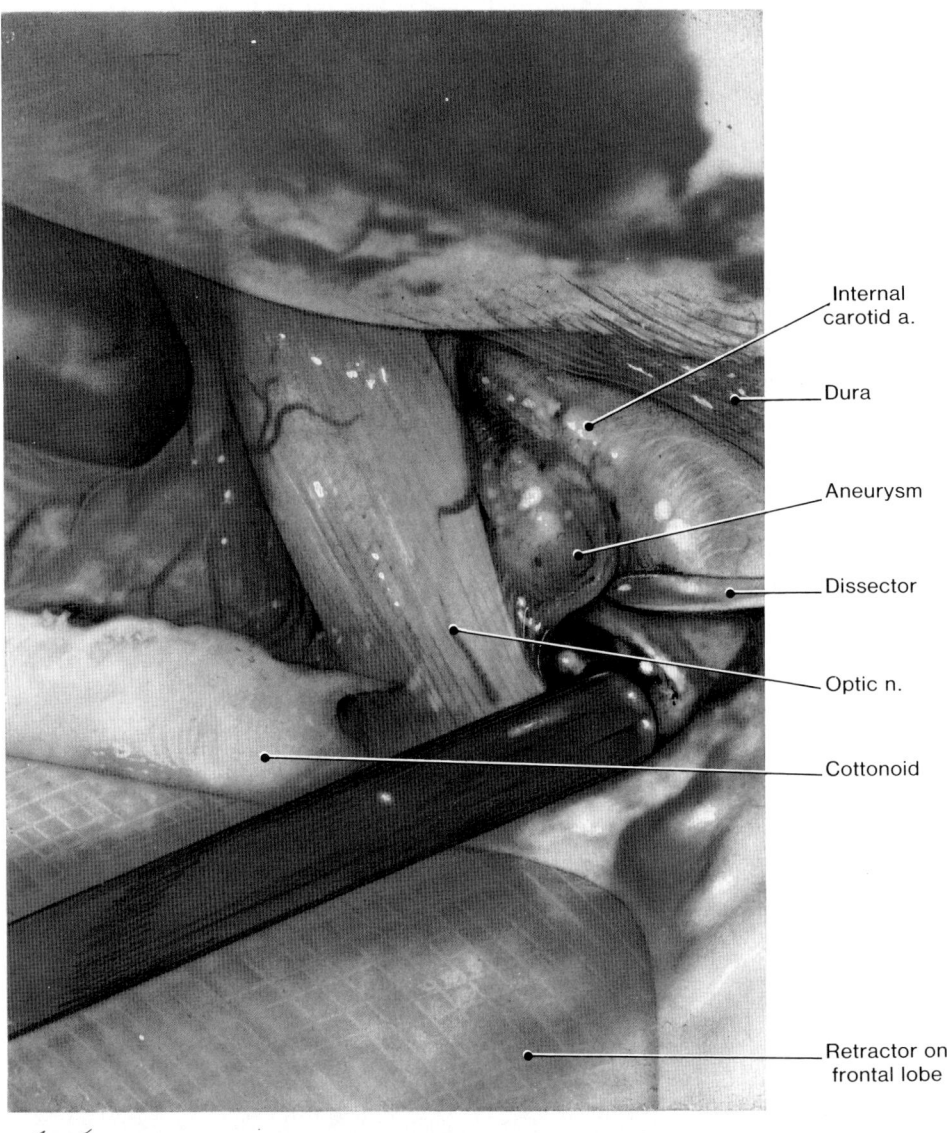

Figure 13.2 Exposure: a carotid-ophthalmic artery aneurysm with a right pterional craniotomy. The aneurysm points medially under the optic nerve, and the proximal neck is hidden by the anterior clinoid process.

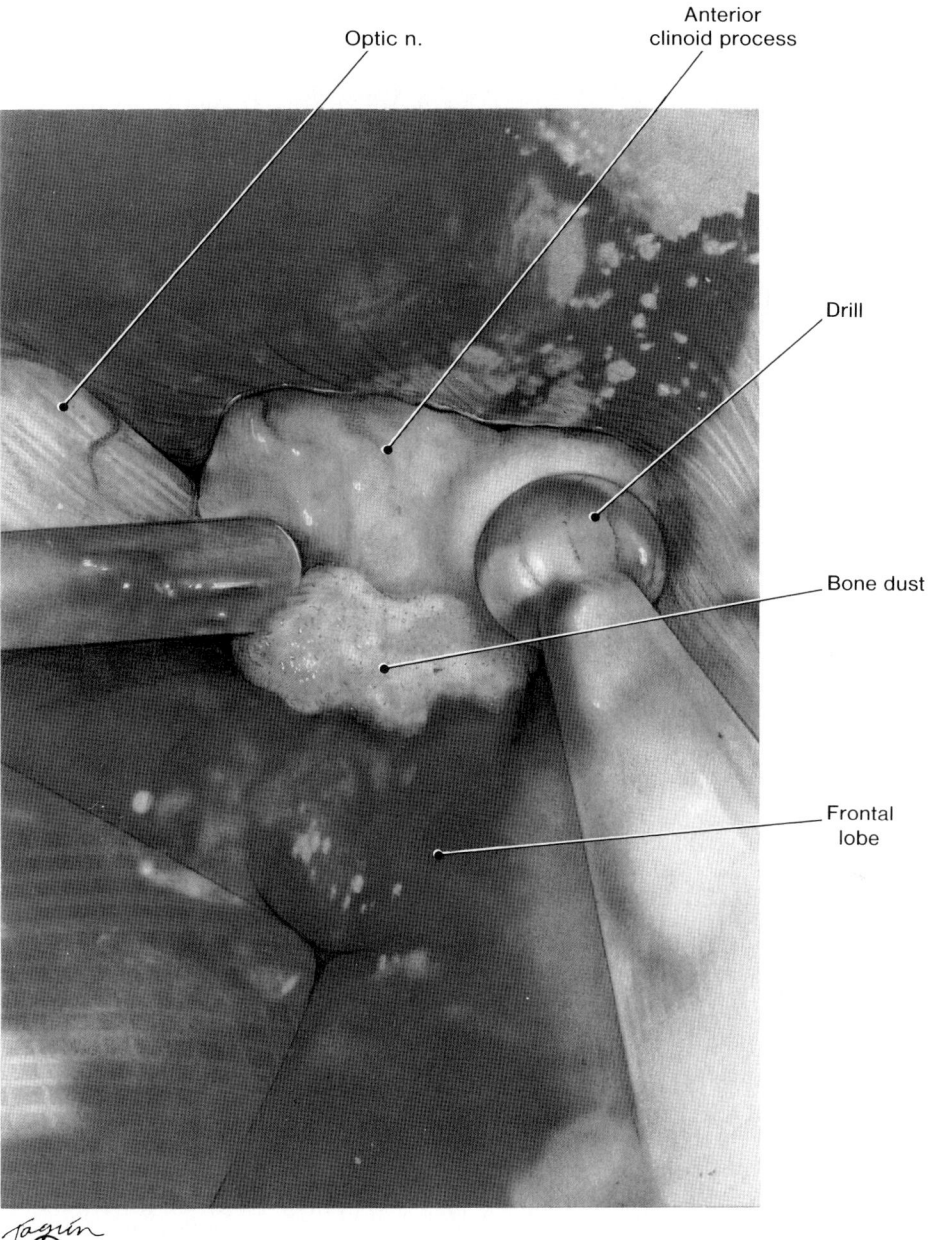

Figure 13.3 Removal of the anterior clinoid process. After the dura is incised and stripped posteriorly, the anterior clinoid process is removed using a diamond drill.

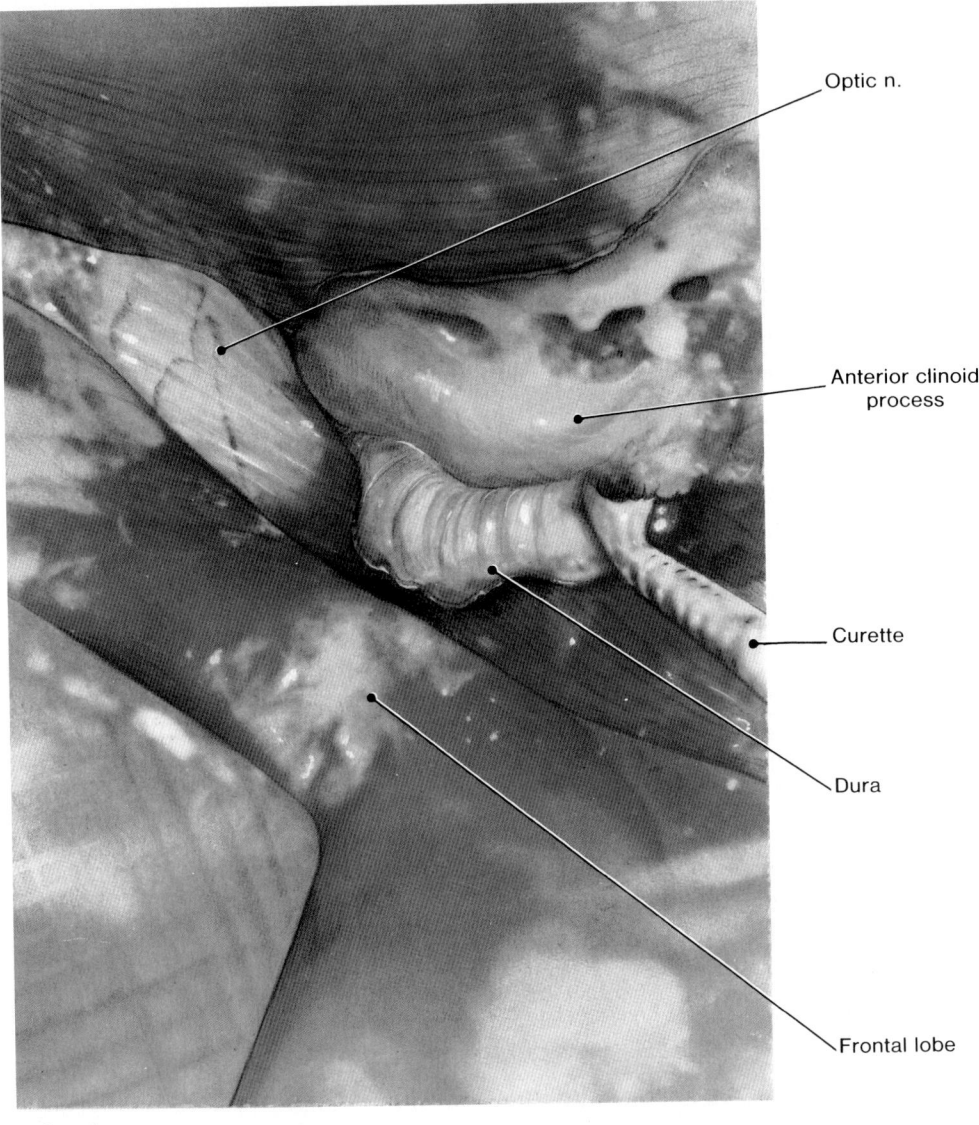

Figure 13.4 Curetting the anterior clinoid process. A 5-0 straight curette is used to gently fracture the bony fragment.

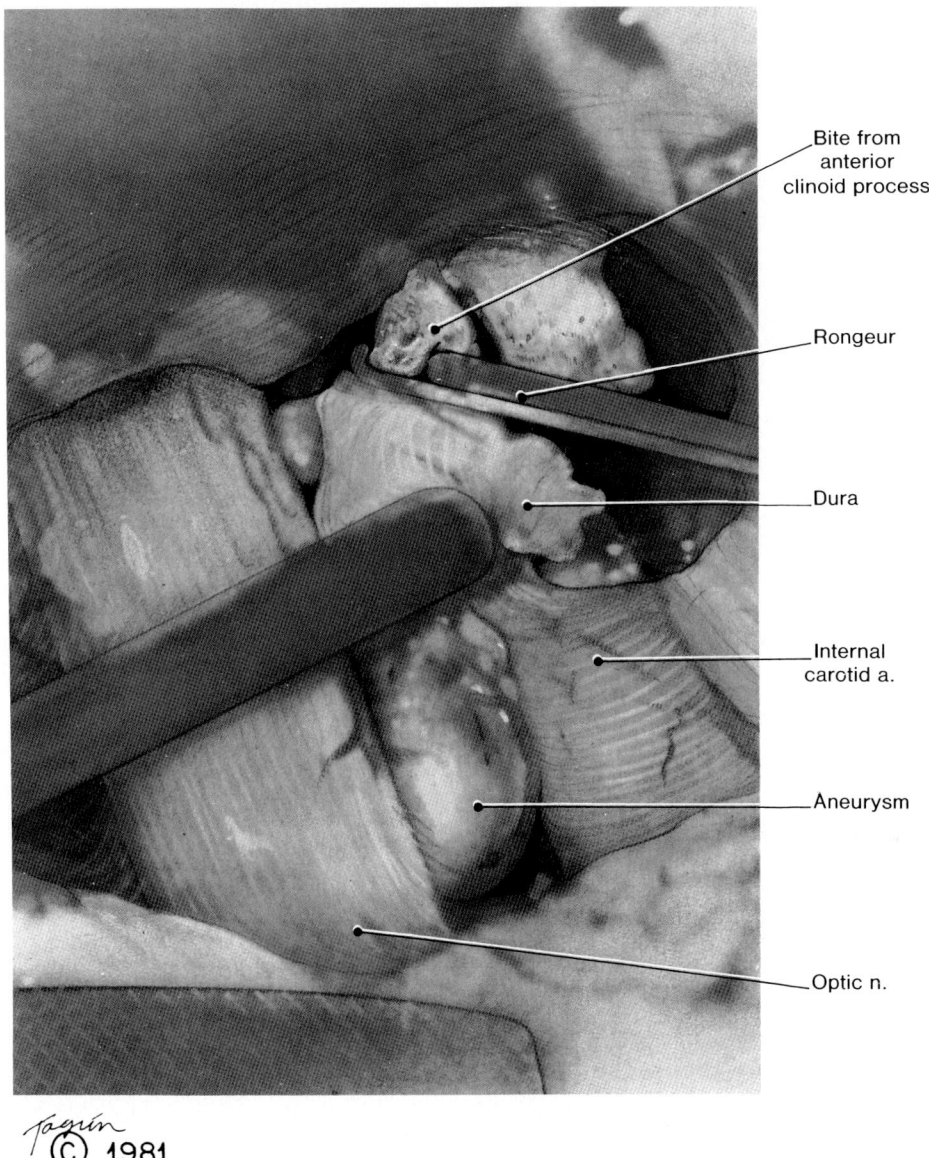

Figure 13.5 Rongeuring anterior clinoid process. A microantrostomy instrument may be used to complete the removal. Bone wax and Surgicel secure hemostasis.

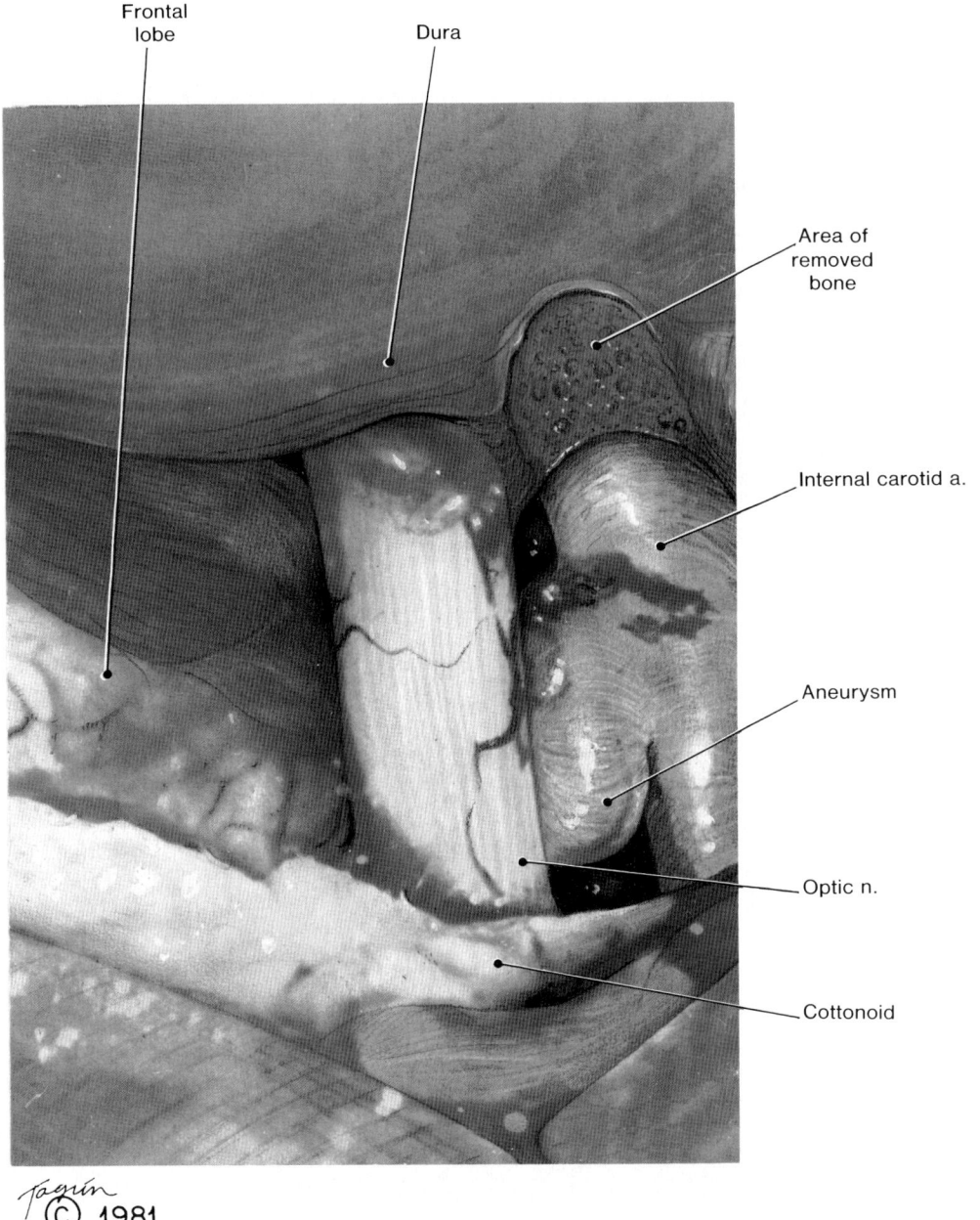

Figure 13.6 Proximal control of internal carotid artery. Removal of anterior clinoid permits dissection of proximal neck and internal carotid artery.

Dissection of the Aneurysm

Once the anterior clinoid process is removed, the protective function of the small dural flap no longer applies and it is removed. The surgeon next obtains proximal and distal control of the internal carotid artery (Fig. 13.6). In many cases, distal control is straightforward. The posterior communicating and anterior choroidal arteries provide a distal boundary for dissection. Proximal control is usually a greater challenge. At this point in the procedure, because of the threat of aneurysmal rupture, the blood pressure is lowered to about 80 mm Hg systolic. This level of hypotension is well tolerated up to 1 hour in most patients. The internal carotid artery is freed proximal to the aneurysm. Often a Rhoton #6 microdissector serves nicely for this dissection. Dense arachnoid bands may be electrocoagulated with the bipolar cautery and cut sharply. Dura may be opened laterally with cauterization and sharp dissection, with the cavernous sinus as an endpoint. Every effort should be made to visualize and spare the ophthalmic artery which usually arises from the internal carotid artery just proximal to the aneurysm neck. If the

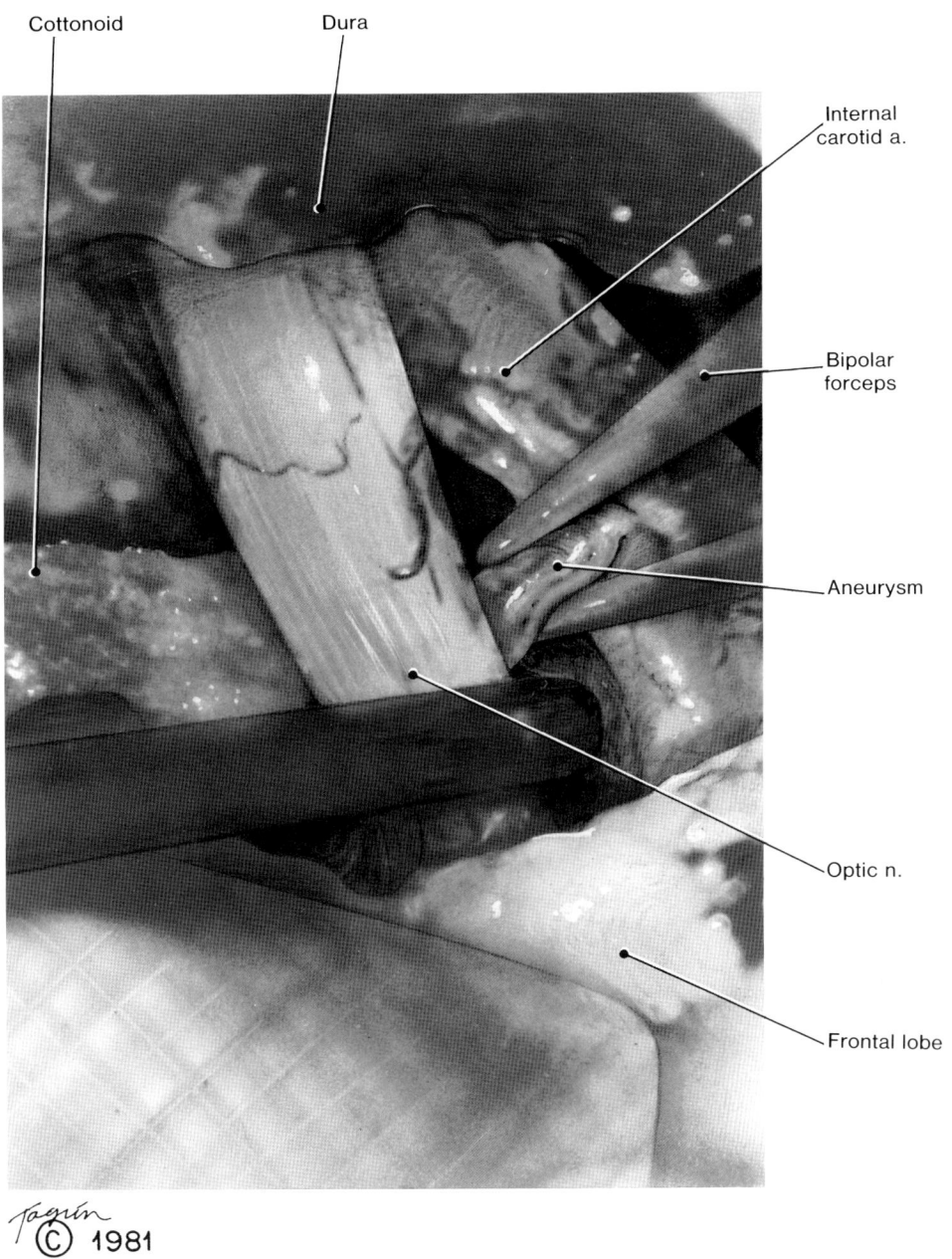

Figure 13.7 Preparation of neck of aneurysm. Gentle application of bipolar cautery at low voltage can define and toughen the neck.

ophthalmic artery is not seen, the proximal neck of the aneurysm must be completely dissected and visualized prior to application of a clip. In many cases, where the aneurysm projects superiorly, gentle deflection of the lesion posteriorly with a sucker will permit passage of a fine dissector proximal to the neck and medially as far as the optic nerve or beneath it. Gentle lateral deflection of the aneurysm may permit dissection of the medial aspect of the aneurysm from the optic nerve. Lesions which point medially beneath the optic nerve will require gentle deflection of the nerve medially and superiorly to isolate the aneurysm neck.

Clipping of the Aneurysm

Clipping of the aneurysm in many cases can be accomplished without substantial manipulation of the sac or neck, and thus moderate hypotension (systolic pressure 70–80 mm Hg) provides adequate reduction of tension in the lesion. Occasionally, a particularly thin-walled lesion or one requiring substantial manipulation for clipping presents a greater danger of rupture. In these circumstances, a brief period of deep hypotension (2–3 minutes at systolic pressure 30–40 mm Hg) will minimize the risk of rupture. For some aneurysms, bipolar coagulation may be needed to shrink the neck before applying a clip (Fig. 13.7). In others, especially those with a broad base, a ligature may help prepare the neck for clipping. Often the available space between the internal carotid artery, the bony skull, and the optic nerve dictate use of the Yasargil clip because of its narrow blade (Fig. 13.8).

In most cases, the sac is deflected distally with a fine suction in order to visualize the neck and ophthalmic artery during clip application. If application of the clip is not satisfactory because of incomplete neck obliteration, encroachment on the optic nerve or occlusion of the ophthalmic artery, the clip is repositioned. If this is not satisfactory, the clip is removed and a different type used. The internal carotid artery and ophthalmic artery must not be compressed or kinked, and the optic nerve should not be excessively deformed. Minor contact between the clip and nerve is common. When significant nerve displacement is caused by the clip, further dissection of the nerve and at times the chiasm may permit a gentle sloping displacement with limited infringement on the nerve. Occasionally, an unusual situation may be encountered where a Drake clip may be used to obliterate the lesion and preserve the optic nerve which passes through its aperture.

Clipping of a Contralateral Aneurysm

A carotid-ophthalmic artery aneurysm may be treated through a contralateral frontotemporal craniotomy (8) (Fig. 13.9). This approach may be indicated when there are bilateral carotid-ophthalmic aneu-

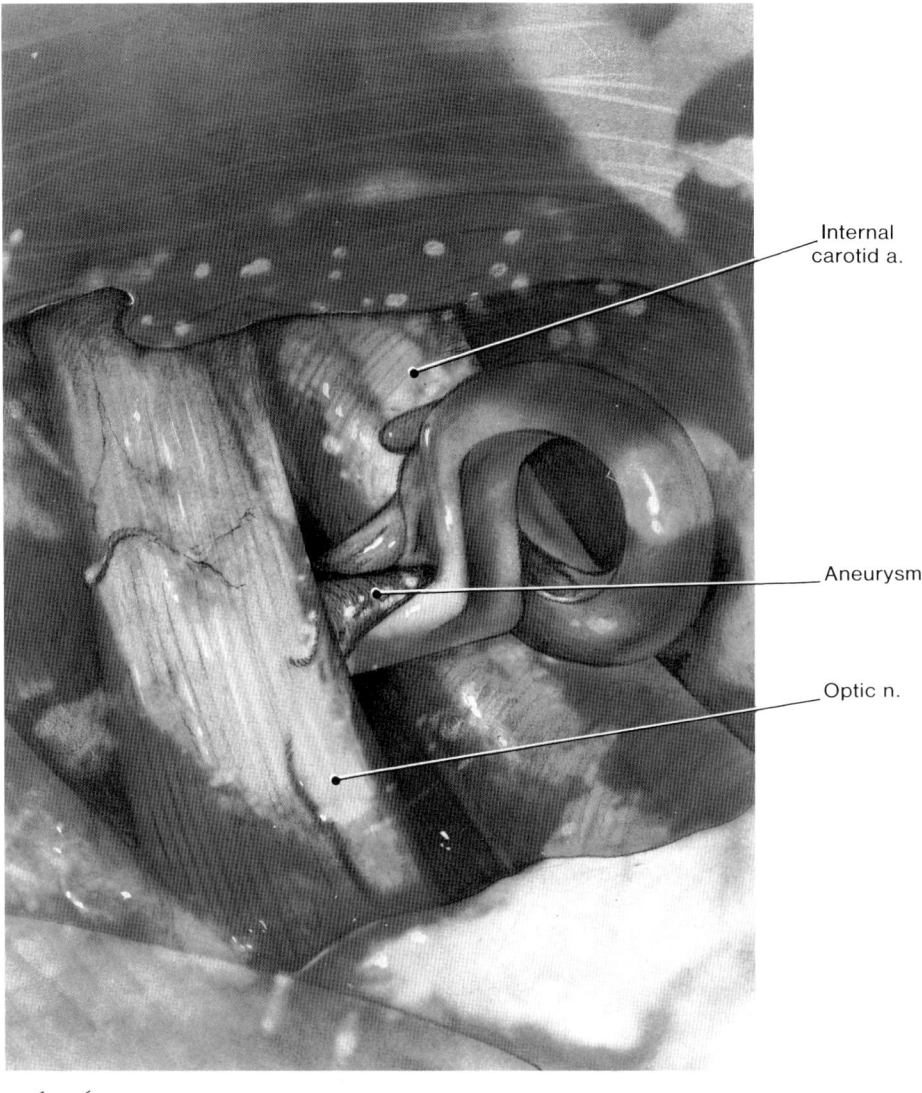

Figure 13.8 Clipping the aneurysm. Often a straight Yasargil clip with its slender blades fits best in the narrow cleft between artery and optic nerve.

rysms or when the aneurysm projects inferiorly and medially. In the exposure of a contralateral lesion, retraction will be deep. Removal of CSF via a subarachnoid catheter may be useful. Extra care must be taken to avoid tearing one or both olfactory nerves at the cribriform plate. As the frontal lobes are elevated, the arachnoid attachments to the optic nerves and chiasm are severed sharply. The contralateral proximal internal carotid artery comes into view inferior to the optic nerve. In this area, the contralateral carotid-ophthalmic aneurysm may be visualized projecting inferiorly and medially from its origin. The neck is freed, and the ophthalmic artery preserved. A straight clip, just long enough to do the job, obliterates the neck. Occasionally, removal of the bony tuberculum sella will be needed to expose the proximal aneurysm neck. Coagulation and reflection of the dura will permit drilling of the obstructing bony prominence. Usually, only a small amount of bone need be removed. Care must be taken to avoid entry into the sphenoid sinus. Careful obliteration of the opening is carried out with bone wax or fat if the sinus is entered.

Indirect Operation

Some aneurysms cannot be effectively obliterated by direct operation. This may be predicted from the angiogram if the lesion projects below the level of the ophthalmic artery into the cavernous sinus. In some cases, the need for an indirect operation can be ascertained only at the time of surgery. For such aneurysms, the safest approach may be cervical carotid occlusion (see Chapter 20 for details of this procedure) (5). Formerly, common carotid occlusion with a gradually occluding clamp was the procedure of choice. However, experience now indicates that the safest approach may be internal carotid occlusion, often with cerebral revascularization (1, 7).

Another method to consider for indirect treatment of unclippable aneurysms is the use of a detachable balloon for carotid occlusion, with or without a bypass graft. The technique has been described and was used in one patient with a giant carotid-ophthalmic aneurysm (2). The possibility of an embolic complication, associated with carotid occlusion, may be reduced by occluding the internal carotid artery intracranially close to or at the neck of the aneurysm. This technique reduces the dead space in which thrombosis and subsequent embolization can occur.

RESULTS

The microsurgical approach to carotid-ophthalmic artery aneurysms has demonstrated good results (see Table 13.1). Of 15 cases, 14 (93%) experienced excel-

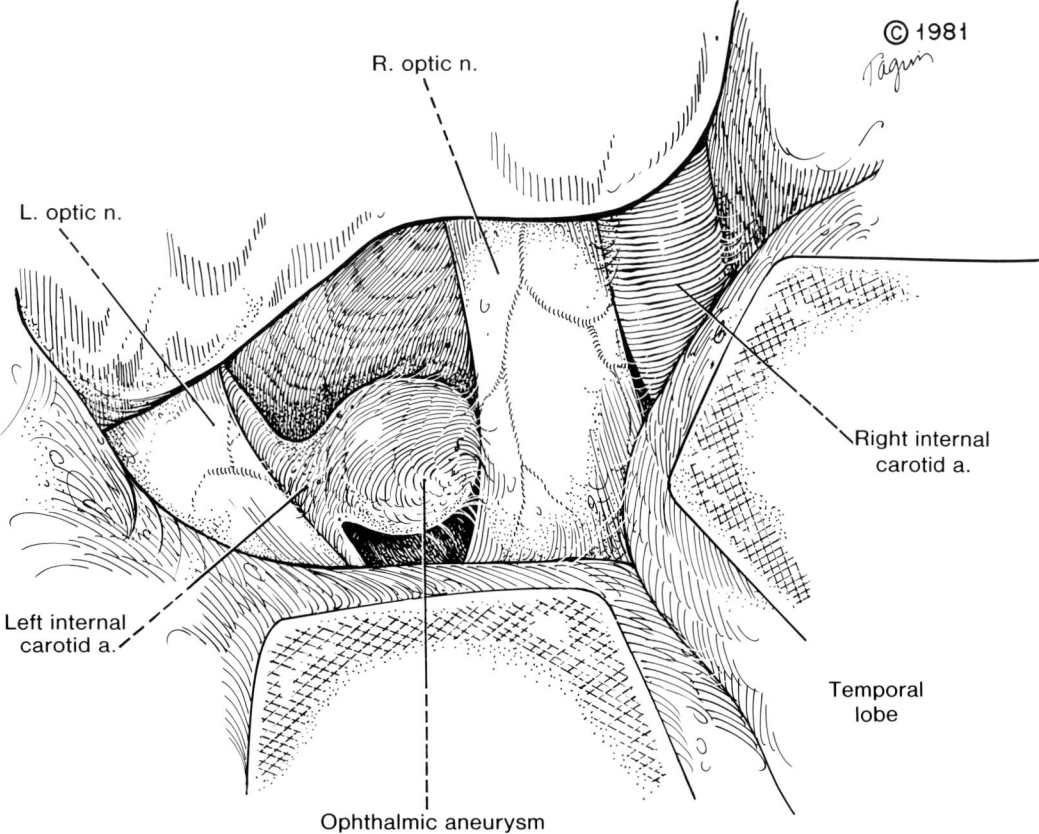

Figure 13.9 Exposure of contralateral ophthalmic aneurysm projecting inferomedially. Here a left carotid-ophthalmic lesion is exposed via a right pterional craniotomy.

lent results (no deficit) or good results (minimal deficit). In one patient, there was ipsilateral permanent blindness after clipping of a giant aneurysm. Although this case is listed as a fair result, the patient resumed the preoperative level of activity.

Visual impairment is a feared complication in the treatment of any sized aneurysm at this site. The effect of treatment on visual symptoms present prior to surgery is unpredictable. Recovery may continue up to 2 years. Factors that have been reported to be associated with a favorable outcome include a relatively short history, use of a direct operative approach, sparing of the ophthalmic artery, avoidance of excessive manipulation of the optic nerve and chiasm, and good decompression of the visual apparatus at the time of surgery (3). The finding of optic pallor does not exclude recovery, nor does an initial postoperative visual deterioration. Factors that have been associated with poor recovery and deterioration of vision after operation include a severe preoperative visual deficit or inability to collapse the aneurysm. Indirect treatment by proximal carotid occlusion may also result in visual recovery in some patients, but the risk of neurological deficits is higher. Whether the use of intraoperative visual-evoked responses can help reduce the chance of postoperative visual impairment has not been studied.

In all 15 of our patients, obliteration of the carotid-ophthalmic artery aneurysms was possible by direct intracranial surgery. Angiographic studies a week or more after surgery revealed total obliteration of the lesions in all 14 studied patients (one patient refused study). Other postoperative complications were uncommon (see Table 13.1). In one patient, uneventful clipping of a carotid-ophthalmic aneurysm was complicated by subgaleal infection and osteomyelitis of the bone flap. There was no new neurological deficit. One patient experienced a transient CSF rhinorrhea. A right frontotemporal craniotomy was utilized for clipping of bilateral ophthalmic aneurysms. Drilling of the tuberculum sella was carried out in order to obtain good visualization of the contralateral carotid-ophthalmic aneurysm origin. Sphenoid sinus mucosa was visualized, and bone wax was utilized to close the small bony opening. Postoperatively, there was substantial CSF rhinorrhea which required a transsphenoidal procedure for obliteration of the leak. The patient's neurological status was unchanged.

Results recorded in the literature are similar (3, 6, 8). Yasargil and Smith reported 92% good-excellent results without mortality (8). For giant lesions presenting with compression of the optic nerves, the outcome was good-excellent in 84% with 5% mortality.

Table 13.1
Carotid-Ophthalmic Aneurysms Treated by Direct Operation

Results	
Excellent	9 ⎫ 93%
Good	5 ⎭
Fair	1[a]
Dead	0
Total	15
Complications	
Unilateral blindness	1
Infected bone flap	1
CSF rhinorrhea	1

[a] Blindness on side of operation. Patient returned to previous level of activity.

REFERENCES

1. Crowell RM: Direct brain revascularization, in Schmidek H, Sweet WH (eds): *Current Techniques of Operative Neurosurgery.* New York, Grune & Stratton, 1978.
2. Debrun G, Fox A, Drake C, Peerless S, Girvin J, Ferguson G: Giant unclippable aneurysms: treatment with detachable balloons. Am J Neurorad 2:167–173, 1981.
3. Ferguson GG, Drake CG: Carotid-ophthalmic aneurysms: the surgical management of those cases presenting with compression of the optic nerves and chiasm alone. Clin Neurosurg 27:263–307, 1980.
4. Ferguson GG, Drake CG: Carotid-ophthalmic aneurysms: visual abnormalities in 32 patients and the results of treatment. Surg Neurol 16:1–8, 1981.
5. Miller JD, Jawad K, Jennett B: Safety of carotid ligation and its role in the management of intracranial aneurysms. J Neurol Neurosurg Psychiatry 40:64–72, 1977.
6. Sengupta RP, Gryspeerdt GL, Hankinson J: Carotid-ophthalmic aneurysms. J Neurol Neurosurg Psychiatry 39:837–853, 1976.
7. Spetzler RF, Schuster H, Roski RA: Elective extracranial-intracranial bypass in the treatment of inoperable giant aneurysms of the internal carotid artery. J Neurosurg 53:22–27, 1980.
8. Yasargil MG, Gasser JC, Hodosh RM, Rankin TV: Carotid-ophthalmic aneurysms: direct microsurgical approach. Surg Neurol 8:155–165, 1977.

Chapter 14 ANTERIOR COMMUNICATING ANEURYSMS

PRESENTATION

Anterior communicating artery aneurysms represent a common and difficult problem in management. These lesions usually present with subarachnoid hemorrhage (SAH). Often the SAH is a minor "warning leak" causing severe headache and a stiff neck, but in many patients there are significant neurological deficits. By virtue of its location, the aneurysm may hemorrhage upward into the third ventricle and hypothalamic region. Damage in these areas may be associated with memory disturbance (particularly for recent events), abulia, inappropriate secretion of antidiuretic hormone, symptomatic hydrocephalus, or autonomic instability with unstable pulse and blood pressure (5). Lateral rupture directly into the parenchyma may involve the internal capsule (7). Delayed complications are common following SAH from these aneurysms. The most frequent problem is vasospasm but hydrocephalus may also cause symptoms.

In a few patients, these aneurysms reach a giant size and compress visual pathways, hypothalamus, or internal capsule (see Chapter 20). The patient may present with progressive visual symptoms, mental disturbance, or hemiparesis.

EVALUATION

The program of evaluation and medical management is outlined in Chapter 10. The timing of angiography and surgery is discussed in Chapter 11. Angiography often requires special views to define the anatomy of the neck of the aneurysm. Oblique views can throw the aneurysm neck into profile (Fig. 14.1D). Sometimes a base view is helpful if other projections fail to depict the lesion adequately. For anterior communicating aneurysms we tend to delay surgery a bit longer (12-14 days after SAH) because of the danger of devastating ischemia from spasm (Fig. 14.1, A-F).

SURGICAL TREATMENT

Initial exposure

We prefer a unilateral frontal craniotomy and gyrus rectus approach for most patients (2, 8). A modified pterional craniotomy provides good exposure (see Chapter 12 and Fig. 14.2A) (9, 10). For right-handed surgeons, a right-sided approach is usually chosen except in some patients when the aneurysm points to the right, or where the left A_1 segment of the anterior cerebral artery is the predominant feeding artery. The patient's head is turned 60° to the vertical to permit a direct view without craning the surgeon's neck. Compared to exposure for ICA aneurysms, the bone flap is taken 2 cm further medially to afford easy subfrontal exposure. It is very important not to try and retract the frontal lobe until the brain is relaxed. The olfactory tract leads the surgeon to the optic nerve and internal carotid artery (Fig. 14.2B). The Greenberg self-retaining retractors are then placed.

Microsurgical Dissection of Feeding Arteries

With a fine hook, the arachnoid is opened over the internal carotid artery and optic nerve (Fig. 14.2B). The surgeon further opens the cistern of the internal carotid artery holding a small suction in the left hand and using the hook, microdissector or microscissors in the right hand. The internal carotid artery is followed distally. In some patients, the origin of the right A_1 segment of the anterior cerebral artery can be visualized and the anterior edge of this vessel followed medially toward the aneurysm (Fig. 14.3). When this is the case, the aneurysm can often be exposed without a large gyrus rectus corticectomy. In most patients, however, the internal carotid artery segment is longer and the anterior cerebral artery origin higher and more posteriorly placed. In such instances, excessive frontal retraction would be needed to see the origin of A_1, and since it is not necessary to expose the entire A_1 segment, it seems wiser to proceed directly to the gyrus rectus corticectomy. A controlled suction device is helpful to provide adequate low-level suction without danger of injury to critical structures. Retraction at this point involves not only elevation of the frontal lobe and olfactory tract, but also a gentle lifting of the lobe away from the interhemispheric fissure. Only when the brain is slack can one obtain and hold this type of critical retraction. The surgeons view is facilitated by the position of the head. If the head is not turned far enough to the left, the surgeon will be bending to the right in an awkward fashion.

A variable number of perforating arteries arise from the A_1 segments, proximal A_2 segment, and the

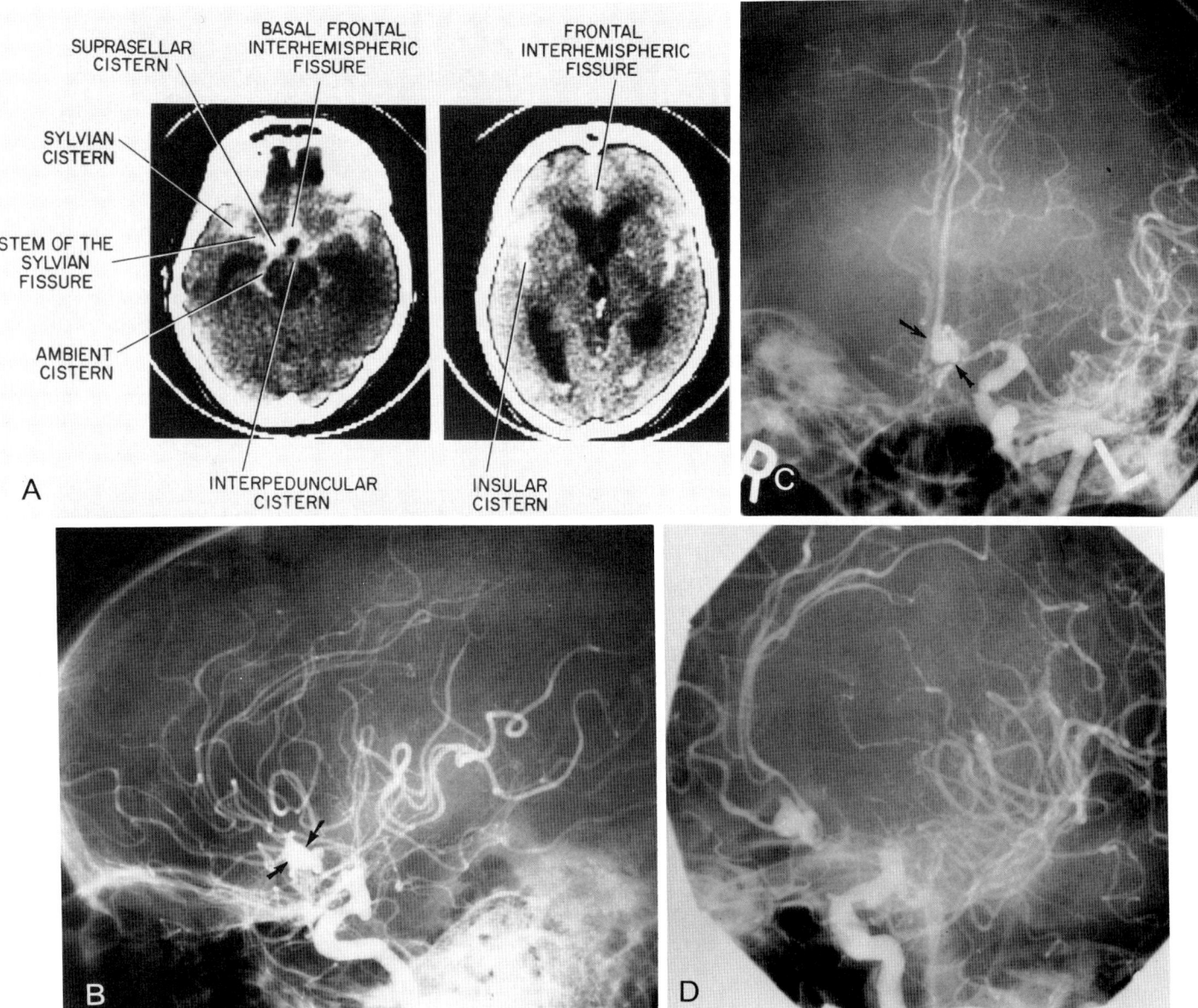

Figure 14.1 Anterior communicating artery aneurysm. CT predicts spasm. Operation delayed 2 weeks after SAH. Drake clip encircles right A_1 segment to obliterate lesion. *A*, CT shows hematoma in basal cisterns 1 day after SAH. Patient intact. *B* to *D*, left carotid angiogram demonstrates a large aneurysm arising from the junction of the left A_1 segment of the anterior cerebral and anterior communicating arteries (*arrows*). Note information about anatomy gained on the oblique view. There is grade 2 spasm of anterior and middle cerebral arteries. No filling of aneurysm on right carotid angiogram. *E*, Left carotid angiogram 8 days after SAH shows more severe left MCA spasm. Head slightly turned so aneurysm is behind the distal internal carotid artery. Right frontal craniotomy deferred until 16 days after SAH. *F* and *G*, postoperative left carotid angiogram shows Drake clip and obliteration of the aneurysm (*open arrow*). The right A_1 segment passes through the Drake clip. No significant spasm. Patient intact.

anterior communicating artery (4, 10). These arteries tend to follow a recurrent course backward along the anterior cerebral artery to enter the anterior perforate substance. Hypothalamic arteries frequently originate from the inferior or posterior aspect of the anterior communicating artery or side of the larger A_1 segment. They are often adherent, but rarely, if ever, originate from the posterior inferior wall of the aneurysm (10). The recurrent artery of Heubner usually arises at or near the junction of the anterior cerebral and anterior communicating arteries and follows a course laterally either anterior or posterior to the A_1 segment to the lenticulostriate arteries. Anomomalus configurations of the anterior cerebral-anterior communicating complex are common (4, 10).

Keeping in mind the possible locations of these

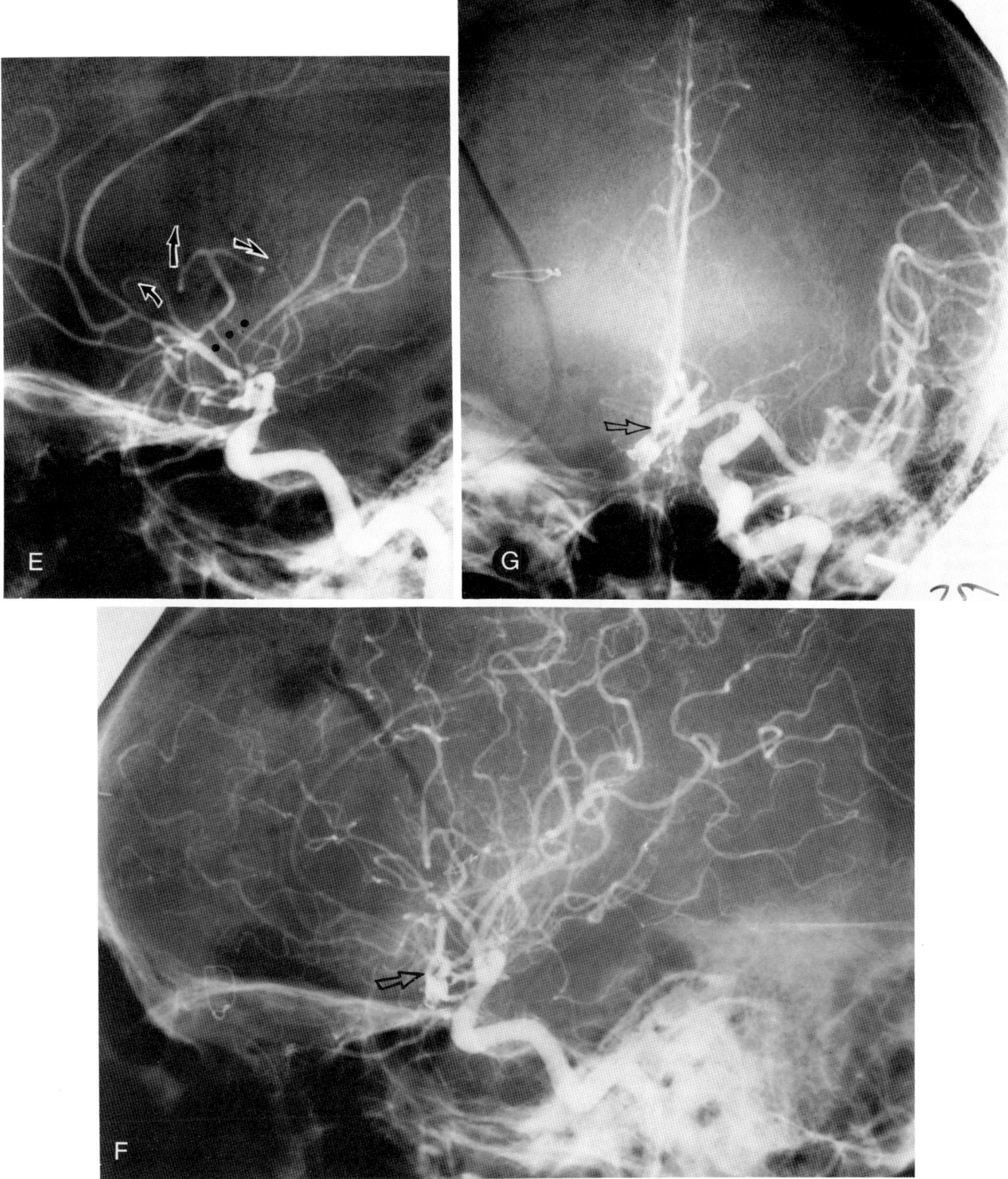

Figure 14.1 (*E* to *G*)

important perforating arteries, a corticectomy is made in the gyrus rectus, just medial to the olfactory tract, beginning at the level of the optic nerve and extending anteriorly for about 1.5 cm (Fig. 14.4). The incision is deepened until the pia-arachnoid over the A₁ segment and then the interhemispheric fissure is reached. This protective layer overlying the aneurysm is left intact. The arachnoid overlying the right

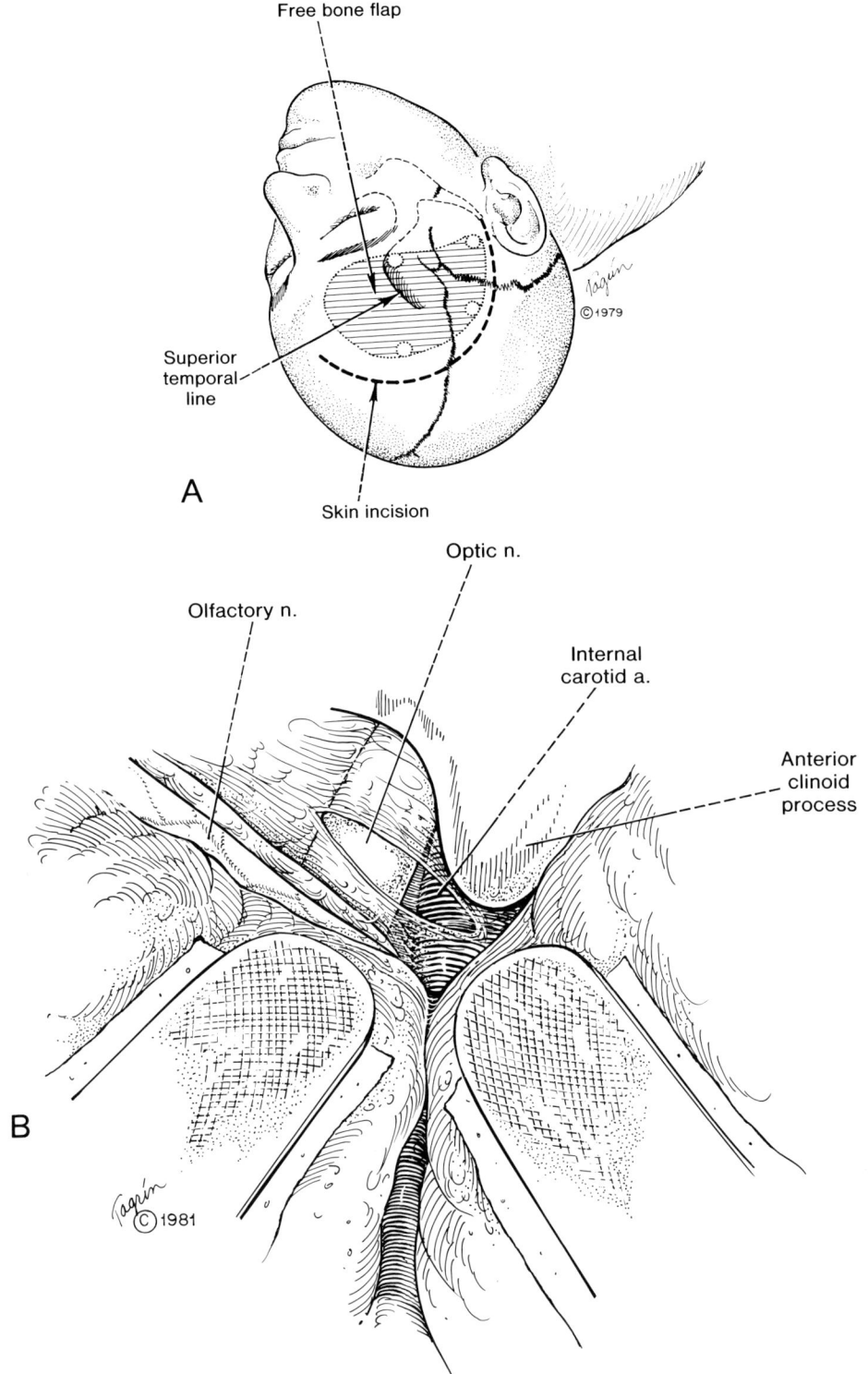

Figure 14.2 *A*, incision and pterional craniotomy. The skin incision is just behind the hairline and the anterior branch of superficial temporal artery. The key burr hole lies just behind the zygomatic process of the frontal bone and inferior to the superior temporal line. Often three burr holes are sufficient. *B*, elevation of frontal lobe. This is done gradually with suction-removal of CSF. The olfactory tract leads back to the optic nerve. Temporal bridging veins are coagulated and cut near the cortex.

A_1 segment is opened (Fig. 14.5). Once the right A_1 anterior cerebral artery is visualized, it is wise in most patients to bring the blood pressure into the range of 80 mm Hg systolic. Branches of this vessel, which may include Heubner's artery, must be preserved. The A_1 segment is followed distally to the

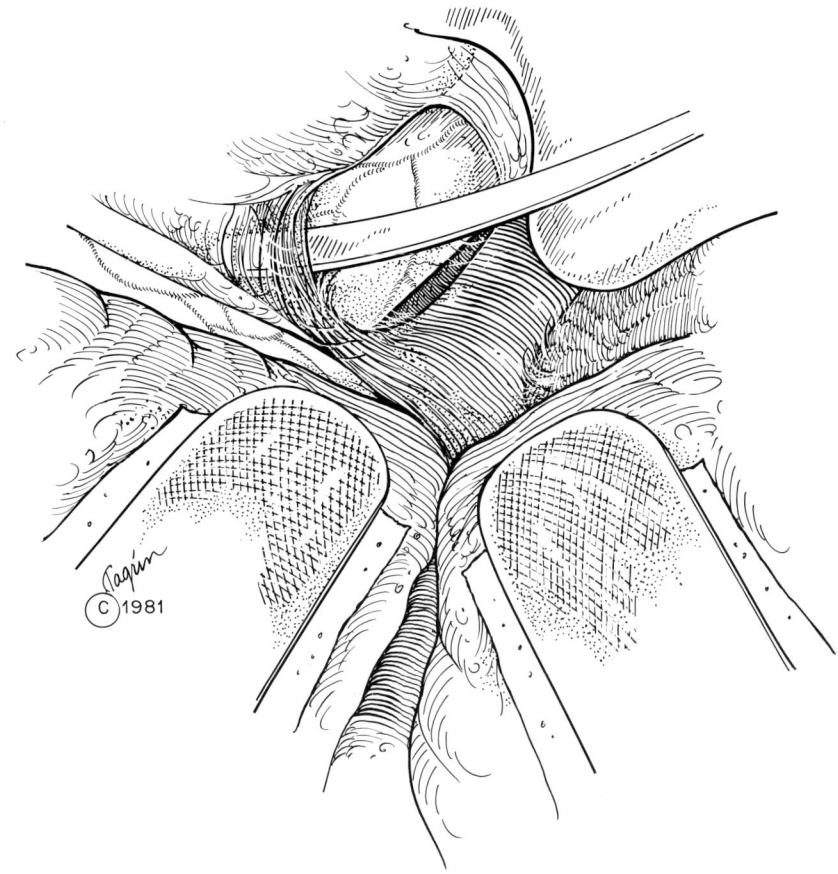

Figure 14.3 Dissection of right A_1 segment. The anterior border of the vessel is freed of arachnoid with a microdissector and microscissors.

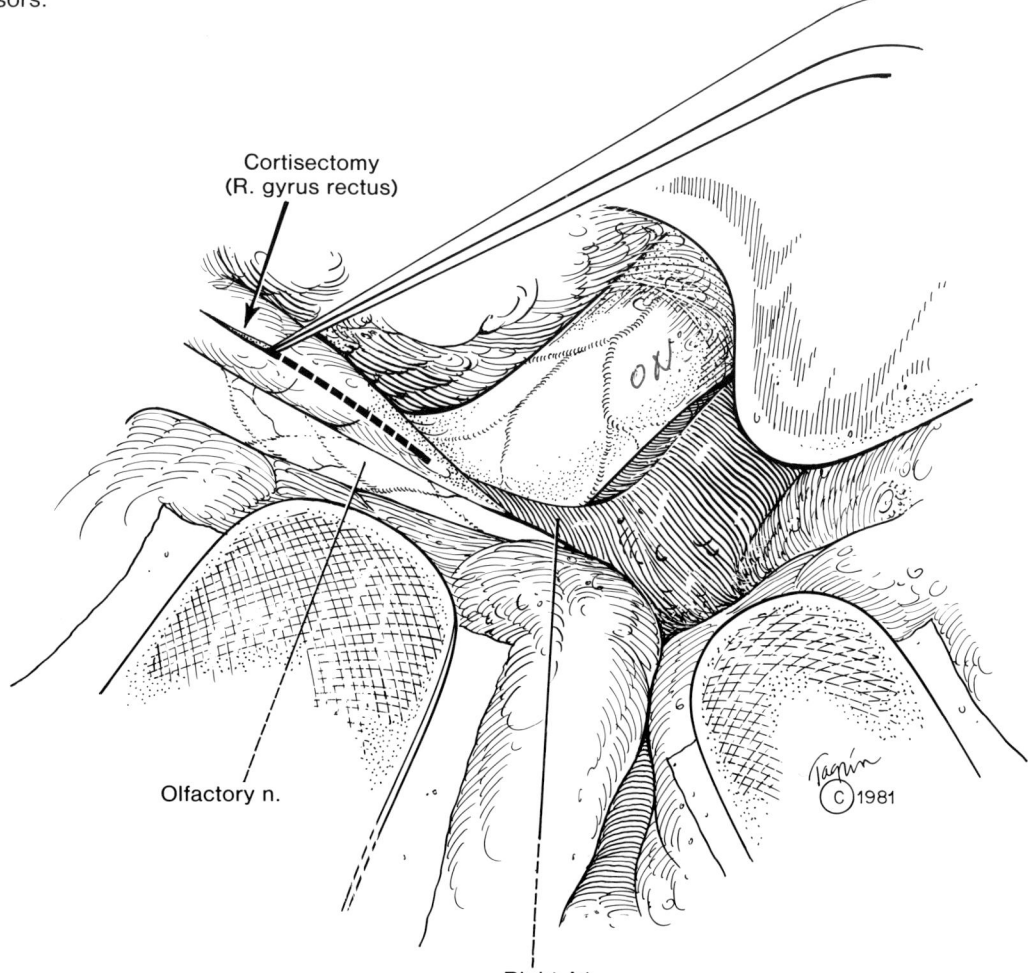

Figure 14.4 Gyrus rectus corticectomy. Bipolar cauterization and incision of pia over 1.0–1.5 cm. Care must be taken to place corticectomy over aneurysm site (usually near the level of the medial edge of optic nerve).

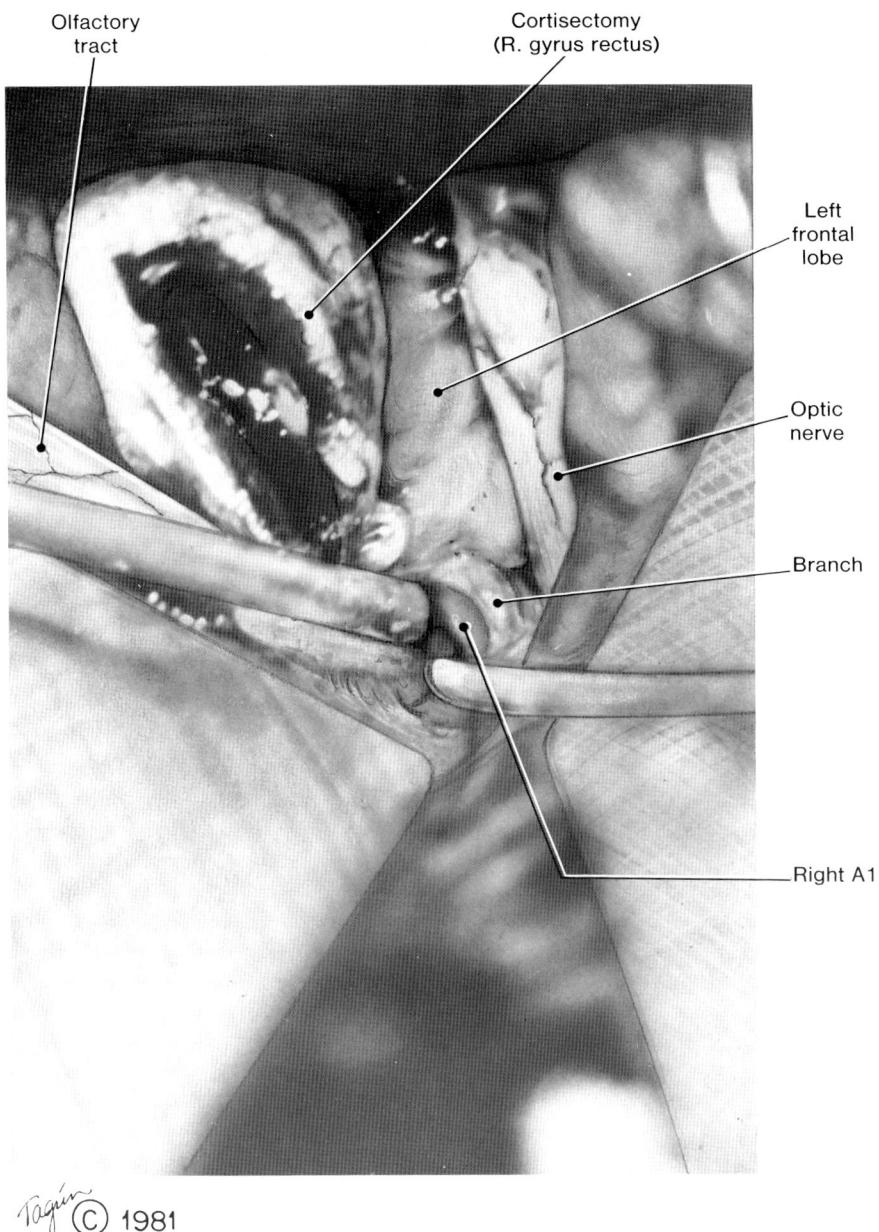

Figure 14.5 Dissection of right A_1 segment through the corticectomy. The microscope has been directed more medially. Suction and bipolar cauterization remove cortex down to interhemispheric pia-arachnoid. With a fine dissector, pia-arachnoid is removed from right A_1 segment and neck of aneurysm.

anterior communicating artery and then to the origin of the right pericallosal artery (A_2 segment). If possible, the aneurysm is avoided at this stage. Dissection proceeds by a combination of blunt dissection with a fine microdissector and microscissors cutting arachnoid after bipolar coagulation. Next, the left A_2 segment is identified in the interhemispheric fissure (Fig. 14.6). The angiogram should be reviewed to determine whether the left A_2 segment is anterior or posterior to its right-sided counterpart. Once the left A_2 segment is identified, it may be followed retrograde to the left A_1 segment. Careful scrutiny of the angiograms and a knowledge of the anatomic variants guide the dissection. Important normal variants include: 1) hypoplastic A_1 segment, 2) reduplicated anterior communicating arteries, and 3) persistent artery to the corpus callosum from anterior communicating artery. Almost always the aneurysm arises from the junction of the larger A_1 and anterior communicating arteries.

As the surgeon seeks to identify the left anterior cerebral artery segments, significant retraction of the aneurysm is often needed. This is best accomplished by leaving pia-arachnoid overlying the lesion, with

Anterior Communicating Aneurysms

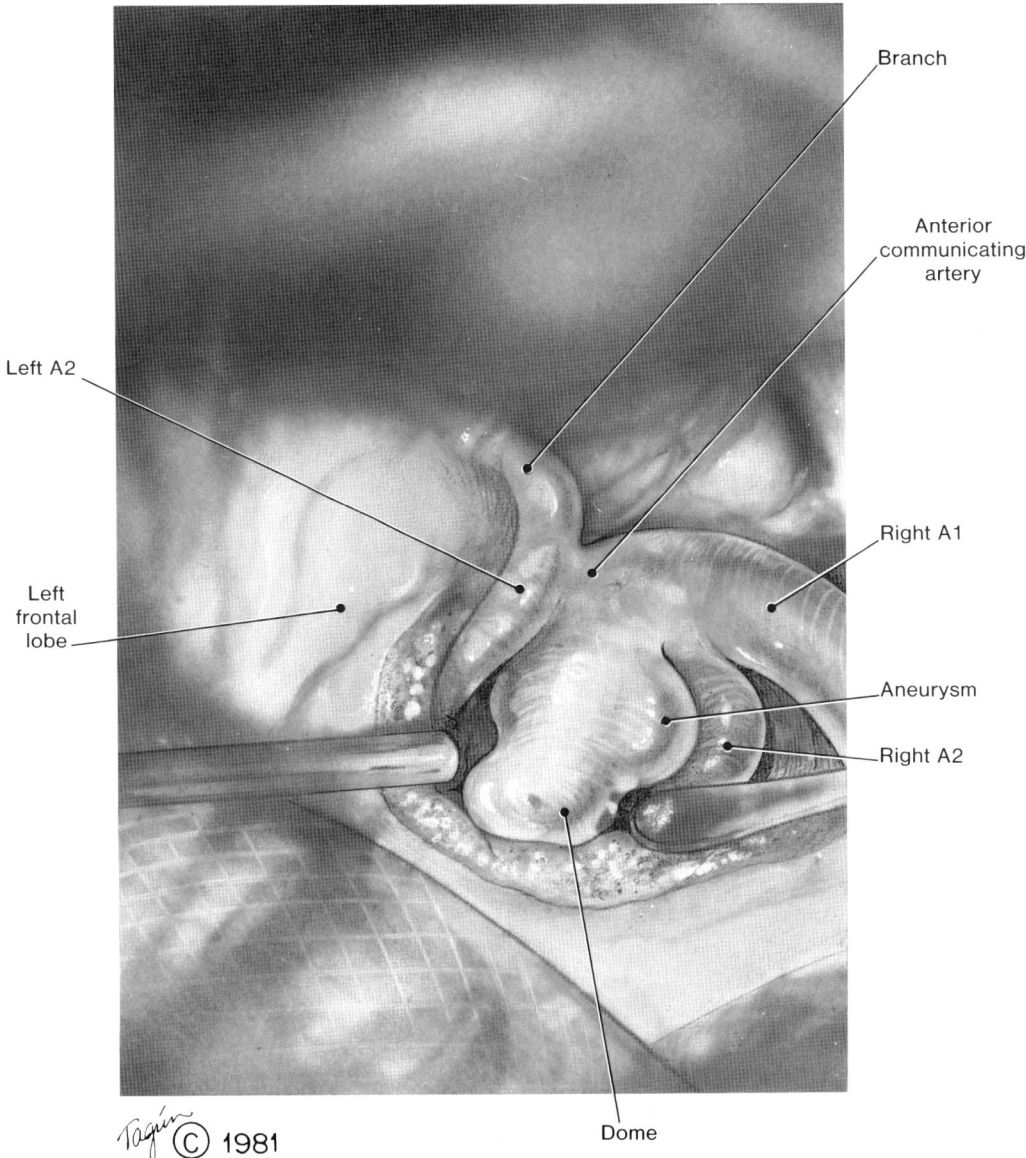

Figure 14.6 Dissection of aneurysm. Proceeding clockwise, the surgeon frees up the right A_1 and A_2 segments of the anterior cerebral arteries, then the left A_2 and A_1 segments. Finally, the aneurysm is encircled, and dome and neck are completely dissected.

retraction applied by the suction through an intervening cottonoid. One seeks to identify and free all major arterial trunks prior to working on the aneurysm. The most common projection of the aneurysm is superiorly into the interhemispheric fissure, and when this is the case, the left A_1 segment may be most accessible ventrally. In this situation, the anterior portion of the aneurysm and frontal lobes are gently reflected superiorly and posteriorly, further opening the arachnoid, permitting sharp dissection of the aneurysm away from the superior surface of the chiasm and both optic nerves. In this way the ventral aspect of the anterior communicating artery and the left A_1 segment may be identified. When the aneurysm points forward, access to the left A_1 segment is easiest from behind the lesion. In either event, encirclement of the lesion is required. Care is taken to preserve the perforating arteries. At this stage it is wise to leave in place any small potentially important arterial branches which are adherent to the dome of the lesion.

Microsurgical Dissection of the Aneurysm

The systolic blood pressure is usually in the 70–80 mm Hg range. Brief, deep hypotension with mean arterial pressure in the 30–40 mm Hg range is often needed. Lesions with paper-thin, angry red patches near the neck will demand this adjunct to prevent rupture. In exceptional cases with markedly thin aneurysm necks, a brief period of deep hypotension to the level of 20–25 mm Hg mean may give the required aneurysm slackness. For these maneuvers, the suction, with or without a cottonoid, is used to reflect the lesion to one side, and a fine dissector or microscissors frees the neck from adherent structures (Fig. 14.6). When visualization permits, sharp dissection is preferable. With the microscope, it is usually possible to identify a cleavage plane right to the edge of the neck. Initially it is wise to dissect a bit up on the wall in case of a tear in the neck which can be disastrous. It may be necessary to reflect the lesion superiorly to assure preservation of the perforating branches of the anterior communicating artery (Fig. 14.7). These vessels are often adherent to the ventral posterior wall of the aneurysm and must be carefully separated from it. In many cases, direct reflection of the aneurysm anteriorly while peering over the right A_2 segment will give the needed view. However, in some instances, with a posteriorly or postero-inferiorly directed lesion, reflection of the aneurysm and the right A_2 superiorly will give a nice view of the ventral aspects of these structures and their plane of separation from the perforators.

In a similar fashion, rotation or reflection of the right A_1 and A_2 segments superiorly and leftward may permit satisfactory visualization of the undersurface of a down-pointing lesion. Whatever the technique, the primary aim is to develop clear cleavage between the ventral-posterior aspect of the aneurysm and the numerous critical perforating arteries emanating from the posterior aspect of the anterior communicating artery. This is particularly important to achieve prior to clipping of the aneurysm because visualization of these perforators during application of the clip is frequently difficult or impossible. Finally, adherent arterial branches overlying the dome of the aneurysm may be dissected free. Such branches may yield to blunt dissection with a right angle hook or ball dissector. In some cases, where accurate visualization of arachnoid bands is possible, sharp dissection with scissors may be preferred. If aneurysmal rupture occurs at this point, the problem

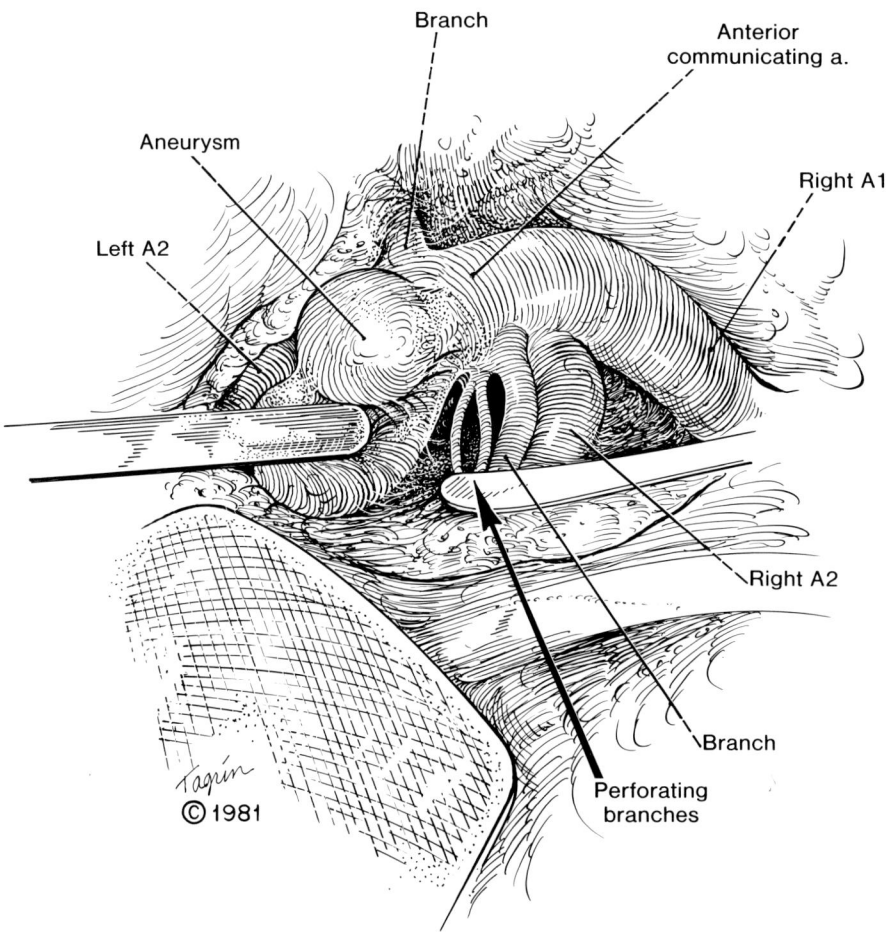

Figure 14.7 Dissection of perforating branches. These crucial vessels emerge from the anterior communicating artery and proceed posteriorly to the hypothalamus. They must be gently freed from the aneurysm and excluded from clipping. Note retraction of the aneurysm with the suction.

Anterior Communicating Aneurysms

can be controlled, since the aneurysm neck has been essentially completely dissected.

Obliteration of the Aneurysm

In the great majority of cases, a metal aneurysm clip is the best solution (Fig. 14.8). Once the lesion has been completely dissected and the relationship of its neck to surrounding critical structures (including the perforating arteries) is defined, the surgeon can judge what technique will best obliterate the lesion. We have usually used a Heifetz or Yasargil clip. The long straight Heifetz clip is particularly effective for upward pointing lesions. Because of the angle of application, the beveled clip applier is frequently used. This clip is also useful for lesions with a wide neck. In some cases, the Sugita clip is used for its narrow blade and wide opening of the jaws. The Yasargil clip is used for lesions with necks smaller than 5 mm. Sometimes a slight curve or even a very abrupt curve will be handy to occlude an aneurysm neck. Often a projecting lobe can be gathered up with the suction tip into the jaws of a Yasargil clip (Fig. 14.9). Release is sometimes difficult with the Yasargil and Sugita clips and may be facilitated by distracting

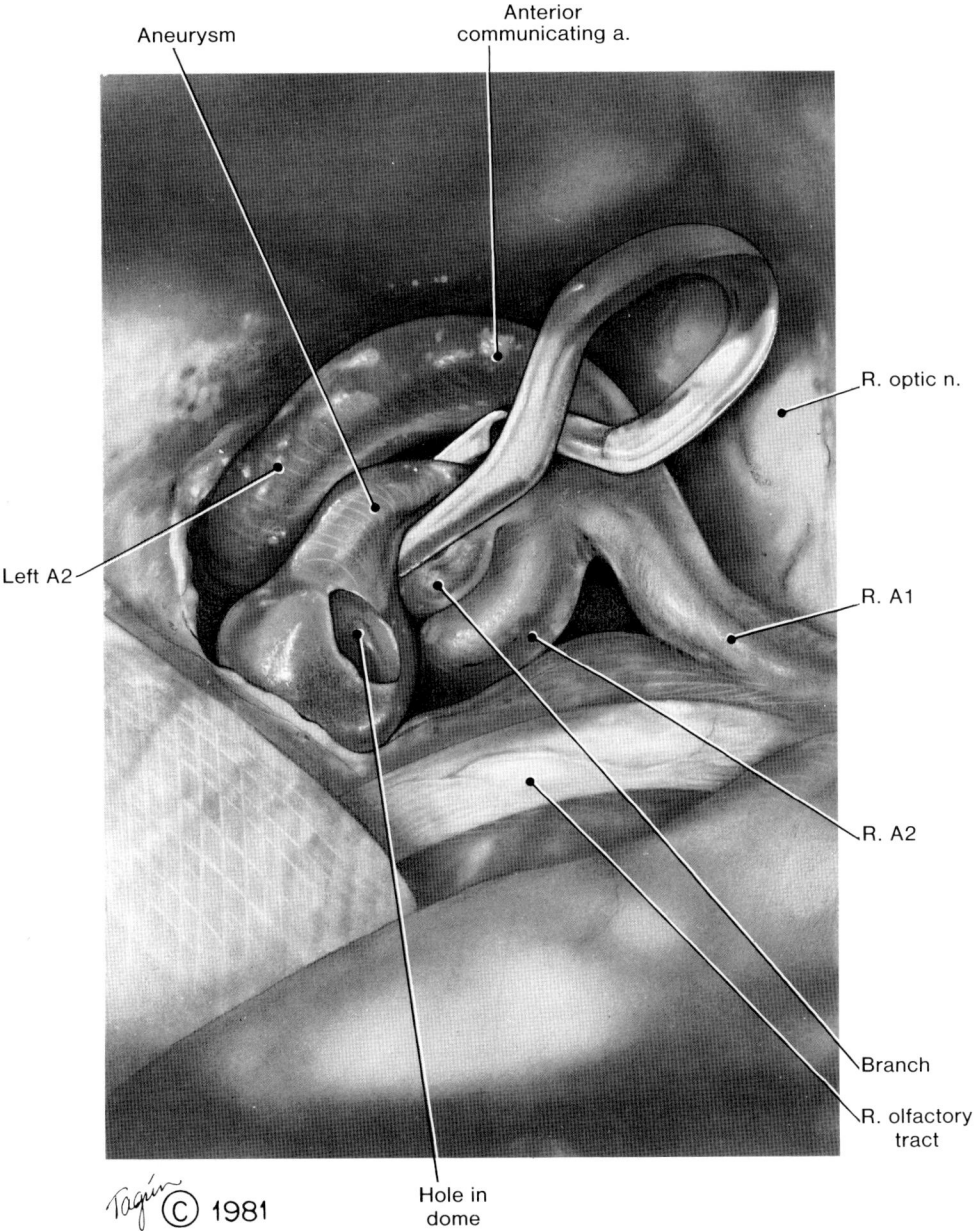

Figure 14.8 Clipping the aneurysm. The entire lesion is obliterated, with preservation of trunk and perforating arteries. The aneurysm is opened to be sure there is complete occlusion of the neck.

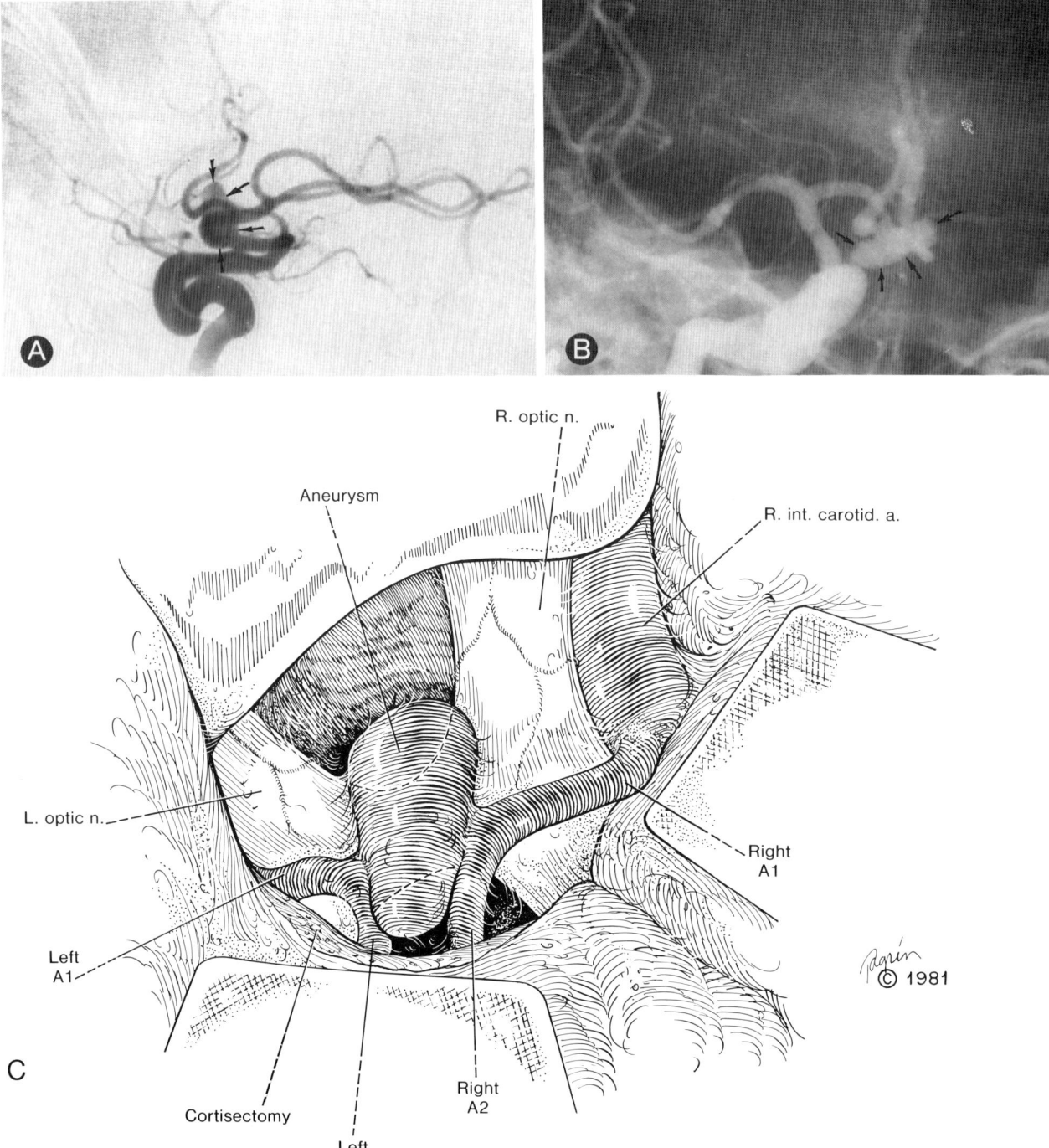

Figure 14.9 Bilobed anterior communicating artery aneurysm: adherence to optic chiasm and posterior bulge. A and B, right carotid angiogram shows projection of aneurysm rostrally and to both sides (*arrows*). Position of lesion near tuberculum sella suggests it may be adherent to basal structures. C, intraoperative illustration shows aneurysm adherent to superior and anterior surfaces of optic chiasm. Under hypotension, sharp and blunt dissection isolated lesion. Perforating arteries coursing posteriorly were spared. D, a suction was used to gather up both bulges of the aneurysm for inclusion in a straight Heifetz clip placed transversely. E and F, postoperative right carotid angiogram shows non-filling of aneurysm and preservation of arteries. The patient was neurologically intact.

the handle blades of the clip applier with the third and fourth fingers placed interiorly. Occasionally a Drake clip may be needed, with the aperture enclosing either the right A_1 or A_2 segment (Fig. 14.1 and 14.10). Bipolar coagulation (Fig. 11.7) or a preliminary ligature (Fig. 11.8) can be used to prepare the lesion for clipping. In some patients, the force of two clips may be needed to assure complete closure of a thick

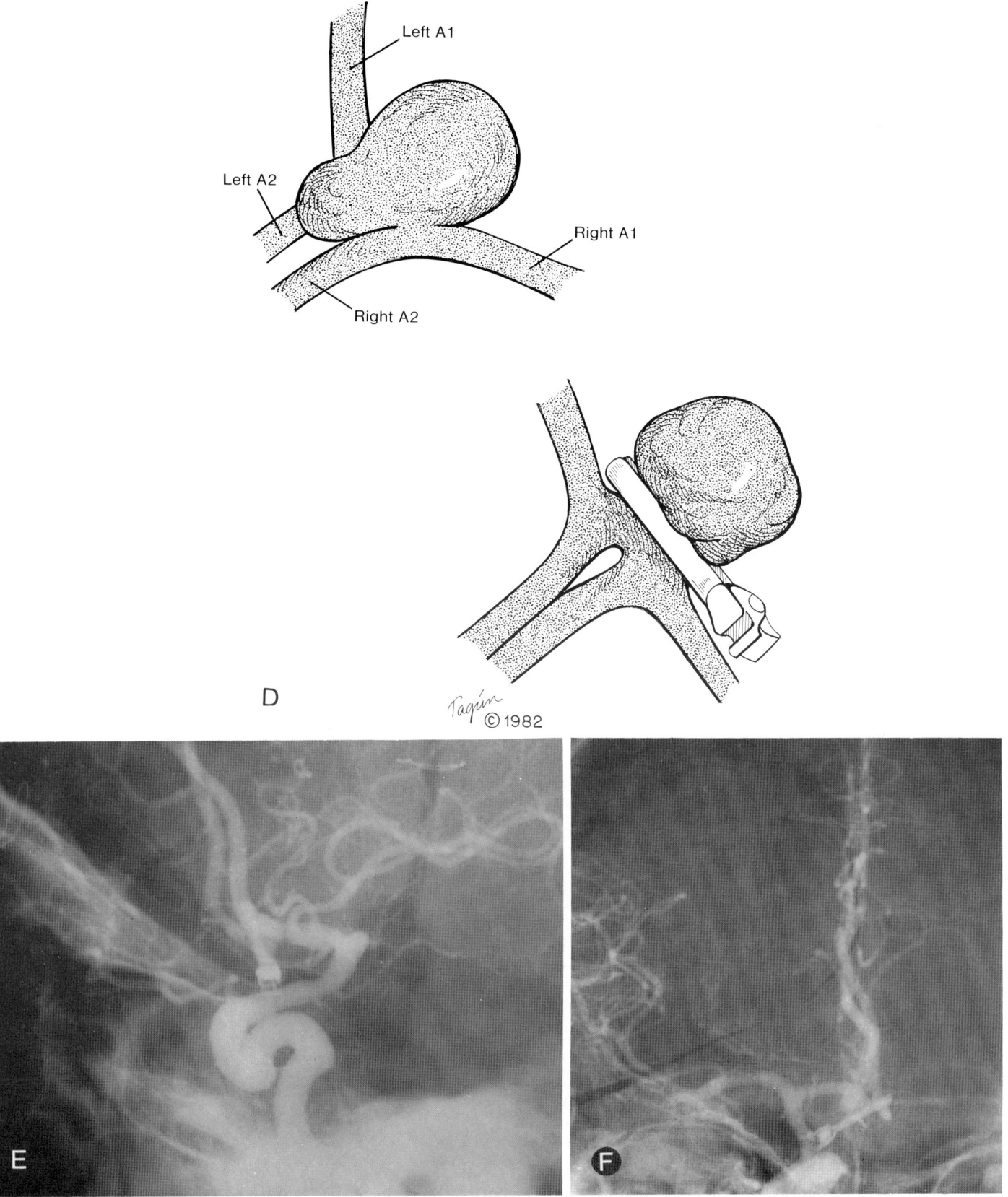

Figure 14.9 (D to F)

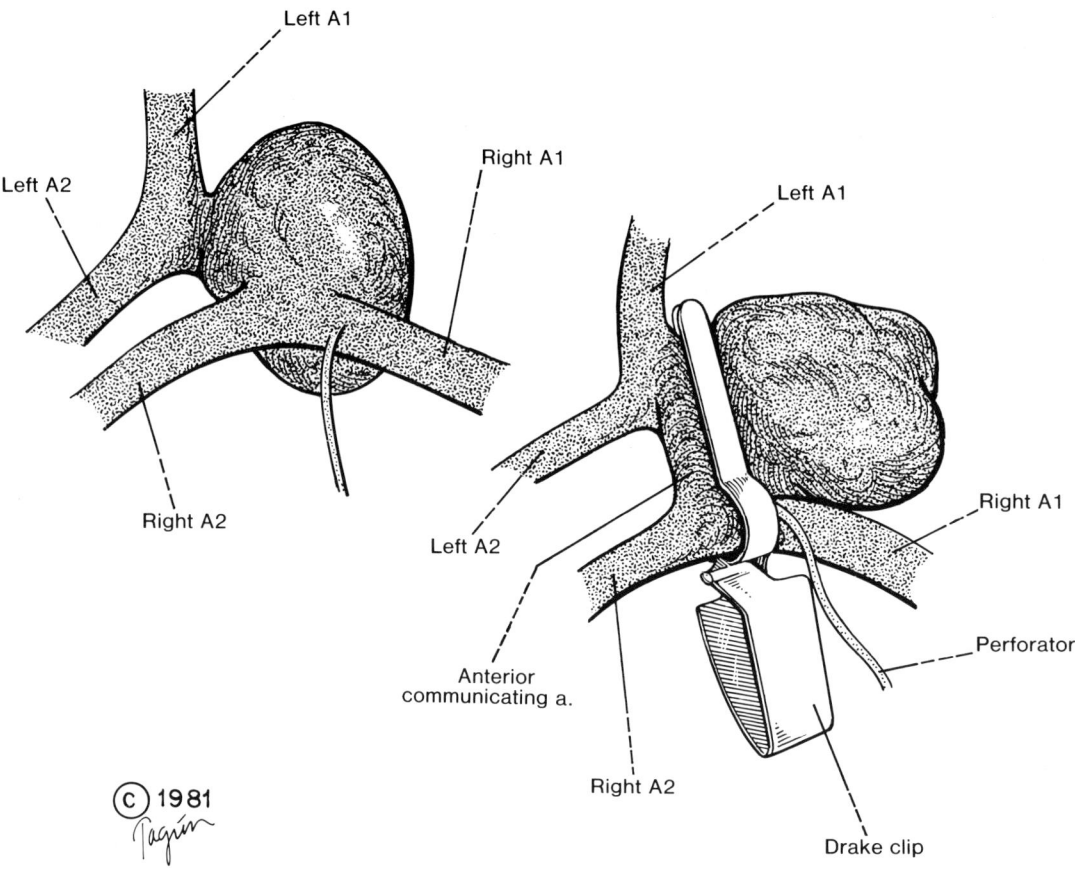

Figure 14.10 Common wall for aneurysm and right A1 artery. Solution of problem: Drake clip spares right A1 segment and perforating arteries.

aneurysmal wall. In other patients, a combination of two clips is necessary for optimum obliteration of the aneurysm neck. We have found a straight clip may occasionally be nicely supplemented with a triangular Heifetz clip to a persistent corner, since the hubs of this pair do not mutually interfere. For giant anterior communicating aneurysms, the Drake clips (up to 24 mm) may provide the only accurate and adequate clipping (see Chapter 20). Both anterior cerebral arteries and the anterior communicating artery with its perforating vessels must be maintained intact. If these criteria are not satisfied, the clip will need to be repositioned as often as necessary to obtain a satisfactory application.

RESULTS

The surgical results in our series are presented in Table 14.1. There were 52 consecutive anterior communicating artery aneurysms treated with microsurgical obliteration. Overall, 38 of the 41 patients (92%) in grades 1–2 preoperatively finished with a result that was either excellent (normal) or good (minor disability) and were able to return to their previous work. In one patient, despite a normal neurological examination, there was persisting disabling anxiety

Table 14.1
Results of Operation

Grade	Excellent	Good	Poor	Death	Total
1–2	28(68%)	10(24%)	2(5%)	1(2%)	41
3–4	—	5(45%)	5(45%)	1(9%)	11
Total	28(54%)	15(29%)	7(14%)	2(4%)	52

which made return to work as a housepainter impossible, despite extensive efforts with drug therapy over a 2-year period. It is possible that this related to impaired frontal lobe function, although there were no other signs of this. In one other case, there was immediate blindness in the right eye following surgery, presumably related to direct intraoperative injury to the optic nerve, clip pressure, or interference with the vascular supply. There was no improvement in vision over a 1-year follow-up. Among the 41 grade 1 and 2 category patients, we encountered a single death, a 47-year-old engineer who underwent uneventful clipping of anterior communicating artery and internal carotid artery aneurysms, only to suffer a fatal postoperative myocardial infarction.

Among 11 patients judged grade 3–4 preoperatively, only five (45%) enjoyed a good result and there were no excellent results. Five additional cases (45%) were judged poor results because of preoperative neurological deficits persisting after surgery (dementia, hemiplegia). There was a single death, a patient who presented deeply comatose with an intracerebral hematoma.

Other neurological complications included temporary left leg weakness due to an embolus to the pericallosal artery. Non-neurological complications included pulmonary embolus, requiring vena cava interruption. In another patient, bilateral femoral head necrosis was noted, apparently related to high dose steroid therapy. Bilateral total hip replacement was curative.

Postoperative angiography was performed in 48 cases. Total obliteration of the aneurysm was demonstrated in every case. "Slipped clips" were not observed. In two instances, the right A_1 segment was narrowed and in another occluded by the clip; none of these patients was symptomatic. Otherwise, normal arterial supply was intact.

Similar results using modifications of the lateral subfrontal approach are recorded in the literature (3, 6, 8, 9). Yasargil and Smith report 87% good-excellent results with 5.1% mortality (10). Hori and Suzuki use a bifrontal craniotomy and interhemispheric approach in most of their patients and have 84% good or excellent results (1). Sengupta et al. analyzed the quality of survival following surgery and found that postoperative intellectual impairment is uncommon, but there were personality changes associated with diminished interest and drive (5). As we also noted in our series, the most important factor relating to outcome was the preoperative clinical condition. Most of the patients in all of these reports had surgery 10 days or longer after the SAH.

REFERENCES

1. Hori S, Suzuki J: Early and late results of intracranial direct surgery of anterior communicating artery aneurysms. J Neurosurg 50:433–440, 1979.
2. Kempe LG: *Operative Neurosurgery, Vol 1: Cranial, Cerebral and Intracranial Vascular Disease.* New York, Springer-Verlag, 1968, pp 54–74.
3. Krayenbuhl HA, Yasargil MG, Flamm ES, Tew JM Jr: Microsurgical treatment of intracranial saccular aneurysms. J Neurosurg 37:678–686, 1972.
4. Perlmutter D, Rhoton AL: Microsurgical anatomy of the anterior cerebral-anterior communicating-recurrent artery complex. J Neurosurg 45:259–272, 1976.
5. Sengupta RP, Chin JSP, Brierly H: Quality of survival following direct surgery for anterior communicating aneurysms. J Neurosurg 43:58–64, 1975.
6. Sundt TM Jr, Whisnant JP: Subarachnoid hemorrhage from intracranial aneurysms. Surgical management and natural history of disease. N Engl J Med 299:116–122, 1978.
7. Suzuki J (ed): *Cerebral Aneurysms. Experiences with 1000 Directly Operated Cases.* Neuron Publishing, Tokyo, 1979.
8. VanderArk GD, Kempe LG, Smith DR: Anterior communicating aneurysms: The gyrus rectus approach. Clin Neurosurg 21:120–133, 1974.
9. Yasargil MG, Fox JL: The microsurgical approach to intracranial aneurysms. Surg Neurol 3:7–14, 1975.
10. Yasargil MG, Smith RD: Management of aneurysms of anterior circulation by intracranial procedures, in Youmans JR (ed): *Neurological Surgery.* WB Saunders, Philadelphia (to be published).

Chapter 15 DISTAL ANTERIOR CEREBRAL ANEURYSMS

PRESENTATION AND EVALUATION

Because they present special surgical problems, aneurysms arising from the distal anterior cerebral artery deserve separate consideration. These lesions generally arise near the genu of the corpus callosum, usually at the bifurcation of the pericallosal and callosomarginal arteries and sometimes at the origin of the frontopolar artery (5). Anatomic variations are common in this area, including communications between the two pericallosal arteries (4). For aneurysms distal to the callosomarginal origin, a diagnosis of a bacterial aneurysm must be considered (see Chapter 21).

Clinical presentation is usually with SAH, though occasionally a giant aneurysm in this area may cause mass effect. Prognosis tends to be worse than for other aneurysms (3, 5). The standard program of evaluation and preoperative management is utilized for these patients (see Chapters 10 and 11). At angiography, base and oblique films generally add little to the information obtained from antero-posterior and lateral views. Surgery is often difficult because of limited interhemispheric access, problems obtaining proximal control of the arterial circulation, and the frequent finding of a broad neck containing atheroma (6).

OPERATIVE TECHNIQUE

Preparation and Positioning

Spinal drainage is a useful adjunct in these patients because of the limited exposure available in the interhemispheric fissure. This space consideration is also a reason for deferring surgery for 10 days or more after SAH. Mannitol, with or without Lasix, is administered at the time of the skin incision to promote a brisk diuresis and subsequent slackening of the brain. Hyperventilation is routine. The preparation and anesthesia technique are described in Chapter 11.

The patient is positioned with the head and neck flexed on the chest, and the orbito-meatal line about 20° above the horizontal. The head is fixed in the three-point headrest with the nose straight ahead to place the midline in a true vertical orientation. With the head in this position, microsurgical access from the vertex may proceed downward to the area of the corpus callosum and the origin of the aneurysm.

Initial Exposure

In general, the approach is via a parasaggittal interhemispheric route. The non-dominant side is chosen whenever possible. Review of the angiogram will outline the venous drainage along the superior saggital sinus. Occasionally extensive bridging veins from the brain to the saggital sinus may bar the way and suggest a left side approach. Veins anterior to the coronal suture can usually be divided with no problem. If the CT scan shows a hematoma in the left frontal lobe, a left parasagittal approach is usually indicated.

For most lesions which lie just at or above the genu of the corpus callosum, a bicoronal incision is used, and a bone flap just in front of the coronal suture and crossing the midline gives adequate exposure (Fig. 15.1A, p. 198). The dura is opened with a horseshoe-shaped flap with the hinge on the midline. Bridging veins from the frontal lobe are divided for access to the interhemispheric fissure. Entry into this area is begun gradually with retraction on the exposed hemisphere with a hand-held retractor. As CSF is removed from the spinal catheter and Mannitol takes its effect, the brain becomes slack. Occasionally, if the brain remains full, ventricular puncture may be used. Dense adhesions of brain to falx may be taken down with electrocoagulation and sharp dissection. The dissection is deepened past the edge of the falx. A self-retaining retractor held by the Greenberg apparatus is introduced on the falx cerebri for medial retraction. Retraction on superior sagittal sinus is avoided. Telfa or a rubber dam covered with cottonoid is introduced over the medial surface of the hemisphere, and lateral retraction by a teflon-coated medium width retractor is applied and also held with the Greenberg apparatus.

Microsurgical Dissection

The surgical operating microscope is positioned and dissection proceeds at 10X or 16X. The exposure is gradually deepened by separating the two cingulate gyri. Generally, this is best accomplished with a #16 suction and microdissector. A small cottonoid in the field may be used to control minor oozing. The cottonoid may protect the brain for gentle suction retraction. In some instances, particularly where extensive subarachnoid hemorrhage has occurred, there may be dense adhesions between the surfaces of arachnoid on the two sides. In this setting, very careful blunt or sharp dissection is used.

The general aim of the initial dissection is to expose the pericallosal artery distal to the aneurysm origin.

Often this effort is aided by following a callosomarginal or other branch artery down to its parent arterial trunk. Frequent and careful reference to the cerebral angiography will assist in tracing the arteries to the pericallosal parent vessel.

Once the pericallosal artery is identified, it is followed retrograde toward its origin (Fig. 15.1B, p. 198). Dissection in this area is particularly perilous because the aneurysm may be densely adherent to the lobes of the brain, and proximal control has not been achieved. Therefore, once the aneurysm has been neared, the blood pressure is lowered to help minimize chances of rupture. When the aneurysm is encountered, every effort is made to avoid the lesion itself and proceed along the side of the pericallosal artery to obtain proximal exposure of this vessel. As the dissection is deepened, the aneurysm is inspected to check the effects of hemispheric retraction.

Ordinarily, the aneurysm will arise from a carina at the origin of a branch vessel from the pericallosal artery, usually the callosomarginal. In this situation, the branch vessel is generally proximal to the aneurysm and its initial segment must also be isolated. No effort is made to dissect the neck of the aneurysm until proximal control of both the pericallosal and the branch vessel have been obtained. Once proximal control is achieved, dissection of the neck is undertaken. Ordinarily, this is accomplished with a fine microdissector or by sharp dissection of adherent portions.

Obliteration of the Aneurysm

Application of bipolar cautery or a ligature may be needed to narrow the neck of the aneurysm for final clipping. Bipolar cauterization appears to be more frequently needed in this location than in many other aneurysmal sites. Yasargil and Carter report that when an atheroma is encountered in the neck of the aneurysm, it may be removed during temporary occlusion of the parent vessel and thus enable definitive clipping (6).

Since the aneurysm origin and arterial carina are approached from end on, special clipping techniques may be required (Fig. 15.1C, p. 199). In order to provide for blades crossing the neck from side to side, a right angle clip may be particularly useful (Fig. 15.2, p. 200). Alternatively, a straight clip may be brought across the neck by grasping the hub at right angles to the blade. Another approach is application of a curved clip, particularly a curved Yasargil, in the same axis as the parent vessel with the curvature flush with the carina of bifurcation. In some cases, a triangular-shaped clip from the Heifetz-Weck series may perfectly occlude the lesion. After application of the clip, careful inspection should confirm complete occlusion of the aneurysm with sparing of the parent and branch arteries. Although pericallosal occlusion is often asymptomatic, it can cause hemiplegia (2). Finally, aspiration of the aneurysm dome will make certain that adequate occlusion of the neck has been accomplished.

RESULTS

In our series of four cases, complete obliteration of the aneurysm was obtained with excellent neurological outcome. There were no complications. Two of these cases involved multiple aneurysms. In one instance it was possible to obliterate an aneurysm of the azygos anterior cerebral A_2 segment along with a middle cerebral artery aneurysm, both approached through a large frontotemporal flap which crossed the midline. In another patient, a total of five aneurysms were clipped through a wide fronto-temporal craniotomy. An increased incidence of multiple aneurysms has been noted when a pericallosal aneurysm is present (4, 6). A higher incidence of azygos A_2 segments has also been found with these aneurysms (1).

The literature records several series with good results from surgical treatment (2, 5, 6). Yasargil and Carter reported 13 cases with no operative mortality and 15% morbidity (6). These authors commented specifically on the difficulties in operating on these aneurysms.

REFERENCES

1. Katz RS, Horoupian DS, Zingesser L: Aneurysms of azygous anterior cerebral artery. Case report. J Neurosurg 48:804–808, 1978.
2. Laitinen L, Snellman A: Aneurysms of the pericallosal artery. A study of 14 cases verified angiographically and treated mainly by direct surgical attack. J Neurosurg 17:447–458, 1960.
3. Nishioka H: Report on the cooperative study of intracranial aneurysms and subarachnoid hemorrhage: Section VII, Part 1. Evaluation of the conservative management of ruptured intracranial aneurysms. J Neurosurg 25:574–592, 1966.
4. Perlmutter D, Rhoton AL Jr: Microsurgical anatomy of the distal anterior cerebral artery. J Neurosurg 49:204–228, 1978.
5. Snyckers FD, Drake CG: Aneurysm of the distal anterior cerebral artery. A report of 24 verified cases. S Afr Med J 47:1787–1791, 1973.
6. Yasargil MG, Carter LP: Saccular aneurysms of the distal anterior cerebral artery. J Neurosurg 40:218–223, 1974.

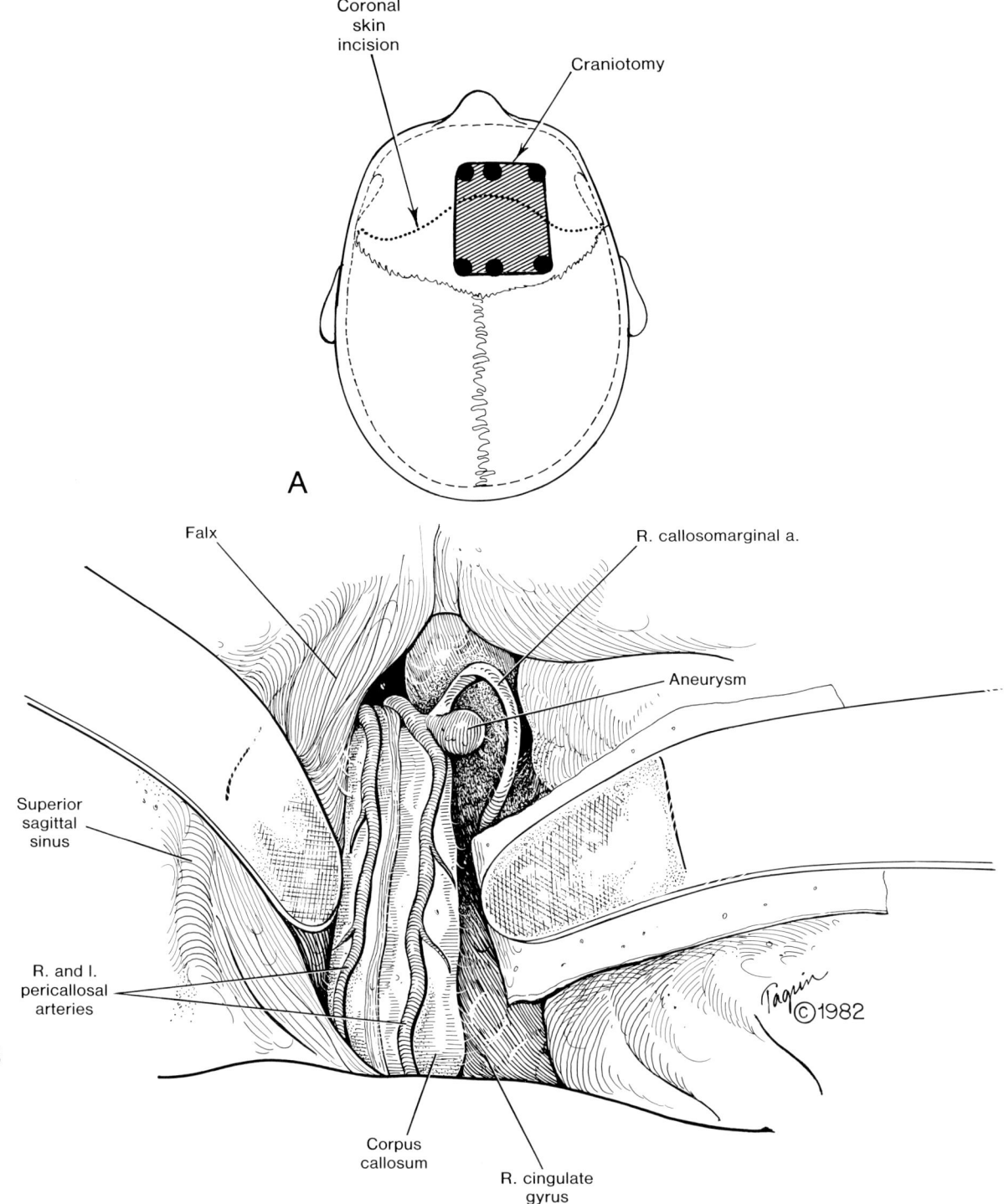

Figure 15.1 Distal anterior cerebral aneurysms. *A*, A coronal incision is used. The bone flap must cross the midline and extend posteriorly to just in front of the coronal suture. *B*, the pericallosal artery is identified by the midline exposure between the medial frontal lobe and the falx. The artery is followed retrograde to expose the aneurysm. *C*, the aneurysm usually arises at a major arterial bifurcation. Either a curved Yasargil clip or a straight clip, with the applicator at right angles to the blades, is used to obliterate these aneurysms and preserve the circulation.

Distal Anterior Cerebral Aneurysms

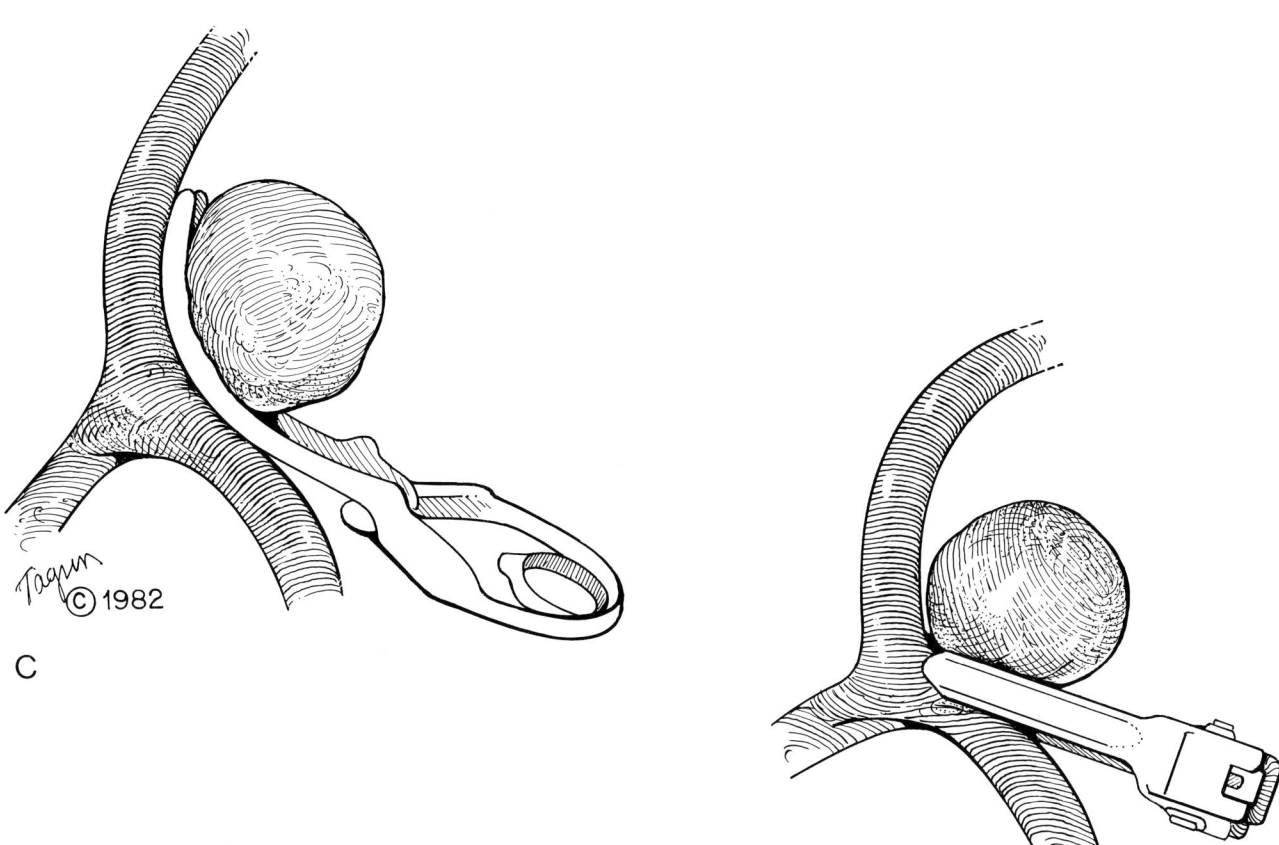

Figure 15.1 (*C*)

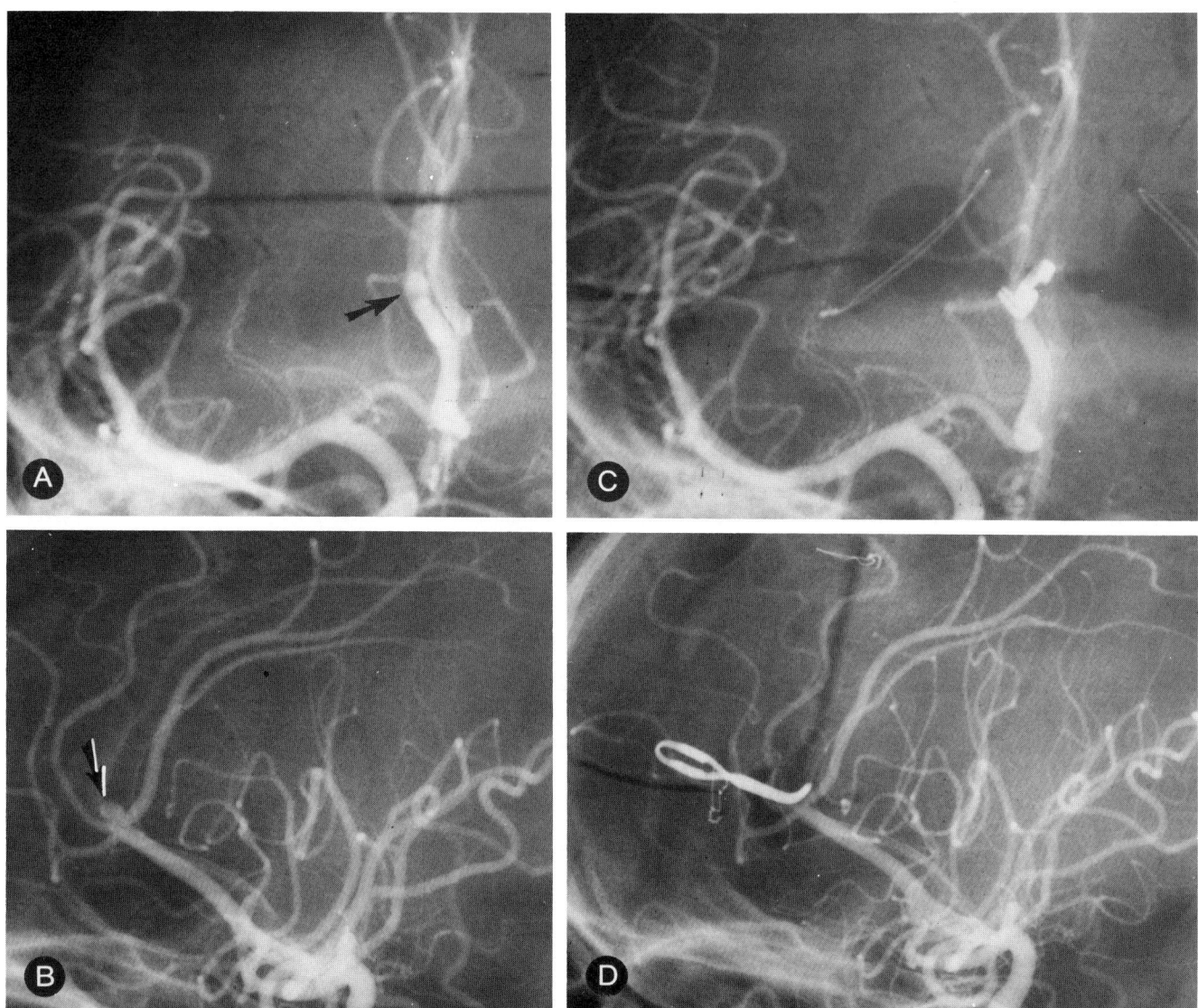

Figure 15.2 Pericallosal aneurysm. *A* and *B*, AP and lateral angiogram done 10 days after SAH showing aneurysm (*arrows*) arising from the genu of the pericallosal artery at the origin of the callosomarginal artery. There is no spasm. *C* and *D*, postoperative angiogram. A Yasargil clip with a right angle on the end has been applied The aneurysm is obliterated and normal arterial circulation preserved. Note the location of the bone flap. The postoperative neurological examination was normal.

Chapter 16 MIDDLE CEREBRAL ANEURYSMS

PRESENTATION AND EVALUATION

Middle cerebral artery (MCA) aneurysms usually arise from the first major division of the middle cerebral artery. Rarely, a more proximal lesion is located on the main trunk of the artery.

These aneurysms usually present with subarachnoid hemorrhage and are more likely to have immediate associated hemiparesis or dysphasia than are aneurysms in the other common locations. This fact may relate to the higher incidence of an associated intracerebral hematoma than is found with other aneurysms. In one report of 156 MCA aneurysms, 49.8% presented with a clot while this was true for only 15.8% of the internal carotid artery aneurysms and 20.2% of the anterior communicating artery aneurysms in the same clinic (7). A giant MCA aneurysm may present with a seizure disorder or with symptoms from direct pressure of the mass. Rarely, TIAs may bring attention to MCA aneurysms.

One may suspect an aneurysm in this site when the initial CT scan shows blood primarily in the area of one Sylvian fissure (Fig. 16.1A). When the angiogram is done, special oblique views may be needed to define the relationship of the aneurysm and the middle cerebral artery branches.

SURGICAL APPROACHES

Middle cerebral aneurysms may be operated either by a subfrontal exposure with splitting of the Sylvian fissure or by transcortical exposure through the superior temporal gyrus. Most neurosurgeons approach MCA aneurysms by opening the Sylvian fissure and following the MCA distally to the aneurysm (4, 7, 8, 11, 12, 14, 16, 17). We have preferred the superior

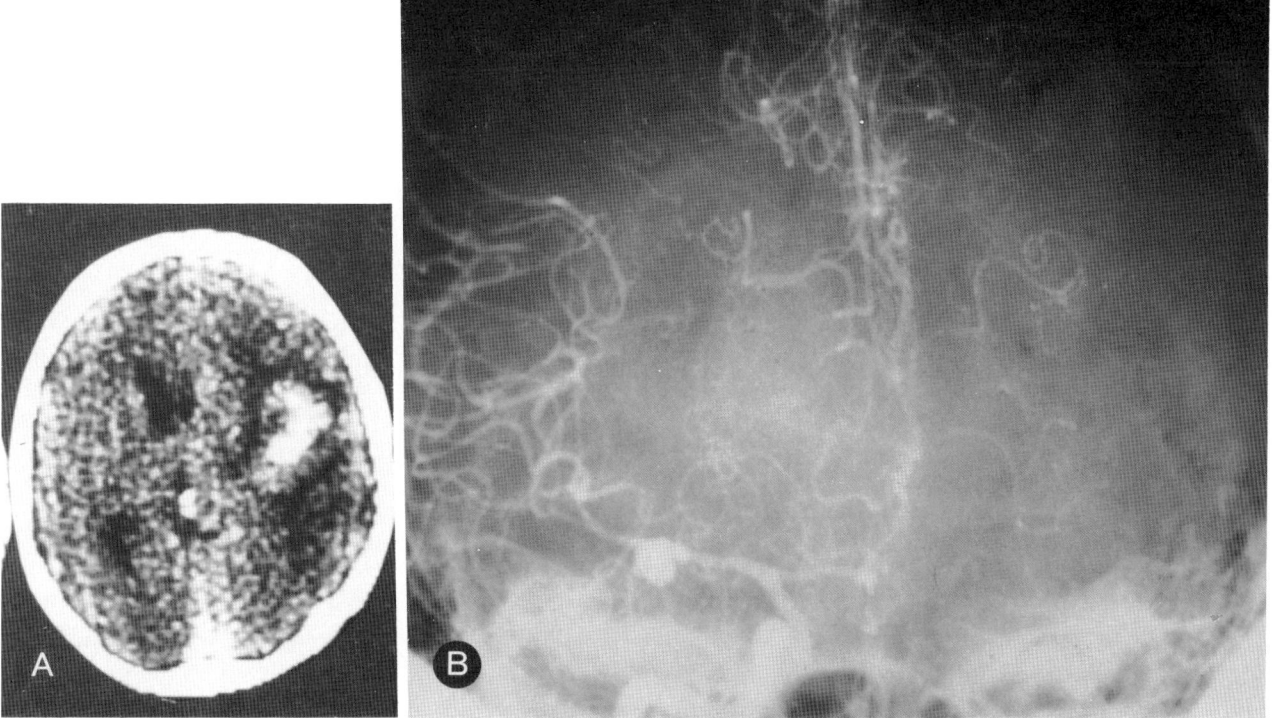

Figure 16.1 Middle cerebral artery aneurysm: evaluation. *A*, CT scan (without contrast) shows a localized hematoma in the anterior aspect of the Sylvian fissure. This finding is highly suggestive of a MCA aneurysm in a patient who presents with SAH. *B*, the angiogram shows considerable spasm. The MCA bifurcation and the aneurysm are much closer to the internal carotid bifurcation than those seen in Figures 16.2 and 16.3. This aneurysm is best approached by a subfrontal exposure, following the MCA distally in the Sylvian fissure.

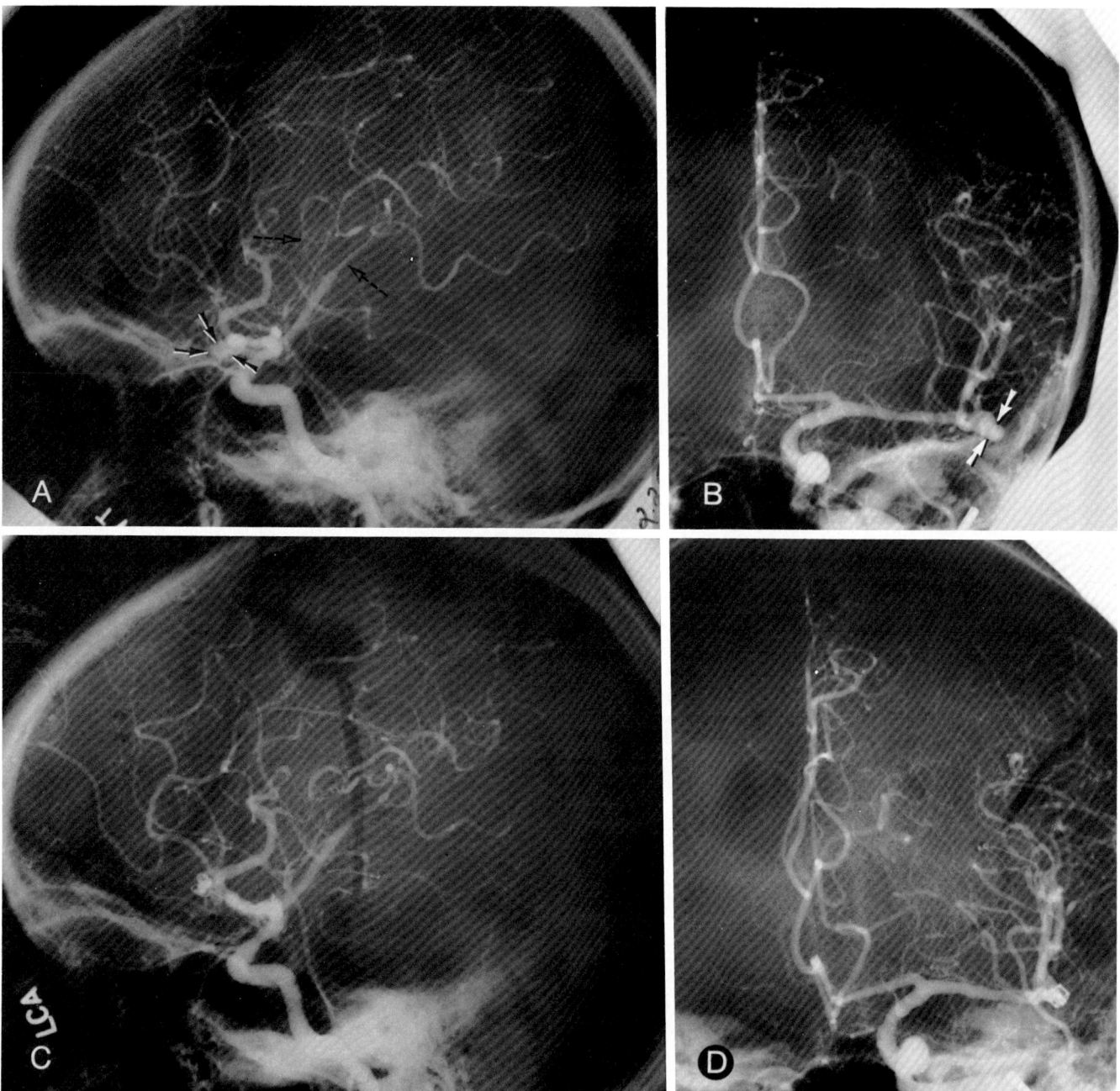

Figure 16.2 Middle cerebral artery aneurysm: clipping via superior temporal gyrus. A and B, the aneurysm projects laterally and anteriorly from the middle cerebral bifurcation (*closed arrows*). The location is ideally suited for a superior temporal gyrus approach. Note the spasm in the distal MCA branches (*open arrows*). C and D, postoperative angiogram shows that the clip obliterates the aneurysm. Some spasm persists.

temporal gyrus approach for the majority of middle cerebral aneurysms. This exposure was first utilized by us in the early 1960s after seeing the illustration by Poppen of an MCA aneurysm exposed through an intratemporal hematoma (9). Subsequently, it was learned that the first detailed description of this technique was by Tönnis and Walter in 1960 (15). Other reports of this approach are those of Berger (1) and Sheppard (13). Kempe uses it when there is a large temporal hematoma (6). Details of the technique and our results have been summarized (3).

We believe that there are several advantages in using the superior temporal gyrus approach to MCA aneurysms. Most MCA bifurcation aneurysms project laterally as a direct continuation of the MCA (Fig. 16.2) or, less commonly, anteriorly, inferiorly,

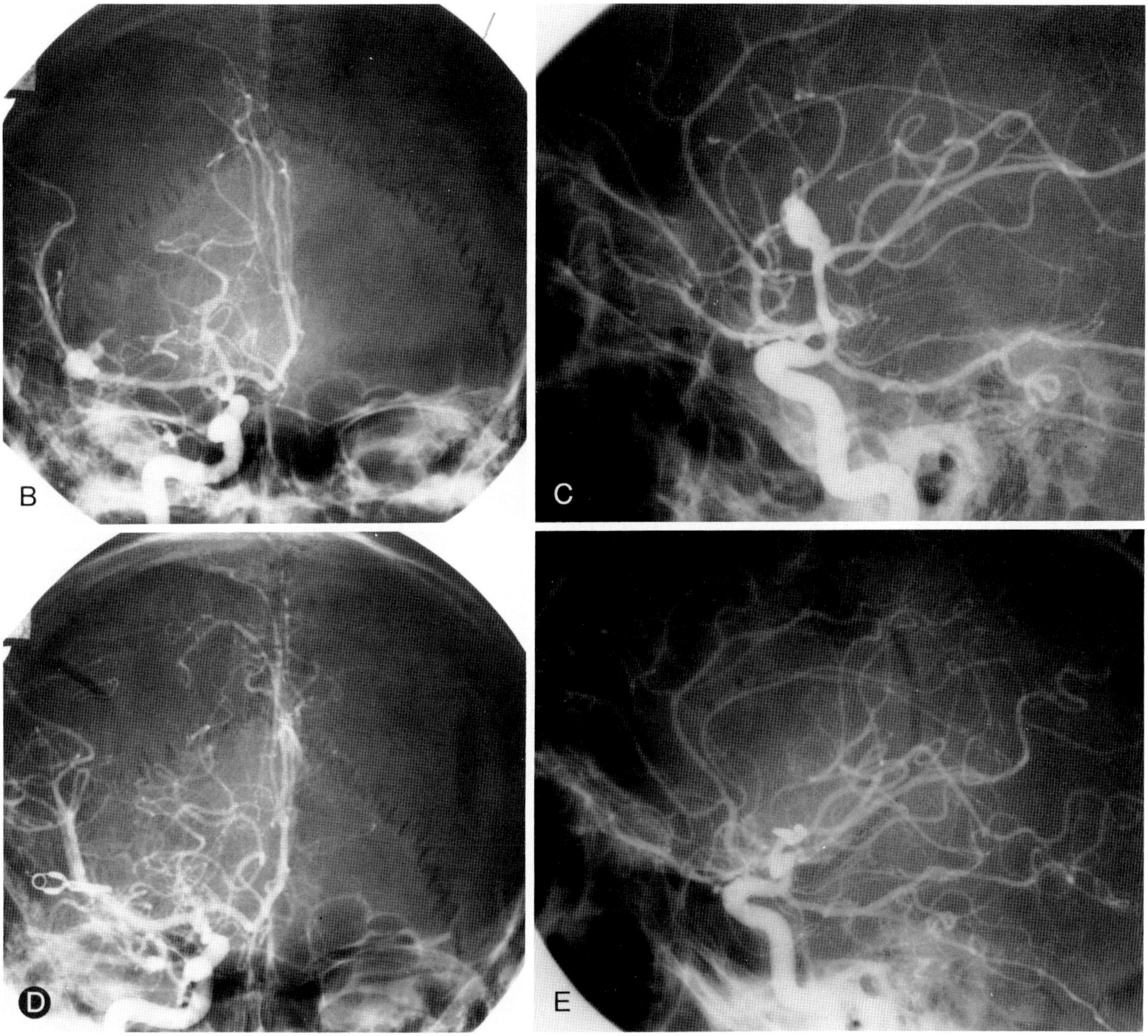

Figure 16.3 Middle cerebral artery aneurysm. *A*, CT scan (without contrast) done at the time of admission after sudden onset of headache, drowsiness, and left hemiparesis. A large hematoma is present in the medial aspect of the Sylvian fissure. *B* and *C*, the angiogram shows the aneurysm pointing superiorly and slightly anteriorly. The MCA is elevated and bowed laterally. Operation was done through a superior temporal gyrus approach. *D* and *E*, postoperative angiograms showing the aneurysm to be clipped and relief of the mass effect.

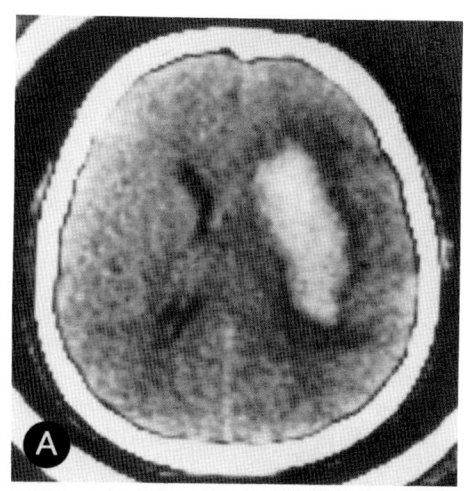

or superiorly (Fig. 16.3). In these patients, the superior temporal gyrus approach allows the surgeon to expose the main trunk of the MCA without disturbing the dome of the aneurysm by following the branches proximally to the base of the aneurysm. Significant retraction is avoided, and retractors are used simply to hold the exposure, which is accomplished by suctioning nonessential brain tissue. This advantage is particularly important in early operations when the brain is swollen and hyperemic or in the presence of a large intracerebral clot. In the latter instance, the clot should be suctioned only as necessary to gain exposure. The clot related to the dome of the aneurysm should be left undisturbed until exposure of the base of the aneurysmal complex is completed. This approach also avoids manipulation of the medial circle of Willis and of the proximal portion of the MCA with its important dorsal perforators. The anatomy of the distal and dorsal aspects of these aneurysms, which includes the relationship of the major divisions and their branches to the neck and dome, can be most difficult to define. In almost one-half of the patients, important lateral lenticulostriate arteries arise from the major divisions shortly after their origin. These small but important vessels run back in a medial direction, usually behind the neck of the aneurysm, to enter the basal ganglia (2, 5, 11). This complex anatomy can be best defined by a circumferential exposure of the base of the aneurysm via the transtemporal approach when combined with thorough removal of the pterion. This circumferential exposure also permits application of the clip from whatever angle seems best.

The superior temporal gyrus approach is not suited for aneurysms of the main trunk of the MCA proximal to the main bifurcation, for aneurysms of the MCA at the point of origin of an early temporal branch, or for patients with a short main trunk of the MCA where the aneurysm arises from an early bifurcation which occurs before the genu (Fig. 16.1). The nine cases of MCA aneurysms in our series which were approached by splitting the Sylvian fissure and following the MCA distally fall into the above categories (3).

The main disadvantage of the transtemporal approach is that the base of the aneurysmal complex is encountered before proximal control of the afferent vessel is assured. However, it is almost always possible to expose enough of the MCA before exposing the dome of the aneurysm so that a temporary clip could be applied in case of premature rupture. The only cases of intraoperative rupture we encountered occurred after such proximal control had been obtained and, with one exception, were satisfactorily handled with suction without having to use a temporary clip on the MCA. Another minor disadvantage of this approach is the need for a slightly larger bone flap than is required for the usual pterional approach. A theoretical disadvantage is the possibility of increasing the risk of epilepsy by the cortical resection.

We are not aware of an increased incidence of seizures in our series, but the followup is relatively short.

In an early experience with middle cerebral aneurysms, some were coated with tissue adhesive. However, during the past 5 years almost all MCA aneurysms have been found to have a neck amenable to clipping.

OPERATIVE TECHNIQUE: SUPERIOR TEMPORAL GYRUS APPROACH

Position

The patient is placed in the supine position with the head turned to the opposite side nearly 90° and tilted slightly backward. In some patients, slight elevation of the ipsilateral shoulder may be necessary. All other aspects of anesthesia, use of the skeletal fixation head rest, and initial preparation and draping are as described in Chapter 11.

Incision and Initial Exposure

The incision starts at the level of the zygoma just in front of the tragus and curves slightly backward above the ear before swinging forward to the edge of the hairline about 2–3 cm lateral to the midline (Fig. 16.4). Technical points regarding this aspect of the operation are discussed in Chapter 12. The branch of the facial nerve to the frontalis muscle and the trunk and frontal branch of the superficial temporal artery are saved with the scalp flap. The muscle is turned down with the skin flap to allow retraction of the muscle down into the temporal region and facilitate exposure of the area of the pterion. The bone flap is then cut in the same manner as for the standard pterional approach, but the cut is extended further back into the temporal bone to expose more of the temporal lobe (Fig. 16.4). The pterion and lateral aspect of the sphenoid ridge are removed in the same manner as for the pterional approach. This step is important because it exposes the anterior aspect of the Sylvian fissure and allows dissection of the aneurysm and clip application from an anterolateral direction in cases where this is preferable. Without removing the pterion, the surgeon is forced to work only from behind, underneath the overhanging bone, which can be a major handicap.

During this phase of the operation, the surgeon can determine how tense the brain is. Lasix and mannitol will have been given as described in Chapter 11 and the pCO2 will be in the low 30's. Usually these measures will reduce brain tension.

The dura is opened over the inferior frontal region approximately 10 mm above the inferior margin of the bone opening. The incision is extended over the anterior temporal region. A second cut is usually made parallel to the Sylvian fissure. The flaps of dura are retracted with sutures (Fig. 16.5).

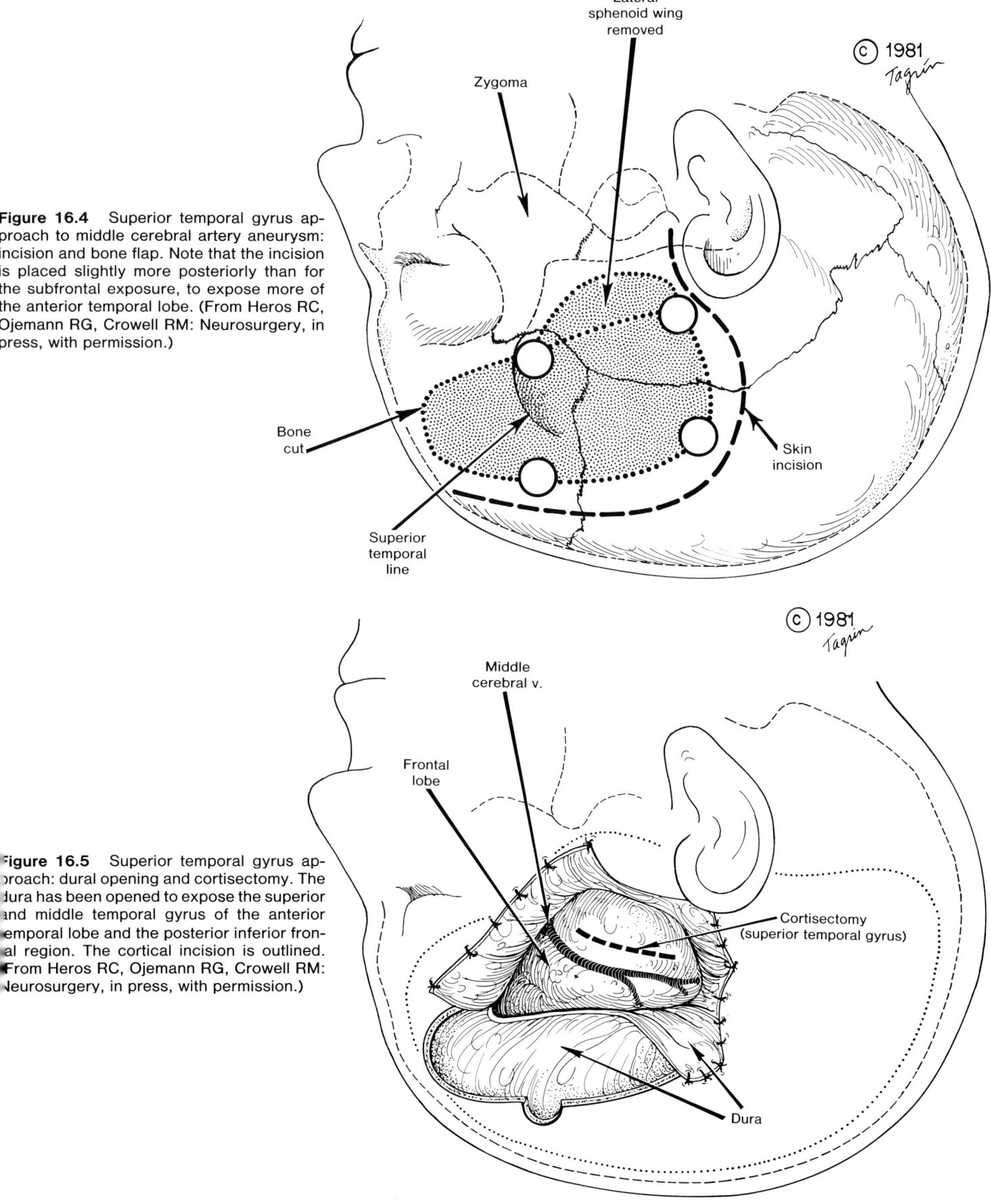

Figure 16.4 Superior temporal gyrus approach to middle cerebral artery aneurysm: incision and bone flap. Note that the incision is placed slightly more posteriorly than for the subfrontal exposure, to expose more of the anterior temporal lobe. (From Heros RC, Ojemann RG, Crowell RM: Neurosurgery, in press, with permission.)

Figure 16.5 Superior temporal gyrus approach: dural opening and cortisectomy. The dura has been opened to expose the superior and middle temporal gyrus of the anterior temporal lobe and the posterior inferior frontal region. The cortical incision is outlined. (From Heros RC, Ojemann RG, Crowell RM: Neurosurgery, in press, with permission.)

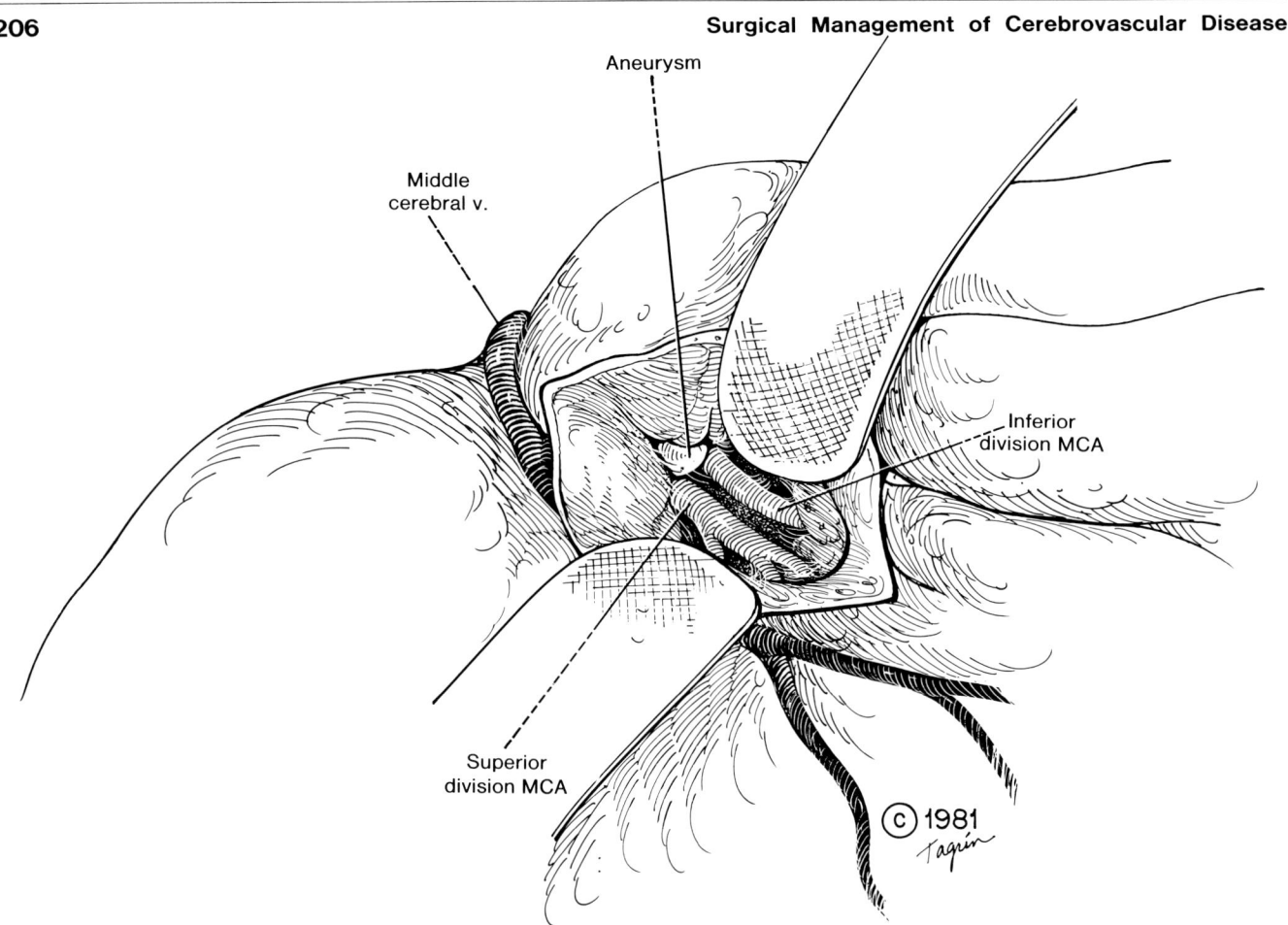

Figure 16.6 Superior temporal gyrus approach: initial exposure of aneurysm. The Sylvian fissure has been entered. The middle cerebral branches are followed anteriorly until the base of the aneurysm is exposed. (From Heros RC, Ojemann RG, Crowell RM: Neurosurgery, in press, with permission.)

Microsurgical Dissection

The operating microscope is brought into place. An incision about 2–3 cm long is made in the superior temporal gyrus starting about 1 cm behind the front of the Sylvian fissure in a direction parallel to the fissure (Fig. 16.5). Using suction and bipolar coagulation as needed, the incision in the superior temporal gyrus is extended medially. Self-retaining retractors are used to aid the exposure. The dissection extends into the vertical segment of the Sylvian fissure over the insula. With microsurgical technique, the branches of the MCA are followed proximally toward the aneurysm (Fig. 16.6). In many cases, subarachnoid hematoma will be adherent to these vessels and will need to be removed. Without disturbing the dome of the aneurysm, one of the two major divisions can usually be followed, on the side away from the aneurysm, to the main stem of the MCA which courses medially and slightly posteriorly. Only enough of the main trunk of the MCA is exposed to allow application of a temporary clip, if needed. Once the distal part of the MCA and the origin of the main divisions are identified, we usually dissect the entire aneurysmal complex, frequently leaving some adherent brain attached to the dome in the area of rupture (Fig. 16.7). Moderate hypotension is instituted at this stage (mean systemic pressure of 50–60 mm Hg in most cases). Complete dissection of the aneurysm allows its safe mobilization to provide full visualization of the neck. This is particularly helpful in the case of large aneurysms, when the anatomy may not be entirely clear until all the aneurysm is exposed. Frequently, a third major branch is encountered and must be dissected away from the neck. At least one of the divisions is usually quite adherent to the aneurysm and must be separated from it with sharp dissection to define the neck. Recurrent lenticulostriate vessels arising from the origin of the main divisions must be identified and separated from the neck. For this final preparation of the neck, we have sometimes found it helpful in cases of large aneurysms to retract the dome using a microdissector, which fits nicely into one of the arms of the Greenberg self-retaining retractor. Once the neck is ready, a clip can be applied from whatever direction seems most appropriate. Frequently, we have had to replace or adjust the clip several times or have used multiple clips, especially for larger aneurysms. The clip posi-

Middle Cerebral Aneurysms

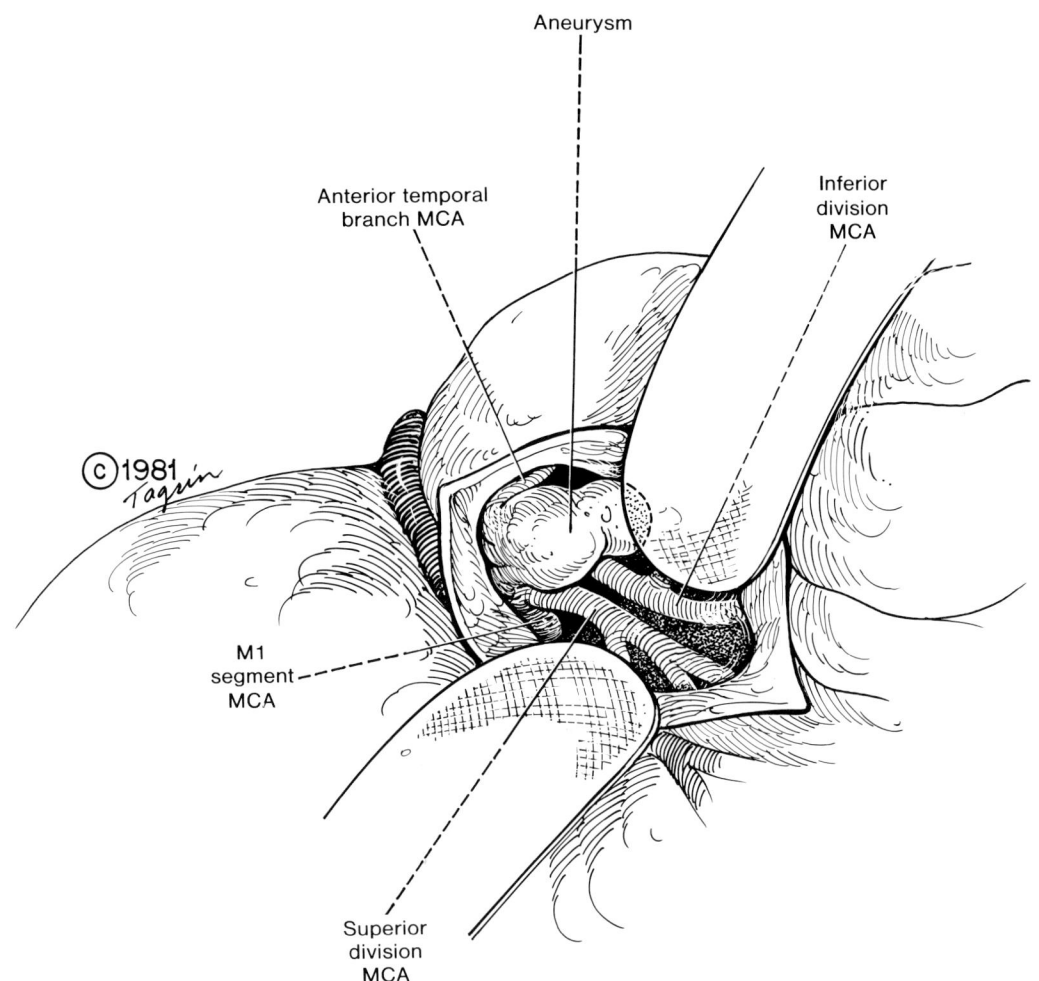

Figure 16.7 Superior temporal gyrus approach: dissection of the aneurysm. The distal M1 segment is identified. Note its medial posterior course. The aneurysm is now dissected from MCA branches and the surrounding tissue after leaving some tissue adherent at the site of the rupture. (From Heros RC, Ojemann RG, Crowell RM: Neurosurgery, in press, with permission.)

tion should be changed if there is any indication of kinking or constriction of the middle cerebral trunk or branches. In avoiding this constriction, a small portion of the neck may not be included in the clip. If this is the case, the region is reinforced with tissue adhesive. Should the aneurysm rupture, steps should be followed as outlined in Chapter 11.

By careful and persistent dissection under the operating microscope, we have found that almost all MCA aneurysms can be clipped. This has also been the finding of Wilson and Spetzler and Lougheed and Marshall (7, 16). The latter authors noted that most MCA branches appearing to arise from the aneurysm were only adherent and could be dissected to the region of the MCA bifurcation (7).

A variation of this approach is described by Rand (10). The dissection to open the Sylvian fissure is started approximately 2-3 cm behind the tip of the temporal lobe. An arterial branch is followed into the fissure toward the aneurysm. When there is extensive hemorrhage, this dissection can be difficult, and on the left side, this approach requires direct retraction on the speech area. Yasargil and Fox also mention this approach (17).

OPERATIVE TECHNIQUE: SUBFRONTAL SYLVIAN FISSURE APPROACH

The position of the patient, incision, craniotomy flap, and dural opening are the same as described for internal carotid aneurysms (Chapter 12). It is important that measures be taken to make the brain as slack as possible.

The frontal lobe is carefully elevated with a teflon-coated hand-held retractor. The olfactory tract is identified and followed posteriorly to the optic nerve. A self-retaining retractor is placed and the operating microscope positioned. Arachnoid is opened over the internal carotid just lateral to the nerve and above the anterior clinoid process. The exposure is followed distal to the internal carotid bifurcation and the self-retaining retractor repositioned. A second smaller retractor is used to gently lift the temporal lobe.

Bridging veins from the temporal lobe to the dura along the edge of the middle fossa are coagulated and divided.

The Sylvian fissure is identified, the thickened arachnoid opened, and the middle cerebral artery followed distally staying on the anterior and inferior surface of the artery away from the perforating arteries. The neck of the aneurysm is exposed from the medial side. Dissection of the branches of the MCA is then begun. How much of the aneurysm is dissected depends on its relationship to the branches. The same techniques described previously are used in dissecting these branches from the aneurysm. Useful instruments include the small microball dissector, microstraight dissector, microcurved Rhoton #6–8 dissectors, microhook, and microscissors.

Aneurysms arising from the trunk of the middle cerebral artery or at the origin of a proximal branch are approached through the Sylvian fissure. Great care must be taken in dissecting the perforating arteries from the neck of the aneurysm before clipping.

RESULTS

We have reported the results in 55 patients with MCA aneurysms treated by the authors and Dr. Roberto Heros (3). Three patients had bilateral aneurysms.

The subfrontal Sylvian fissure approach was used in 10 operations on nine patients. The aneurysms in this group were generally smaller and originated either at an early bifurcation (Fig. 16.1B) or at the origin of a lenticulostriate vessel. There were no deaths and only one patient worsened as a result of surgery. This patient had a small aneurysm clipped under systemic hypotension. A massive intracerebral hemorrhage developed when the systemic pressure was inadvertently raised with a vasopressors to about 170 mm Hg systolic to check for hemostasis. It was postulated that this hemorrhage occurred as a result of the dysautoregulation that follows a period of significant hypotension. One must be very careful to avoid raising blood pressure beyond normal levels to check for hemostasis.

The superior temporal gyrus approach gave similarly good results. Among 49 patients operated via this route, 10 were performed for unruptured aneurysms, and the other operations were done for aneurysms that had bled from several hours to 3 months before surgery. The median day of surgery was the 15th day after SAH. The average age in the group of patients undergoing operation via the superior temporal gyrus was 48.6 years. Table 16.1 correlates the postoperative results with the preoperative grade. Good preoperative status (grade 0, 1, 2) was associated with good results in 31 of 32 cases, and grade 3 patients had 90% good or fair results. Half of the moribund patients achieved fair to good outcome, while three of eight died. Table 16.2 correlates the postoperative result with the estimated size of the

Table 16.1
Middle Cerebral Artery Aneurysms Approached through the Superior Temporal Gyrus: Preoperative Grade and Results[a]

Preoperative Grade (Hunt)	Number of Cases	Results[b]			
		Good	Fair	Poor	Dead
0, 1, 2	32	31	1	0	0
3	9	3	5	1	0
4	4	1	2	1	0
5	4	0	1	0	3
Total	49	35	9	2	3

[a] Modified from Ref. 3.
[b] Good: normal or minimal neurological deficit that resolved in less than 3 months. Fair: ambulatory and independent but with permanent mild to moderate neurological deficit. Poor: permanent moderate to severe neurological deficit.

Table 16.2
Middle Cerebral Artery Aneurysms Approached through the Superior Temporal Gyrus: Size and Results[a]

Size (mm)	Number of Cases	Results[b]			
		Good	Fair	Poor	Dead
<7	2	2	0	0	0
7–15	23	17	3	1	2
15–25	16	11	5	0	0
>25	8	5	1	1	1
Total	49	35	9	2	3

[a] Modified from Ref. 3.
[b] Good: normal or minimal neurological deficit that resolved in less than 3 months. Fair: ambulatory and independent but with permanent mild to moderate neurological deficit. Poor: Permanent moderate to severe neurological deficit.

aneurysm. The giant lesions did worse than the other groups. In 19 cases, we did not perform postoperative angiography; these included 16 instances of smaller aneurysms in which the surgeon felt confident about a satisfactory clipping and the three cases in which the aneurysm was only wrapped. The other 30 cases had postoperative angiography. Except for varying degrees of vasospasm, the only significant findings were partial occlusion of one arterial division in one case and visualization of about 20% of the neck of the aneurysm in another. In addition, the MCA was found to be occluded in one patient with a giant aneurysm who had an intraoperative tear of the main trunk of the MCA. The surgeon attempted to repair the tear by suturing, but the patient awoke hemiplegic. In all the other postoperative angiograms, the aneurysm was found to be obliterated and all the major divisions well filled.

Operative complications included the above-mentioned hemiplegia, a subdural empyema, and a subdural hematoma. The only fatalities occurred in three patients who were in deep coma before surgery and were operated on an emergency basis to evacuate a large intracerebral hematoma. Two of these patients did not have preoperative angiography and their suspected aneurysm was confirmed at surgery. A fourth patient operated in this condition made a fair recovery. In these four patients, the aneurysm was clipped during the operation.

Eight patients had symptomatic thrombophlebitis; two of these had pulmonary emboli which, fortunately, were not fatal. Of these patients, one had an unruptured aneurysm. The others had recently experienced a subarachnoid hemorrhage and were being treated with epsilon-aminocaproic acid. Their surgery had been delayed an average of 27 days after SAH, usually because of preoperative vasospasm.

Only two patients in this series sustained a permanent neurological deficit as a result of postoperative vasospasm. This deficit was mild in one case and moderate in the other. Probably the most important factor in the low incidence was the policy of not operating before the 10th day after SAH, and deferring surgery in those patients with angiographic evidence of severe vasospasm. This policy has resulted in relatively "late" surgery, with the median day of surgery being the 15th day after SAH in the group of patients with a ruptured aneurysm. The only "early" operations performed in this series were in patients who required urgent evacuation of a temporal lobe hematoma and, in accordance with our usual policy, had the aneurysm clipped during this procedure. Lougheed and Marshall also found that with the use of the microscope in 18 patients with middle cerebral artery aneurysm, there were no operative mortalities and no patient was worse (7).

REFERENCES

1. Berger E: Targeted approach to middle cerebral artery trifurcation aneurysms. Excerpta Med Int Congr Ser 418:199, 1977.
2. Grand W: Microsurgical anatomy of the proximal middle cerebral artery and the internal carotid artery bifurcation. Neurosurgery 7:215-218, 1980.
3. Heros RC, Ojemann RG, Crowell RM: The superior temporal gyrus approach to middle cerebral aneurysms: technique and results. Neurosurgery (to be published).
4. Höök O, Norlén G: Aneurysms of the middle cerebral artery. A report of 80 cases. Acta Chir Scand Suppl 235:1-39, 1958.
5. Jones TH, Crowell RM: Microsurgical anatomy of the middle cerebral artery stem (M_1 segment) (in preparation).
6. Kempe L: Operative Neurosurgery. New York, Springer-Verlag, 1968.
7. Lougheed WM, Marshall BM: Management of aneurysms of the anterior circulation by intracranial procedures, in Youmans JR (ed): Neurological Surgery. Philadelphia, WB Saunders, 1973, vol 2, pp 742-750.
8. Peerless SJ: The surgical approach to middle cerebral and posterior communicating aneurysms. Clin Neurosurg 21:151-165, 1974.
9. Poppen JL: An Atlas of Neurosurgical Techniques. Philadelphia, WB Saunders, 1960, pp 158-161.
10. Rand RW: Microneurosurgery in cerebral aneurysms, in Rand (ed): Microneurosurgery. St. Louis, CV Mosby, 1978, ed 2, pp 318-319.
11. Rhoton AL, Saeki N, Perlmutter D, Zeal A: Microsurgical anatomy of common aneurysm sites. Clin Neurosurg 26:248-306, 1979.
12. Robinson RG: Ruptured aneurysms of the middle cerebral artery. J Neurosurg 35:25-33, 1971.
13. Shepard RH: Operation for aneurysms of the middle cerebral artery, in Rob C, Smith R (eds): Operative Surgery. Fundamental International Techniques. London, Butterworth and Company, 1979, ed 3, pp 252-257.
14. Suzuki J, Kodama N, Fujiwara S, Ebina T: Surgical treatment of middle cerebral artery aneurysms: From the experiences of 174 cases, in Suzuki J (ed): Cerebral Aneurysms: Experiences with 1000 Directly Operated Cases. Tokyo, Tokyo Press Company, Ltd, 1979, pp 278-283.
15. Tönnis W, Walter W: Ein neuer operativer Zugang zu den sackförmigen Aneurysmen der basalen Hirngefäße. Wien Med Wochenschr 110:145-147, 1960.
16. Wilson CB, Spetzler RF: Operative approaches to aneurysms. Clin Neurosurg 26:232-247, 1979.
17. Yasargil MG, Fox L: The microsurgical approach to intracranial aneurysms. Surg Neurol 3:7-14, 1975.

Chapter 17 BASILAR BIFURCATION ANEURYSMS

PRESENTATION AND EVALUATION

Aneurysms arising from the top of the basilar artery are the most common posterior circulation aneurysms. The usual presentation is subarachnoid hemorrhage (SAH). Symptoms do not differ significantly from those associated with SAH from anterior circulation aneurysms. On occasion, a basilar tip aneurysm may present with a third nerve palsy, progressive neurological dysfunction from direct pressure, or chronic headache.

On the angiogram the aneurysm usually projects upward in line with the basilar artery trunk, but less commonly it projects posteriorly between the peduncles or anteriorly against the clivus. The angiogram may be misleading in several respects. A leash of perforating arteries may appear to arise from the aneurysm, but in fact they originate from the proximal posterior cerebral (P_1) arteries and sweep up and back around the dome of the aneurysm (1, 2). The P_1 arteries, which may also appear to arise from the aneurysm, originate from the basilar artery. Though P_1 may appear on the angiogram to be well away from the side of the lesion in some cases, this is often the result of a thick aneurysmal wall or mural thrombus, and most commonly the P_1 vessels are tightly applied to the aneurysm. When occlusion of the basilar artery is being considered in the treatment plan, the posterior communicating arteries must be visualized. At times vertebral injection with concomitant ipsilateral carotid compression will be needed to visualize this vessel (Allcock test).

Often the sac of the aneurysm is considerably larger than the portion filled with contrast because of mural thrombus. Comparison of the CT scan with the angiographic appearance will help in clarifying this point.

Preoperative review of the angiographic studies directs the surgical approach. The height of the basilar bifurcation in relation to the dorsum sella is crucial. Usually, the bifurcation is at or just above the level of the posterior clinoid process, and thus may be exposed subtemporally with moderate temporal lobe retraction. Occasionally, the bifurcation is high above the dorsum, and correspondingly greater retraction is required. When the basilar apex is below the level of the dorsum sella, section of the tentorium posterior to the fourth nerve entry point may be needed. Exposure of a low-lying basilar apex will occasionally require a combined subtemporal and suboccipital approach with tentorial section (see Chapter 18).

OPERATIVE TECHNIQUE

A subtemporal approach offers good exposure of most basilar bifurcation aneurysms (1–3, 5). This is done from the right side, except in some patients where the aneurysm points to the right or when the patient has a left oculomotor palsy or right hemiparesis.

Preoperative treatment and induction of anesthesia follow the guidlines outlined in Chapter 11. The patient is placed in the lateral decubitus position. A spinal subarachnoid catheter is placed. The head is fixed in a 3-point headrest with the temporal squama parallel to the floor and the vertex dipped 15° below the horizontal. A linear incision provides sufficient exposure to turn a small temporal bone flap (Fig. 17.1). Bone is removed down to the floor of the middle fossa to minimize brain retraction. Lumbar drainage, hyperventilation, and osmotic diuresis provide a slack brain.

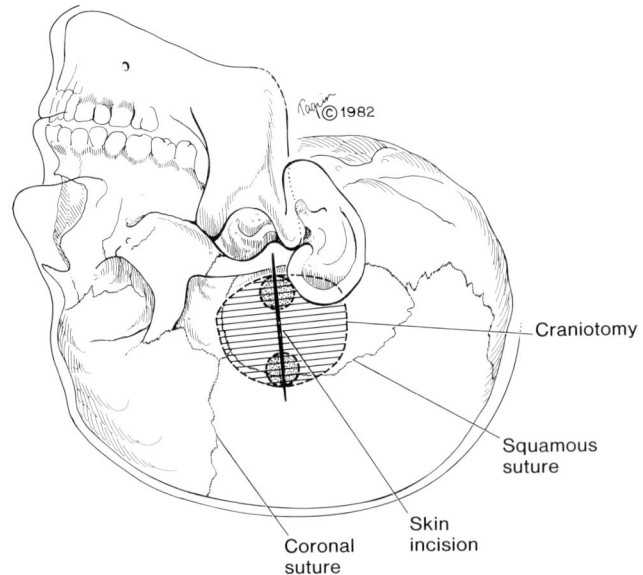

Figure 17.1 Operative technique: temporal craniotomy. A straight incision gives enough room. The approach is usually on the right, unless there is a preoperative left third nerve palsy or right hemiplegia. The craniotomy should be extended to the floor of the middle fossa.

Basilar Bifurcation Aneurysms

The dura is opened to provide access to the floor of the middle fossa (Fig. 17.2). Telfa (or a sheet of rubber dam and cottonoid) is gently introduced under the temporal lobe down to the uncus. A broad Teflon-coated retractor blade gently elevates the temporal lobe, exposing the free edge of the tentorium. For these maneuvers, it may become necessary to coagulate and divide bridging veins from the inferior temporal lobe to the transverse sinus. This is best done early in the exposure to avoid annoying bleeding. Only those veins likely to be torn are sacrificed, lest venous drainage of the lobe be compromised excessively. The third nerve should be visualized beneath the covering of arachnoid (Fig. 17.3). This is the central landmark for exposure. If the side of the brainstem and the fourth nerve are directly in view, or if the brainstem seems to curve and recede posteriorly, the line of sight is too far posterior. Once the retractor blade and its underlying protecting mat are in place, these may be fixed to the Greenberg retractor. Excessive retraction should be avoided, for it may cause temporal lobe infarction. On one occasion we stopped an operative effort and deferred it a week because of inadequate slackness to the brain.

Microsurgical Dissection

With the initial exposure established, the operating microscope is moved into position. Under the microscope the retractor may be adjusted. The tip of the retractor blade should lie just on the uncus. The third nerve will rise with the temporal lobe during elevation. In cases of a high basilar bifurcation, more extensive dissection of the third nerve may be required. In most patients, however, simply working inferior to the third nerve avoids excessive manipulation and reduces the chance of third nerve palsy. A 4-0 Neurolon suture is placed in the edge of the

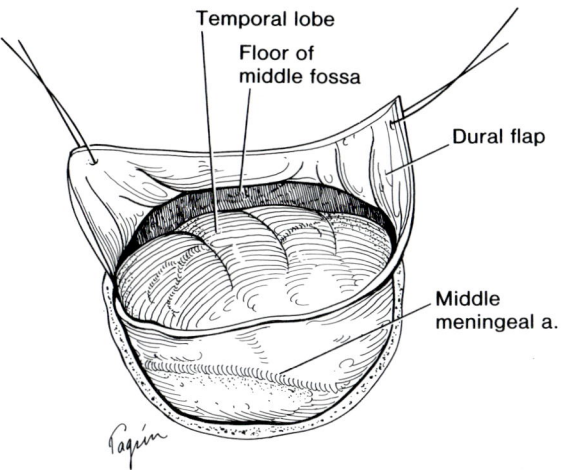

Figure 17.2 Dural opening. This is taken to the floor of the middle fossa to minimize brain retraction.

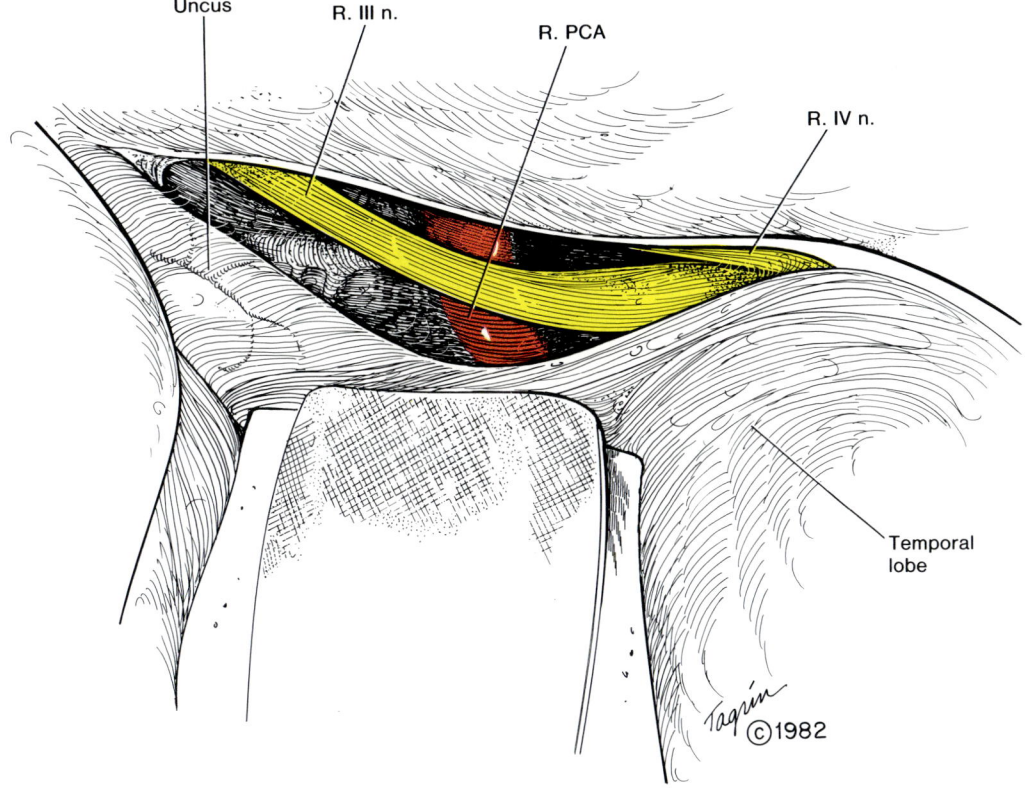

Figure 17.3 Subtemporal approach. Bridging veins are sacrificed and the temporal lobe gently elevated. The free edge of tentorium comes into view with the third and fourth cranial nerves and the posterior cerebral artery (PCA), beneath a sheet of arachnoid.

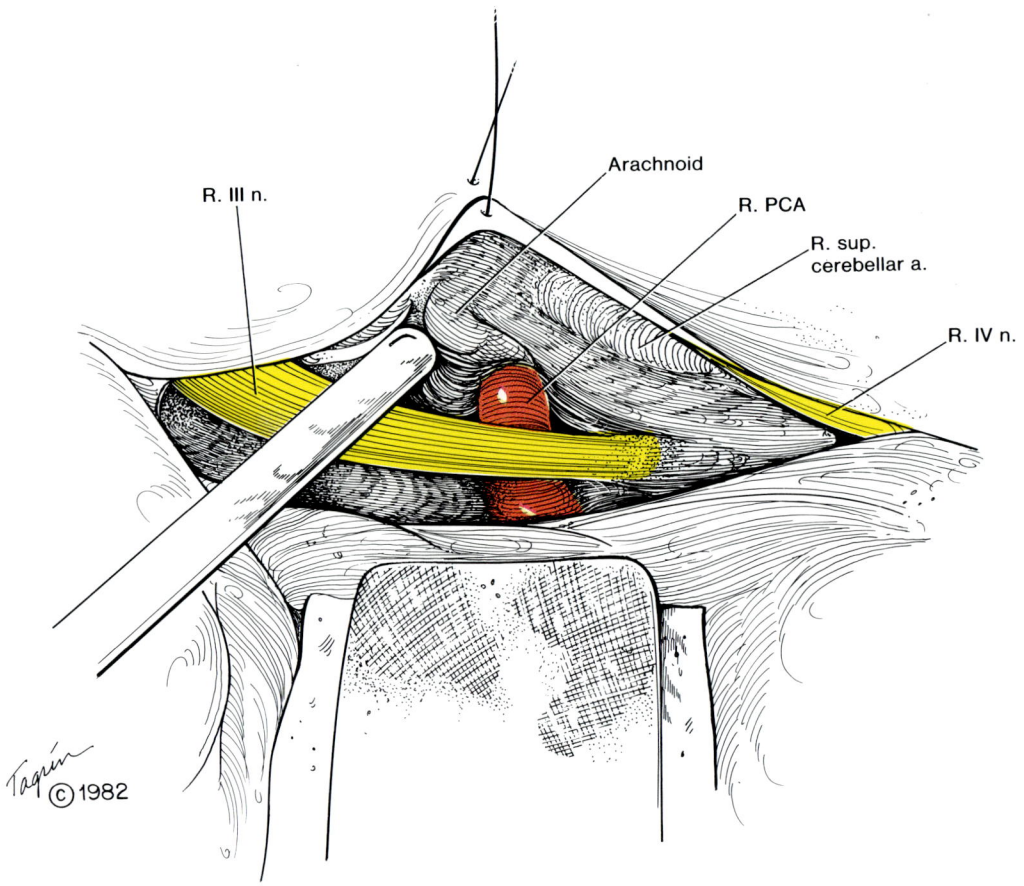

Figure 17.4 Dissecting the right PCA. The edge of the tentorium has been opened and retracted. The arachnoid is opened with a hook, and the right PCA followed back toward its origin. The third nerve is left attached to the uncus.

tentorium just anterior to the insertion of the fourth nerve. This retraction suture is inserted in the middle fossa dura, taking care to avoid venous channels, and is tied to provide retraction of the tentorial edge. This maneuver provides further visualization of the brainstem and basilar bifurcation.

With a sharp hook, the arachnoid is opened over the P_1 segment of the posterior cerebral artery (PCA) and the origin of the superior cerebellar artery (SCA) (Fig. 17.4). A fine suction (#16 gauge) is used, at reduced vacuum tension to remove CSF from the cisterns. Using a fine dissector, the surgeon follows the SCA and P_1 segment to the basilar tip area. The posterior communicating artery is carefully preserved as a source of collateral circulation and the origin of important perforating arteries.

Unless the aneurysm points anteriorly, the next maneuver is to dissect anterior to the neck and distal basilar artery to expose the P_1 segment on the opposite side (Fig. 17.5). This critical landmark establishes the relative anatomic positions of the two P_1 segments and the basilar trunk, thus setting up the remainder of the dissection. Reference to the Townes projection of the angiogram will assist in identification of the position of the two P_1 segments. A precise visualization of upward or downward tilting of the left P_1 segment is essential for accurate clipping of the aneurysm without occluding this vessel and its critical perforators. In the case of a large lesion, it is possible to mistake the opposite SCA for the PCA with potential disastrous consequences. Once the P_1 segment on the left is identified, the proximal neck of the aneurysm may be prepared anteriorly with gentle dissection.

With this anatomy firmly in mind, the most critical dissection may be undertaken along the posterior aspect of the neck (Fig. 17.6). Here the mean arterial pressure is held in the 35–40 mm Hg range to aid dissection. In most cases, a 16-gauge suction may be used to deflect the neck of the aneurysm forward as a fine microdissector gently sweeps perforators and brainstem posteriorly. A gentle, insistent dissecting technique will be rewarded by a view of the posterior aspect of the left P_1 segment alongside the origin of the third nerve. To avoid an unduly narrow pathway with potentially dangerous traction on the aneurysm and perforators, it is useful to dissect a significant length of the perforating arteries away from the aneurysm. With these structures slack on either side of the dissection plane, an instrument or clip is less

Basilar Bifurcation Aneurysms 213

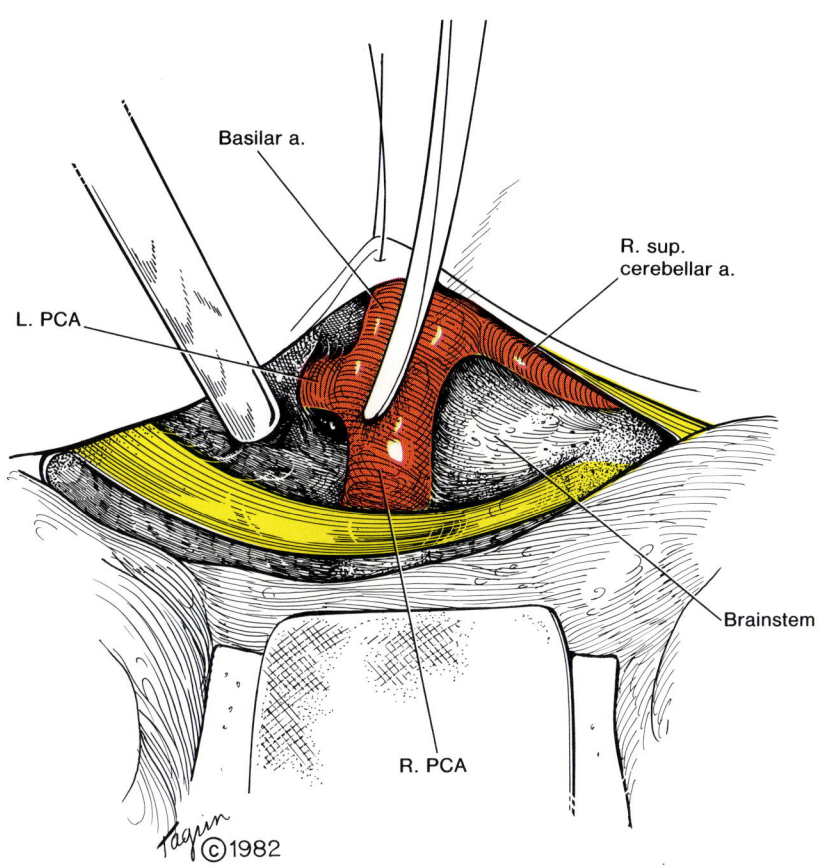

Figure 17.5 Dissecting anteriorly. Unless the aneurysm points forward, one can safely work across the basilar apex and aneurysm neck to define left P_1 segment, thus establishing the key landmarks.

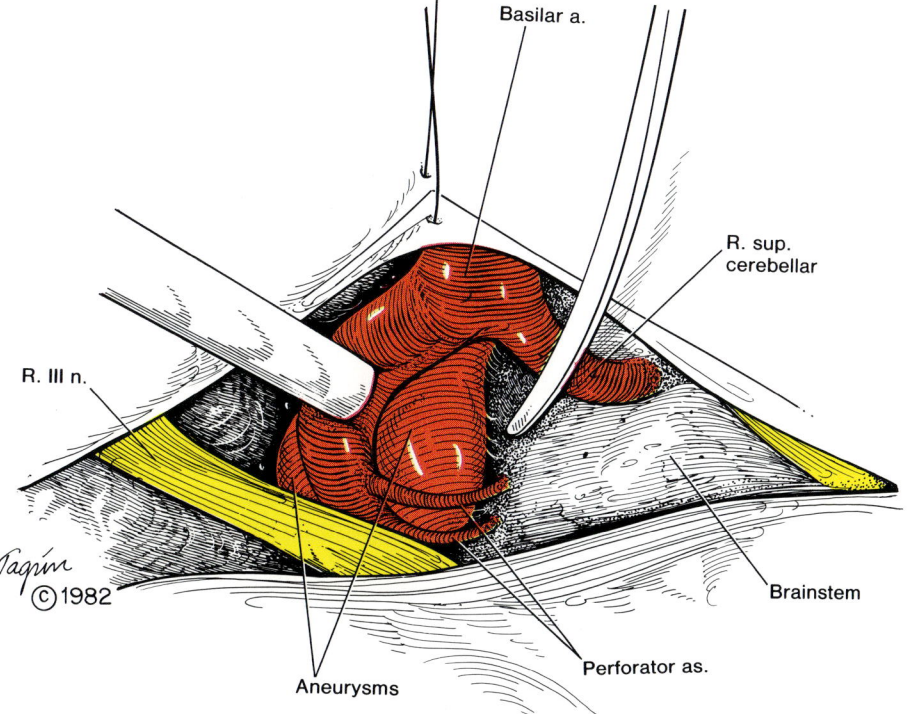

Figure 17.6 Dissecting posteriorly. For most basilar aneurysms, this is the most difficult step. A fine microcurved dissector is convenient to sweep brainstem and perforating arteries away from the neck and proximal dome.

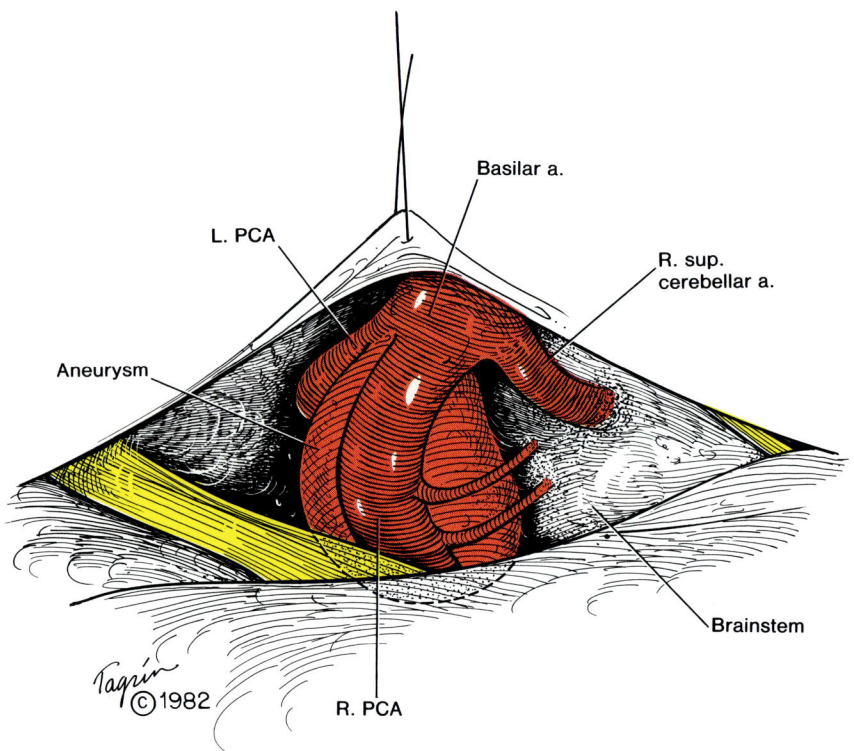

Figure 17.7 Dissection completed. Once the anterior and posterior walls of neck are freed, a clip is selected. In this situation, where right PCA bars the way, a Drake clip is a good choice, to avoid excess manipulation or kinking of the vessel.

likely to tear or rupture the aneurysm. Under direct microsurgical vision, it must be precisely ascertained that the perforating arteries have been safely dissected away from the aneurysm (Fig. 17.7). Sacrifice of any of these perforating vessels is likely to lead to brainstem infarction and serious neurological deficit. Occasionally, one or two tiny perforators may be occluded without deficit, but it is safest to try to preserve them all.

Obliterating the Aneurysm

Most of these aneurysms are occluded with a clip and usually a fenestrated Drake clip is the best choice (Fig. 17.8). For most basilar tip aneurysms, the shoulder and arm of the PCA on the right embrace the neck and lateral dome. In this situation, much retraction of the lesion and substantial dissection from the PCA can be obviated by the use of a fenestrated Drake clip. The clip demands precision; it must be exactly the right length, and it must be applied precisely. The blade length must correspond exactly to the neck width. If it is too long, it overlaps and occludes the left P_1 segment; if it is too short the lesion is incompletely obliterated. If the aperture is not exactly positioned, the aneurysm may bulge into the fenestration, remaining unclipped, or the blade may grasp the right P_1 segment with resulting occlusion. Measurement on the Townes view and rough measurement of the breadth of the lesion at surgery will help in selecting the proper clip. In general, the tendency is to select a clip which is longer than needed. The Drake-Kees clips are supplied in even lengths from 6 to 24 mm. In addition, a fenestrated clip from Heifetz-Weck is available. The latter may be trimmed with a wire cutter and seems to break clean in a more satisfactory manner should an intermediate length be required. A file is used to smooth the cut end.

For selected cases, some other clip may be preferable. When the space for each blade is limited and P_1 can be dissected from the aneurysm completely, a Yasargil or Sugita clip with their narrow blades (less than 1 mm) may provide the solution. For other lesions with a broader neck from which the P_1 segment can easily be dissected, a straight Heifetz clip may serve well (Fig. 17.9). In general, straight clips appear to be most useful in this location.

Occasionally, a ligature may be the best answer. In these cramped quarters, the technique of ligature passage without a ligature carrier may offer a satisfactory alternative. In this method, the aneurysmal neck is deflected to one side and with the bipolar forceps, a 3-0 silk ligature is passed deep to the lesion. Then the aneurysm is deflected in the opposite direction and under direct vision the suture is retrieved

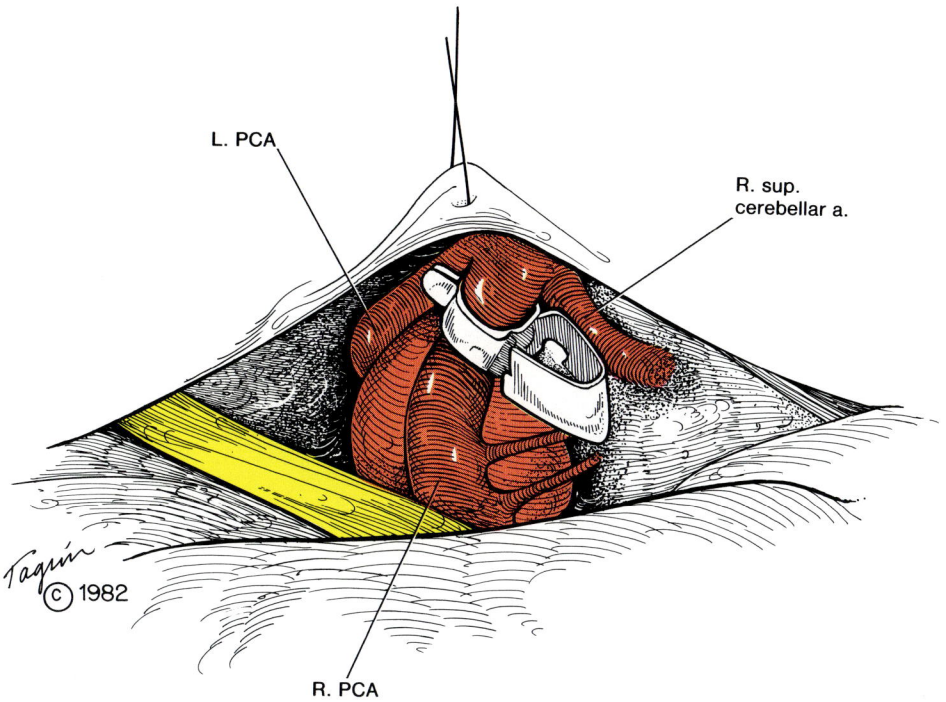

Figure 17.8 Aneurysm clipped. An 8-mm Drake clip has been applied. The clip just barely crosses the neck, and properly so, for a longer one might occlude the left P_1 segment or a shorter one inadequately obliterate the lesion. The fenestration encircles the right P_1 segment (but no aneurysm tissue).

from its position along the other side of the neck. The ligature may then be tied down for complete obliteration of the lesion or to set the stage for final clipping.

After obliteration, the position of the clip or ligature must be checked carefully. If the position of the clip is not desirable, it must be adjusted for precise obliteration of the lesion and preservation of normal arteries. In some cases, temporary clipping may be utilized for further dissection of the aneurysm followed by reposition of the clip. The clip is advanced with a gentle wiggling or axial rotation of the blades to decrease frictional drag on the lesion. During clip advancement, the tip of the clip should be inspected under direct vision so that it advances just to the point of touching the opposite PCA. After the clip is allowed to close, this tip position is again checked on both sides of the lesion. The left P_1 segment and its perforators must be free (Fig. 17.10). The entire neck of the aneurysm must be gathered into the obliterating clip blades. If this objective has been achieved, aspiration of the aneurysm with a 25-gauge spinal needle assures complete obliteration of the lesion. Should there be a tiny dog-ear of unclipped aneurysm which defies clipping, application of muscle may be best to reinforce the lesion. In view of the proximity of the brainstem, cranial nerves, and perforating arteries, we have avoided the use of tissue adhesives with their potentially toxic effects.

Special Problems

Though posterior pointing basilar tip aneurysms seem most forbidding, good results have been achieved with such cases. After initial dissection across the anterior neck to the PCA, the difficult job is dissecting out the posterior neck from the interpeduncular cistern (Fig. 17.11). The approach is much the same as with the upward pointing lesions, except that more extensive posterior retraction on the peduncle is required. It is of greatest importance that the pia-arachnoid of the peduncle and all the perforators travel together posteriorly. Adequate dissection of the aneurysmal neck and perforators will minimize the chance of rupture or inadvertent tear as the clip is being placed. Complete dissection to the opposite edge of the neck, with visualization of the P_1 segment, is mandatory to avoid inaccurate clipping.

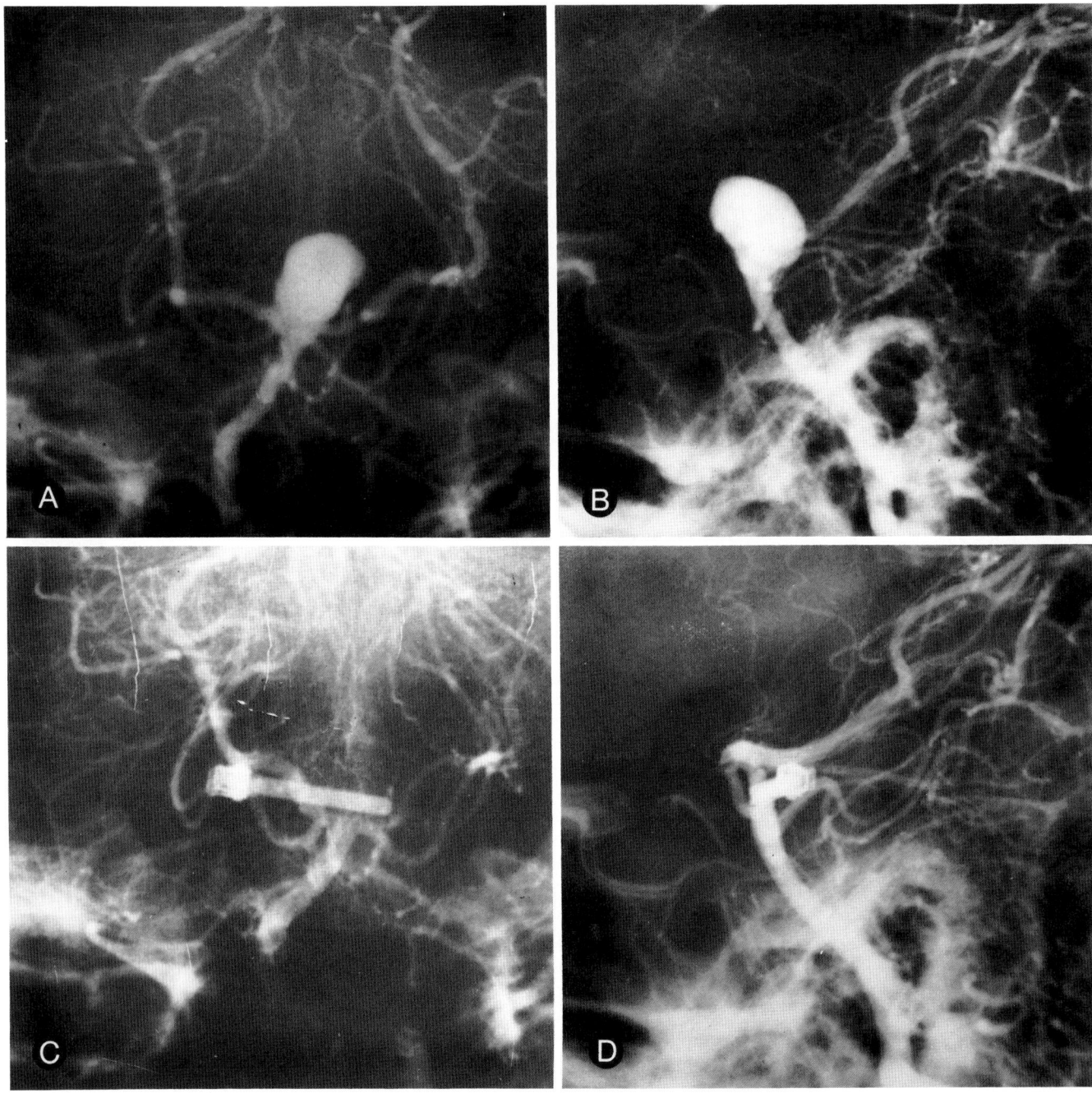

Figure 17.9 Obliteration of large basilar tip aneurysm. *A* and *B*, preoperative angiogram shows lesion pointing superiorly and posteriorly, at the level of the posterior clinoid process. *C* and *D*, postoperative angiogram shows obliteration of lesion with presevation of normal arteries. The clip was applied without section of tentorium. Severe perioperative visual hallucinations gradually subsided and examination reverted to normal.

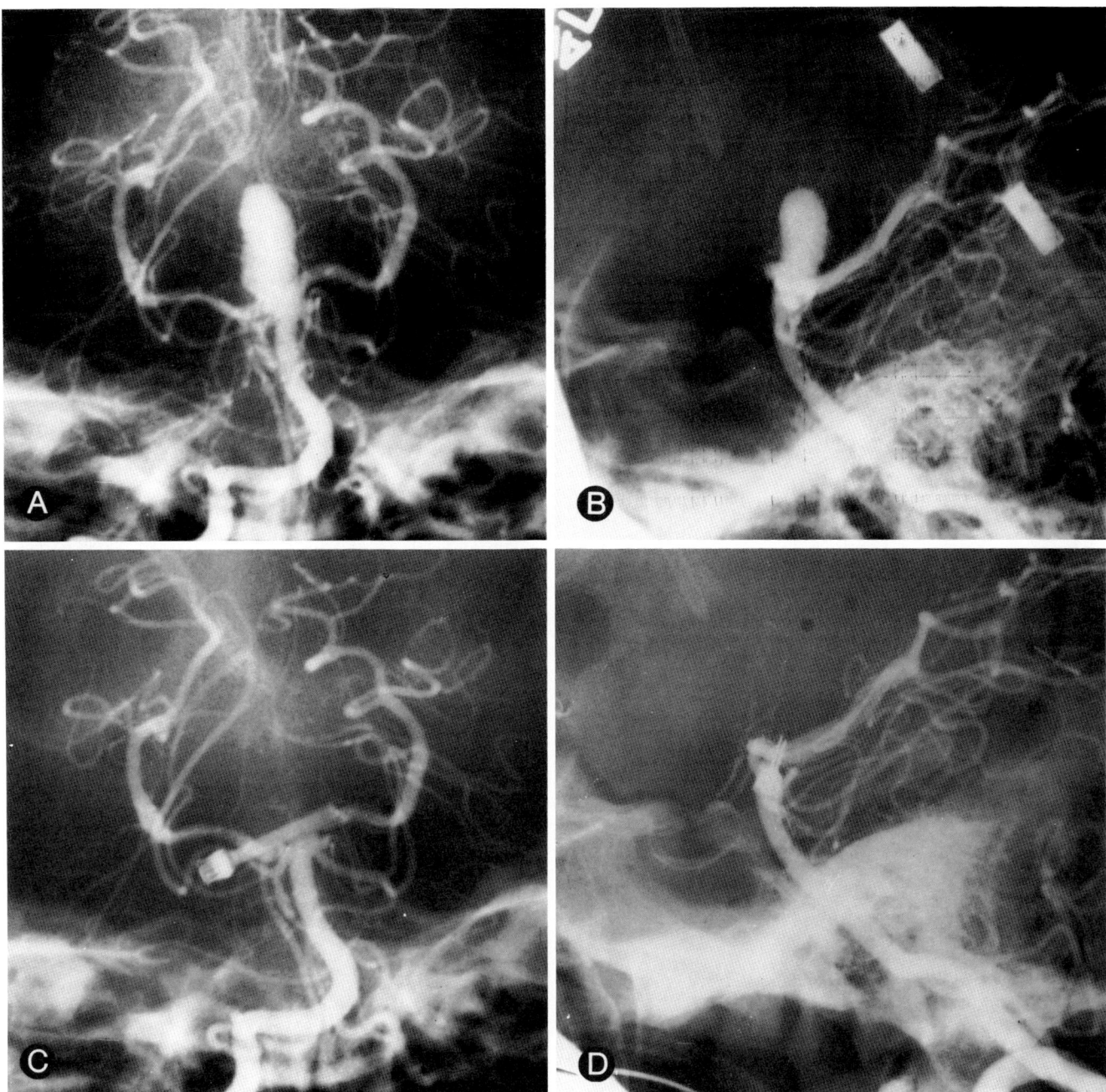

Figure 17.10 Importance of perforating arteries. *A* and *B*, angiograms show a large aneurysm directed upward. The patient had abulia and hemiparesis. Difficult surgery done on day 27; two small perforators from left P_1 could not be excluded from the clip. *C* and *D*, aneurysm obliterated, P_1 arteries normal. Severe obtundation persists, probably due to occlusion of two perforant arteries.

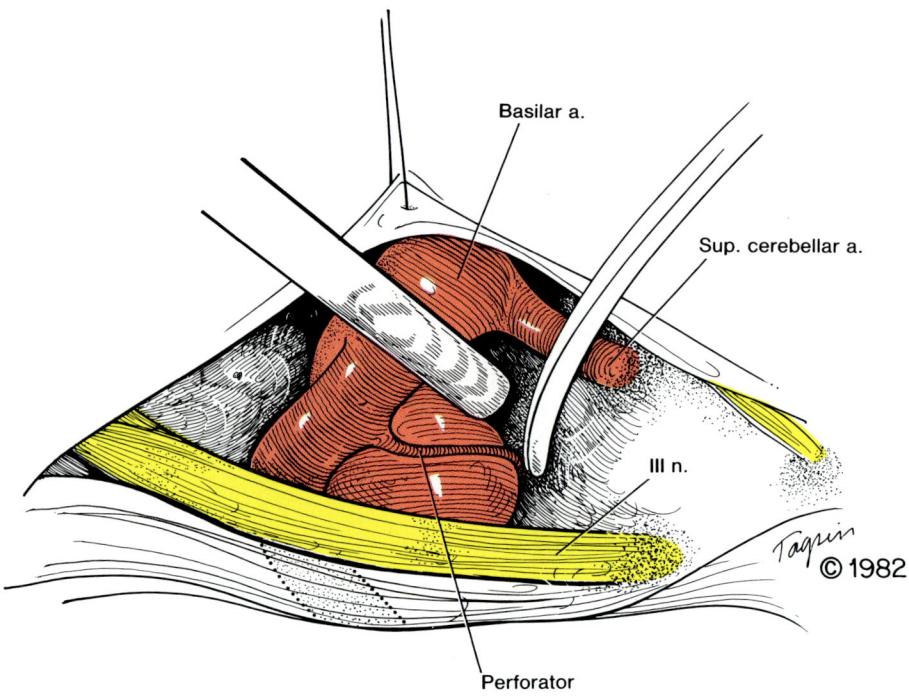

Figure 17.11 Aneurysm pointing back into brainstem. The anterior neck is dissected first. Then brainstem and perforators are swept away from the posterior neck of the aneurysm.

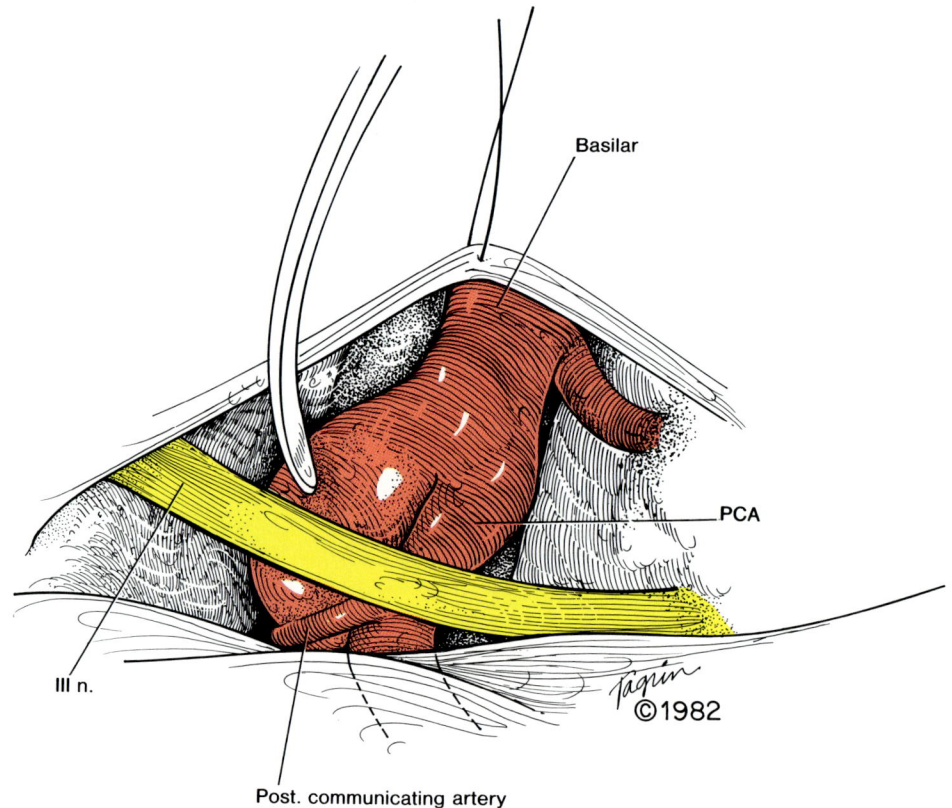

Figure 17.12 Aneurysm adherent to clivus. It may be best to free the posterior aspect first. Then gentle dissection, preferably outside the hematoma, may free the anterior neck.

Basilar Bifurcation Aneurysms

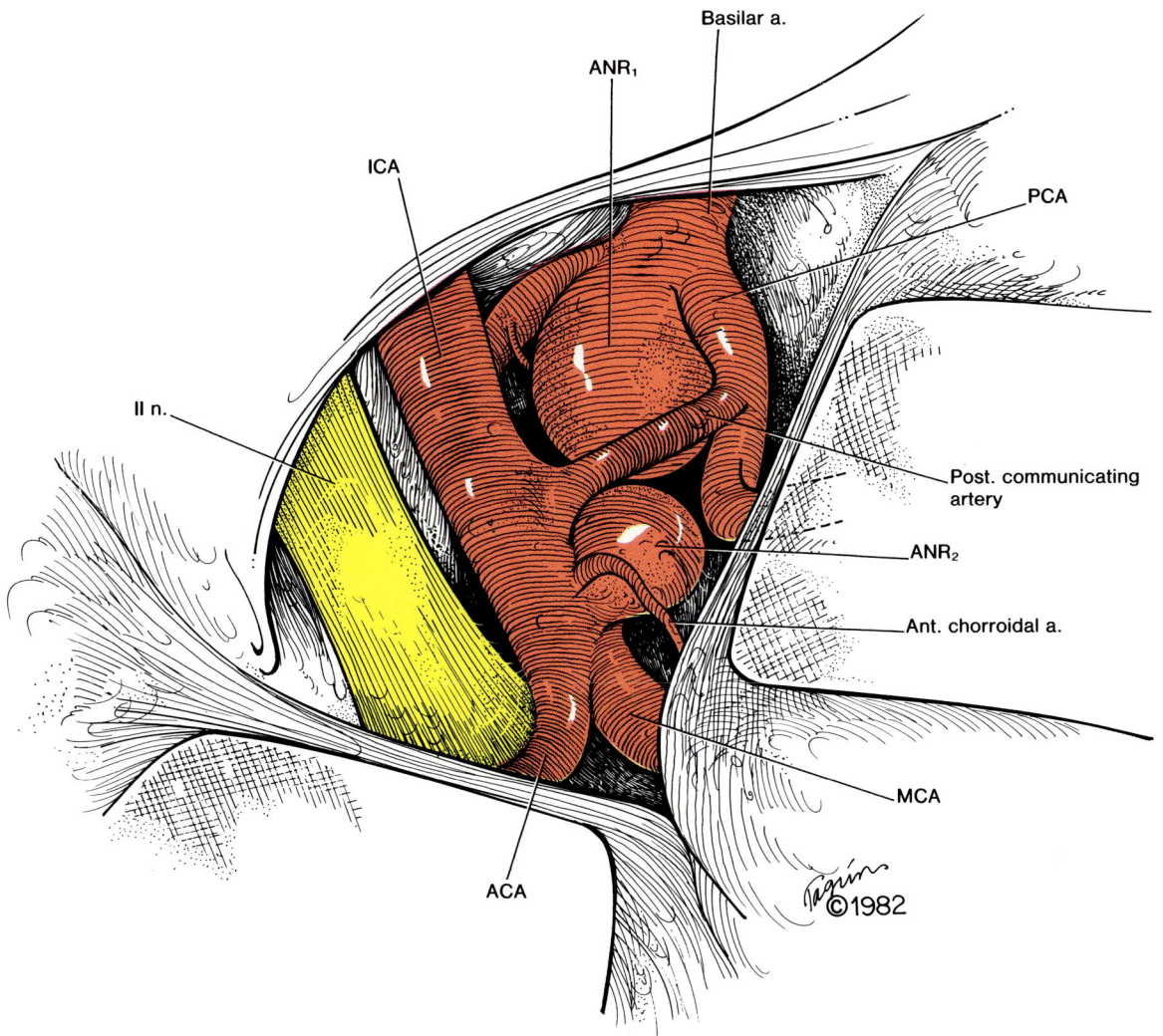

Figure 17.13 Pterional approach. Through a right pterional craniotomy, one can deal with both a basilar apex aneurysm, and a right ICA-anterior choroidal aneurysm. Note the difficulty in visualizing perforating arteries from the P_1 segments.

The anterior pointing lesions, least common of all, present an entirely different problem (Fig. 17.12). Frequently, these aneurysms are adherent to the clivus. If there is clot present anteriorly, it is wise to proceed outside the clot, providing a bit of extra margin for the dissection. If there is a red angry area on the anterior aspect of the lesion, it may be preferable to prepare the posterior aspect of the lesion first. The perforating vessels are usually less adherent in this type of aneurysm, if they are attached to the lesion at all. For large and giant lesions, the bulk interferes with accurate visualization, particularly of the left P_1 segment. Indenting the lesion with a suction under hypotension may facilitate dissection of the neck and application of clip. The clip application may be difficult because the bulk of the lesion forces the clip down into the basilar artery itself. To solve this problem, application of the clip well up on the aneurysm may permit sliding of the clip down into perfect position as the blades are closed. A preliminary ligature around the neck of the lesion or inclusion of P_1 in the blades of the clip, where the posterior communicating artery is large, may permit obliteration of the neck. Successful treatment of the giant lesions is much more difficult than in the case of smaller lesions.

A pterional approach may sometimes be used for treatment of basilar bifurcation aneurysms (4, 6) (Fig. 17.13). After fashioning a pterional craniotomy with removal of the lateral sphenoid ridge, the Sylvian fissure is opened for visualization of the internal carotid artery. Deeper dissection permits access to the basilar tip, either between the carotid artery and the optic nerve or lateral to the carotid artery, whichever cleft is larger. The approach may afford a nice view of the perforators originating from the left P_1 segment. There are several disadvantages which render the approach less useful for most basilar tip

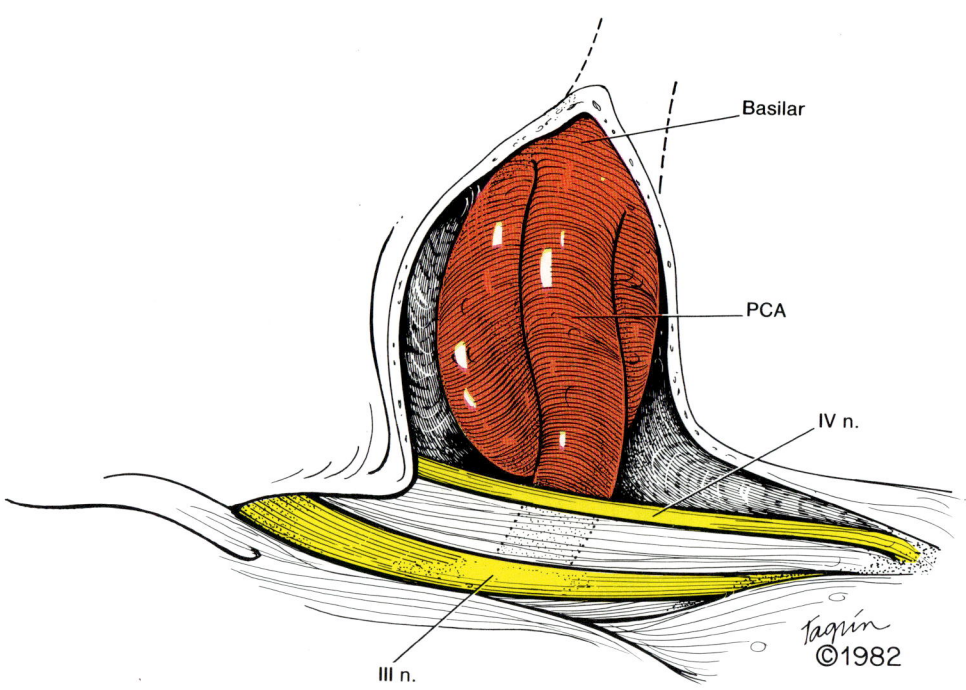

Figure 17.14 Low-lying basilar aneurysm. Section of the tentorium, posterior to incorporation of the fourth nerve, permits access to almost all low-lying basilar apex aneurysms.

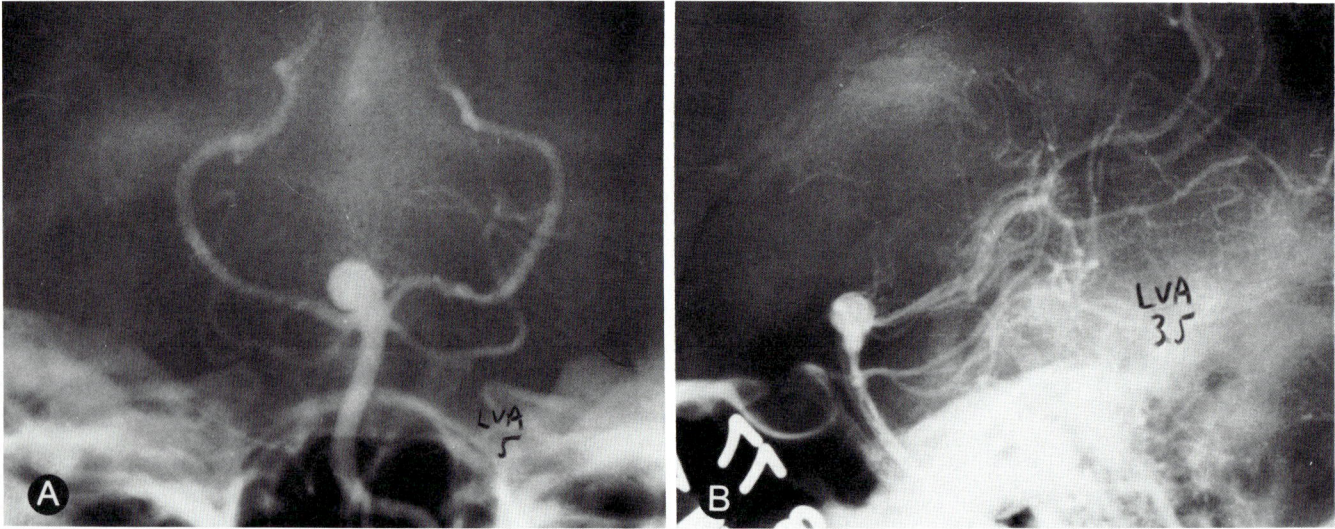

Figure 17.15 Importance of posterior communicating artery. *A* and *B*, angiograms show small apex basilar aneurysm. *C* and *D*, postoperative angiograms show obliteration of the aneurysm and left P_1 segment by excessively long clip. *E*, left PCA fills well via posterior communicating artery. This vessel was seen on preoperative angiography, thus allowing sacrifice of the left P_1 segment with little risk. No new deficits were noted after surgery.

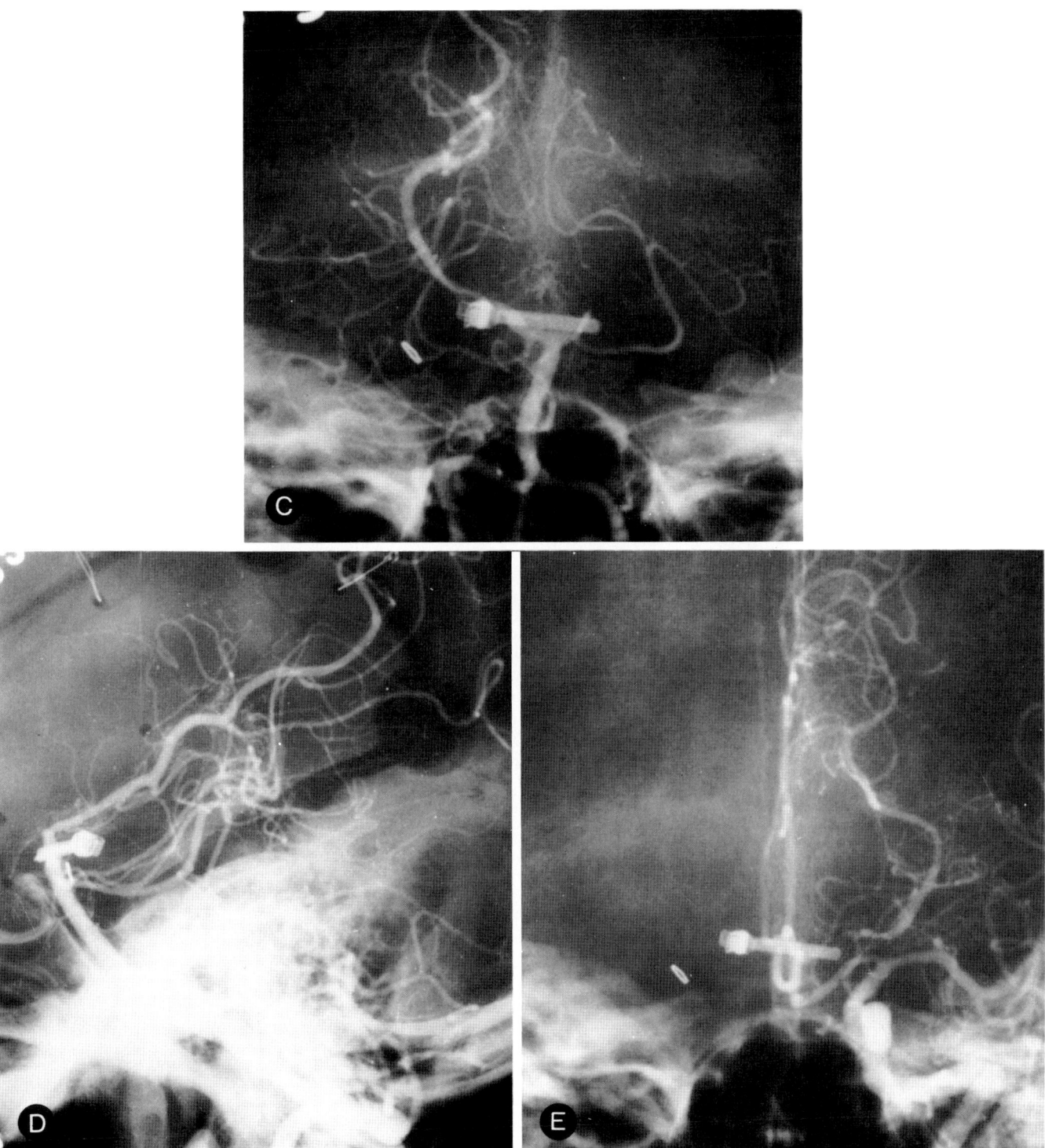

Figure 17.15 (*C* to *E*)

lesions: the angle of clip application, oblique rather than direct lateral, is more difficult to visualize anatomically; the space available is less in most cases; in some patients, the aneurysm is obscured by the posterior clinoid process; and most importantly, the perforators on both sides may be completely obscured by the lesion itself. However, this approach is particularly advantageous when another aneurysm of the carotid or anterior communicating system is to be dealt with at the same operation. The subfrontal part of the exposure through the Sylvian fissure has access to the anterior circulation, while the posterior temporal portion of the opening then permits a subtemporal dissection to the basilar tip.

A low-lying basilar bifurcation may require special technique. This situation can be anticipated when the angiogram shows the basilar bifurcation at or below the posterior clinoid process. Often adequate exposure can be obtained by section of the tentorium (Fig. 17.14). The incision is placed posterior to the entry of the fourth cranial nerve to avoid injury to this structure. Clips or bipolar cauterization control bleeding from venous channels in the tentorium.

RESULTS

Over a 5-year period, 20 patients were operated for a basilar bifurcation aneurysm. These patients ranged in age from 26 to 59 years, with an average of 45 years. Fifteen of the patients were females and five were males. The presenting complaint was subarachnoid hemorrhage in 15 patients, chronic headache in three patients, and progressive neurological dysfunction in two patients. For those patients with subarachnoid hemorrhage, the average time from ictus until surgery was 11 days. In five instances, symptomatic cerebral vasospasm was present. Multiple lesions were documented in three patients, two of whom had additional arteriovenous malformation of the brain.

Results, excluding giant aneurysms, are presented in Table 17.1. Of those presenting in good neurological condition (grade 1–2), seven of 11 experienced excellent results, and two patients were judged to have good results (81.8%). There were two poor outcomes. In one patient with a large aneurysm pointing upwards, intraoperative rupture required protracted hypotension with a mean arterial blood pressure of about 40 mm Hg for 90 minutes. The patient experienced a syndrome of abulia and mild hemiparesis without CT evidence of infarction. In another case, excessive right temporal lobe retraction led to temporal edema and infarction with resultant hemiparesis.

Table 17.1
Results[a]

Grade	Excellent	Good	Poor	Dead
1–2	7	2	2	0
3–4	1	4	2	0
Total	8	6	4	0

[a] Giant lesions excluded.

In patients with poor presenting condition (grade 3–4), there was a single excellent result, four good, and one poor. In one instance, two perforating arteries could not be freed from the wall of the aneurysm, and their occlusion led to further neurological deterioration. In one patient, the left posterior cerebral artery was occluded with a clip with no new neurological deficit (Fig. 17.15). Preoperative angiography had shown a good posterior communicating artery. These results for all grades of patients are similar to those reported by others (1–6).

The most frequent complication was an ipsilateral third nerve palsy which occurred in 16 of the 20 cases. In 10 cases, this resolved completely over a period of 3 months or less. In four cases, a partial third nerve palsy persisted. Eight of the 16 third nerve palsies were complicated by other abnormalities of extraocular movement. Neurological deterioration with various signs was noted in the four patients listed in the poor outcome group. There were no deaths in this series of cases.

REFERENCES

1. Drake CG: The surgical treatment of aneurysms of the basilar artery. J Neurosurg 29:436–446, 1968.
2. Drake CG: The treatment of aneurysms of the posterior circulation. Clin Neurosurg 26:96–144, 1979.
3. Peerless SJ, Drake CG: Management of aneurysms of posterior circulation, in Youmans JR (ed): Neurological Surgery 2nd Ed (to be published).
4. Samson DS, Hodosh RM, Clark WK: Microsurgical evaluation of the pterional approach to aneurysms of the distal basilar circulation. Neurosurgery 3:135–141, 1978.
5. Wilson CB, Hoi Sang U: Surgical treatment for aneurysms of the upper basilar artery. J Neurosurg 44:537–543, 1976.
6. Yasargil MG, Antic J, Laciga R, Jain KK, Hodosh RM, Smith RD: Microsurgical pterional approach to aneurysms of the basilar bifurcation. Surg Neurol 6:83–91, 1976.

Chapter 18 BASILAR TRUNK AND VERTEBRAL ANEURYSMS

BASILAR TRUNK-SUPERIOR CEREBELLAR ARTERY ANEURYSMS

These aneurysms arise at the distal crotch of the origin of the superior cerebellar artery and usually project laterally, occasionally forward (7). Most patients present with subarachnoid hemorrhage (SAH). There may be a third nerve palsy since this nerve lies in a close relationship to the aneurysm. .

The subtemporal approach illustrated in Chapter 17 for low-lying basilar bifurcation aneurysms is used to expose these lesions. Peerless and Drake have described the operative exposure in detail (7). The approach is from the side of the fundus of the aneurysm. The tentorium is retracted with a suture to aid exposure. In some patients, the tentorium needs to be divided. Care must be taken to prevent injury to the fourth cranial nerve. By first working down the sides of the aneurysm from the front, the dome is avoided. Depressing the sac against the peduncle will reveal the neck of the aneurysm emerging from the basilar artery and the superior cerebellar artery below. The P_1 segment may be seen, but if the aneurysm is of any size, the artery will be hidden above and behind. Working behind the aneurysm, it can be separated from the peduncle using a microdissector. The waist and neck of the aneurysm are freed from the P_1 segment. With the aneurysm displaced forward, the neck is visualized and any perforating branches separated. Care must be taken not to injure the third nerve which frequently winds around the neck. If application of a clip is difficult because of the nerve, a ligature may be used or the neck shrunk with coagulation. The superior cerebellar artery may emerge from the side of the neck and one must be careful not to kink it with the ligature or clip.

The largest operative experience has been reported by Peerless and Drake (7). They had a high percentage of excellent and good results.

BASILAR TRUNK-ANTERIOR INFERIOR CEREBELLAR ARTERY ANEURYSMS

These aneurysms arise at the carina or origin of the anterior inferior cerebellar artery (AICA) over the clivus (Fig. 18.1) (1, 3, 5, 7). Patients usually present with SAH. There is a close relationship of the aneurysm to the abducens nerve so a sixth nerve weakness may be present.

The surgical approach is either through a subtemporal transtentorial exposure or through a suboccipital craniectomy (2, 4, 7). The origin of AICA is usually the border zone for exposure of the basilar trunk from above or below. In general, those lesions over the lower third of the clivus are exposed from the suboccipital opening while those above are approached through the tentorium. The choice of the approach depends on the location of the aneurysm in relation to the clivus, its size and projection, and a consideration of the disadvantages of each approach (from above, possible injury to the fifth, sixth, seventh, and eighth cranial nerves and dominant temporal lobe; from below, the chance of injury to the tenth and eleventh cranial nerves). For example, a high-lying AICA aneurysm which points laterally is best approached from above.

In some patients, lesions between AICA and the vertebrobasilar junction may be hard to expose from below. Here, a combined subtemporal-transtentorial-suboccipital exposure can permit rotation of the brainstem with excellent visualization of the lower basilar trunk (Fig. 18.2) (6). Since section of the transverse sinus is employed, preoperative angiographic visualization of the contralateral sinus is necessary. In view of the deep temporal retraction required, a right-sided approach is used.

For a transtentorial approach, a substantial posterior temporal craniotomy permits subtemporal exposure to the tentorial edge (7). Care must be taken to preserve the vein of Labbé because of the possibility of venous infarction. The mid-temporal lobe is elevated. The tentorium is opened behind the insertion of the fourth nerve and is incised 1–2 cm posterior to the petrous ridge. The tentorium can be folded forward and sutured to the floor of the middle fossa. This exposes the fourth and fifth cranial nerves and the petrosal vein which is divided. The same retractor may then elevate both the temporal lobe and the edge of the cerebellum just lateral to the fifth nerve. The exposure is through an opening between the fifth nerve medially and the seventh and eighth nerves laterally. The sixth nerve and basilar artery are exposed and the aneurysm is seen as the basilar artery is followed inferiorly. The aneurysm, which generally points laterally, is carefully dissected near the origin, with care to avoid injury to the sixth nerve which is often adherent to the dome. The AICA must be freed from the lesion and carefully observed during final clipping.

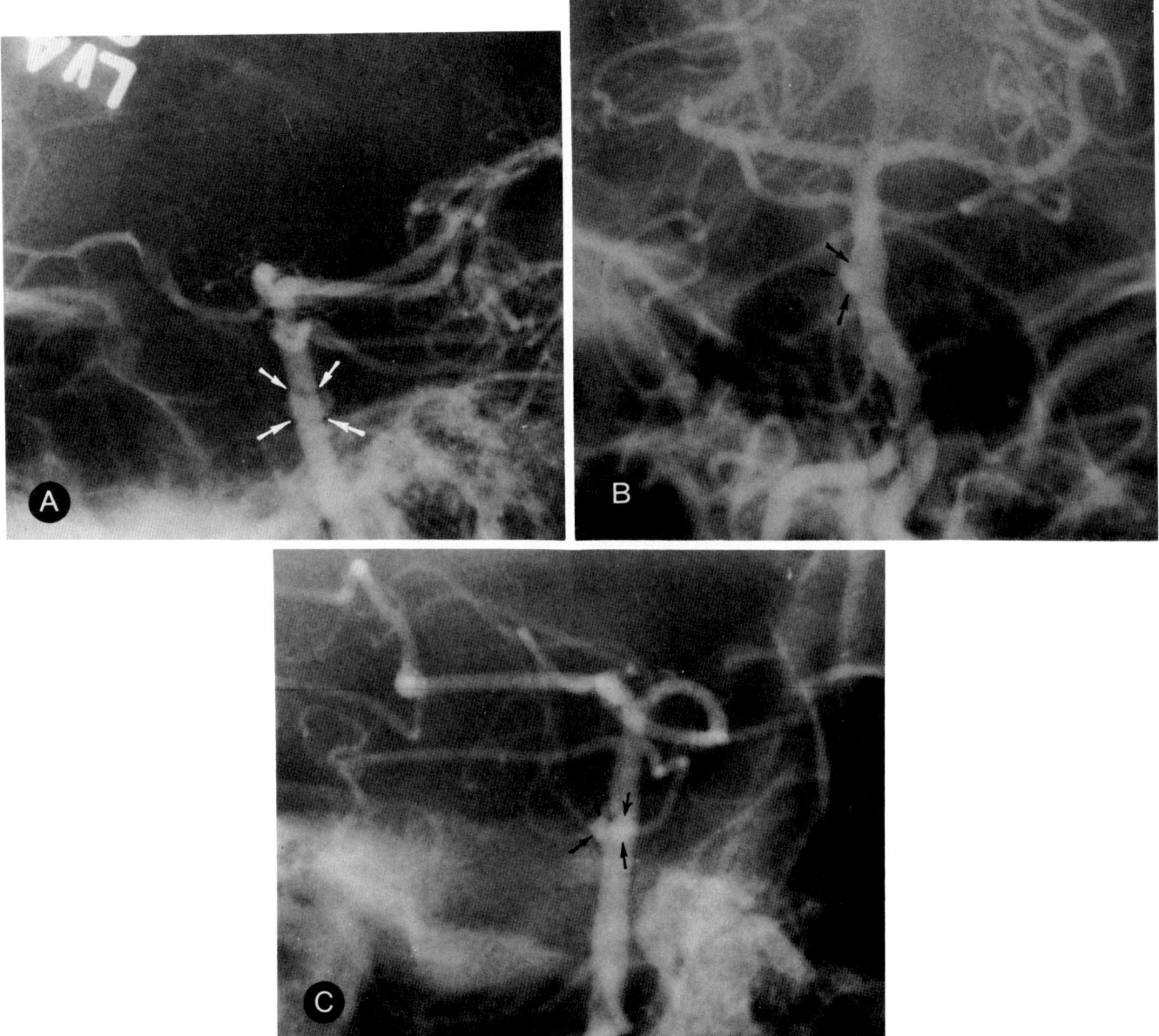

Figure 18.1 Basilar-AICA aneurysm. *A* and *B*, lateral and AP angiograms demonstrate the aneurysm (*arrows*) pointing posteriorly and to the right. *C,* oblique view reveals bilobular nature of the lesion (*arrows*). Patient was grade I after subarachnoid hemorrhage. Refused operation. No change on angiography 1 year later.

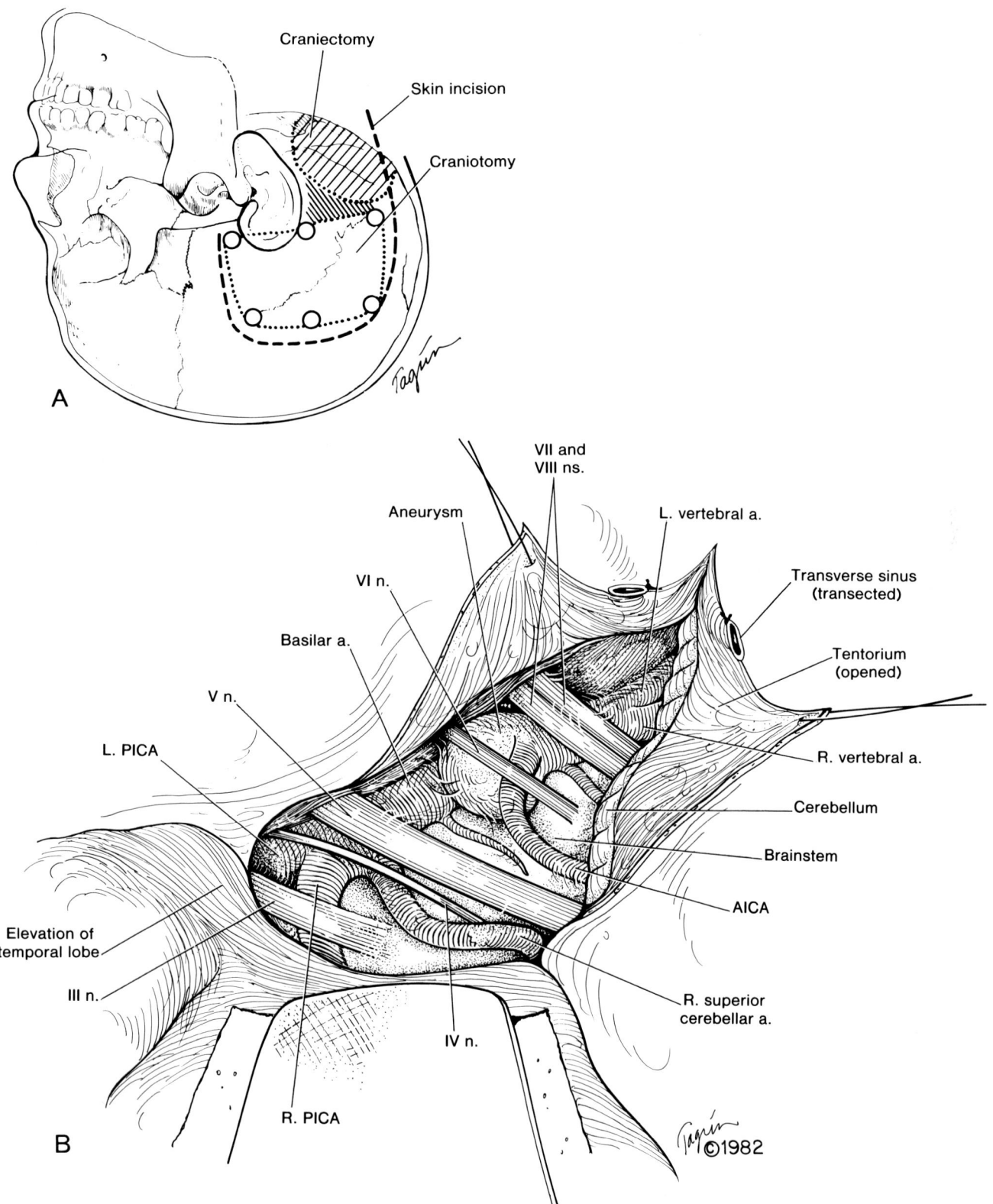

Figure 18.2 Approach to basilar trunk. A combined subtemporal-suboccipital approach is used. The tentorium is sectioned widely to expose the length of the basilar artery.

Peerless and Drake have reported 27 patients who were grade one or two at the time of operation. There were 18 excellent, three good, and four poor results, and two deaths.

VERTEBRAL-POSTERIOR INFERIOR CEREBELLAR ARTERY ANEURYSMS

Presentation and Evaluation

These aneurysms usually arise at the distal carina at the origin of the posterior inferior cerebellar artery (PICA) from the vertebral artery (Fig. 18.3A). Since the vertebral artery may have a tortuous course and the origin of PICA may vary, these aneurysms can occur from near the intracranial entry of the vertebral artery to near the vertebrobasilar junction. They tend to point superiorly and slightly posteriorly and lie against the medulla. Occasionally the aneurysm arises distal to the origin of the PICA. These aneurysms usually have an intimate relationship to the vagus and hypoglossal nerves.

Most patients with this aneurysm present with SAH. The headache is more likely to be localized to the neck and occipital region than with anterior circulation aneurysms. SAH with a sixth nerve or lower cranial nerve palsy is often due to this aneurysm. Giant aneurysms may present with symptoms and signs suggesting cerebellopontine angle tumor. The true size may only be seen with the CT scan. When a PICA aneurysm is suspected or bilateral carotid angiography is negative in SAH, it is important that both vertebral arteries be visualized to include the origin of both PICAs, even if separate injections of the two vertebral arteries are needed.

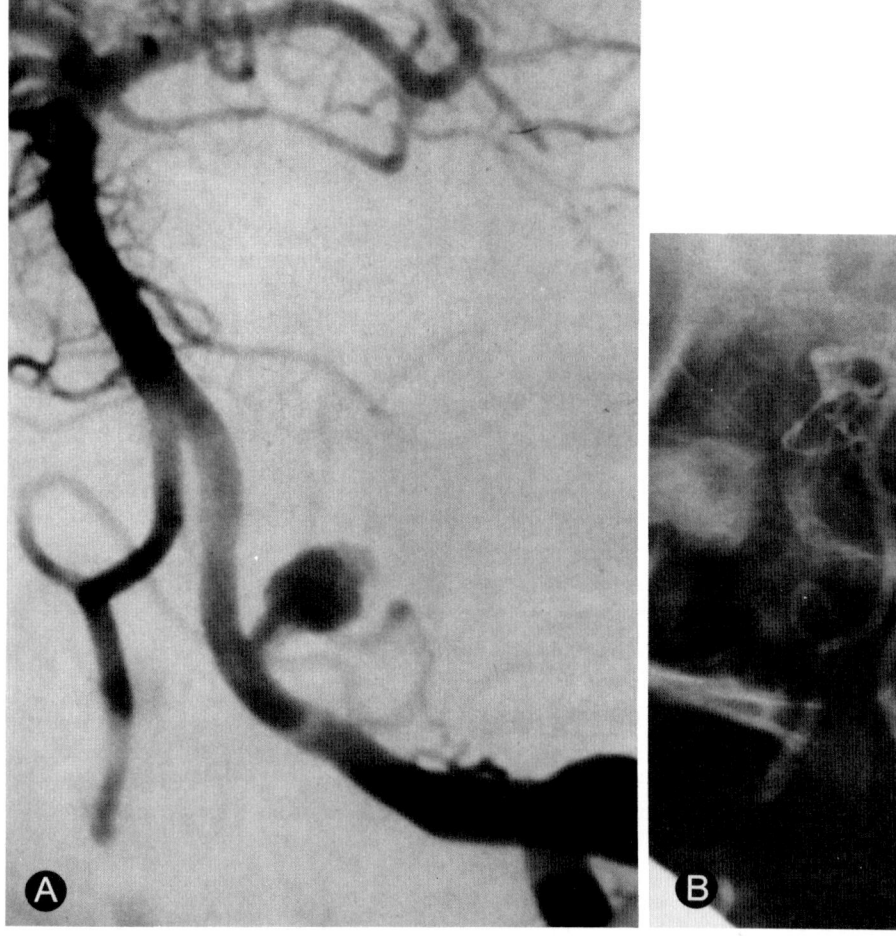
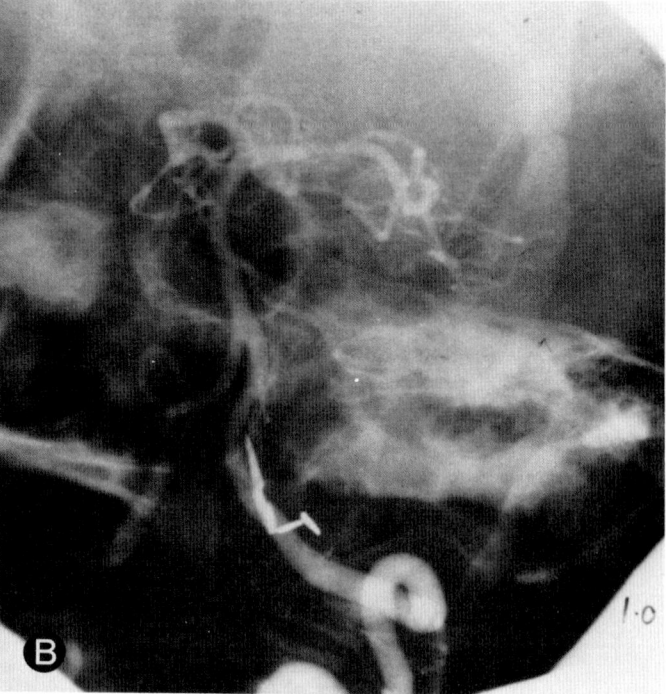

Figure 18.3 Vertebral-PICA aneurysm. A, preoperative angiogram showing aneurysm arising from distal crotch of origin of PICA from the vertebral artery. B, postoperative angiogram demonstrates obliteration of the aneurysm and preservation of PICA.

Operative Technique

These aneurysms are approached through a unilateral suboccipital craniectomy (2, 4, 7, 8). The side of the approach is selected after careful review of the angiogram since aneurysms of one vertebral artery may lie on the opposite side because of the extensive torturousity of the artery (8).

The patient may be placed in the lateral "parkbench," prone, or sitting position. We prefer either the prone or lateral position. The lateral position with the nose turned 20° below the horizontal provides good access and is comfortable for the seated surgeon. If the patient is placed on the operating room (OR) table with the head toward the "foot," then the surgeon's legs fit comfortably beneath the OR table.

We prefer a midline incision with a hockey stick extension to the side of the lesion (Fig. 18.4A). This will provide access for the suboccipital craniectomy with removal of the lateral foramen magnum. It is important to carry the craniectomy laterally in order to provide the requisite line of sight to the premedullary subarachnoid space. Usually it will be necessary to remove the arch of C1. The dura is opened with flaps placed laterally to give maximum exposure in this area. The cisterna magna is opened and drained of CSF (Fig. 18.4B). This permits gradual medial and superior retraction of the slack cerebellum.

The cerebellum is lifted off the medulla with a narrow retractor blade placed on the base of the tonsil (18.4C). The eleventh nerve is exposed. The vertebral artery is identified emerging from under the dentate ligament and the loop of PICA is seen. The vertebral artery is traced distally. The origin of PICA, almost always just proximal to the lesion, stands as a good landmark. Eventual exposure is gained with patience and gentle dissection (Fig. 18.4D). The access to the lesion and PICA is between filaments of the tenth and eleventh nerves which must be protected meticulously against the possibility of injury which can cause disabling hoarseness and dysphagia. In addition, any arterial branches to the medulla should be spared. As the rest of the aneurysm is brought into view, it is best to work on either side of PICA and up the sides of the vertebral artery beyond the neck (Fig. 18.4E). Usually that portion of the dome of the aneurysm adherent to the medulla can be left undisturbed and only the neck isolated (Fig. 18.4F). On occasion, depending on the projection of the aneurysm, it may be necessary to dissect it out of a medullary indentation. Bipolar coagulation may be needed to define the neck. Some care will be needed during this maneuver to avoid injury to the twelfth cranial nerve on the far side of the neck. A small straight Yasargil clip or a Drake clip encircling PICA may be used to finish the job.

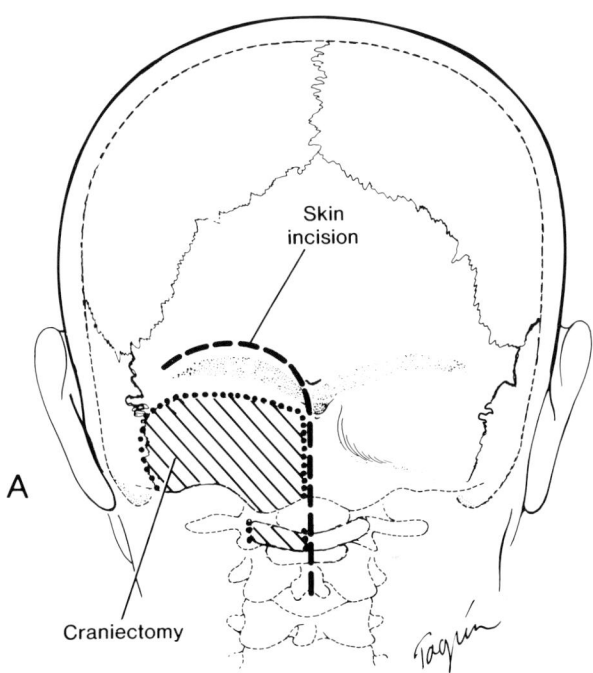

Figure 18.4 A to F, approach to vertebral-PICA aneurysms. A, patient placed in lateral or prone position. A midline incision with a "hockey stick" extension is used. The area of bone removal is shown.

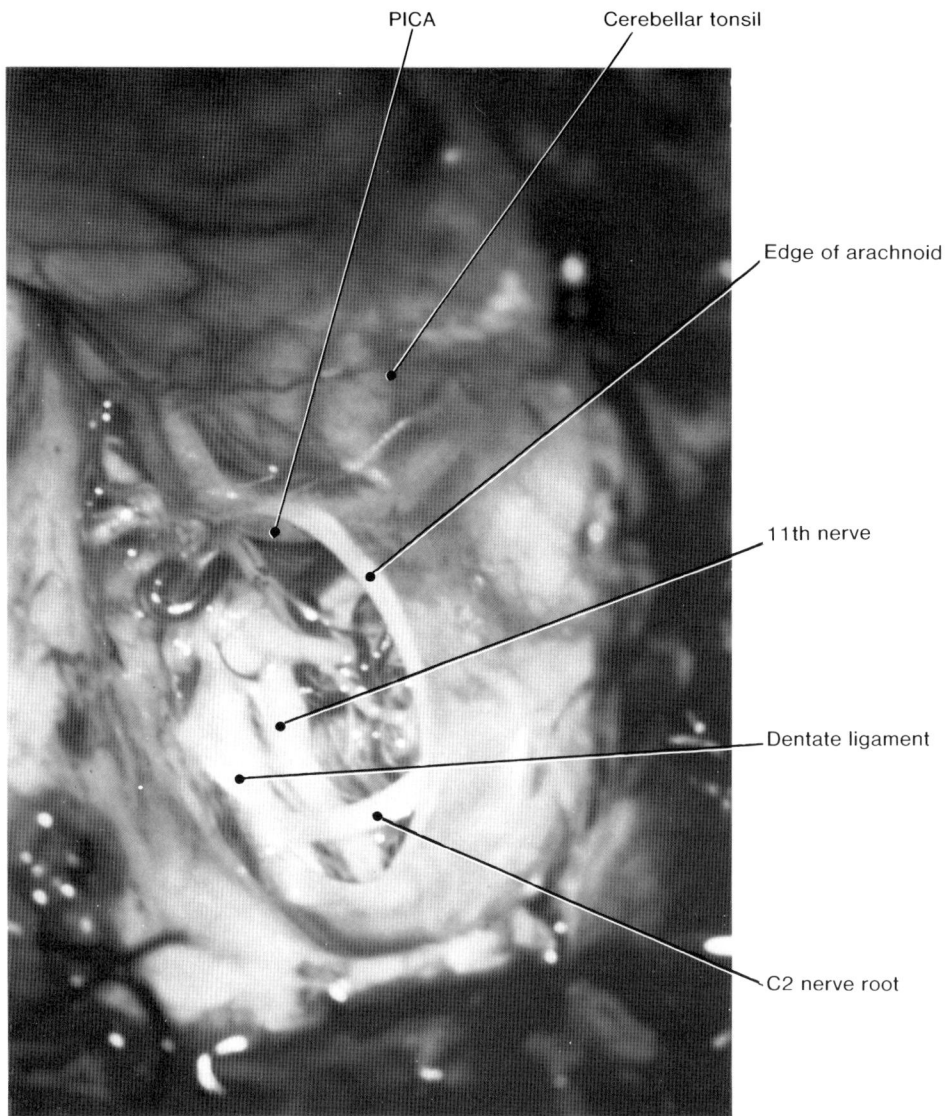

Figure 18.4 *B*, the arachnoid of the cisterna magna has been opened. The cerebellar tonsil is seen with PICA looping around the inferior edge. The rostral insertion of the dentate ligament and the eleventh nerve are seen.

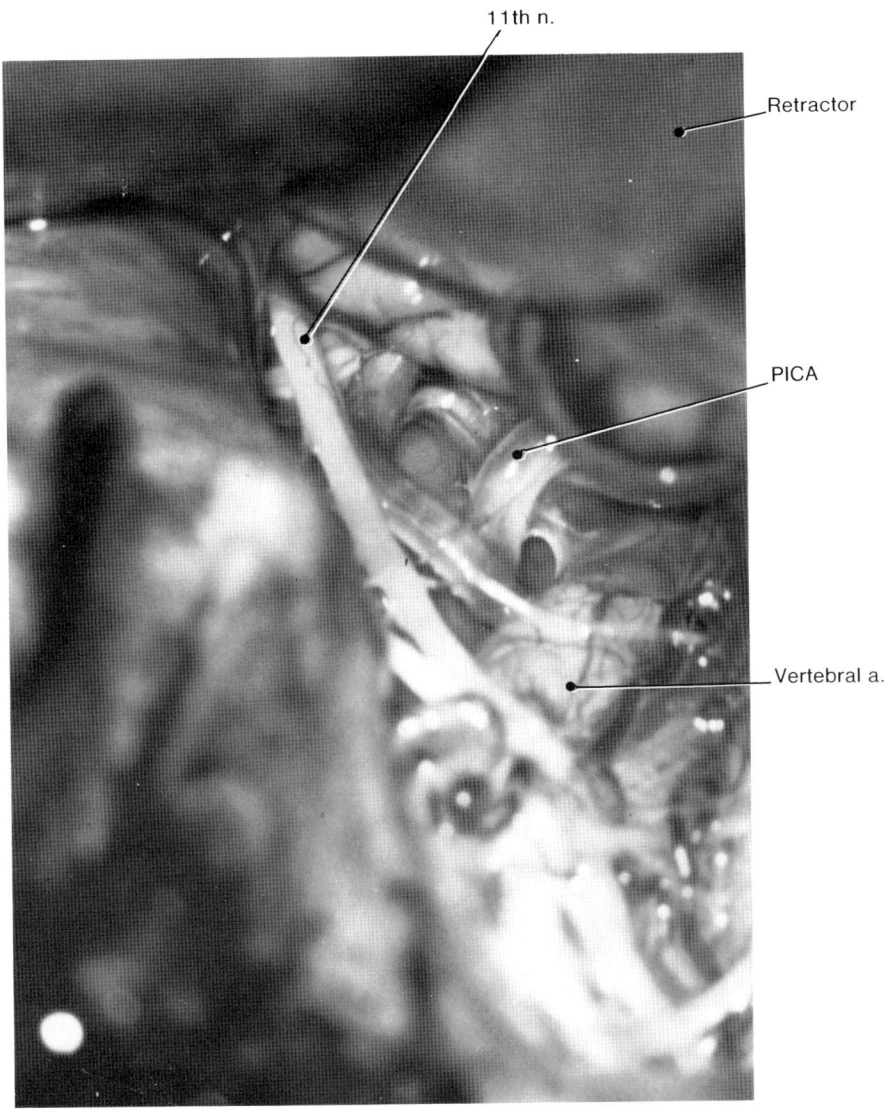

Figure 18.4 *C*, the cerebellum is lifted with a narrow retractor blade placed on the tonsil. The vertebral artery is identified and the loop of PICA seen.

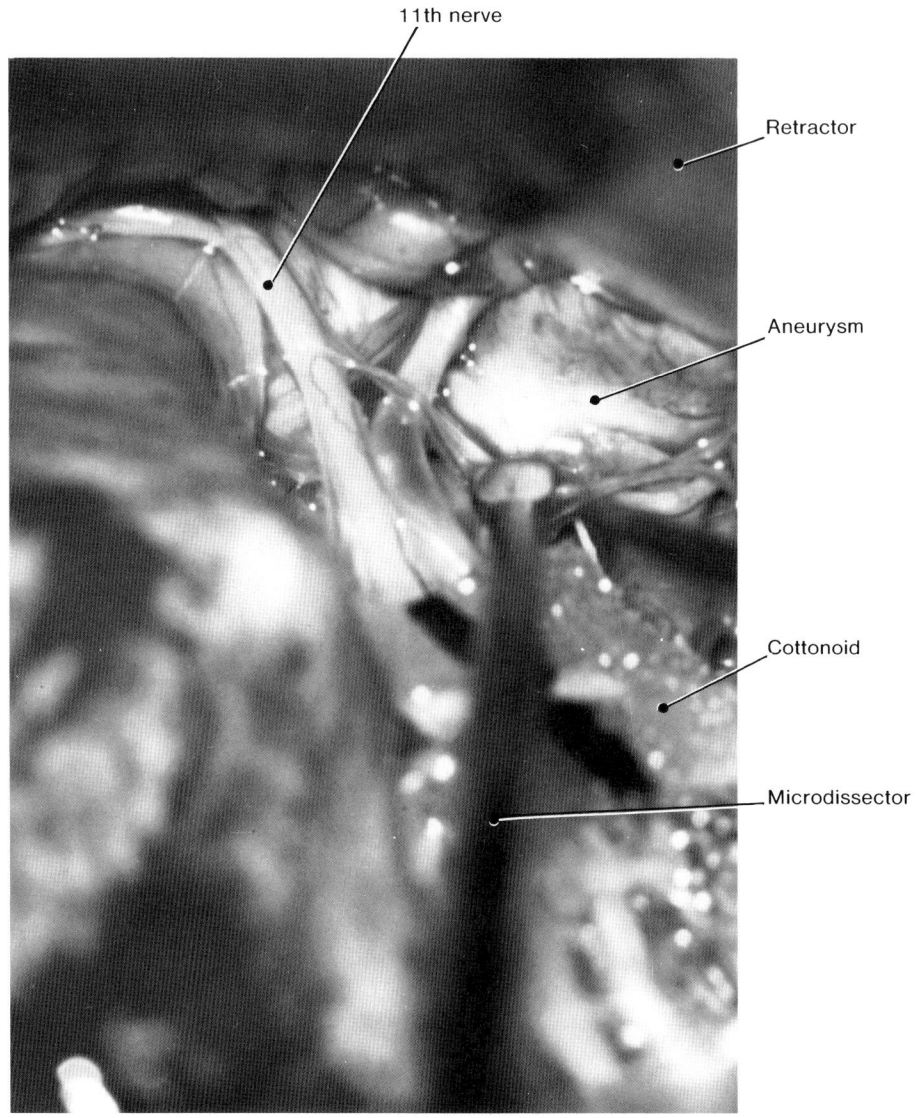

Figure 18.4 *D*, the wall of the aneurysm is visualized. The lateral PICA loop has been depressed and is covered with a cottonoid. Rootlets of the vagus nerve crossing the posterior surface of the aneurysm are being freed with the straight dissector.

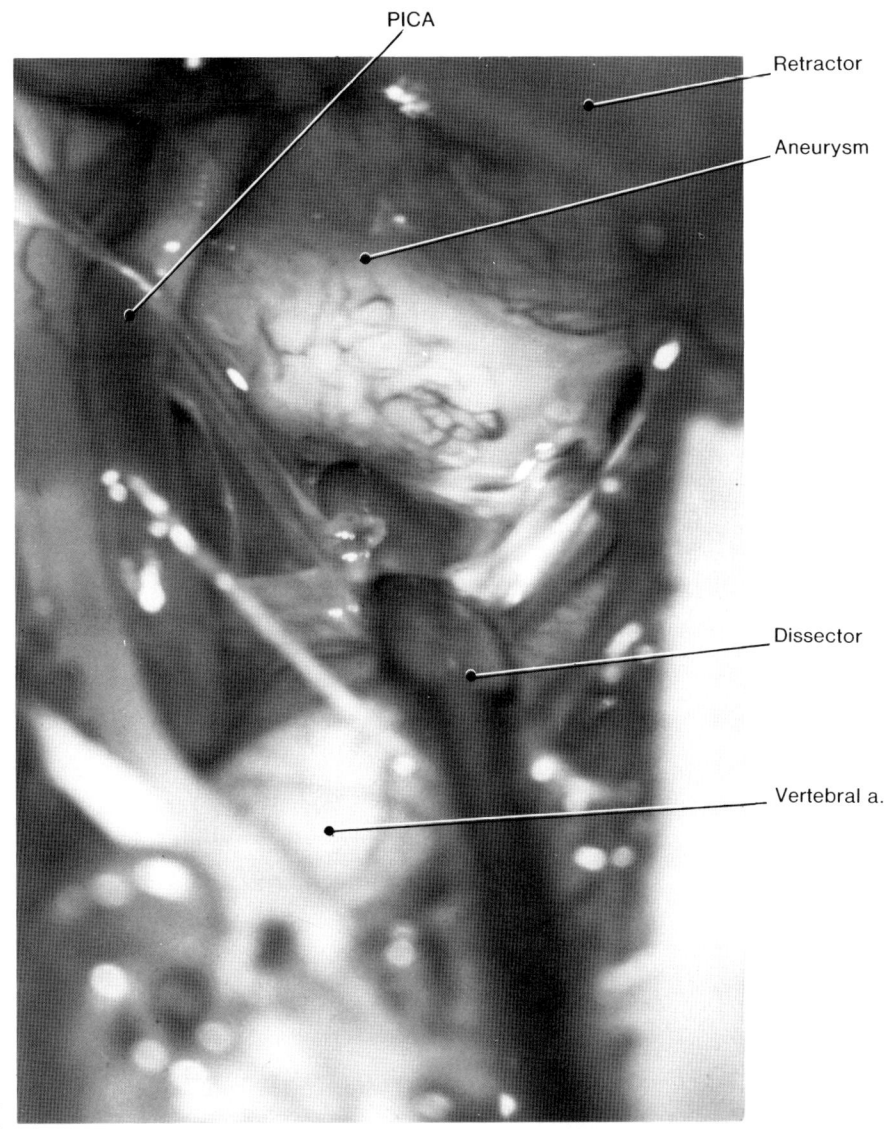

Figure 18.4 *E*, the neck of the aneurysm is exposed. Dissection with the microstraight dissector progresses on each side of PICA and along the vertebral artery.

Results

In four patients that we treated, three had an excellent clinical result. In three of the four cases, some dysphagia and/or dysphonia occurred immediately postoperatively. Complete recovery of this dysfunction occurred in two of the individuals. In one patient, the problem with airway protection seemed severe enough to warrant elective tracheostomy and gastrostomy 2 days after clipping the aneurysm. In another patient, severe dysphonia was noted postoperatively. While on the road to apparent recovery 2.5 weeks after surgery, the patient was found dead in bed. No evidence of oropharyngeal obstruction was present, but strong suspicion of airway compromise must be entertained. When there is severe lower cranial nerve impairment postoperatively, we proceed promptly to tracheostomy.

In one patient, angiographic study postoperatively disclosed a "slipped" clip with roughly half the lesion still filling, but the patient refused further surgery. She remains well 3 years after operation. In one patient, the bleeding lesion appeared to be at least partially fusiform with dissection of hemorrhage in

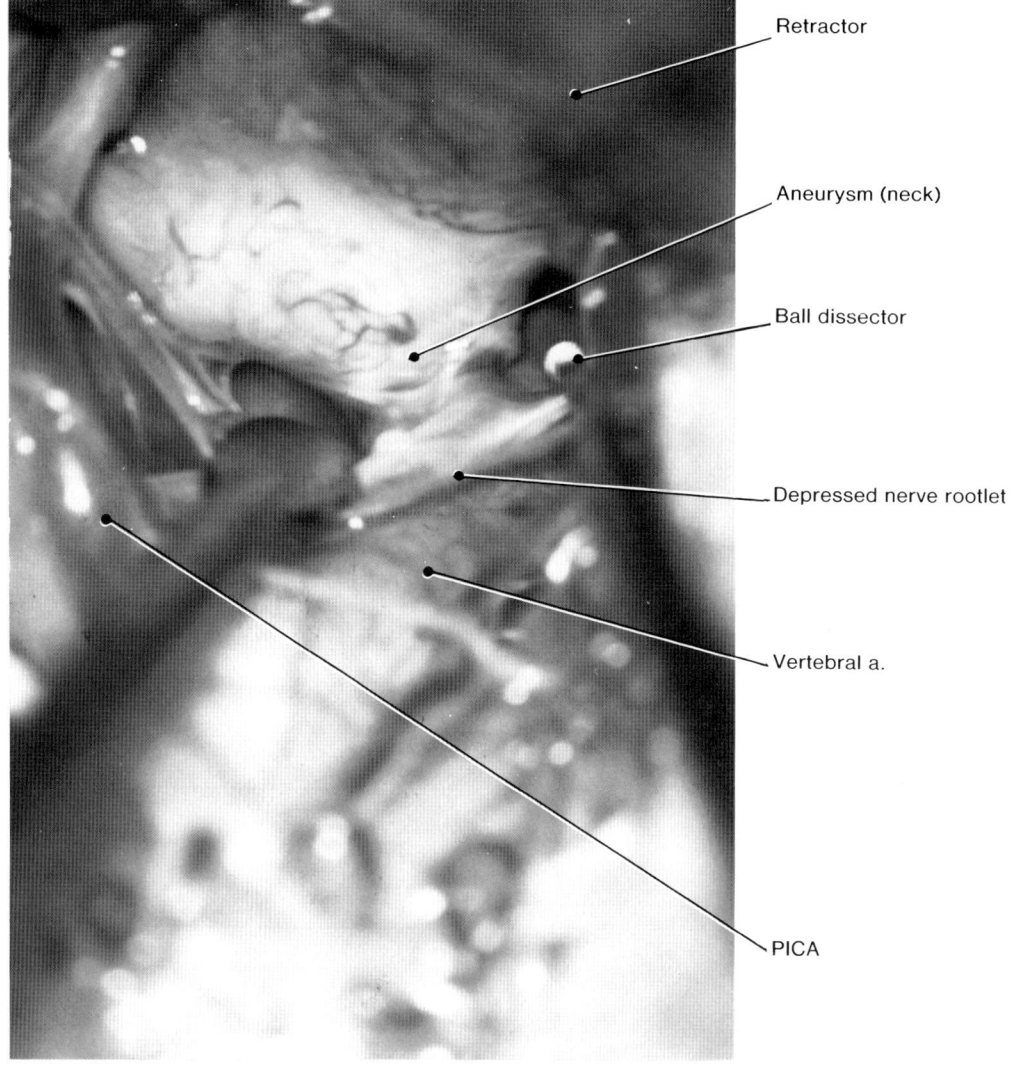

Figure 18.4 *F,* some of the rootlets of the vagus nerve have been depressed exposing the lateral side of the neck (straight microdissector) and the medial side of the neck (microball dissector). The aneurysm is ready for clipping.

the sheath of the vertebral artery. In view of a dominant contralateral vertebral artery, this lesion was trapped with sparing of PICA and an eventually excellent outcome after recovery of moderate dysphonia and dysphagia.

Peerless and Drake have reported a series of 69 patients who were grade one or two at the time of operation. There were 59 excellent and eight good results and two deaths (7).

REFERENCES

1. Chou SN, Oritz-Suarez HJ: Surgical treatment of arterial aneurysms of the vertebrobasilar circulation. J Neurosurg 41:671–680, 1974.
2. Drake CG: The surgical treatment of aneurysms of the basilar artery. J Neurosurg 29:436–446, 1968.
3. Drake CG: The surgical treatment of vertebral basilar aneurysms. Clin Neurosurg 16:114–169, 1969.
4. Drake CG: The treatment of aneurysms of the posterior circulation. Clin Neurosurg 26:96–144, 1979.
5. Hammon WM, Kempe LG: The posterior fossa approach to aneurysms of the vertebral and basilar arteries. J Neurosurg 37:339–347, 1972.
6. Kasdon DL, Stein BM: Combined supratentorial and infratentorial exposure for low-lying basilar aneurysms. Neurosurgery 4:422–426, 1979.
7. Peerless SJ, Drake CG: Management of aneurysms of posterior circulation, in Youman JR (ed): Neurological Surgery, 2nd Ed (to be published).
8. Rhoton AL Jr: Anatomy of saccular aneurysms. Surg Neurol 14:59–66, 1980.

Chapter 19 MULTIPLE, UNRUPTURED, AND ASYMPTOMATIC ANEURYSMS

MULTIPLE ANEURYSMS

Evaluation and Management

In clinical and angiographic series of intracranial aneurysms, multiple lesions are found in approximately 15% of the patients (5-7). Bilateral symmetrical aneurysms are most common on the internal carotid and middle cerebral arteries. The incidence of multiple aneurysms is a compelling reason to perform four vessel angiography in all patients known to have one aneurysm.

Although TIAs or seizures may occasionally draw attention to multiple aneurysms, the usual presentation is subarachnoid hemorrhage (SAH). In this situation, the initial problem facing the clinician is determination of which aneurysm ruptured. On the basis of angiographic criteria, Wood was able to correctly pinpoint the site of bleeding in 90% of the cases, as confirmed at surgery or autopsy. (13) In this study, the bleeding lesion was associated with larger size, multiple lobes, local mass effect, or local spasm. CT scanning makes the identification of the bleeding source more accurate. Demonstration of local subarachnoid hematoma in relation to an aneurysm is strong evidence of its rupture (Fig. 16.1). On the other hand, subarachnoid clot demonstrated by CT may be misleading. A hematoma in the interpeduncular cistern may come from an internal carotid-posterior communicating artery aneurysm instead of a basilar artery aneurysm. Clinical, CT, and angiographic data should be weighed carefully in the determination of the site of bleeding.

Once the source of SAH has been ascertained, therapy for this lesion proceeds according to the plan described in Chapters 10 and 11. If, during the procedure to obliterate the bleeding aneurysm, one or more asymptomatic lesions are easily exposed and can be clipped with little or no increased risk to the patient, this is done (9). This approach also provides the surgeon with the opportunity to examine several aneurysms, particularly if at surgery the presumed bleeding aneurysm shows no local signs of hemorrhage. If none of the lesions examined at surgery seem to have bled, then one must conclude that the source is elsewhere, and if another aneurysm is known to exist, this lesion should be treated.

If the bleeding lesion has been clipped, and one or more aneurysms exists outside the operative field, therapy for these lesions is guided by the criteria outlined for asymptomatic aneurysms, since the likelihood of bleeding from the unruptured aneurysm is low (see page 237). If the patient has no significant neurological deficit after surgery, we have usually waited about 6 weeks between operations to allow sufficient recovery from the first procedure. If, however, the patient has a neurological deficit after the initial surgery, a greater period of time between procedures should be considered.

Operative Technique

For multiple aneurysms, the scalp and bone flap may be modified to provide access to as many lesions as possible. A frontotemporal bone flap may be carried posteriorly into the temporal region to provide both a subfrontal access to the internal carotid circulation and a subtemporal approach to the basilar bifurcation. A coronal incision with the bone flap extending across the midline and low into the pterional area can provide access to both internal carotid and middle cerebral lesions, as well as to a distal anterior cerebral aneurysm (Fig. 19.1). A generous frontotemporal flap may provide access to both internal carotid arteries and even both middle cerebral arteries if CSF is drained extensively. It should be emphasized, however, that inadequate exposure should not be accepted to avoid another procedure (Fig. 19.2). When an asymptomatic aneurysm cannot be dealt with safely through the exposure, being used for a symptomatic aneurysm, it is better practice to defer its therapy for another day when optimum surgical exposure can be obtained.

A major decision when multiple lesions are exposed in an operative field is the question of which lesion to clip first. In principle, one prefers to eliminate the ruptured aneurysm. It is important to maintain exposure to the other lesions in question. If a ruptured superficial lesion is clipped, this may bar the path to a more deeply placed aneurysm. In this situation, it may be wiser to deal with the more deeply placed lesion first, even if it is unruptured.

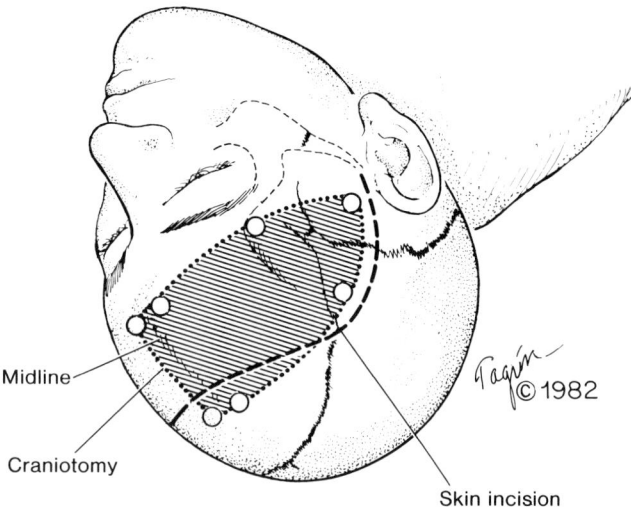

Figure 19.1 Exposure for multiple aneurysms. Coronal skin incision and large bone flap extending across midline provide access to circle of Willis and distal anterior cerebral artery.

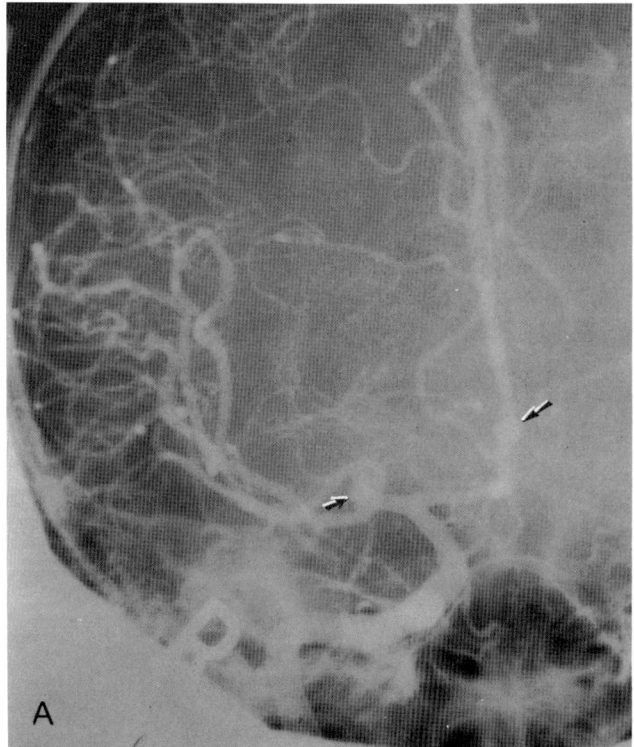
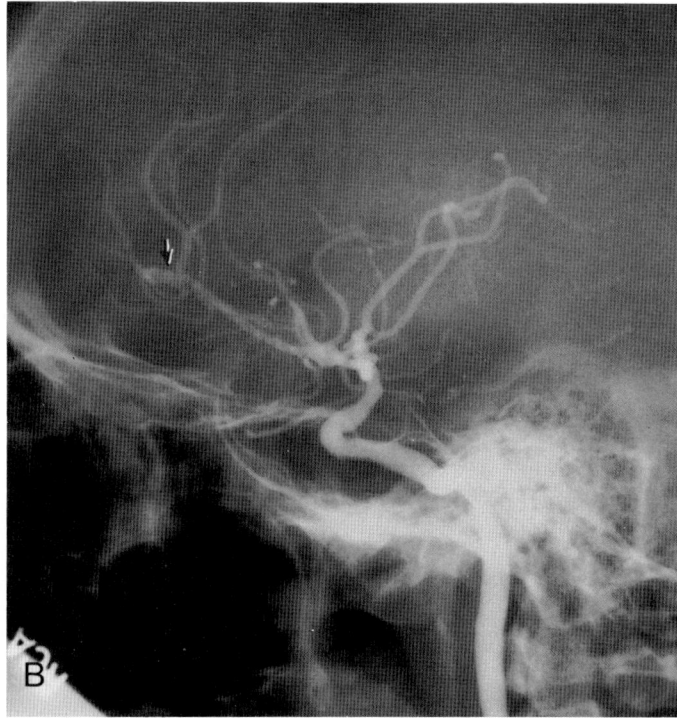

Figure 19.2 Operative approach to multiple aneurysms. *A* to *E*, right A-P and lateral; left AP, lateral, and oblique views show four aneurysms (*arrows*): bilateral middle cerebral artery bifurcations, anterior communicating artery, and pericallosal artery. There is also evidence of hydrocephalus. There is no indication as to which aneurysm bled. Comment: This 46-year-old man had SAH with drowsiness but no focal signs. Angiography was done on the 9th day after SAH. The CT scan did not localize the site of the hemorrhage. To approach these lesions a large left frontal temporal flap that crossed the midline was used. First, the left middle cerebral aneurysm was exposed and clipped via a sylvian fissure approach. This was not the site of hemorrhage. The right middle cerebral aneurysm was seen by going over the optic chiasm and under the frontal lobe to the opposite carotid bifurcation and then exposing the middle cerebral bifurcation. This exposure was not easy and the aneurysm was clipped with difficulty. Next, the anterior communicating aneurysm was exposed and clipped. This was the lesion that had bled. The dura was opened to the right of midline, the right frontal lobe was retracted laterally, and microdissection done to expose the aneurysm at the junction of the pericallosal and callosomarginal arteries. *F* to *I*, right AP and oblique, left AP and lateral carotid angiograms showing obliteration of all aneurysms except the one on the right middle cerebral artery where the clip either had slipped or had not been satisfactorily placed. Reoperation was done through a right frontal temporal approach. *J*, postoperative right carotid angiograms showing obliteration of the remaining aneurysm. The patient made a good recovery with the only deficit being a loss of smell.

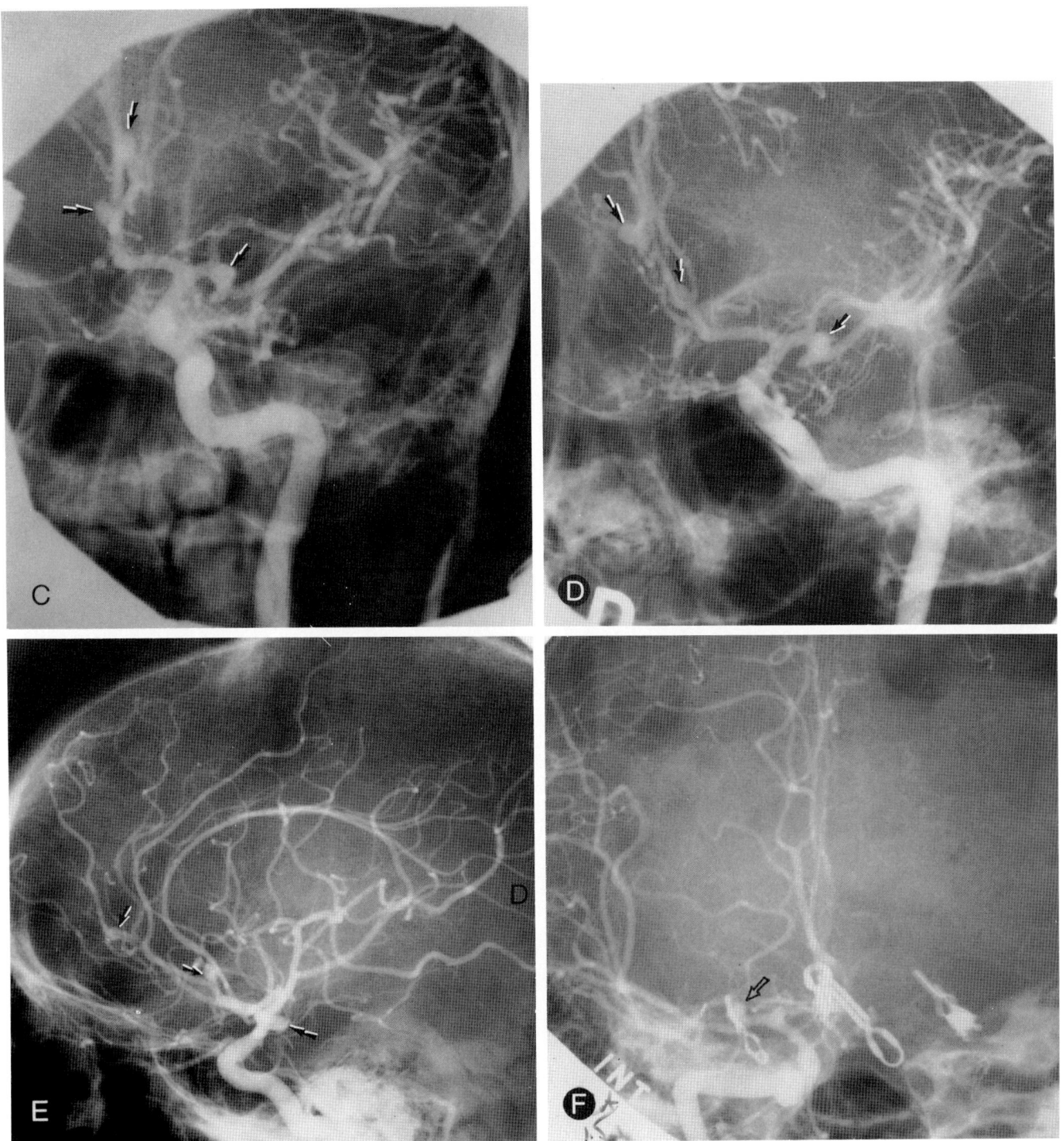

Figure 19.2 (C to F)

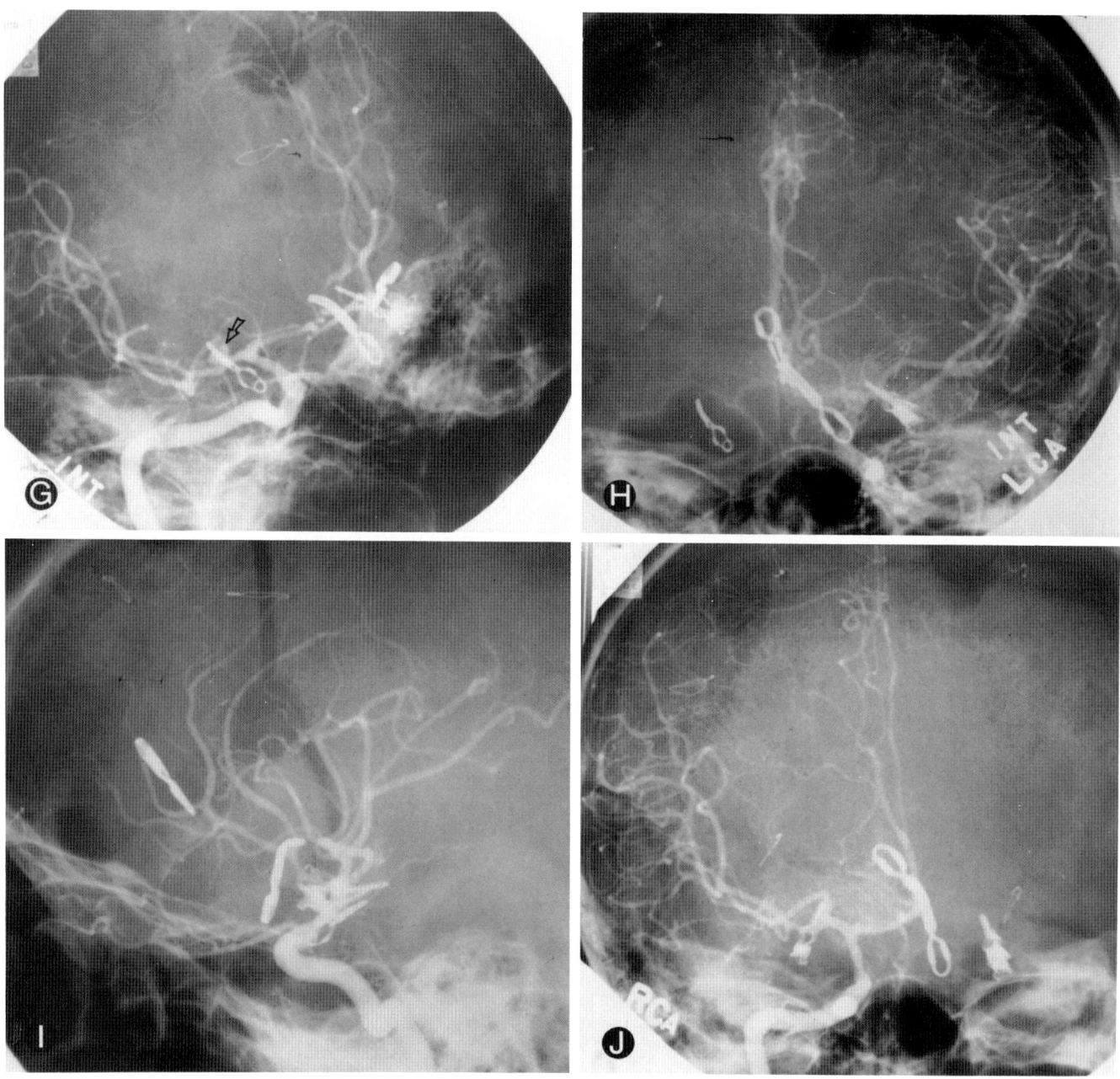

Figure 19.2 (G to J)

UNRUPTURED SYMPTOMATIC ANEURYSMS

Occasionally, an unruptured intracranial aneurysm presents with a focal neurological deficit, seizures, TIAs, or headache. The largest group of patients is those in which the first indication of an intracranial aneurysm is compression of a cranial nerve. The most common lesion to present in this fashion is the internal carotid-posterior communicating artery aneurysm with local compression of the third nerve. Enlargement of such a lesion may cause pain in the orbit with a partial or complete third nerve palsy, which usually (but not always) causes a fixed and dilated pupil. Compression of the optic nerves or chiasm may be caused by an enlarging carotid ophthalmic or anterior communicating artery aneurysm.

Headaches may indicate the presence of cerebral aneurysm. The precise mechanism for the headaches is obscure. In some patients, pain probably relates to the relationship of the aneurysm to the dura. In others it has been suggested that prerupture enlargement of the aneurysm may lead to headaches.

Intracranial aneurysm may present with transient ischemic attacks or cerebral infarction (11). Proving a causal relationship is difficult, and will depend on demonstration of emboli in the distal territory of the parent artery. Presumably the mechanism in these cases is mural thrombus within the aneurysm becoming dislodged with subsequent distal embolization. The exact risk of stroke after TIA by such mechanism is unknown.

Seizure may be the first warning of an intracranial aneurysm (Fig. 19.3). Such lesions are generally large with protrusion into frontal or temporal lobes. Gliotic reaction to the mass lesion produces an epileptogenic focus. The appearance of seizures may be related to increasing size of the lesion.

Evaluation includes CT with and without contrast and angiography. When the patient is medically stable and the aneurysm accessible, surgical therapy is usually indicated to prevent further neurological deterioration and to guard against the risk of subarachnoid hemorrhage. This combination of threats to the nervous system is usually sufficiently grave to warrant undertaking the low risk associated with surgical treatment. In some older patients, medical instability and a difficult lesion could favor a conservative approach, with follow-up angiography after 1 year. Surgical treatment is reconsidered if the aneurysm has enlarged.

ASYMPTOMATIC ANEURYSMS

In some cases, an intracranial aneurysm comes to light as an incidental finding on CT scanning or cerebral angiography. The combination of carotid stenosis and intracranial aneurysm is discussed in Chapter 1. With the advent of minimally invasive digital subtraction angiography, it is likely that many more such incidental lesions will be discovered in patients with minor symptomatology. Unruptured multiple aneurysms, discovered during identification of a separate ruptured lesion, likewise are regarded as asymptomatic aneurysms.

What is the threat from such asymptomatic aneurysms? Every bleeding aneurysm was once an asymptomatic aneurysm. Growth and rupture of asymptomatic lesions has been documented (2, 6). Some 26,000 subarachnoid hemorrhages occur yearly and half these patients die before they reach medical attention. In this sense, the asymptomatic aneurysm appears to be the precursor of a major threat to life. However, autopsied cases demonstrate that many intracranial aneurysms, particularly the very small ones, never cause a bleeding episode during life. Heiskanen presented the follow-up results of 61 patients with SAH in whom there were at least two intracranial aneurysms where only the ruptured aneurysm had been clipped (3). During a 10-year follow-up period, seven patients (1.1% per year) bled from a previously unruptured aneurysm and four died. Six additional patients suffered rebleeding more than 10 years after the first SAH and three died. On an average follow-up period of 16 years, the incidence of SAH was 1.3% per year and slightly over one-half of these patients died from the hemorrhage.

The problem then becomes a matter of discriminating between those asymptomatic lesions which pose a substantial threat of rupture and those which do not. Several efforts have been made to achieve this discrimination on the basis of size of aneurysm on angiography. Data from the Mayo Clinic indicates that lesions 10 mm or greater pose a threat sufficient to warrant operation, but these statistics are based on selected cases (12). The Cooperative Study suggested that lesions 7 mm or larger in diameter may be regarded as threatening (4). As operative risk diminishes, some have suggested that lesions as small as 3 mm in diameter may warrant operative handling (6). An aspect not considered in these papers is the question of the character of the lesions; certainly a multi-lobular lesion poses a greater threat of hemorrhage. Other important considerations are age and medical status. In a younger patient with good health, the tendency to operate will be stronger. Another point is the surgical difficulty posed by the lesion. The tendency to operate is greater if the lesion is relatively accessible. In general, we suggest surgical therapy for most asymptomatic aneurysms 7 mm or greater (1, 6–8, 10) (Fig. 19.4). Using these guidelines, excellent results have been achieved, with morbidity of under 5% and no mortality (1, 9, 10).

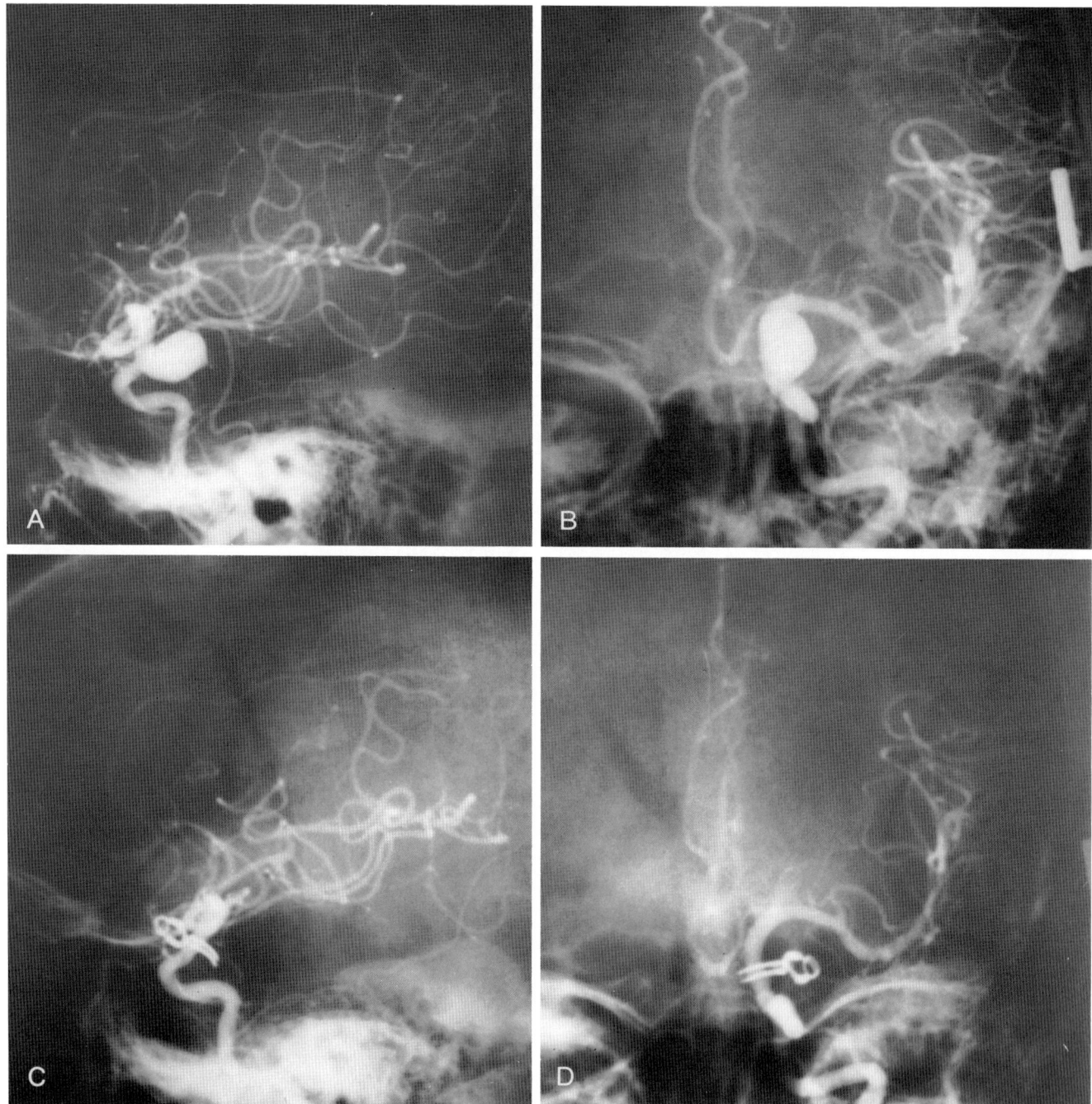

Figure 19.3 ICA aneurysm presenting with seizures. *A* and *B*, left carotid angiogram shows large ICA posterior communicating aneurysm. Comment: At surgery, patient's lesion was adherent to medial temporal lobe. Obliteration of aneurysm by ligation and clipping. *C* and *D*, postoperative angiogram confirms clipping. The patient experienced severe dysphasia beginning 4 days after operation which gradually cleared.

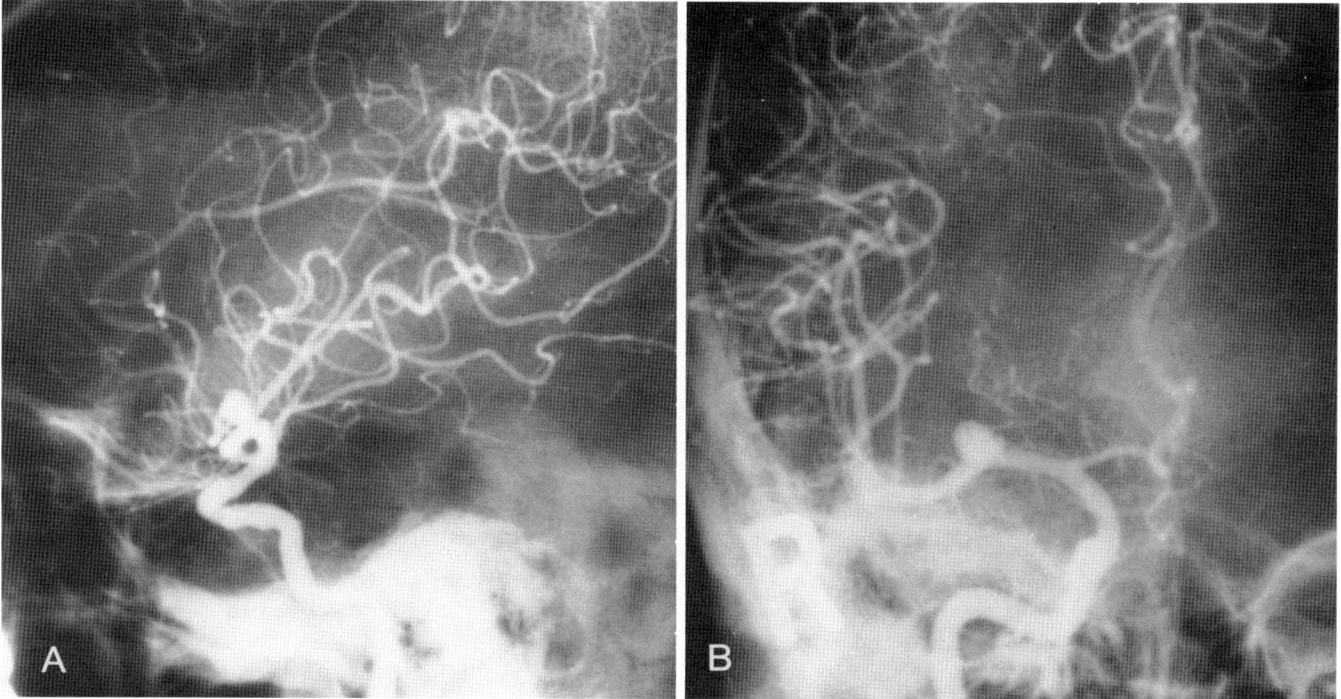

Figure 19.4 Asymptomatic aneurysm. A and B, right carotid angiogram demonstrates 7-mm aneurysm of the middle cerebral artery. Comment: The angiogram was done because the patient had nonspecific headaches, her mother had an aneurysm, and the patient was very anxious regarding SAH. The aneurysm was clipped. Postoperative angiography confirmed obliteration of the lesion. Neurological examination was normal.

REFERENCES

1. Drake CG, Girvin JP: The Surgical Treatment of Subarachnoid Hemorrhage with Multiple Aneurysms, in Morley TP (ed): *Current Controversies in Neurosurgery*. Philadelphia, W. B. Saunders, 1976, pp 274-278.
2. Heiskanan O, Martilla I: Risk of rupture of a second aneurysm in patients with multiple aneurysms. Neurosurgery 32:295-299, 1970.
3. Heiskanen O: Risk of bleeding from unruptured aneurysms in cases with multiple intracranial aneurysms. J Neurosurg 55:524-526, 1981.
4. Locksley HB: Report on the Cooperative Study of Intracranial Aneurysms and Subarachnoid Hemorrhage. Section V, Part II. Natural history of subarachnoid hemorrhage, intracranial aneurysms and arteriovenous malformations. J Neurosurg 25:321-368, 1966.
5. McKissock W, Richardson A, Walsh L, Owen E: Multiple intracranial aneurysms. Lancet 1:623-626, 1964.
6. Mount LA, Brisman R: Treatment of multiple aneurysms-symptomatic and asymptomatic, Clin Neurosurg 21:166-170, 1974.
7. Moyes PD: Surgical treatment of multiple aneurysms and of incidentally discovered unruptured aneurysms. J Neurosurg 35:291-295, 1971.
8. Ojemann RG: Management of the unruptured intracranial aneurysm. N Engl J Med, 304:725-726, 1981.
9. Salazar JL: Surgical treatment of asymptomatic and incidental intracranial aneurysms. J Neurosurg 53:20-21, 1980.
10. Samson DS, Hodosh RM, Clark WK: Surgical management of unruptured asymptomatic aneurysms. J Neurosurg 46:731-734, 1977.
11. Stewart RM, Samson D, Diehl J, Hinton R, Ditmore QM: Unruptured cerebral aneurysms presenting as recurrent transient neurologic deficits. Neurology 30:47-51, 1980.
12. Wiebers DO, Whisnant JP, O'Fallon WM: The natural history of unruptured intracranial aneurysms. N Engl J Med 304:696-698, 1981.
13. Wood EH: Angiographic identification of the ruptured lesion in patients with multiple cerebral aneurysms. J Neurosurg 21:182-198, 1964.

Chapter 20 GIANT ANEURYSMS

PATHOLOGY

Intracranial aneurysms larger than 25 mm in diameter are considered giant aneurysms (11). These lesions comprise about 5% of all intracranial aneurysms (8). They arise most commonly from the internal carotid artery, middle cerebral artery, and basilar apex, with occasional appearance in the region of the anterior communicating artery and in other locations in the posterior circulation.

As the lesion and its neck expand, there is sequential broadening of the parent artery and splaying of branch vessels arising in that zone. Atherosclerosis within the neck and the fundus of the lesion is common and may become calcified in later stages. The addition of mural thrombus to segments of the aneurysm may cause progressive discrepancy between the external dimensions and residual lumen; this discrepancy can be detected by comparing CT and angiography (6, 9). Mural thrombus may convey a measure of protection from rupture in some portions of the aneurysmal wall, but other areas may be paper-thin.

Giant aneurysms may present with symptoms due to compression from the mass without rupture. However, evidence indicates that subarachnoid bleeding is a common threat from these lesions (2, 8).

SURGICAL MANAGEMENT

Treatment has been perilous and sometimes ineffective. Carotid ligation for anterior circulation lesions was proposed many years ago (12), but despite this treatment, aneurysmal growth and rehemorrhage still occur. Attempts at obliteration of the neck have sometimes led to disastrous results. Techniques for wrapping, coating, piloinjection, and electrothrombosis have been suggested, but these approaches have not been established (2, 8).

Recent technical developments have improved the picture. Microsurgery now provides the opportunity for safe occlusion of the aneurysm neck in as many as one-third of the cases (2, 4, 13, 15, 18). Where this proves impossible, ligation of the extracranial or intracranial feeding artery may be safe and effective (2, 4, 12, 13, 17, 18). Determination of cerebral blood flow with the parent vessel occluded can indicate whether collateral circulation will protect the distal vascular territory (10, 18). Where collateral circulation is inadequate, cerebral revascularization with extracranial to intracranial bypass grafting can supply the required circulation (16, 17). Occasionally, where proximal ligation does not thrombose the lesion, trapping may be required. Only occasionally will wrapping be indicated. Endaneurysmorrhaphy can rarely be performed safely. For some lesions, techniques of elective cardiac arrest may be useful, particularly if heparinization can be avoided (14).

Intracranial Operation on the Aneurysm

Wherever possible, direct exposure with obliteration of the aneurysm neck and protection of the parent vessel and branches is desirable (2, 18). A significant number of these aneurysms have a neck that is suitable for ligation or clipping. Unfortunately, even the most sophisticated angiography with multiple special views often cannot decide this issue. Laminated mural thrombus near the neck can give the appearance of a satisfactory slender, "clippable" neck where none in fact exists. Scrutiny of the angiograms in comparison with CT, particularly coronal and sagittal reconstruction, may accurately depict this situation (6, 9). Even when the angiogram does not suggest a neck, one may still be present, or can be created at the time of direct intracranial exploration. Therefore, most giant intracranial aneurysms deserve exploration, on the chance that a neck can be found and obliterated (2). Moreover, when this tactic is possible, the lesion may be partially or completely excised, thus relieving compression of local structures. In other situations, where ligation is impossible or bilateral carotid aneurysms exist, direct obliteration of the lesion can avoid the potential hazard of sacrificing important cerebral circulation.

Giant aneurysms present special problems for direct operation. By virtue of their bulk, complete dissection is usually impossible. This means that examination of the entire neck of the lesion may be particularly difficult. Once the neck is dissected, obliteration often defies the surgeon's efforts. Sometimes one is fortunate enough to encounter a neck which will straightaway accept the clip. Often the neck is broad and a large aneurysm clip will be needed. The Drake clip, with its blade length of up to

24 mm, is particularly handy for giant aneurysms. A "piggyback" technique, with side-by-side overlapping clips, may be needed for especially broad necks (Fig. 20.1).

Irregular atherosclerosis in the neck of some lesions defies the clip. Though some zones of neck oppose, others may remain open between nubs of atherothrombotic material in the jaw of the clip. In this situation, preliminary ligature may then permit satisfactory obliteration of the neck with a clip (Fig. 20.2). In some instances, gentle preliminary crushing of the neck with a mosquito hemostat will prepare a seat in which the clip may lodge. The neck of the aneurysm and its associated interior atherosclerosis should be carefully inspected prior to these maneuvers. Sometimes, hard atheroma is present, which could fracture, causing a tear of the wall or distal embolization. In such cases, ligation of the feeding artery may be a better treatment.

In some patients, the bulk of the aneurysm tends to drive a clip or ligature back into the vessel of origin. In others the mass may be the cause of symptoms. Therefore, debulking maneuvers may be helpful or essential. Temporary techniques include placement of a figure of eight ligature or clips on the dome which can be removed. Other techniques permit no retreat; insertion of a large bore needle into the residual lumen with continuous suction aspiration of blood (3), or opening the lesion for direct removal of laminated clot down to the residual lumen. Occasionally, soft material may be removed readily. More commonly, laminated dense fibrotic clot is thick and adherent to the aneurysm wall and must be removed with forceps or by sharp dissection. It is easy to tear the aneurysm wall. By finding and dissecting a plane between the clot and wall, one can remove the clot with greater safety. Once launched on such a course, one is committed to dissection and obliteration of the aneurysm. Therefore, it is mandatory to ascertain prior to opening the aneurysm that satisfactory obliteration will be possible. Adjuncts for these maneuvers are temporary clips and deep hypotension (mean pressure 40 mm Hg) with short intervals down to 20 mm Hg. In addition, hypothermia, use of barbiturates or controlled cardiac arrest may be considered.

Extracranial Occlusion of the Carotid Artery

The principle of ligating the artery of origin to thrombose an aneurysm has long been applied to the treatment of giant internal carotid aneurysms by using cervical carotid ligation (5, 12). Experience has indicated that with common carotid ligation ischemia is less likely but so is thrombosis of the lesion. Internal carotid artery occlusion is more likely to thrombose the lesion but the risk of ischemia is higher. Fortunately, technological advance has provided the means for assessing the risk of distal ischemia in individual cases and for augmenting collateral blood supply where necessary. Determination of regional cerebral blood flow during temporary occlusion of the internal carotid artery can indicate the risk of ischemic stroke after ligation (10). If collateral circulation appears inadequate, then STA-MCA bypass grafting (or long vein revascularization) may augment middle cerebral collateral supply to permit carotid ligation (4, 16, 17). With this approach, almost all patients should tolerate extracranial internal carotid artery occlusion. This is probably accomplished best with the patient awake following implantation of the Crutchfield clamp.

The technique for application of the clamp is illustrated in Fig. 20.3, A to F. The exposure is the same as outlined for carotid endarterectomy (see Chapter 2). After checking the Crutchfield clamp, it is applied around the internal carotid artery just above the bifurcation so that a stump will not be left. In the rare circumstance where common carotid occlusion is to be used, the clamp is placed on the distal common carotid artery so that when it is closed, only enough room is left at the bifurcation for flow between the external and internal carotid arteries. It is important to avoid a pocket where thrombus might form. The intraarterial pressure distal to the clamp is recorded as the clamp is gradually closed and then opened (Fig. 20.3G) The clamp is initially closed just enought to start a reduction in the distal intraarterial pressure.

After recovery from anesthesia, the clamp is abruptly closed with assessment of the patient's response. Unless angiography indicates severe impairment of collateral flow, we believe abrupt occlusion should be attempted because it reduces the risk of embolization. If the patient tolerates occlusion nicely, then the stem of the Crutchfield clamp may be removed on the following day. If signs of ischemia develop, then the clamp may be loosened within the first 6–8 hours following occlusion. After that period of time, exploration of the artery would be needed to exclude local thrombus before safe restoration of flow through the internal carotid artery can be done. In order to diminish the chance of distal embolization, either from the aneurysm or from the propagated thrombus after ligation, administration of heparin during occlusion and for a week thereafter is probably a worthwhile step, unless the patient has had a recent SAH or craniotomy within the preceding 5 days. If, in spite of the preoperative testing, the patient does not tolerate occlusion of the internal carotid artery, then a decision has to be made between gradual internal occlusion, common carotid occlusion, or use of a bypass graft prior to occlusion. In general, a bypass graft is preferred, followed by either abrupt or gradual occlusion of the internal carotid artery.

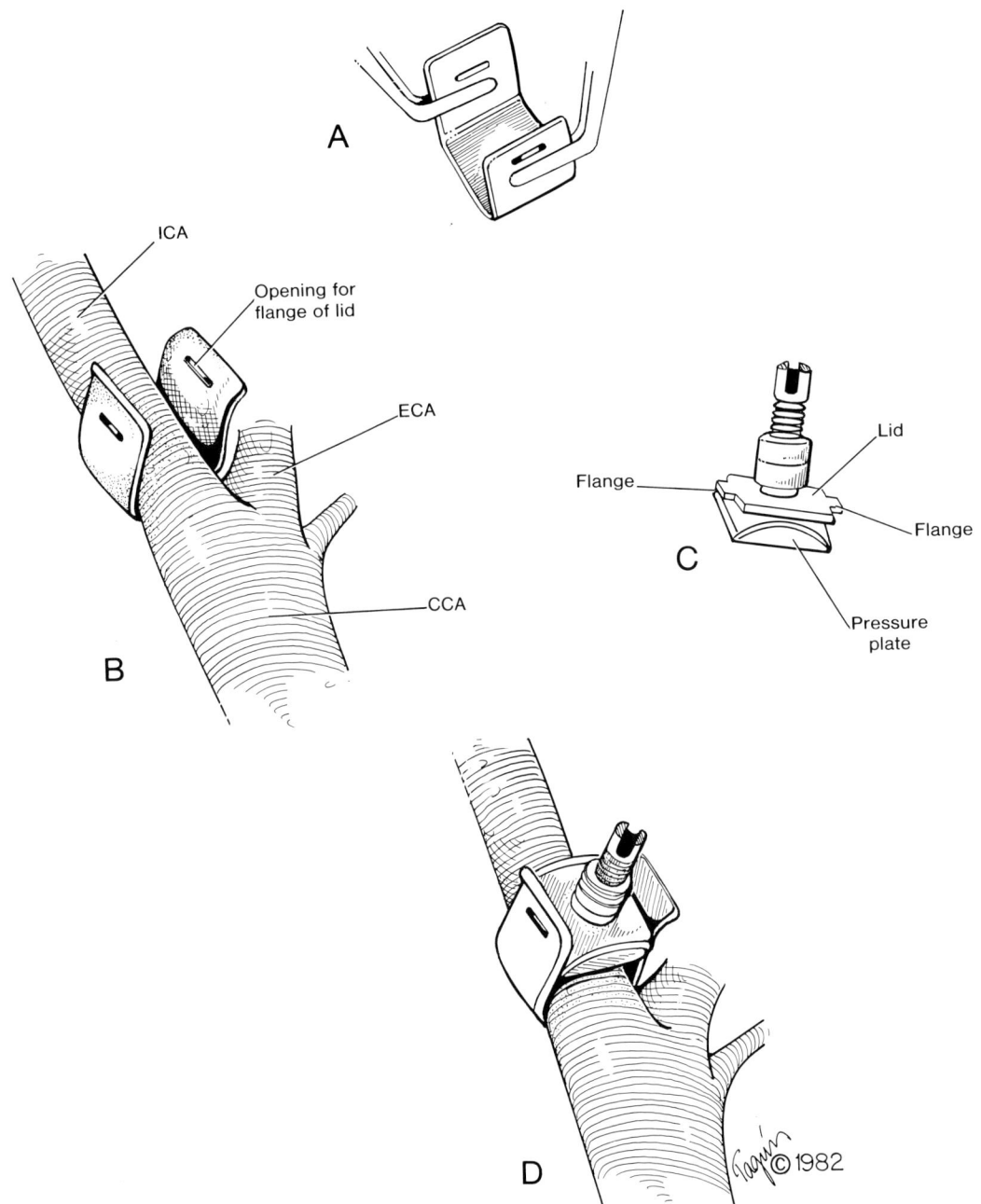

Figure 20.1 Placement of Crutchfield clamp. *A*, the U-shaped portion of the clamp may be held open with right angle clamps to permit removal or replacement of the lid assembly (see *C*). *B*, with the lid assembly removed, the U-shaped portion of the clamp is gently positioned about the initial portion of the internal carotid artery. *C*, the lid assembly consists of a screw through the lid to a pressure plate. Flanges on the lid fit into slots in the U-shaped portion. *D*, the lid assembly is fitted into place, with flanges engaging slots as shown. Right angle clamps open the U-shaped portion as shown in *A*. *E*, the control assembly consists of a screwdriver, handle, and locks. This assembly is pushed through a lateral stab wound with the cap in place to protect the tip of the screwdriver. *F*, the U-shaped portion is rotated to receive the control assembly. Turning the screw occludes the artery. *G*, recording of intraarterial pressure when clamp must be left partially open. Note that pressure in this patient starts to drop between 4 and 5 turns. The pressure with complete occlusion is about 40 mm. The clamp is left at a point where a slight reduction in pressure has occurred.

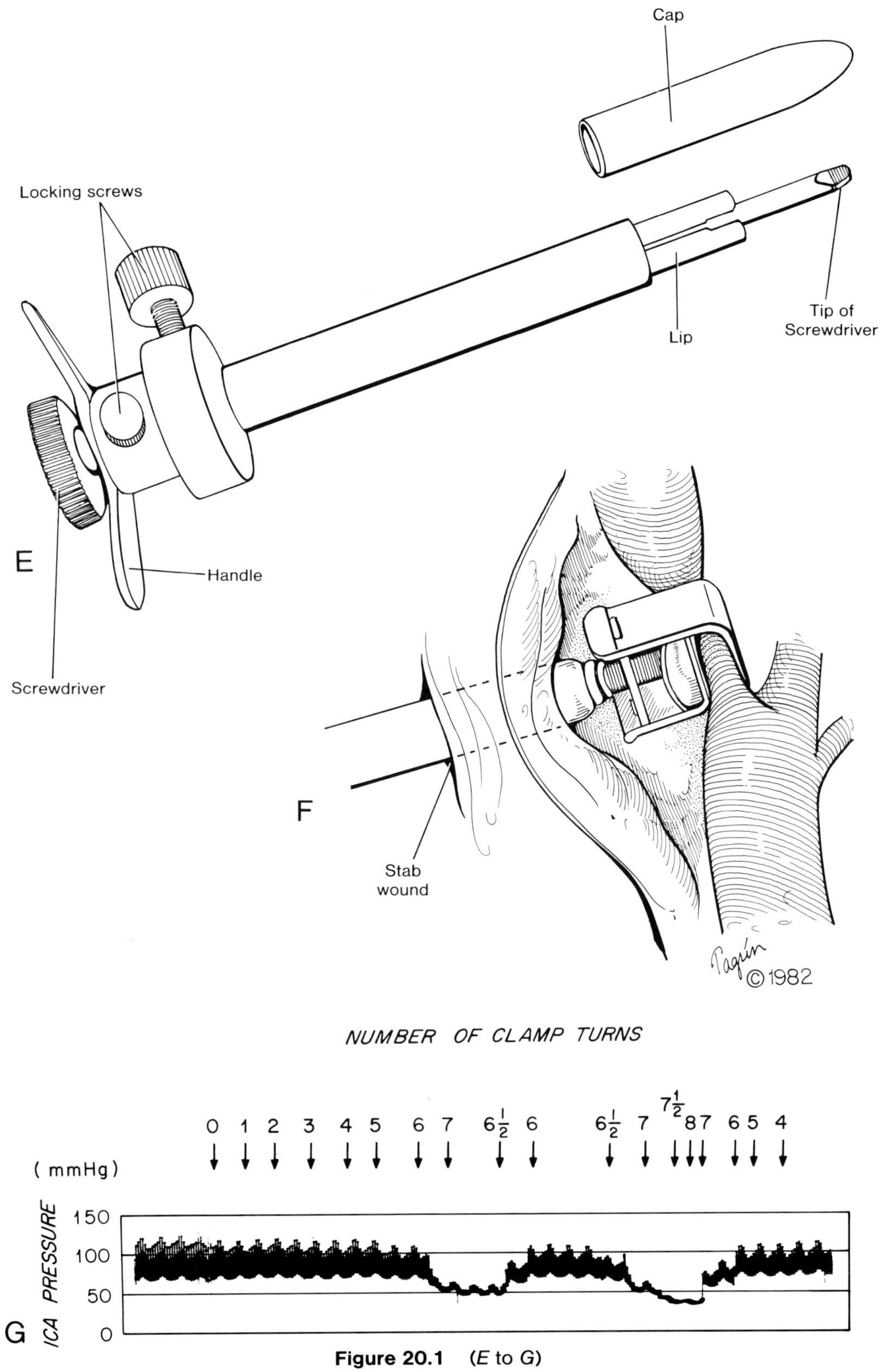

Giant Aneurysms 243

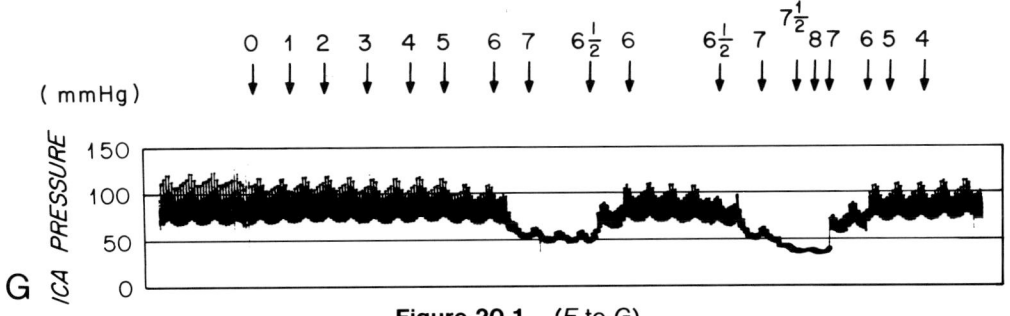

Figure 20.1 (E to G)

Intracranial Arterial Occlusion

Drake and colleagues have ingeniously occluded virtually every major intracranial artery for the treatment of distal unclippable aneurysms (2). A nice balance of distal flow and pressure is sought; pressure low enough to thrombose the aneurysm, collateral flow high enough to avoid infarction. In some patients, augmentation of collateral blood supply prior to intracranial arterial occlusion is needed. For middle cerebral lesions, this will mean superficial temporal artery-middle cerebral artery bypass. However, even this added circulatory supply may be insufficient. Therefore, placement of a snare ligature about the parent artery has been suggested for middle cerebral artery ligation with the patient fully awake (2). This provides a monitor of cerebral perfusion. If the patient tolerates tightening of the snare ligature for 30 minutes, then the ligature may be permanently occluded and buried. If the patient does not tolerate the ligature, then it may be released for restoration of flow.

Intracranial arterial occlusion has also been applied to the internal carotid artery and the A1 segment of the anterior cerebral artery. Snare ligature occlusion of the intracranial vertebral, basilar, proximal posterior cerebral, and superior cerebellar artery may also be carried out to achieve thrombosis of lesions arising from these vessels (2). Augmentation of posterior circulation may be considered to permit one-stage occlusion of the parent vessel under anesthesia.

Occasionally, proximal ligation will not lead to thrombosis of the aneurysm when there is particularly brisk collateral circulation. In this setting, continued symptoms relative to mass effect or subarachnoid hemorrhage may demand a further effort to thrombose the lesion and remove its mass. Since the proximal parent artery has already been occluded in such cases, abrupt occlusion of the parent artery just distal to the aneurysm ("trapping") may be accomplished safely if other collateral circulation (including established bypass) can be protected during surgery.

Detachable Balloon Technique

The development of the intravascular detachable balloon technique has provided the possibility of occluding certain giant aneurysms indirectly while preserving carotid flow. However, initial experience with this procedure indicates that it is safer to use the balloon for occlusion of the carotid artery when the aneurysm cannot be clipped (1). The technique allows the occlusion to be done close to the neck of the aneurysm (Fig. 20.4). The major advantage of balloon occlusion of the internal carotid artery over using a clamp is that the balloon may be placed higher with reduction of the dead space in which thrombosis can occur. We agree with Debrun et al. that thromboembolism is the most common cause of complications with proximal ligation of the carotid artery (1). If it is determined that a STA-MCA bypass is required because of inadequate collateral circulation, the balloon occlusion can be done within 24–48 hours of the operation.

MANAGEMENT OF SPECIFIC ANEURYSMS

Giant Paraclinoid Internal Carotid Aneurysms

Giant ophthalmic aneurysms are the most common of the larger aneurysms arising from the internal carotid artery, but occasionally aneurysms arise from the posteriolateral portion of this artery and in some the neck is so wide the origin is unclear (2, 7). Patients may present with progressive visual loss, subarachnoid hemorrhage, or transient ischemic attacks.

These lesions have been managed with overall good results, but even application of a variety of modern approaches has not averted serious complications in some cases. Twenty-five giant paraclinoid aneurysms of the internal carotid artery were treated at Massachusetts General Hospital and Presbyterian University Hospital in Pittsburgh and have been summarized by Dr. Roberto Heros and colleagues (Table 20.1) (7). Seventeen aneurysms were explored intracranially. Of these, 13 were directly clipped and one was wrapped with gauze and glue. Of the other three, two were treated by internal carotid ligation after STA-MCA bypass and one by common carotid ligation. Postoperative angiography was done on seven of the 14 cases in which the aneurysm was clipped. In all procedures there was satisfactory obliteration of the aneurysm and preservation of the internal carotid artery. Narrowing of minor degree was present in some cases. In all the patients who did not have postoperative angiography, the aneurysm was opened and collapsed at surgery. There was one death in the immediate postoperative period due to hemorrhage when a clip slipped. There were no disabling neurological complications outside the visual system.

A pterional approach is used, but the frontal exposure is slightly larger to allow a wider range of angles for clip application. In preparation for possible EC-IC bypass the frontal branch of the STA is carefully preserved, though not dissected free. The dura over the anterior clinoid and optic canal roof is reflected back over the optic nerve and aneurysm, and then the anterior clinoid and the posterior end of the roof of the optic canal are removed with the high speed drill and small rongeurs and curettes (see Chapter 13).

Rather than using deep systemic hypotension, we prefer to use temporary cervical or intracranial internal carotid artery occlusion to soften these aneurysms at the time of clip application. Frequently, a second clip needs to be placed on the internal carotid artery below the posterior communicating artery to trap the aneurysm temporarily.

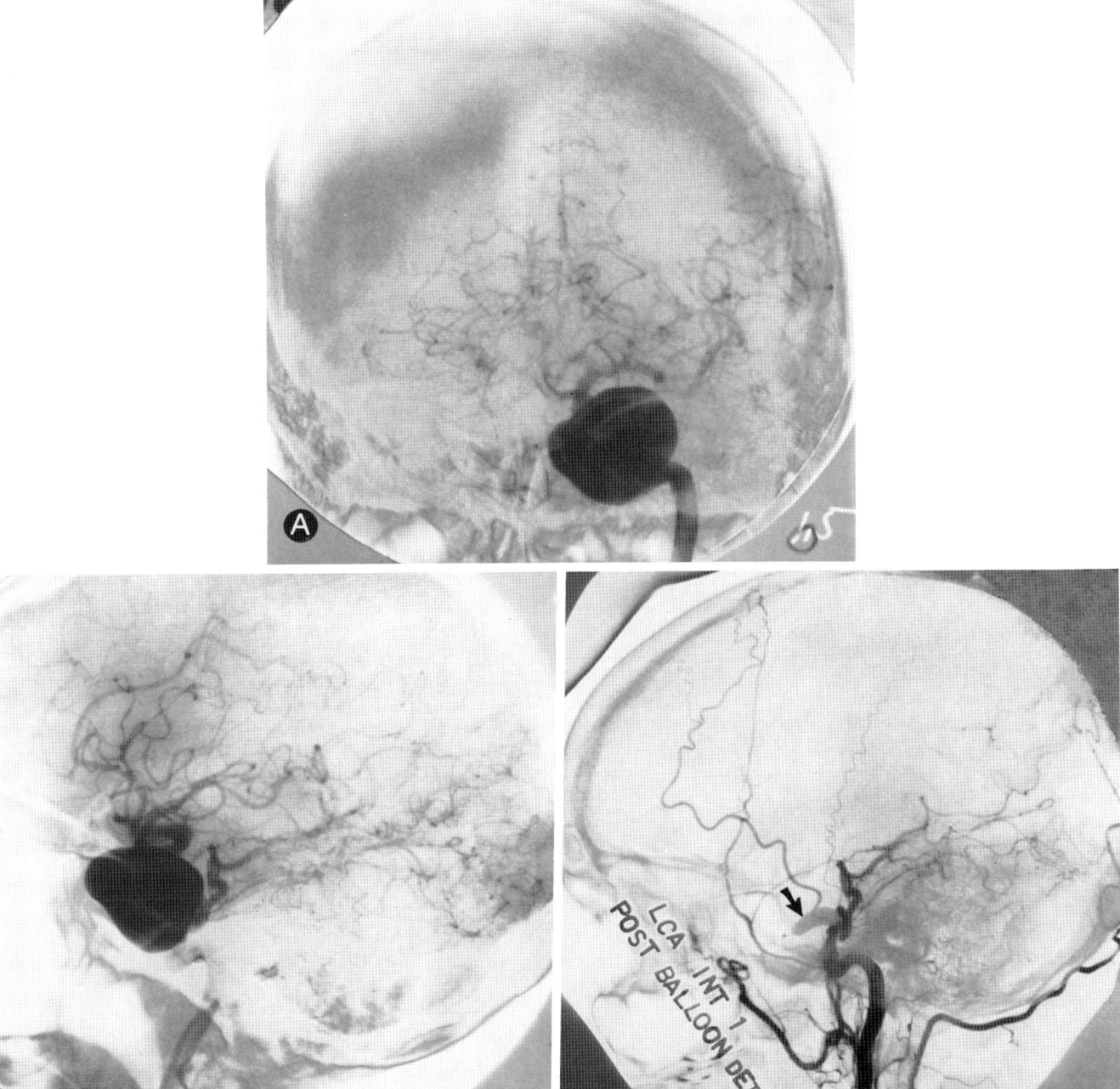

Figure 20.2 Balloon occlusion of internal carotid-trigeminal artery aneurysm. *A* and *B*, AP and lateral left carotid angiogram showing giant internal carotid aneurysm arising in relationship to a trigeminal artery. *C*, angiogram after treatment by Dr. Gerard Debrun using a detachable balloon (*arrow*). The aneurysm and distal internal carotid artery are occluded but flow is preserved through the trigeminal artery into the posterior circulation. (These pictures are reproduced through the courtesy of Dr. Gerard Debrun.)

Table 20.1
Giant Paraclinoid Aneurysms: Surgical Results (Modified from Ref. 7)[a]

	Number of Patients	Neurological Condition		Visual Condition			Dead
		Good	Poor	Same	Better	Worse	
Direct operation[b]	14	13	0	7	3	3	1[d]
CCA ligation	4	4	0	2	1	1	1[e]
ICA ligation							
With EC-IC bypass	5	2	2	2	2	0	1[f]
Without EC-IC by-pass	1	1	0	0	1	0	0
Trapping[c]	1	1	0	1	0	0	0
Totals	25	21	2	12	7	4	3

[a] All patients were Hunt grades 0–2 preoperatively.
[b] All treated by clipping of the aneurysmal neck except for one that was treated by reinforcement with gauze and glue.
[c] Patient previously treated by CCA ligation required "trapping" because of continuing aneurysmal growth.
[d] Died from hemorrhage 4 hours after operation when clip slipped.
[e] Died 1 year after CCA ligation from recurrent subarachnoid hemorrhage.
[f] Died from embolic complication.

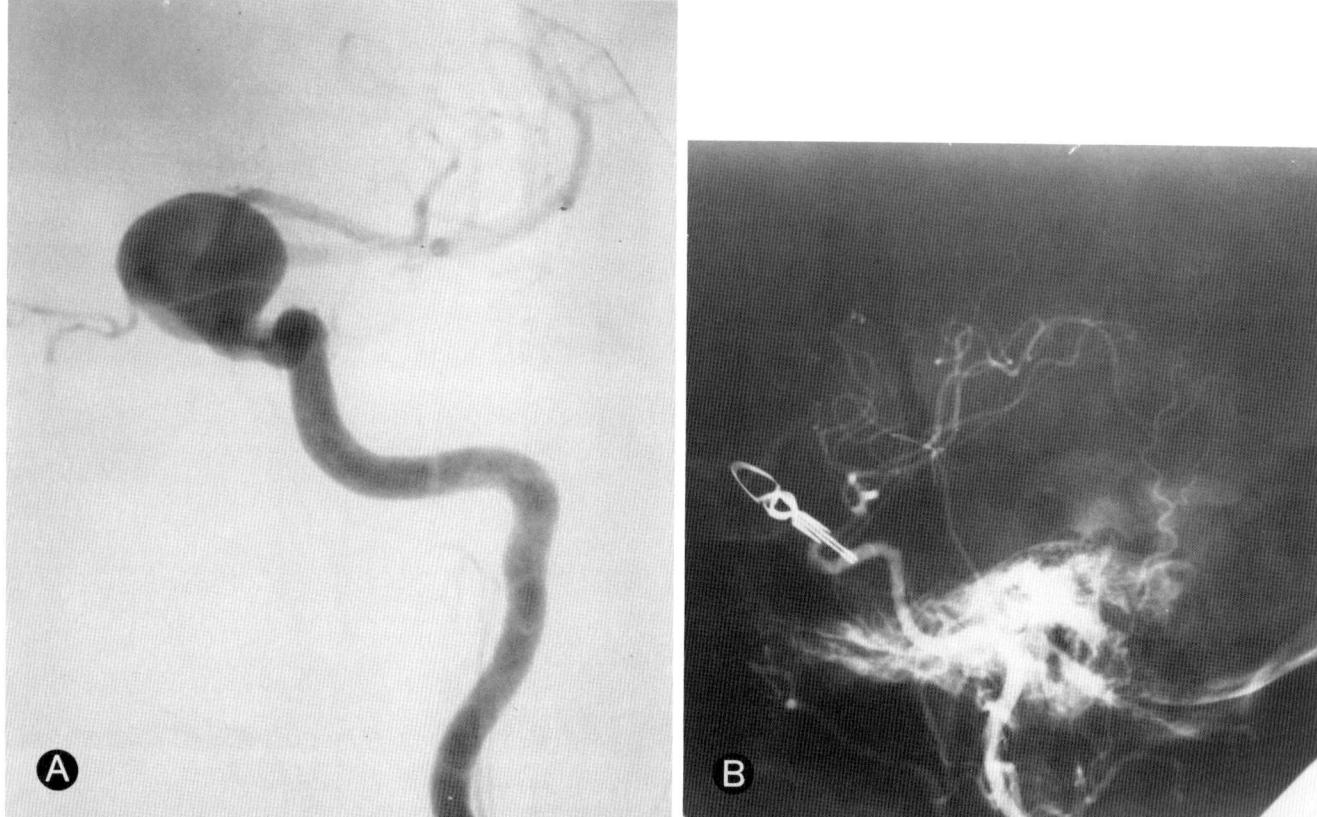

Figure 20.3 Giant ophthalmic artery aneurysm. A, the aneurysm projects superiorly compressing the optic nerve. B, postoperative angiogram shows one of the tricks to use in occluding the aneurysm. A long clip has been placed across the neck of the aneurysm preserving internal carotid circulation. A second clip holds the blades of the first clip closed. Prior to placing the second clip, the blades of the long clip would open with each pulsation of systolic blood pressure.

For occlusion of the aneurysm, we have found the long Drake or Yasargil clips most useful (Fig. 20.1 and 20.2). Frequently, the blades must be applied blindly under the optic nerve toward the pituitary fossa. It is important to have a soft aneurysm to avoid perforation of the aneurysm as the clip is advanced to collapse the broad neck. Often the blades of the clip pulsate, at least during systole, when the temporary clip on the internal carotid artery is removed. Often multiple clips are needed to assure closure. Occasionally, tissue adhesive on the clip helps prevent slipping.

Eleven patients were treated by a trapping procedure or by either common carotid ligation or internal carotid ligation in the neck. Of the group of five patients treated by internal carotid ligation preceded by an EC-IC bypass graft, three patients developed embolic complications, which in one patient resulted in death. One of the four patients treated by ligation of the common carotid artery died 1 year later from a recurrent subarachnoid hemorrhage.

The treatment of choice for paraclinoid aneurysms is direct clipping. With persistence and careful technique, the majority of these lesions can be clipped safely. This form of treatment should be attempted whenever it appears feasible, whether or not the patient is symptomatic, provided there are no medical contraindications to surgery. In patients with symptomatic paraclinoid aneurysms that cannot be clipped directly, internal carotid occlusion is preferable. Use of a Crutchfield clamp is standard, but in some centers, occlusion with a detachable balloon catheter may be considered.

Intracavernous Aneurysms

While not all intracavernous aneurysms are giant, it is convenient to include them in this section because they are usually treated by some type of carotid occlusion (Fig. 20.5). However, not all of these aneurysms need be treated. The natural history is that they maintain their size for many years and they rarely rupture to cause a carotid cavernous fistula (see Chapter 24) or bulge intracranially to cause subarachnoid hemorrhage (1). However, when they cause pain or occular muscle palsy, these symptoms may be reversed by treatment with carotid occlusion (4).

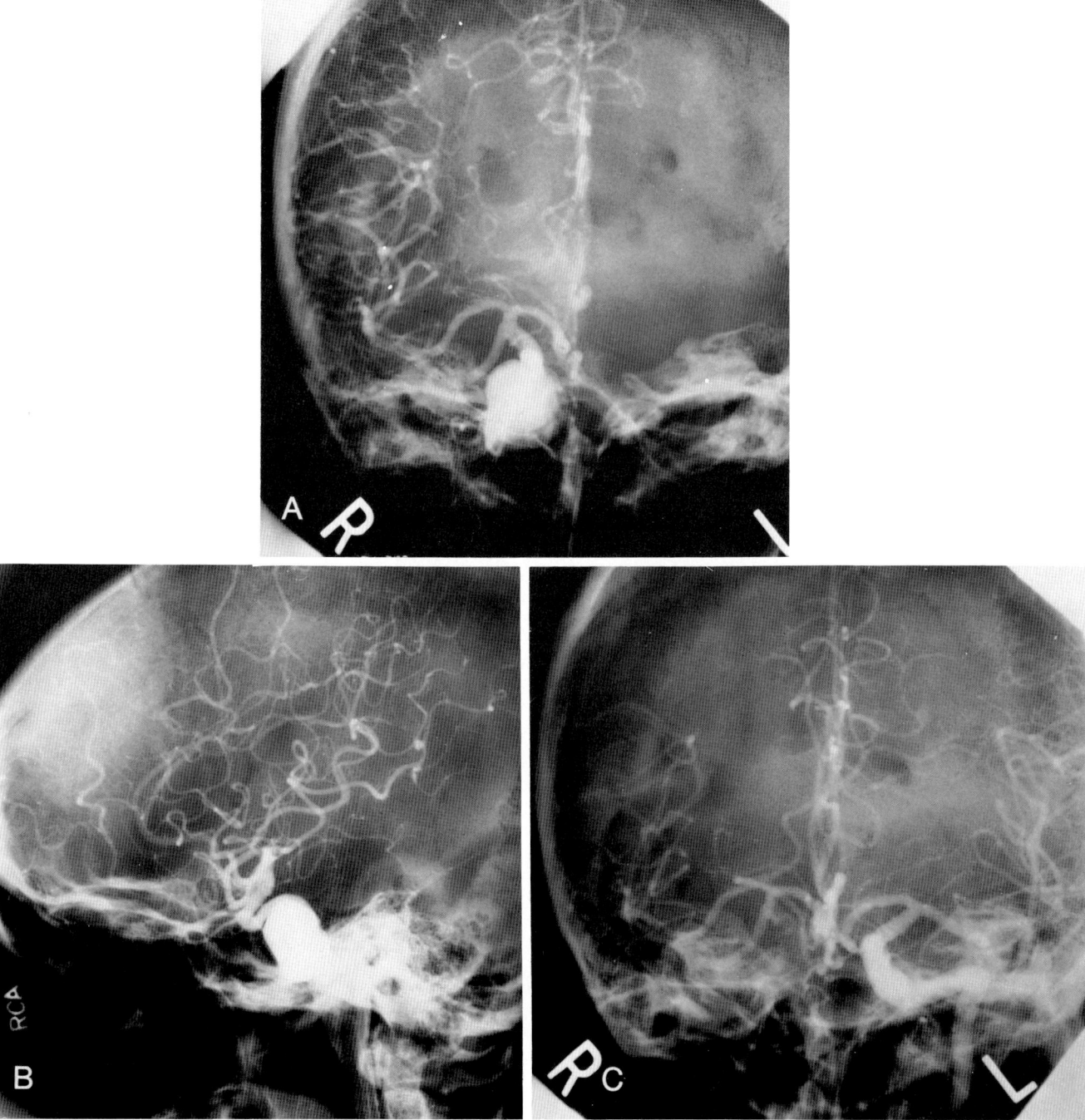

Figure 20.4 Giant intracavernous aneurysm. *A* and *B*, AP and lateral right carotid angiograms show the giant aneurysm within the cavernous sinus. *C*, left carotid angiogram with cross-compression shows excellent cross-circulation. *D*, after internal carotid occlusion the vertebral angiogram shows flow into the distal right internal carotid and middle cerebral arteries. *E*, patient's external carotid angiogram shows collateral filling from the ophthalmic to internal carotid artery but no filling of the aneurysm. Comment: The patient presented with pain around the eye and a third nerve palsy. She was treated with abrupt internal carotid occlusion under local anesthesia with EEG monitoring. All symptoms resolved.

Giant Aneurysms

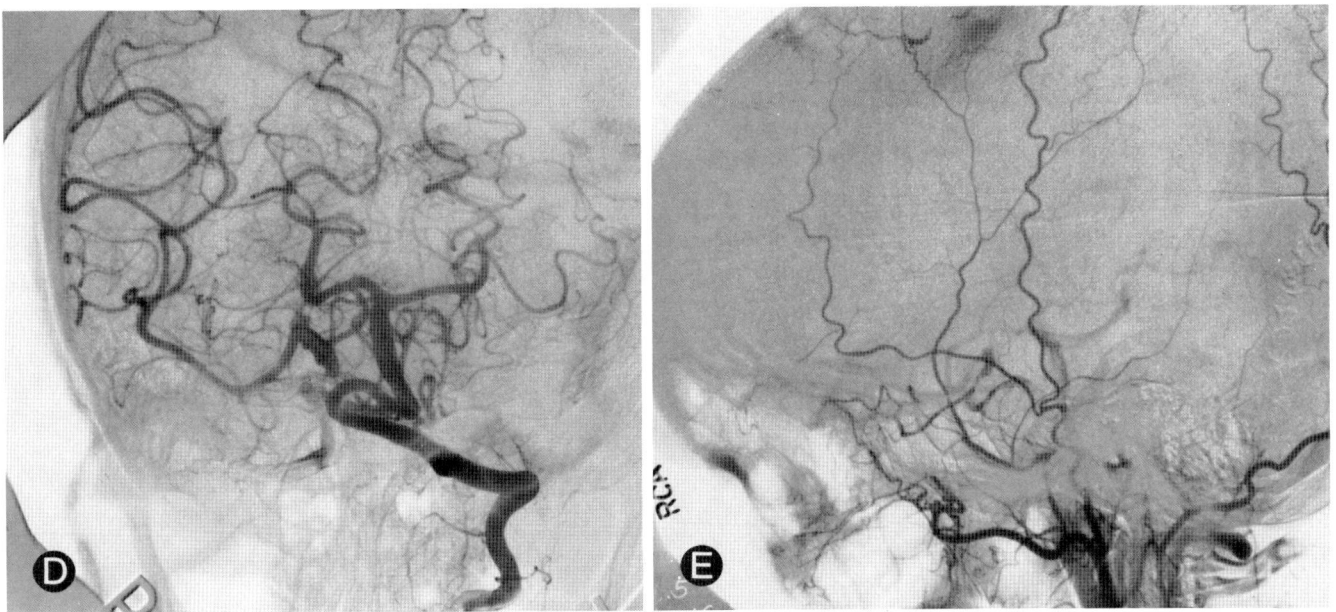

Figure 20.4 (*D* and *E*)

Giant Internal Carotid-Posterior Communicating Aneurysms

These aneurysms usually project posteriorly and can compress the temporal lobe and brain stem. They may cause headache and third nerve palsy, and when they enlarge superomedially, the visual pathways are compressed. Drake found that most of these lesions have a neck that can be clipped (2) (Fig. 20.2).

Giant Anterior Communicating Aneurysms

These aneurysms may present with compression of the visual apparatus, frontal lobes, or hypothalamus and clinically act like a suprasellar tumor. They may also cause headache and subarachnoid hemorrhage. Fortunately, many of these aneurysms will have a neck that can be occluded (Fig. 20.6). Often removal of much of the mass is very important in the treatment of symptoms caused by these aneurysms.

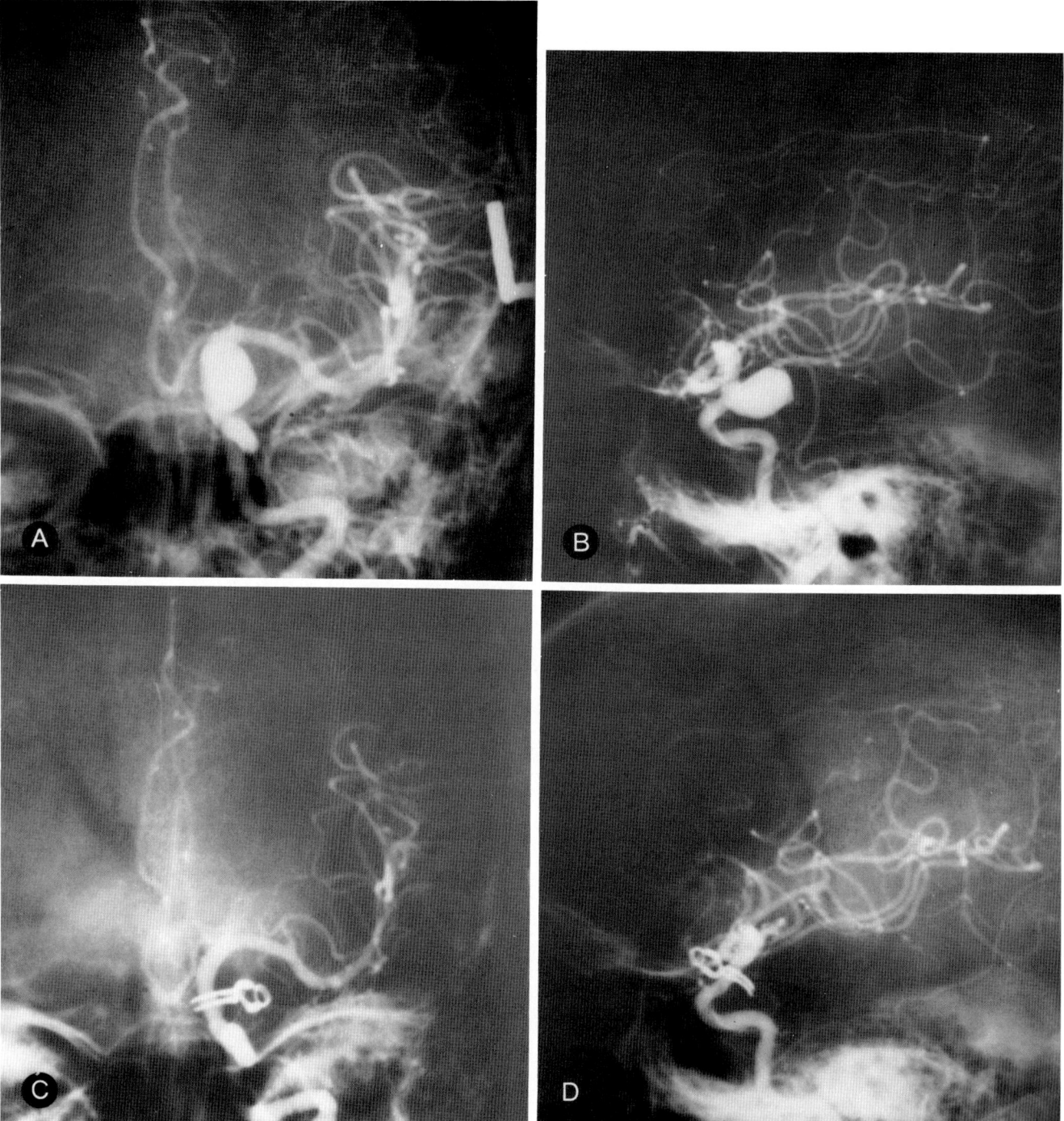

Figure 20.5 Giant internal carotid-posterior communicating aneurysm. *A* and *B*, AP and lateral angiograms show the giant aneurysm. On the lateral view a thrombus is seen in the superior aspect of the aneurysm. *C* and *D*, postoperative angiogram. The neck of the aneurysm would not hold a clip until it was narrowed with a ligature.

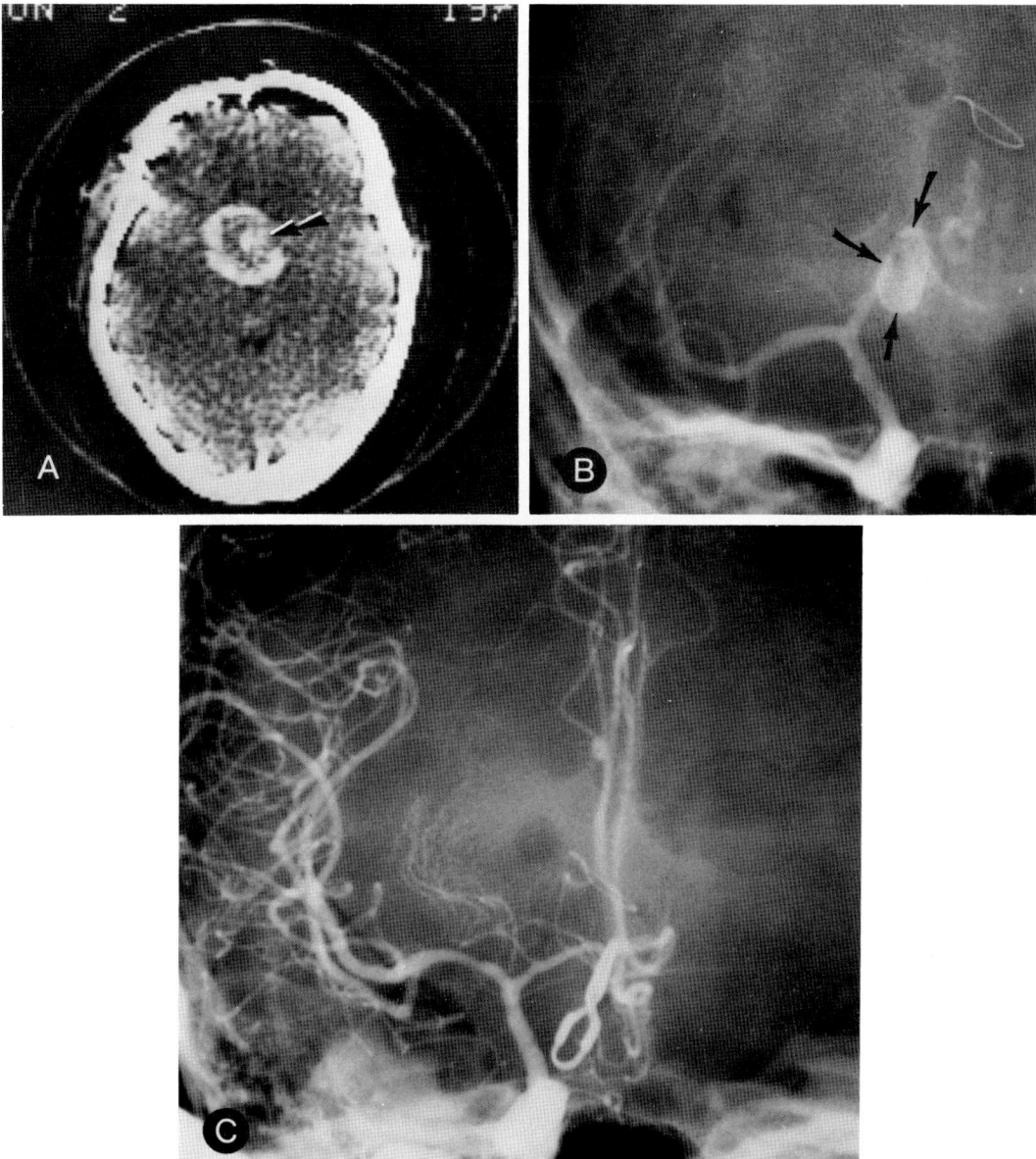

Figure 20.6 Giant anterior communicating aneurysm. *A,* CT scan shows area of enhancement (*arrow*) within a ring lesion. This is characteristic for a giant, partially thrombosed aneurysm. *B,* right carotid angiogram demonstrates the aneurysm (*arrows*). Note the discrepancy in the size of the lesion seen on the CT scan and angiogram. *C,* postoperative angiogram showing the aneurysm to be occluded and the mass effectively reduced. Comment: Patient seen at another hospital with evidence of optic chiasm compression. Exploration was done based on the CT scan and without angiography. At our reoperation, the aneurysm was clipped and debulked. This was followed by relief of symptoms.

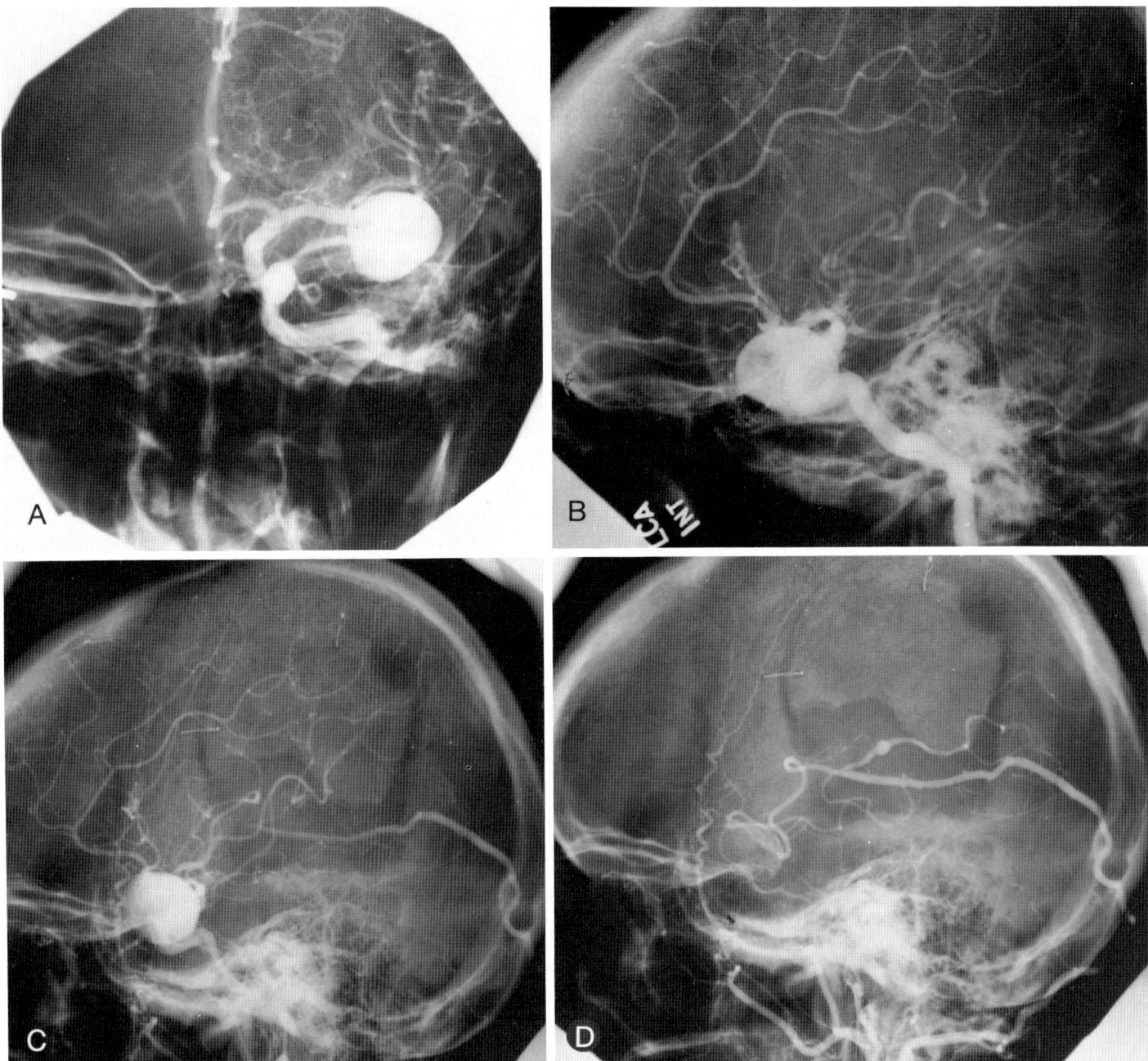

Figure 20.7 Giant middle cerebral aneurysm. *A* and *B*, AP and lateral angiogram outline the giant aneurysm. *C* and *D*, functioning bypass graft demonstrated. Comment: Patient treated with bypass graft and internal carotid occlusion. The superficial temporal artery was not adequate and, therefore, a vein bypass was done from the occipital artery to the middle cerebral artery. Subsequent CT scan showed thrombosis of much of the aneurysm.

Giant Middle Cerebral Aneurysms

The most common clinical presentation consists of headache, seizures, hemiparesis, and dysphasia, when the dominant side is involved, but subarachnoid hemorrhage can also occur (2).

Most of these aneurysms should be explored and an attempt made to define a neck that can be clipped. In a few patients it is best to wrap the aneurysm. In four patients where the aneurysm could not be clipped, Drake utilized proximal middle cerebral artery occlusion with a functioning EC-IC bypass (2). At operation, a tourniquet was placed on the M1 segment as close to the aneurysm as possible. The middle cerebral artery was then occluded in subsequent days with the patient awake and using artificial hypertension as necessary. On occasion, a bypass graft has been combined with internal carotid occlusion when adequate exposure of the proximal middle cerebral artery was not possible (Fig. 20.7).

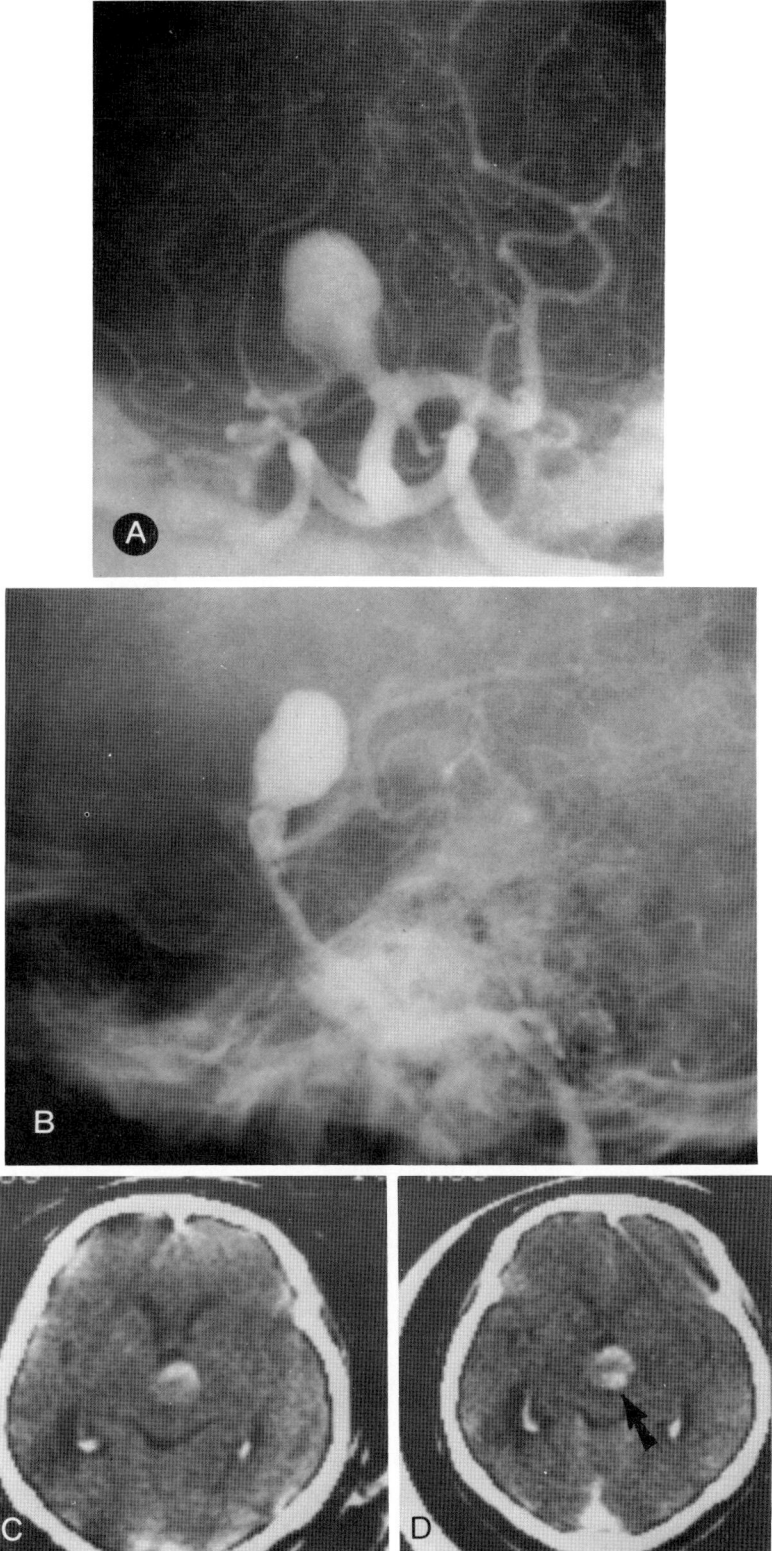

Figure 20.8 Giant P_1 segment aneurysm. *A* and *B*, AP and lateral vertebral angiogram shows the large aneurysm projecting superiorly from the P_1 segment. *C,* non-contrast CT scan shows true size of the partially thrombosed aneurysm. *D,* contrast CT scan shows area of enhancement (*arrow*) in relation to overall size of aneurysm.

Giant Basilar Bifurcation Aneurysms

The clinical picture of those aneurysms projecting upward and posteriorly includes personality changes, loss of recent memory, ataxia, dementia (often with hydrocephalus), bulbar signs, or quadriparesis. Projection to one side causes a third nerve palsy. If the aneurysm extends far enough forward, field defects can be found.

The largest experience has been reported by Drake (2). It is important that preoperative angiography define the size and potential of collateral circulation through each posterior communicating artery. The aneurysm should be exposed using the approach outlined in Chapter 17. In many patients, the neck of the giant aneurysm can be clipped (Fig. 20.8). If not, occlusion of the basilar artery just proximal to the aneurysm should be considered.

REFERENCES

1. Debrun G, Fox A, Drake C, Peerless S, Girvin J, Ferguson G: Giant unclippable aneurysms: Treatment with detachable balloons. Am J Neuroradiol 2:167–173, 1981.
2. Drake CG: Giant intracranial aneurysms: Experience with surgical treatment in 174 patients. Clin Neurosurg 26:12–95, 1979.
3. Flamm ES: Suction decompression of aneurysms. Technical note. J Neurosurg 54:275–276, 1981.
4. Gelber BR, Sundt TM Jr: Treatment of intracavernous and giant carotid aneurysms by combined internal carotid ligation and extra-to intracranial bypass. J Neurosurg 52:1–10, 1980.
5. Giannotta SL, McGillicuddy JE, Kindt GW: Gradual carotid artery occlusion in the treatment of inaccessible internal carotid artery aneurysms. Neurosurgery 5:417–421, 1979.
6. Handa J, Nakano Y, Aii H, Handa H: Computed tomography with giant intracranial aneurysms. Surg Neurol 9:257–263, 1978.
7. Heros RC, Nelson PB, Ojemann RG, Crowell RM, Debrun G: Large and giant paraclinoid aneurysms. Choice of surgical technique, complications and results (in press).
8. Hosobuchi Y: Direct surgical treatment of giant intracranial aneurysms. J Neurosurg 51:743–756, 1979.
9. Lavyne MH, Kleefield J, Davis KR, Ojemann RG, Crowell RM: Giant intracranial aneurysms of the anterior circulation: Clinical characteristics and diagnosis by computed tomography. Neurosurgery 3:356–363, 1978.
10. Miller JD, Jawad K, Jennett B: Safety of carotid ligation and its role in the management of intracranial aneurysms. J Neurol Neurosurg Psychiat 40:64–72, 1977.
11. Morley TP, Barr HWK: Giant intracranial aneurysms: Diagnosis, course, and management. Clin Neurosurg 16:73–94, 1969.
12. Odom GL, Tindall GT: Carotid ligation in the treatment of certain intracranial aneurysms. Clin Neurosurg 15:101–116, 1968.
13. Onuma T, Suzuki J: Surgical treatment of giant intracranial aneurysms. J Neurosurg 51:33–36, 1979.
14. Silverberg GD, Reitz BA, Ream AK: Hypothermia and cardiac arrest in the treatment of giant aneurysms of the cerebral circulation and hemangioblastoma of the medulla. J Neurosurg 55:337–346, 1981.
15. Sonntag VKH, Yuan RH, Stein BM: Giant intracranial aneurysms: A review of 13 cases. Surg Neurol 8:81–84, 1977.
16. Spetzler, RF, Schuster H, Roski R-A: Elective extracranial-intracranial arterial bypass in the treatment of inoperable giant aneurysms of the internal carotid artery. J Neurosurg 53:22–27, 1980.
17. Spetzler RF, Roski RA, Schuster H, Takaoka Y: The role of EC-IC bypass in the treatment of giant intracranial aneurysms. Neurol Res 2:345–359, 1980.
18. Sundt TM Jr, Piepgras DG: Surgical approach to giant intracranial aneurysms. Operative experience with 80 cases. J Neurosurg 51:731–742, 1979.

Chapter 21 INFECTIOUS INTRACRANIAL ANEURYSMS

INTRODUCTION

Since William Osler described in 1885 an aortic aneurysm associated with bacterial endocarditis, the term "mycotic" aneurysm has been used to designate any aneurysm which develops following infection in the wall of an artery (40). Until a few years ago, almost every publication concerning intracranial "mycotic" aneurysms reported a bacterial cause for the aneurysm, usually in association with endocarditis. Reports of aneurysms related to meningitis and cavernous sinus thrombophlebitis, as well as true mycotic (fungal) aneurysms have subsequently appeared (37). The designation, bacterial intracranial aneurysm, should be used for those aneurysms that result from bacterial infection (8). It is suggested that all types of aneurysms due to infection be grouped under the heading of infectious intracranial aneurysms (37).

Several publications have reviewed the subject of bacterial intracranial aneurysms (8, 9, 12, 17, 37). In one, 85 cases found at angiography, operation, or autopsy between 1954 and 1978 were summarized (8). In another, we analyzed infectious intracranial aneurysms documented by angiography and reported in the 20 years from 1959 through 1978 (37). This included 53 patients with bacterial intracranial aneurysm associated with definite or probable endocarditis (1, 3, 5-9, 13, 15, 17, 18, 20-24, 28, 29, 31, 32, 34-37, 41, 43, 45, 51, 54, 55), five cases due to meningitis (15, 39, 49, 50), seven related to cavernous sinus thrombophlebitis (25, 46, 49, 51), and five fungal aneurysms (2, 11, 16, 26, 53). Subsequently, further reports of patients with bacterial aneurysms documented by angiography have appeared bringing to 81 the total number of cases through 1980 (4, 12, 14, 19, 27, 33, 44, 47, 48, 52).

BACTERIAL INTRACRANIAL ANEURYSMS

Clinical Manifestations

The majority of bacterial intracranial aneurysms occur in patients with subacute bacterial endocarditis, some of whom have associated congenital or rheumatic heart disease. In a few patients with bacterial intracranial aneurysms, a diagnosis of endocarditis is not established. Usually there has been a history of infection such as pharyngitis, infected laceration, or drug addiction.

Bacterial aneurysms are due to infected emboli reaching the cerebral circulation and are most often located on a distal branch of an intracranial artery, usually a middle cerebral artery branch. This location tends to differentiate bacterial aneurysm from the more common developmental aneurysm usually found on the circle of Willis or proximal cerebral arteries.

Neurological problems are frequent in patients with bacterial endocarditis and may be the presenting symptoms. Neurological symptoms were found by Jones et al. in 29% (110 of 385) and Pruitt et al. in 39% (84 of 218) of patients with bacterial endocarditis (20, 42). The majority of patients have evidence of cerebral embolism with infarction, but hemorrhage (subarachnoid or intracerebral) and infarction followed by hemorrhage may occur. A few patients have had brain abscess or meningitis. Occasionally, headache has been noted without evidence of hemorrhage (22).

Intracranial bacterial aneurysms occur in 4-10% of patients with bacterial endocarditis (8). The incidence may be even higher since some aneurysms are asymptomatic. Multiple aneurysms occur in about 20% of the patients with an aneurysm, but the true figure is unknown since very few patients have had full angiography. The lesions may occur at any age.

When a patient with endocarditis develops a bacterial aneurysm, the most common presentation is subarachnoid or intracerebral hemorrhage. Patients without a previous diagnosis of bacterial endocarditis may have the onset of hemorrhage from a bacterial aneurysm as the first manifestation of the disease. Another clinical group first presents with symptoms and signs of cerebral ischemia, but an aneurysm is discovered with angiography. A few patients with cerebral infarction later develop a subarachnoid or intracerebral hemorrhage from an aneurysm (42). Recurrent hemorrhage occurs but the incidence is unknown.

In our review of 81 patients with documented bacterial aneurysms due to endocarditis, 65 had enough clinical information to determine the probable initial neurological event that led to the angiogram (Table 21.1). This was definite or probable hemorrhage in 42, infarction in 16, infarction followed by hemorrhage in five, and headache without hemorrhage in two. In 16 patients with a ruptured bacterial aneurysm, reported by Pruitt et al., eight had a history suggesting embolization and infarction prior to the hemorrhage (42). At angiography, an occluded vessel was often found in association with the aneurysm.

The most frequent organism cultured in patients

with bacterial aneurysms due to endocarditis has been streptococcus (Table 21.2). However, staphylococcus has become a common organism in the reports during the past few years. In some cases no organisms can be isolated from the blood culture due to prior antibiotics. In spite of the improvement in the recovery rate from infectious endocarditis with antibiotic treatment, the incidence of neurological complications of the disease has not been significantly reduced (22, 25). It is important to note that aneurysms can develop and hemorrhage can occur in a patient who is receiving adequate antibiotic treatment.

Diagnostic Studies

When there is evidence to suggest subarachnoid hemorrhage in a patient with bacterial endocarditis, a CT scan followed by cerebral angiography should be done. It has been suggested that the presence of cerebral embolization during the course of bacterial endocarditis is a strong indication for cerebral angiography (32).

The CT scan should be done with and without contrast enhancement. It may localize the aneurysm either directly or by demonstrating adjacent hematoma. The extent of intracerebral or intraventricular hemorrhage is determined. CT may also show edema, infarction, abscess and/or hydrocephalus.

Angiography is the definitive study to outline the location of the aneurysm and its relationship to the parent vessels (Figs. 21.1 to 21.4). If the diagnosis of associated subarachnoid hemorrhage is in doubt or if meningitis is suspected, a lumbar puncture is indicated after the CT scan has been done.

There is a striking predilection for involvement of the middle cerebral artery. No less dramatic is the tendency for involvement of a distal intracranial branch regardless of which artery is involved (Table 21.3). In the 71 patients in whom the site of the angiographically proven bacterial aneurysm was definitely established on the initial angiogram, 64 had at least one aneurysm on a distal branch of an intracranial artery, and in 55 a middle cerebral artery branch was involved. Very few patients have had complete

Table 21.1
Clinical Presentation in Patients Found to Have Bacterial Intracranial Aneurysms (Summary of Reported Cases through 1980)

Hemorrhage	42
Infarction	16
Infarction followed by hemorrhage	5
Headache without hemorrhage	2
No data	16

Table 21.2
Bacteriology (Summary of Reported Cases through 1980)

Streptococcus	36
Staphylococcus	15
Pseudomonus	2
Enterococcus	1
Corynebacterium	1
Cardiobacterium	1
Multiple organisms	4
No growth	10
No data	11

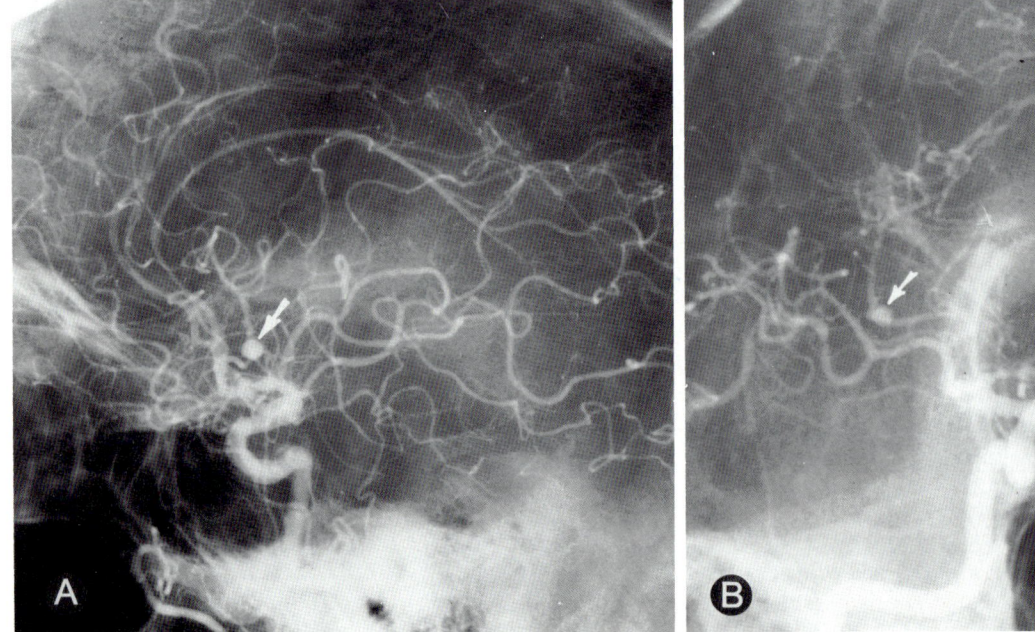

Figure 21.1 Bacterial intracranial aneurysm: distal middle cerebral artery branch. *A*, lateral angiogram showing aneurysm (*arrow*) on ascending frontal parietal branch of the MCA. *B*, oblique angiogram defines the relationship of the aneurysm (*arrow*) to the parent artery. Comment: The patient presented with an intracerebral hemorrhage and was found to have SBE.

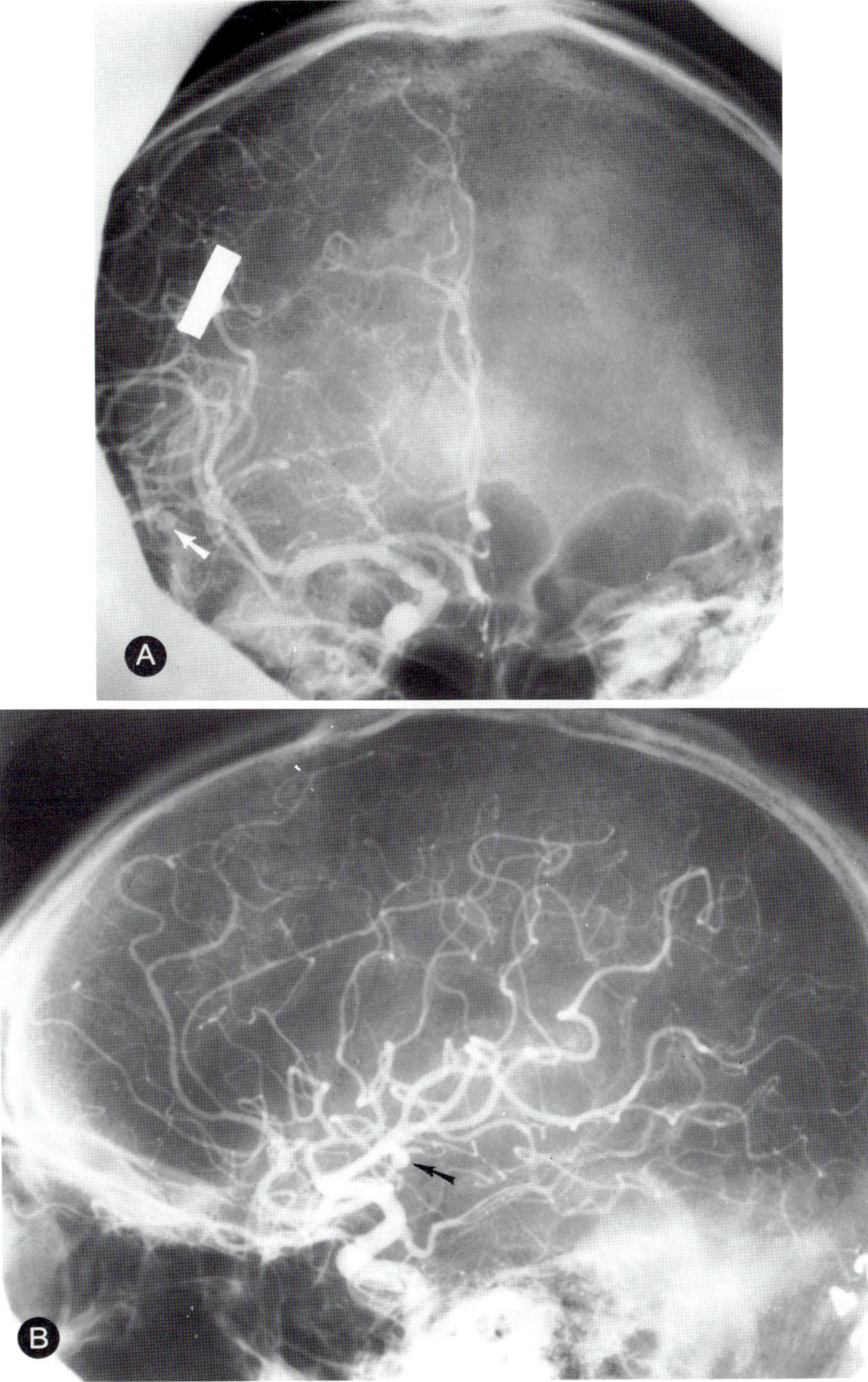

Figure 21.2 Bacterial intracranial aneurysm: distal middle cerebral artery branch. A and B, AP and lateral angiogram shows aneurysm on a superior temporal branch of the middle cerebral artery. Comment: The patient presented with a history of pharyngitis and then SAH. There was no evidence of SBE. The aneurysm was excised at operation. Pathological findings were consistent with an infectious lesion.

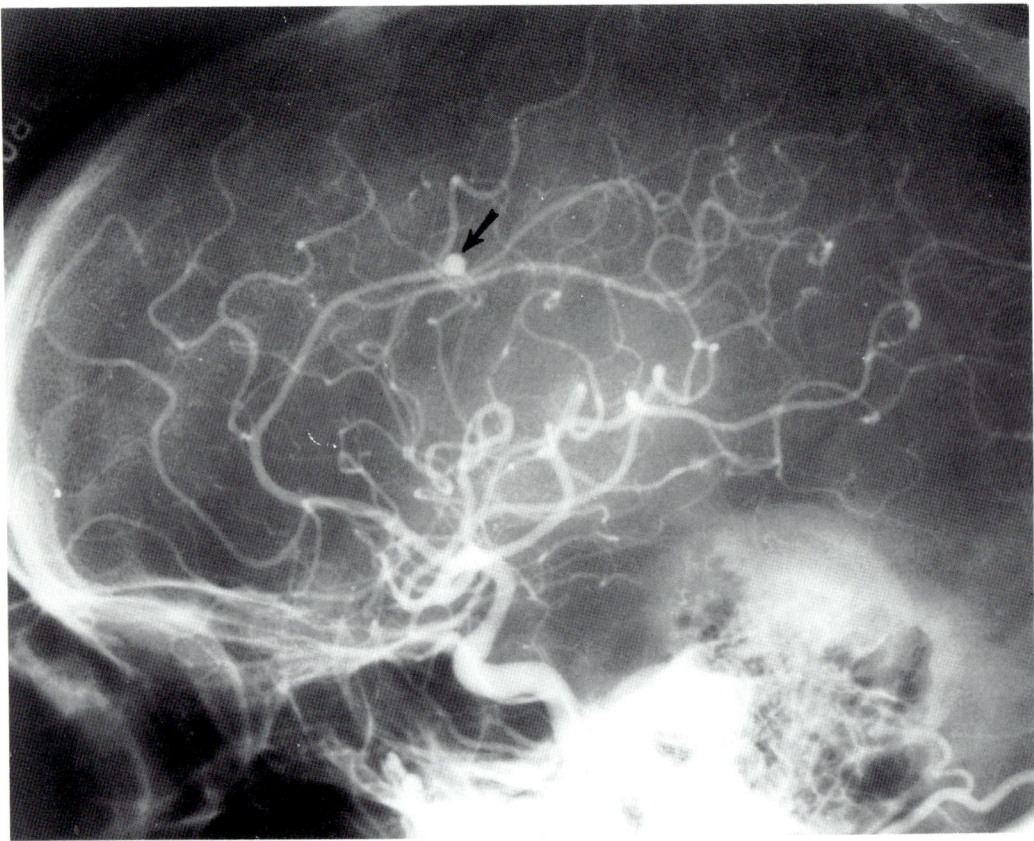

Figure 21.3 Bacterial intracranial aneurysm: distal anterior cerebral artery branch. The lateral angiogram shows the aneurysm (*arrow*) several centimeters distal to the site of the usual developmental pericallosal aneurysm. Comment: The patient had SBE. The lesion healed with antibiotic therapy.

Table 21.3
Findings on Initial Angiogram (Summary of Reported Cases through 1980)

Aneurysm location	
Single	61
Distal middle cerebral artery	44
Distal anterior cerebral artery	3
Distal posterior cerebral artery	4
Proximal intracranial artery	7
Not specified: middle cerebral artery	3
Multiple	15
Distal middle cerebral artery only	4
Distal middle cerebral artery and other vessels	7
Combinations not including distal MCA	2
Not specified	2
No aneurysm seen	5
Occluded artery in addition to aneurysm	13

angiography so the true incidence of multiple aneurysms is unknown.

Follow-up angiography was reported in 27 patients, who had not had surgery, within a few days to 8 months after the first study but usually within 2–8 weeks. A few patients had more than one follow-up study. In eight patients, a new aneurysm was found with three having had a normal initial angiogram. At the time of the last angiographic study, the aneurysm was no longer visualized in eight, was smaller in five, unchanged in four, larger in six, and in four a new aneurysm was found but no further study was reported. Seven other patients had postoperative angiography. The original aneurysm was gone in all cases but one patient had a new distal middle cerebral aneurysm that had ruptured.

Decisions Regarding Management

A program of treatment for patients with bacterial intracranial aneurysm can be outlined based on a review of the literature (7, 8, 12, 37, 38, 42, 43). Medical treatment should include the appropriate intravenous antibiotics the use of steroids and other medical measures to reduce cerebral edema when indicated. The use of antifibrinolytic agents has not been studied in this illness.

The place of surgical treatment has been discussed in several reports. Bingham reviewed 45 cases of bacterial intracranial aneurysms of all types where it was thought that adequate antibiotic treatment had been given and where angiography had been done

(7). He concluded that there did not appear to be a clear-cut advantage of surgery plus antibiotics over antibiotics alone. Twenty patients received only antibiotic treatment but three died from hemorrhage while under treatment. In the 25 patients who had combined antibiotic and surgical treatment, six died, but most of these were poor risk patients. He noted that the mortality associated with a definitive surgical procedure for bacterial intracranial aneurysm on distal arterial branches appeared to be quite low if one eliminated the poor risk surgical candidates from death due to cardiac or other medical problems and from fatal hemorrhage due to a second previously undiagnosed aneurysm. He recommended an operation only if the aneurysm enlarged or did not change in size after 6 weeks of antibiotic therapy. Bohmfalk et al. reviewed reports of 17 patients who had surgical removal of bacterial aneurysms of distal arterial branches (8). There was no mortality. These authors also noted six patients in the literature who did not develop hemorrhage until after completion of their antibiotic treatment for endocarditis. Cantu et al. reported an autopsy series of five patients with death due to rupture of a bacterial aneurysm, and all were receiving intensive antibiotic therapy at the time of the hemorrhage (9). Pruitt et al. reported nine patients who were adequately treated with antibiotics prior to aneurysmal ruptures (42). Frazee et al. concluded that patients with a diagnosis of bacterial endocarditis who develop sudden severe headache, focal neurological signs or symptoms of seizures should undergo serial angiography every 7 to 10 days throughout their hospitalization (12). If an aneurysm is identified, it should be excised whenever possible.

The results from a review of the literature of 81 patients who had angiography because of a neurological symptom and were found to have a bacterial aneurysm are outlined in Table 21.4. Of 30 patients treated with antibiotics, where the outcome was known, 13 died. Elective surgery was done in 29 patients; two patients died but both had recovered from surgery only to die from rupture of a second unrecognized aneurysm. As would be expected, the results were worse when emergency surgery was required, usually because an intracranial hematoma had caused a serious neurological deficit.

Our recommendations are as follows: 1) A single bacterial aneurysm on a distal middle cerebral artery branch associated with subarachnoid or intracerebral hemorrhage should be excised if the patient's medical condition is stable. 2) For bacterial aneurysm on the proximal arterial trunks, unruptured aneurysms or those involving arteries whose excision is very likely to cause a serious neurological deficit, a program of antibiotics and serial angiography is indicated. How often the angiogram should be done has not been established and recommendations have ranged from one to several weeks. We suggest 10-14 days. If the aneurysm is larger at follow-up angiography, surgery is indicated. If it is the same size or smaller, the antibiotic treatment is continued. Angiography is repeated at an appropriate interval and again when antibiotic treatment is completed. If the aneurysm does not disappear after treatment or at any time becomes larger, surgery is usually indicated.

The literature does not give a definitive answer as to what to do with the patient when multiple bacterial aneurysms are found. A review of 15 reported cases of multiple bacterial aneurysms, due to all causes including meningitis, revealed that 11 were treated nonsurgically and none died as a direct result of this treatment (12). Analysis of reports of 10 patients with multiple bacterial aneurysms seen on angiography and related to established or probable endocarditis revealed that seven were treated by antibiotics alone with only one death (37). This was in a patient who also was a heroin addict and had brain abscess and infarction. There is no explanation for these findings of a low mortality rate with antibiotic therapy alone as compared to the higher mortality rate for nonsurgically treated patients with a single aneurysm. However, we have already noted the fact that two patients who had recovered from elective surgery for removal of a single aneurysm subsequently died because of hemorrhage from a second unrecognized aneurysm. Frazee et al. proposed that if multiple aneurysms are unilateral, they should be excised at one operation wherever possible, and if they are bilateral, the largest or the one presumed to have bled should be excised and then the patient followed by angiography (12). Another suggestion is to treat the patient with antibiotics, repeat the angiogram at 2-week intervals and when therapy is completed. If the lesions become larger or do not disappear after treatment, surgery may be indicated.

In planning the surgical treatment, it is important to remember that these aneurysms have an inflammed, friable wall which may easily fragment. For peripheral lesions, the aneurysm can be excised with the small vessel from which it arises, usually with little or no neurological deficit. The less common proximal or less accessible lesions may present a more serious technical problem. Treatment with an-

Table 21.4
Treatment and Results (Summary of Reported Cases through 1980)

	Recovered[a]	Died	No information	Total
Antibiotics	17	13	1	31
Elective surgery[b]	27	2	0	29
Emergency surgery[b]	8	6	0	14
No treatment	1	1	1	3
No data	0	0	4	4

[a] Some patients who recovered from their neurological illness subsequently died from a cardiac cause and some were left with a neurological disability.
[b] Patients who had surgery also received antibiotics.

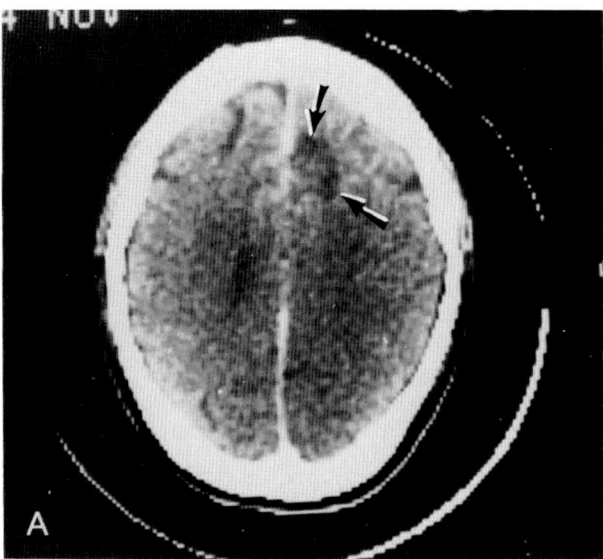
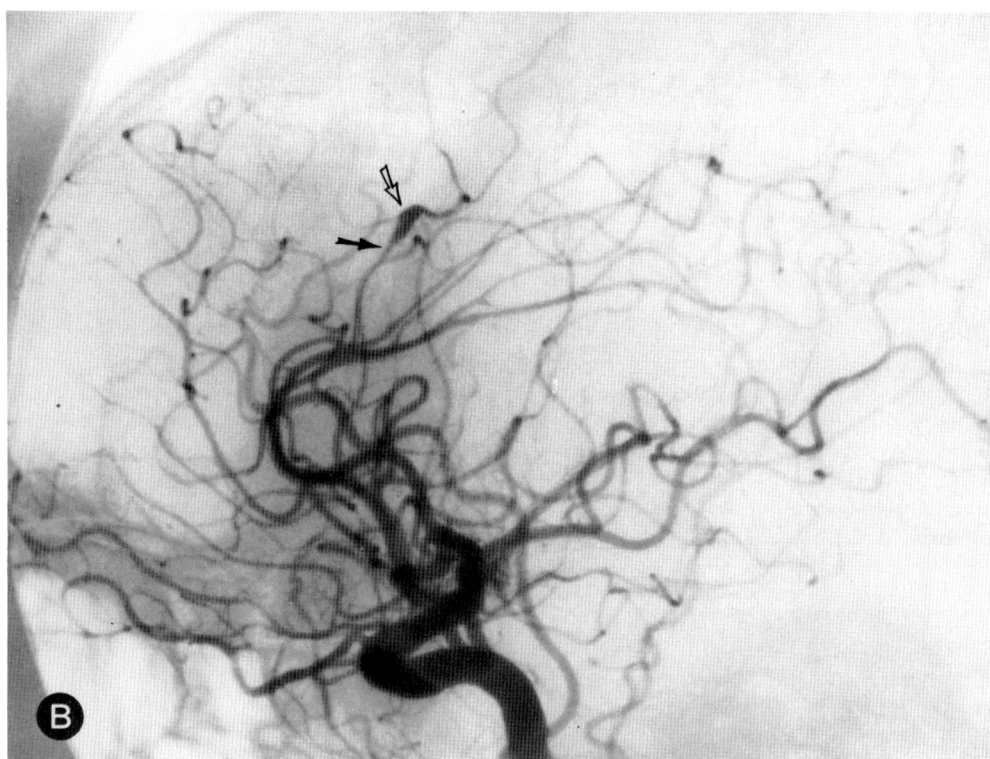

Figure 21.4 Bacterial intracranial aneurysm and associated brain abscess. *A,* initial CT scan when patient presented with a febrile episode (URI) and a rapidly progressive disturbance in mental function. A low density area with minimal adjacent enhancement is seen (*arrows*). *B,* angiogram shows a fusiform lesion (*open arrow*) on a distal branch of the anterior cerebral artery (*closed arrow*) consistent with a bacterial aneurysm. The low density area seen on CT was aspirated and an abscess confirmed. The patient was treated with antibiotic therapy. There was no evidence of SBE. *C,* CT scan 2 weeks later shows smaller abscess with well-defined capsule which enhances. *D,* angiogram shows the aneurysm to be smaller (*open arrow*) and marked narrowing of the parent vessel (*closed arrow*). Complete recovery followed a full course of antibiotic treatment.

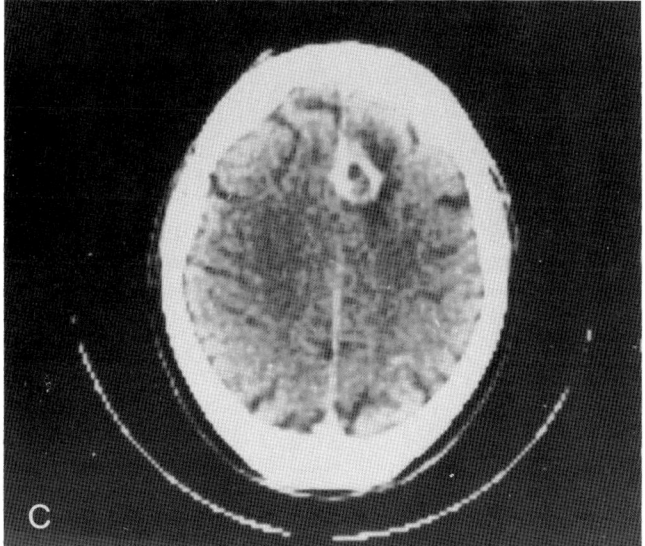
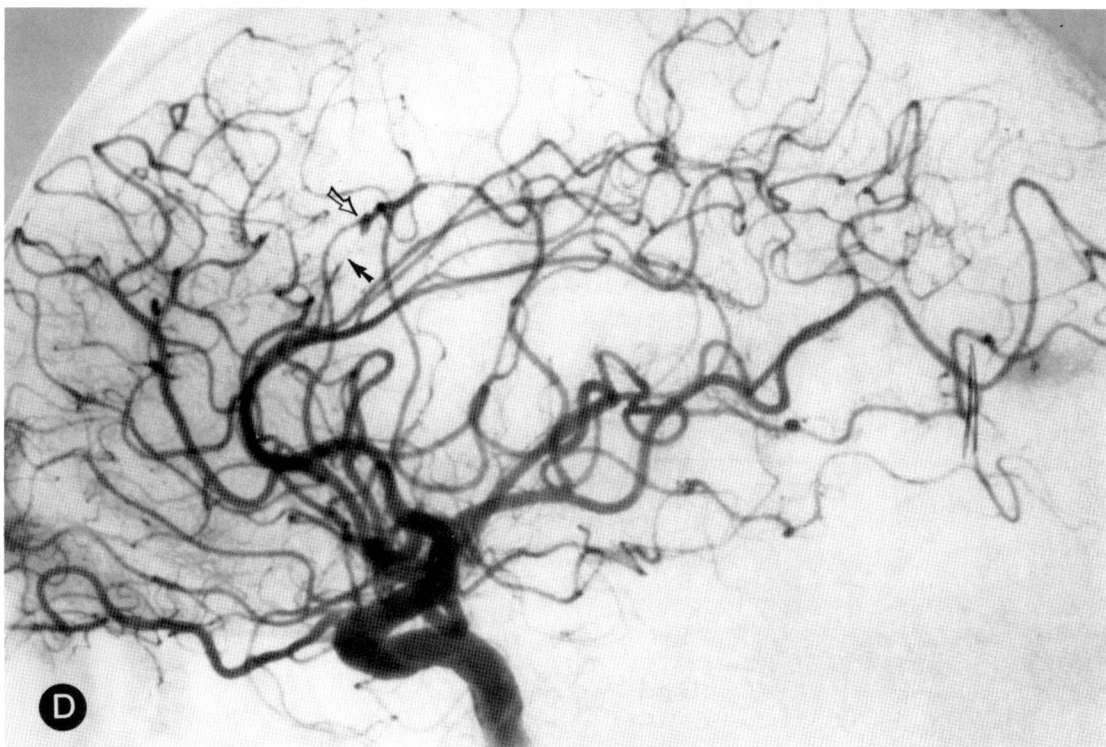

Figure 21.4 (C and D)

tibiotics may allow the arteritis to resolve with fibrosis in the wall of the aneurysm and parent artery. The lesion can then be handled more safely at surgery (43). If surgery is needed for a proximal lesion or aneurysm involving a critical artery, a bypass graft may be required as the initial procedure. This has been reported in two patients (10).

At the time of surgery, the neurosurgeon may encounter not only an intracerebral hematoma or an area of infarction but also a brain abscess (Fig. 21.4). In the series of cases reported through 1980, five patients had associated brain abscess.

BACTERIAL INTRACRANIAL ANEURYSMS ASSOCIATED WITH MENINGITIS

Arterial lesions have been described in meningitis caused by a variety of organisms. Extensive arterial changes can occur with a panarteritis which may lead to thrombosis, but on occasion the wall is weakened and an aneurysm forms. Five patients with aneurysms associated with meningitis and documented by angiography have been reported (15, 37, 39, 49, 50).

In two cases, hemorrhage occurred from the aneurysm, two presented with seizures and neurological deficit, and one developed a cavernous sinus syndrome due to another aneurysm. There is a striking difference between the location of these aneurysms and those associated with endocarditis: four of the six aneurysms involved the distal anterior cerebral artery branches and the one patient with a distal middle cerebral aneurysm had osteomyelitis of the adjacent skull.

Treatment considerations are the same as outlined for bacterial aneurysm associated with endocarditis.

BACTERIAL ANEURYSMS OF THE INTERNAL CAROTID ARTERY ASSOCIATED WITH CAVERNOUS SINUS THROMBOPHLEBITIS

Seven patients have been reported through 1978 where cavernous sinus thrombophlebitis was associated with development of an aneurysm of the internal carotid artery (25, 37, 46, 49, 51). In five patients, the thrombophlebitis followed an infection near the eye or on the face while one had an abscess of the ankle and the other pneumonia. In some patients, septicemia was found with no evidence of endocarditis. *Staphylococcus* was found in all five patients where a culture report was available. Persistent evidence of exophthalmus and ophthalmoplegia led to angiography.

Two patients were treated by common carotid ligation and one by a trapping operation. Angiography prior to operation had shown enlargement of the aneurysm in two of these patients.

FUNGAL INTRACRANIAL ANEURYSMS

The reports of 13 patients with fungal or "true" mycotic aneurysms have been reviewed (30). The most common causative organisms are *Aspergillus*, which spreads from sinuses or follows cranial surgery, *Phycomycetes*, seen in patients with diabetes mellitis or systemic illness, and *Candida*, seen with endocarditis and systemic infections.

The fungal aneurysm is usually located on a proximal major intracranial artery. However, in one case where the aneurysm was due to emboli from endocarditis, involvement was in the distal middle and anterior cerebral arteries. Associated thrombosis in contiguous or remote basal arteries is common.

Treatment of the local sinus condition or systemic illness with antifungal medication and a attempt at direct surgical therapy have been tried. There is no reported case with survival.

REFERENCES

1. Agnoli A, Bettag W: Endokarditis und subarachnoidalblutung. Z Neurol 199:295–305, 1971.
2. Ahuja GK, Jain N, Vijayaraghavan M, Roy S: Cerebral mycotic aneurysm of fungal origin. J Neurosurg 49:107–110, 1978.
3. Alajouanine T, Castaigne P, Lhermitte F, Cambier J: The cerebral arteritis of bacterial endocarditis: its late complications. J Am Med Assoc 170:1858, 1959.
4. Almazan V, Pulpon A, DeTeresa L, Catalan E, Burgui L, Artaza-Andrade M: Mycotic aneurysm secondary to bacterial endocarditis. Arch Inst Cardiol Mex 48:1224–1232, 1978.
5. Amine AR: Neurosurgical complications of heroin addiction: brain abscess and mycotic aneurysm. Surg Neurol 7:385–386, 1977.
6. Bell WE, Butler C II: Cerebral mycotic aneurysms in children. Two case reports. Neurology 18:81–86, 1968.
7. Bingham WF: Treatment of mycotic intracranial aneurysms. J Neurosurg 46:428–437, 1977.
8. Bohmfalk GL, Story JL, Wissinger JP, Brown WE Jr: Bacterial intracranial aneurysm. J Neurosurg 48:369–382, 1978.
9. Cantu RC, LeMay M, Wilkinson HA: The importance of repeated angiography in the treatment of mycotic-embolic intracranial aneurysms. J Neurosurg 25:189–193, 1966.
10. Day AL: Extracranial-intracranial bypass grafting in the surgical treatment of bacterial aneurysm. Report of two cases. Neurosurgery 9:583–588, 1981.
11. Davidson P, Robertson DM: A true mycotic (Aspergillus) aneurysm leading to fatal subarachnoid hemorrhage in a patient with hereditary hemorrhagic telangiectasia. Case report. J Neurosurg 35:71–76, 1971.
12. Frazee JG, Cahan LD, Winter J: Bacterial intracranial aneurysms. J Neurosurg 53:633–641, 1980.
13. Gilroy J, Andaya L, Thomas VJ: Intracranial mycotic aneurysms and subacute bacterial endocarditis in heroin addiction. Neurology 23:1193–1198, 1973.
14. Grinberg M, Lage SH, de Almeida GG, Stolf N, DeCourt LV: Infectious endocarditis, cerebral mycotic aneurysm and meningeal hemorrhage. Arq Bras Cardiol 32:257–261, 1979.
15. Harrison MJG, Hampton JR: Neurological presentation of bacterial endocarditis. Br Med J 2:148–151, 1967.
16. Horten BC, Abbott GF, Porro RS: Fungal aneurysms of intracranial vessels. Arch Neurol 33:577–579, 1976.
17. Hourihane JB: Ruptured mycotic intracranial aneurysm. A report of three cases. Vasc Surg 4:21–29, 1970.
18. Ishikawa M, Waga S, Moritake K, Handa H: Cerebral bacterial aneurysms: report of three cases. Surg Neurol 2:257–261, 1974.
19. Jara FM, Lewis JF Jr, Magilligan DJ Jr: Operative experience with infective endocarditis and intracerebral mycotic aneurysm. J Thorac Cardiovasc Surg 80:28–30, 1980.

20. Jones HR Jr, Siekert RG, Geraci JE: Neurologic manifestations of bacterial endocarditis. Ann Intern Med 71: 21-28, 1969.
21. Katz RI, Goldberg HI, Selzer ME: Mycotic aneurysm. Case report with novel sequential angiographic findings. Arch Intern Med 134:939-942, 1974.
22. Kaufman SL, White RI Jr, Harrington DP, Barth KH, Siegelman SS: Protean manifestations of mycotic aneurysm. Am J Roentgenol 131:1019-1025, 1978.
23. King AB: Successful surgical treatment of an intracranial mycotic aneurysm complicated by a subdural hematoma. J Neurosurg 17:788-791, 1960.
24. Laguna J, Derby BM, Chase R: Cardiobacterium hominis endocarditis with cerebral mycotic aneurysm. Arch Neurol 32:438-439, 1975.
25. Lansky LL, Maxwell JA: Mycotic aneurysm of the internal carotid artery in an unusual intracranial location. Dev Med Child Neurol 17:79-88, 1975.
26. Mahaley MS, Spock A: An unusual case of intracranial aneurysm, in Smith JL (ed): *Neuro-ophthalmology*. St. Louis, CV Mosby, 1968, vol 4, pp 148-166.
27. Maly Z: Paraventricular hemorrhage from a mycotic aneurysm. Cesk Neurol Neurochir 41:394-396, 1978.
28. Matson DD: Intracranial arterial aneurysms in childhood. J Neurosurg 23:578-583, 1965.
29. McNeel D, Evans RA, Ory EM: Angiography of cerebral mycotic aneurysms. Acta Radiol Diagn 9:407-412, 1969.
30. Mielke B, Weir B, Oldring D, von Westarp C: Fungal aneurysm: Case report and review of the literature. Neurosurgery 9:578-582, 1981.
31. Morin MA, Talalla A: Angiography for mycotic aneurysm. N Engl J Med 281:1249-1250, 1969 (letter).
32. Moskowitz MA, Rosenbaum AE, Tyler HR: Angiographically monitored resolution of cerebral mycotic aneurysms. Neurology 24:1103-1108, 1974.
33. Nishimura T, Aoki N, Aruga T, Hashimoto I, Imanaga H, Kubota M, Mizutani H, Tanishima K: A case of mycotic aneurysm after open heart surgery. No Shinkei Geka 7:371-375, 1979.
34. Ng KK, Wong WK, Skene-Smith H: Ruptured mycotic intracranial aneurysm. Australas Radiol 19:255-257, 1975.
35. Noonan JA, Wilson CB, Spencer FC, Talbert WM Jr: Cerebral and cardiac complications from bacterial endocarditis. A Successfully managed case with unusual complications. Am J Dis Child 116:666-674, 1968.
36. North-Coombes D, Schonland MM: Cerebral mycotic aneurysm. A case report. S Afr Med J 48:1808-1810, 1974.
37. Ojemann RG: Infectious intracranial aneurysms, in Fein J, Flamm E (eds): *Cerebral Vascular Disease* (in Press).
38. Ojemann RG: Treatment of Bacterial Intracranial Aneurysms, in Schmidek H (ed): *Current Techniques in Operative Neurosurgery* (in press).
39. Ojemann RG, New PFJ, Fleming TC: Intracranial aneurysms associated with bacterial meningitis. Neurology 16:1222-1226, 1966.
40. Osler W: Gulstonian lectures on malignant endocarditis. Lancet 1:415-418, 459-464, 505-508, 1885.
41. Pool JL, Potts DG: *Aneurysms and Arteriovenous Anomalies of the Brain*. New York, Harper and Row, 1965, pp 60-62.
42. Pruitt AA, Rubin RH, Karchmer AW, Duncan GW: Neurologic complications of bacterial endocarditis. Medicine 57:329-343, 1978.
43. Roach MR, Drake CG: Ruptured cerebral aneurysms caused by micro-organisms. N Engl J Med 273:240-244, 1965.
44. Sato T, Sakuta Y, Suzuki J, Takaku A: Successful surgical treatment of intracranial mycotic aneurysm with brain abscess. Acta Neurochir 47:53-61, 1979.
45. Schold C, Earnest MP: Cerebral hemorrhage from a mycotic aneurysm developing during appropriate antibiotic therapy. Stroke 9:267-268, 1978.
46. Shibuya S, Igarashi S, Amo T, Sato H, Fukumitsu T: Mycotic aneurysms of the internal carotid artery. Case report. J Neurosurg 44:105-108, 1976.
47. Shillito J Jr: Strokes in children. Clin Neurosurg 23:185-219, 1976.
48. Simmons KC, Sage MR, Reilly PL: CT of intracerebral hemorrhage due to mycotic aneurysm. Case report. Neuroradiology 19:215-217, 1980.
49. Suwanwela C, Suwanwela N, Charuchinda S, Hongsaprabhas C: Intracranial mycotic aneurysms of extravascular origin. J Neurosurg 36:552-559, 1972.
50. Sypert GW, Young HF: Ruptured mycotic pericallosal aneurysm with meningitis due to Neisseria meningitidis infection. Case report. J Neurosurg 37:467-469, 1972.
51. Tanemura H, Sakai N, Yamamori T, Yamada H: Intracranial mycotic aneurysm. Report of a case. Neurol Surg (Tokyo) 5:871-875, 1977.
52. Valadares JB, deSouza MT, Hankinson J, Hall K, Sengupta R: Multiple intracranial mycotic aneurysms. Case report. *Arq Neuropsiquiatr* 37:311-318, 1979.
53. Visudhiphan P, Bunyaratavej S, Khantanaphar S: Cerebral aspergillosis. Report of 3 cases. J Neurosurg 38:472-476, 1973.
54. Yarnell PR, Stears J: Intracerebral hemorrhage and occult sepsis. Neurology 24:870-873, 1974.
55. Ziment I, Johnson BL Jr: Angiography in the management of intracranial mycotic aneurysms. Arch Intern Med 122:349-352, 1968.

Chapter 22 ARTERIOVENOUS MALFORMATIONS OF THE BRAIN

Arteriovenous malformation (AVM) of the brain is a cluster of direct communications between arteries and veins of congenital origin. While there are documented cases of rapid progressive enlargement of AVMs, this is a rare finding (35, 42). In most cases, the lesion remains unchanged or the enlargement is very slow over many years (10, 24, 42). There is a well-known association with intracranial saccular aneurysm, which usually occurs on a major feeding artery to the AVM (30). When bleeding occurs in the setting of associated aneurysm and AVM, it is usually the aneurysm which has ruptured (10).

The prevalence of AVM is relatively small, accounting for about 10% of all intracranial hemorrhages. Nonetheless, AVM represents the third most common cause of intracranial bleeding after saccular aneurysm and spontaneous intraparenchymal bleeding.

Pathological studies show that AVMs are composed of dilated, thin-walled arteriovenous channels which lack internal elastic lamina (10, 30). The feeding and draining vessels appear to be normal but may be hypertrophied. Careful scrutiny of pathological material has shown the presence of xanthochromia in virtually all specimens, suggesting that some degree of hemorrhage is a very common feature. Most of the cerebral AVMs are roughly conical in shape, with the apex touching the ventricular surface and the base at the cortex. This location reflects the embryological origin of the AVMs as a persistence of normally regressing channels linking the surface with the lining of the primitive neural tube. AVMs may be found throughout the brain, including all the lobes of the cerebrum, the corpus callosum, basal ganglia, cerebellum, and brainstem.

CLINICAL PRESENTATION

Intracranial AVMs present with intracranial bleeding in some 50% of the cases (10). Ordinarily, the hemorrhage is largely intraparenchymal, although extension into the ventricular system is common, and associated subarachnoid hemorrhage not unusual. The impact of intracranial bleeding is variable. According to the Cooperative Study, approximately 10% will die from the first hemorrhage, and of the survivors, roughly 14% are disabled (30).

The second most common presentation is a convulsive disorder, sometimes difficult to control by ordinary medical measures. AVMs may also cause cerebral dysfunction by virtue of mass effect, increased venous pressure, or vascular steal phenomena. Rarely, AVMs lead to intractable headache, which may sometimes be cured by surgical excision.

Waltimo compared the size of the malformation with the onset of symptoms (41). In 25 patients with an AVM volume in excess of 7 cm^3, 18 (72%) presented with seizures and seven (28%) with hemorrhage, while in 20 cases with an AVM volume of less than 7 cm^3, five (25%) presented with seizures and 15 (75%) with hemorrhage. He also reported that frontal malformations had a tendency to present with seizures and occipital malformations with hemorrhage.

The risk of rebleeding from AVMs has been discussed by several authors (10, 17, 30, 38, 42). The largest source of information is the Cooperative Study, but the period of follow-up was not long: an average of 6.5 years (3–10 years) (30). Kjellberg, quoted by Drake, has derived from these data a rebleed rate of 3.7% per year for AVMs which had ruptured, with a 0.9% rate of death per year from that hemorrhage (10). In the same analysis, patients presenting with seizures experienced hemorrhage at a rate of approximately 1% per year, with no deaths. Studies with longer follow-up have indicated that recurrent bleeding from intracranial AVM constitutes a major hazard to life (14, 22, 29, 38). This includes the report by Forster et al. who reviewed Olivecrona's series with a mean follow-up of 15 years and found that in 35 patients who were managed conservatively, 17% died from hemorrhage and 20% were severely disabled (11). They also found that the patient who had epilepsy but who had never bled had a 1 in 4 chance of hemorrhage in 15 years; the patient who had bled once had a 1 in 4 chance of bleeding again in 4 years, and the patient who had bled twice had a 1 in 4 chance of bleeding again within 1 year. Troupp's long-term follow-up of 137 untreated AVMs indicated that only 27 patients were well, 14 were in fair condition, 28 disabled, 23 were dead from the AVM, 10 were dead from other causes, and 19 were lost to follow-up (39). There seemed to be a worse prognosis in parietal central and infratentorial lesions in this series. Waltimo has produced evidence to suggest that devastating hemorrhage is more common from smaller and moderate-sized lesions than from large ones (42).

While the long-term outlook seems threatening for patients with AVM, the risk of treatment must be less than that of the outlined natural history. Surgical excision has traditionally been the treatment of choice (26). Other treatment modes are being developed, including intravascular techniques and the use of high energy irradiation.

EVALUATION

In the patient with sudden onset of headache and neurological deficit, the diagnosis of AVM must be considered. Likewise, focal motor seizures or focal neurological deficit will raise the question of AVM, along with other intracranial abnormalities. Occasionally, intractable headaches, particularly with migraine or its equivalent, will raise suspicion of intracranial AVM.

In all cases of suspected AVM, computed tomography, with and without contrast enhancement, may be diagnostic. In the setting of intracranial bleeding, CT can pinpoint the location, dimensions, mass effect, and extension of the hemorrhage. The location of the hemorrhage may indeed suggest a diagnosis of AVM, particularly in a younger patient without a history of hypertension or anticoagulant therapy (Figs. 22.1 and 22.2, A and B). After the administration of contrast material, dilated venous channels draining the AVM may be visualized (Fig. 22.2, C to E).

This finding is highly suggestive of the diagnosis. Its absence does not exclude the possibility of AVM, in that the resolution of even fourth-generation scanners may be inadequate to detect certain small lesions, or the lesion may be compressed by the hematoma. The unenhanced scan may show high density in some patients who have not bled, particularly where there is a thrombosed AVM or in those that have calcification.

For the patient with hemorrhage as the initial presentation, other studies should include a coagulation profile (prothrombin time, partial thromboplastin time and platelet count) together with routine admission studies (EKG, serum electrolytes). For the patient with convulsive seizures, an EEG will be useful for characterization of the discharge focus and follow-up during medical therapy.

For most patients suspected of harboring an AVM, the definitive diagnosis is made with cerebral angiography. An adequate angiogram will demonstrate not only the lesion, but also all feeding arteries and draining veins. High-speed angiographic technique, with four exposures per second in the arterial phase, is recommended for depiction of the dynamics of

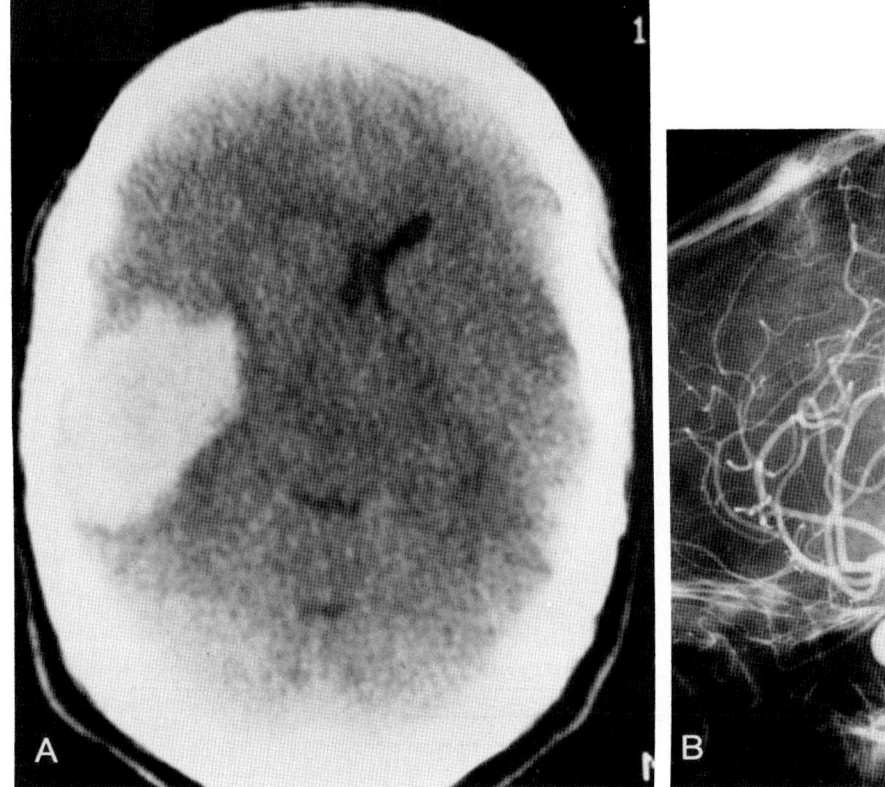
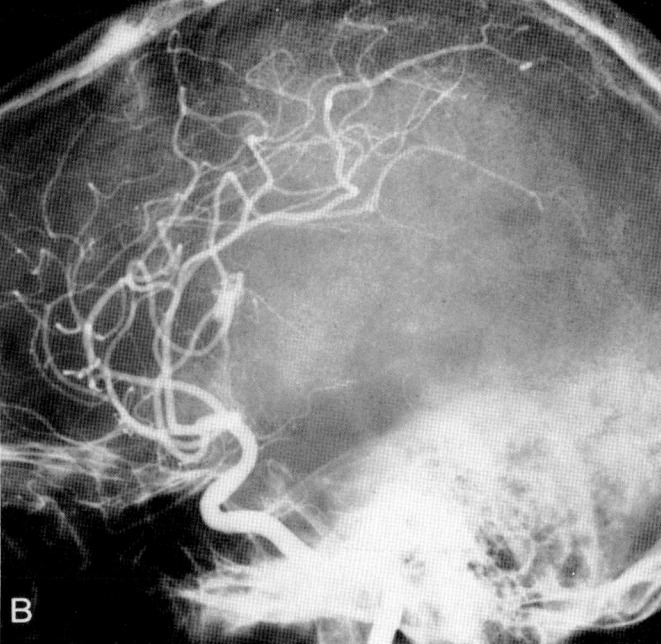

Figure 22.1 CT scan and history suggest AVM. *A*, CT scan shows a large left posterior temporal hematoma with no blood in the cisterns. *B*, angiogram demonstrates a small anterior Sylvian AVM with evidence of a large temporal mass effect. Comment: In a 37-year-old man with the sudden onset of right hemiparesis, the location of hematoma, absence of blood in the cisterns, and lack of history of hypertension or coagulation disorder made AVM the most likely diagnosis. The patient made a full recovery following surgery.

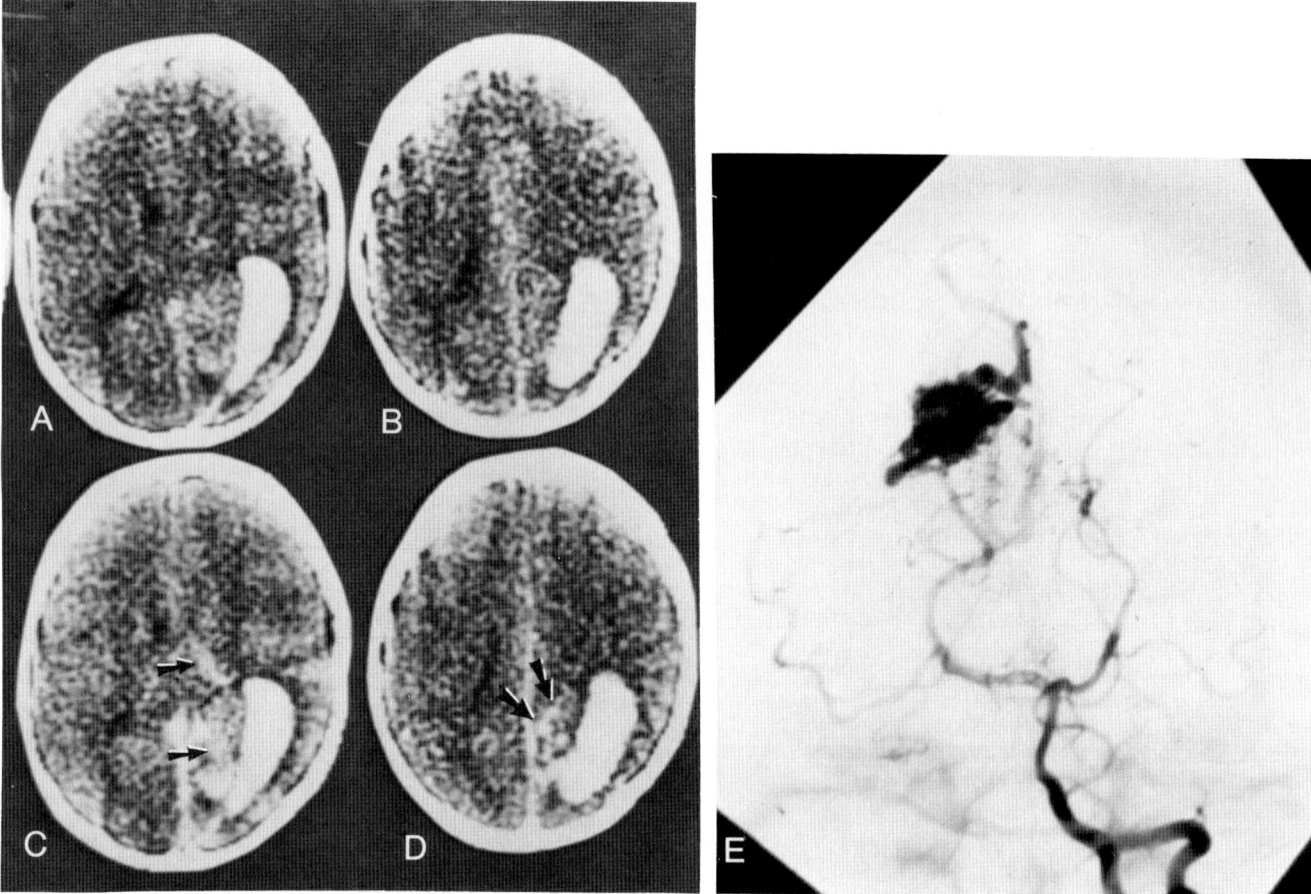

Figure 22.2 CT after contrast shows AVM. *A* and *B*, scans done before contrast injection show a right occipital lobe hematoma. *C* and *D*, after contrast injection, dilated vessels of the AVM are outlined (*arrows*). *E*, angiogram confirms the diagnosis of a right occipital AVM. Comment: The location of the hematoma in a young patient with the sudden onset of neurological deficits suggests a diagnosis of AVM. This is confirmed on the CT scan.

feeding arteries and draining veins. The external carotid circulation should be studied, because it may supply branches to a lesion involving the cortex, especially those abutting the tentorium (6).

Occasionally, a patient with an intraparenchymal hemorrhage and no obvious cause (hypertension, brain tumor, anticoagulation) will not show an arteriovenous malformation on angiography, although the location of the hemorrhage on the CT scan suggests this possibility. This situation may arise from obliteration or compression of the AVM by the local hematoma. The cause may be defined by angiography performed 3 weeks or more after the hemorrhage (Fig. 22.3). At this interval, some of the hematoma will have resolved, and an AVM may now fill when studied angiographically.

Another uncommon situation is the patient who presents with a seizure or onset of mild neurological deficit suggesting brain tumor, and the CT scan shows a hyperdense lesion without contrast which persists indefinitely, which may enhance, and where angiography remains negative (Fig. 22.4). At operation, a well-demarcated lesion is found, usually with evidence of old hemorrhage, and on microscopic examination a thrombosed AVM is seen (13, 33). We have encountered five such lesions, one each in the frontal and temporal regions, two in the cerebellum, and one in the brain stem. None had any major feeding arteries. All had hyperdense lesions on the non-contrast CT, presumably due to the area of thrombosis. In several patients, repeat CT scans had been done over several months.

SURGICAL EXCISION

Unless there is an intracerebral or subdural hematoma that demands early intervention, the operation on an AVM can wait until there is full recovery from the effects of the SAH or intracerebral bled. Since there is little risk of early rehemorrhage, epsilon-aminocaproic acid is not used and efforts are directed to reducing the effects of cerebral edema. The surgeon may wish to wait at least 3-4 weeks after the hemorrhage to allow maximum recovery. However, one does not want to postpone the opera-

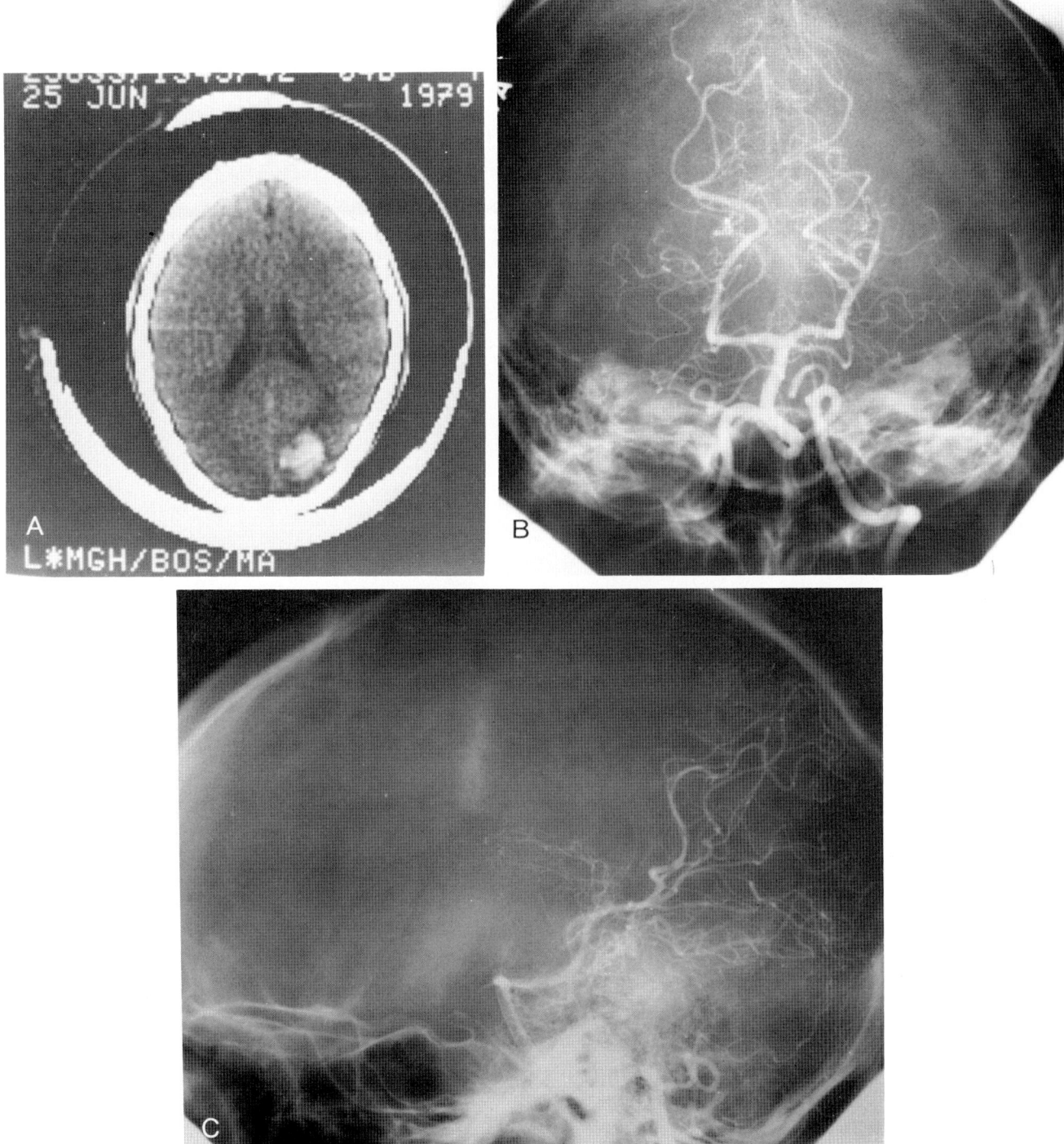

Figure 22.3 Demonstration of AVM on delayed angiogram. *A,* CT scan shows a right occipital lobe hematoma. *B* and *C,* AP and lateral vertebral angiogram reveals no abnormality. The carotid studies were also normal. *D* and *E,* AP and lateral vertebral angiogram 3 weeks later shows filling of a small AVM and an early draining vein (*arrows*). Comment: This 19-year-old boy had the sudden onset of headache. The second angiogram was done at a planned interval of time.

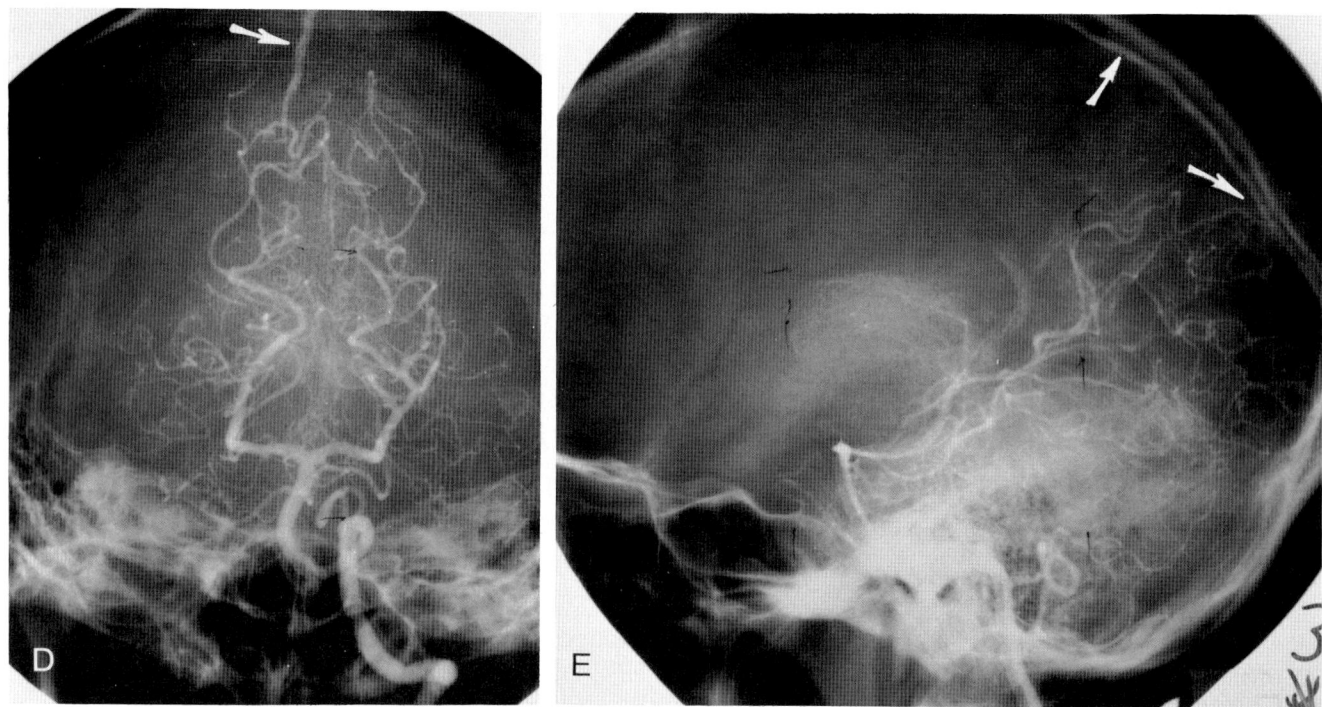

Figure 22.3 (*D* and *E*)

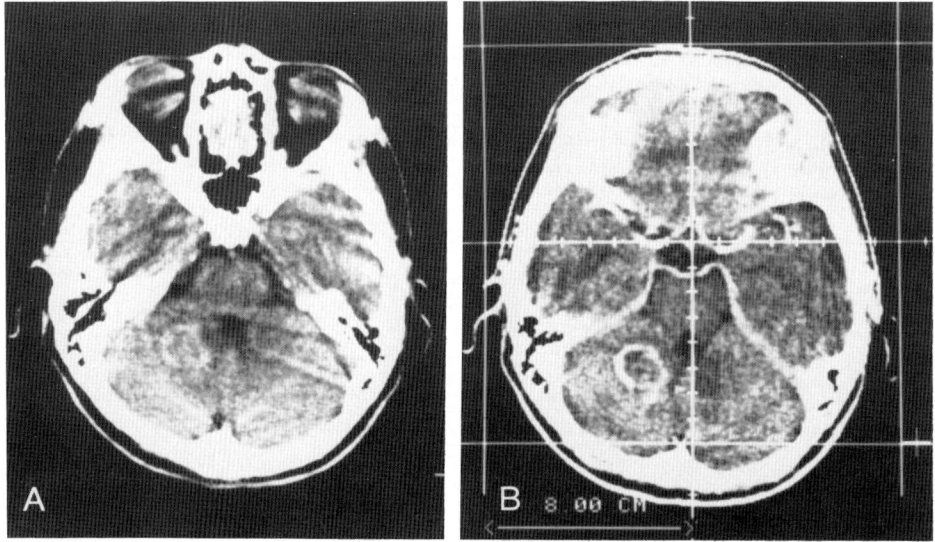

Figure 22.4 Symptomatic occult (thrombosed) AVM. *A*, CT scan done without contrast. Note hyperdense paraventricular lesion in the right cerebellar hemisphere. *B*, CT done after intravenous contrast injection shows enhancement in the periphery of the lesion. Comment: Patient presented with onset of difficulty using her right hand and slight unsteadiness of gait and had right cerebellar signs on examination. The cerebellar dysfunction persisted and she developed nausea. Angiogram was normal. At operation, a localized lesion was found and excised. There had been a small old hemorrhage. Pathological examination revealed a thrombosed AVM.

tion too long since the presence of a hematoma may aid in the dissection of the AVM. In some patients, preoperative embolization will be a useful preoperative adjunct (see "Embolization" p 271).

In some very large lesions, with a substantial sump effect stealing from the brain, total obliteration may result in catastrophic cerebral edema (10, 36, 41, 43). This phenomenon may be related to shunting of blood, formerly destined for the AVM, back into the cerebrum, which is unable to autoregulate the sudden increase in volume of blood. The new flow patterns may thus lead to severe edema and even hemorrhage and death. In this setting, a staged elimination of the lesion, a two-stage operation or embolization and then excision may be the safest approach.

Technique

The general aspects of the anesthesia and the measures to reduce brain tension prior to opening the dura are the same as recorded in Chapter 11 for aneurysms. Hypotension has not been utilized routinely, but on occasion it may be important in controlling hemorrhage from the fragile vascular walls.

In most patients, operation is designed to pursue the conical AVM from its base at the surface to its apex at the ventricle. Use of the operating microscope and bipolar coagulation have made possible the separation of margins of cerebral AVMs from banks of neighboring gyri. Furthermore, microsurgery has been helpful in identification of the gliotic plane that surrounds the AVM in the white matter.

Most often, AVMs that bleed do so into the parenchyma, particularly subcortical white matter. In the case of large hematomas, the bleeding zone and subsequent cavitation are evident on the CT scan. Even in cases where the CT does not show such a hematoma, a thin zone of prior bleeding with improved dissection plane is often present. Identification of this plane of cleavage with the operating microscope is the key to further dissection. A thin xanthochromic edge with slightly increased fullness to the tissue will be characteristic of the zone of optimum dissection. As one proceeds along the margin of the lesion, knuckles of red AVM will be seen protruding beyond this gliotic capsule. Generally, a red draining vein can lead to the main nidus of the AVM. In silent brain, one can dissect with a 16-gauge sucker, just superficial to the layer of gliosis in order to avoid annoying bleeding. One should stay close to the lesion, however, lest the plane of dissection wander into important brain tissue. Use of a fine dissector, suction, or the bipolar forceps serves to define the gliotic plane. In eloquent zones, one must stay right on the surface of the AVM, sparing critical pia and neighboring gray matter. When one encounters small feeding vessels, these are electrocoagulated with bipolar cautery and then cut. Larger feeding arteries may also need to be clipped and coagulated. On some very large arteries aneurysm clips are used.

If bleeding should occur, light pressure on a cottonoid usually suffices to control the oozing. Sometimes bipolar cauterization will be needed, or even application of small bits of Surgicel. Occasionally, with more vigorous hemorrhage, an aneurysm clip may be used to seal the rent. A common characteristic of small tiny feeding arteries is their fragility. Very light bipolar coagulation with a delicate grasping movement may be used, or even tangential application of the forceps, together with constant saline irrigation to prevent sticking of the forceps. The dissection is planned to permit early access to major feeding arteries for their occlusion. At least one major draining vein is preserved for occlusion as the final step in the excision. When there is any doubt about the suitability of occluding a draining vein, it is temporally clipped, and the effect on the AVM carefully assessed to be sure there is no swelling before permanent occlusion is applied.

As much retraction as possible is done against the AVM, but retraction of brain tissue may be required to obtain the requisite space to work, since the AVM cannot be debulked interiorly. For large lesions, substantial retraction may be required as provided by the Greenberg self-retaining retractor.

The surgical approach is governed by the size and precise location of the lesion. For many convexity lesions, a standard craniotomy flap, with generous margins around the lesion, will provide the required access. Whenever the lesion approaches the midline, it is well to take the craniotomy flap across the midline to permit flexibility as one opens the dura near the superior sagittal sinus. Every effort should be made to preserve important bridging veins emptying into the superior sagittal sinus. Lesions in important areas, such as the angular gyrus, will require utmost care to avoid injury (Fig. 22.5). Dissection must stay right on the surface of the AVM. Large lesions in eloquent zones carry the highest morbidity for surgical excision, but this has been reduced with microsurgical techniques (Fig. 22.6).

In dealing with a lesion on the falx or the tentorium, it may be necessary to excise part of these structures with the AVM, or utmost care utilized in separation by electrocoagulation of the lesion from the falx or tentorium. This is a difficult business; the CT scan is useful in suggesting whether a thin rim of brain tissue along the midline will make the dissection easier in these regions.

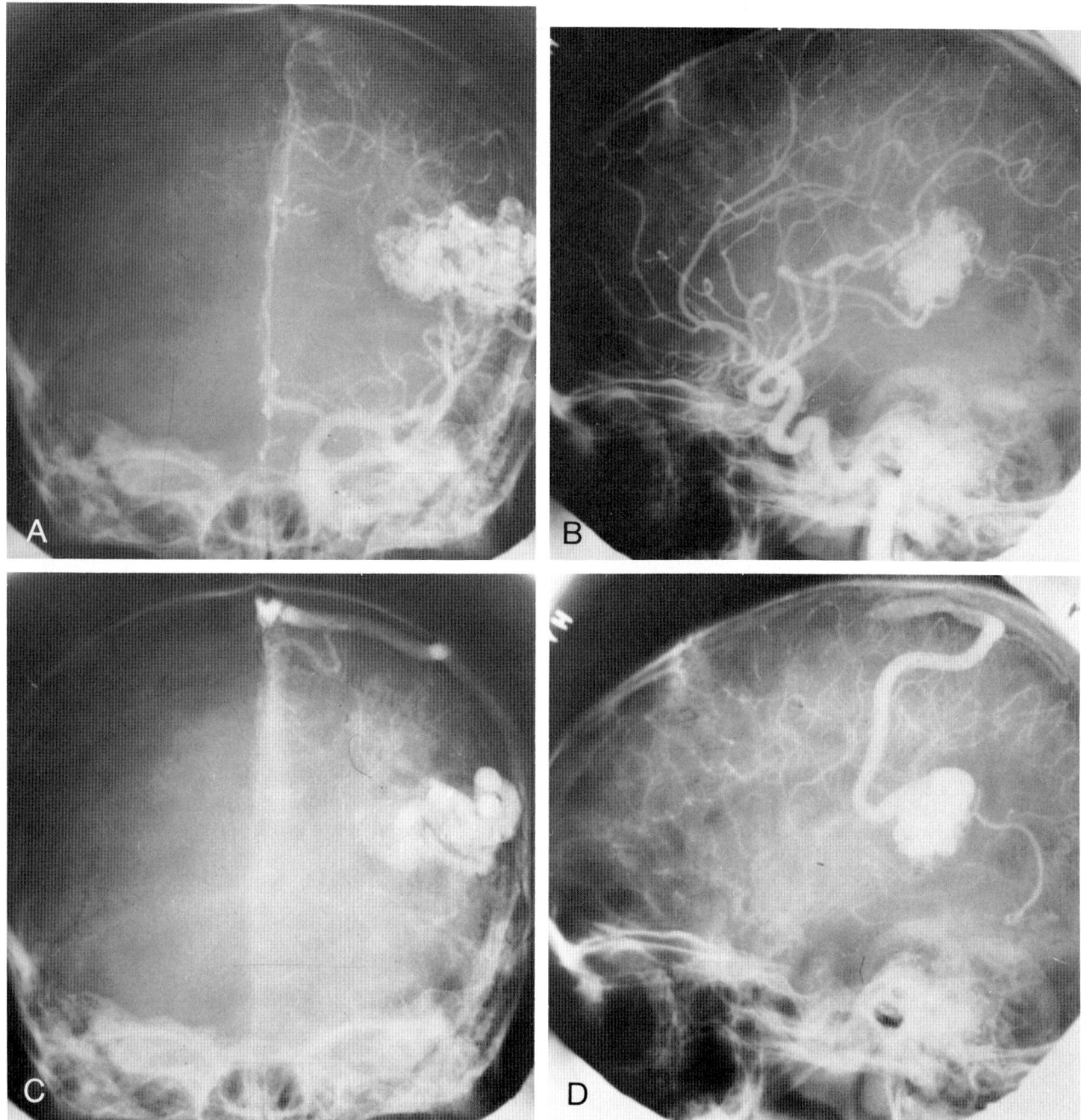

Figure 22.5 Total excision of AVM in Wernicke's area. *A* to *D*, left carotid angiogram shows a localized convexity AVM in the region of left angular gyrus with the venous drainage toward the midline. *E* and *F*, there is some arterial supply to the medial portion of the malformation from the posterior cerebral artery. *G* to *I*, total excision of the AVM has been accomplished with preservation of the major arterial vessels supplying important brain distal to the AVM. Comment: The patient was a 13-year-old boy who had seizures that were difficult to control. Postoperatively, seizure control was easily accomplished and the neurological examination was normal.

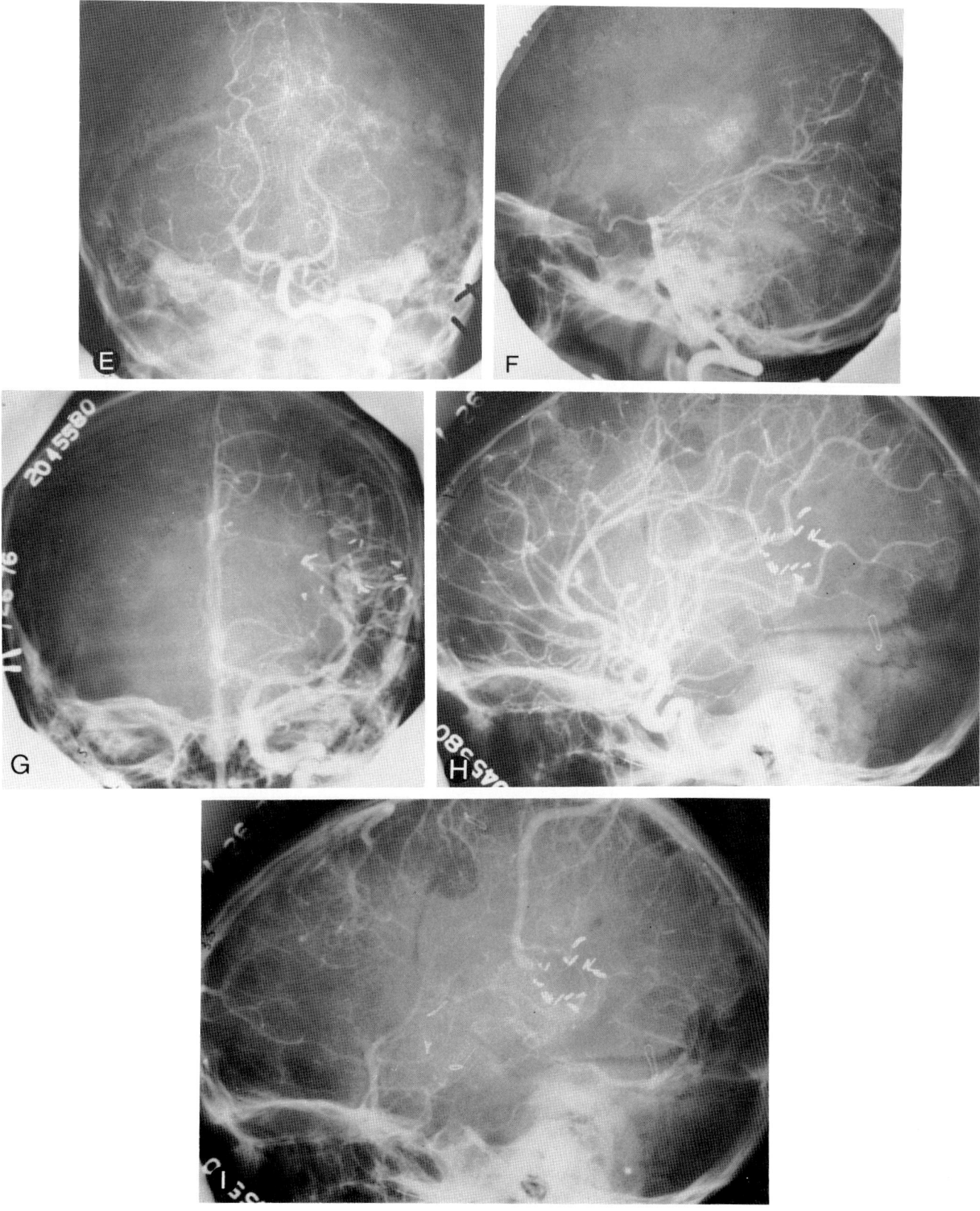

Figure 22.5 (*E* to *I*)

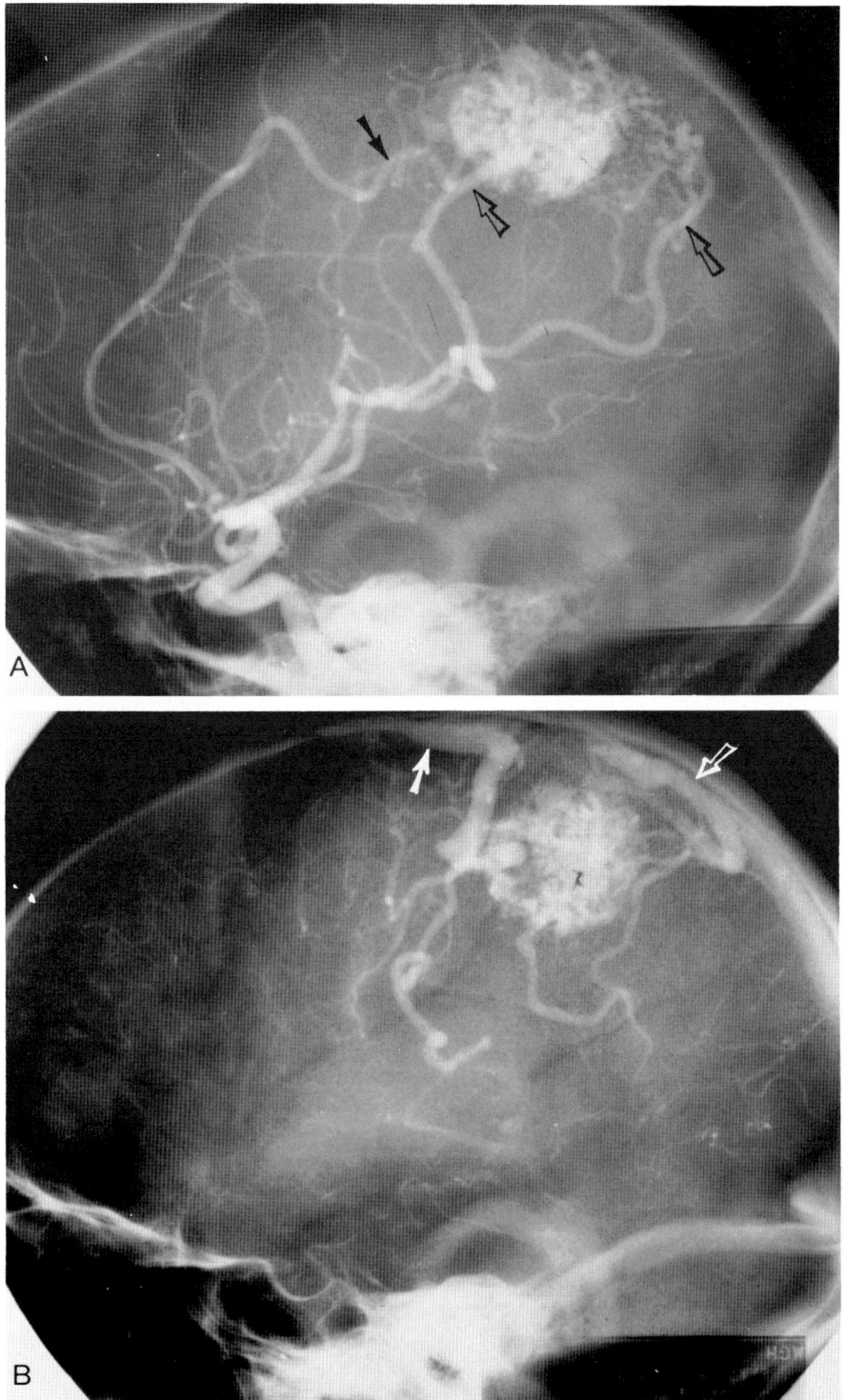

Figure 22.6 Parietal parasagittal AVM. *A* to *C*, preoperative right carotid angiogram shows in *A* and *C* the feeding branches from the anterior (*closed arrows*) and middle (*open arrows*) cerebral arteries. *B*, venous drainage is both anterior and posterior from the lesion. *D*, the vertebral angiogram reveals supply from anastomosis to posterior parietal branches. *E* and *F*, postoperative angiogram shows complete excision of the AVM. Note preservation of the distal circulation in the middle cerebral artery branch to the Rolandic area (*middle arrow*). Comment: This 32-year-old man had a mild hemorrhage from this AVM. Postoperatively, the neurological examination was normal.

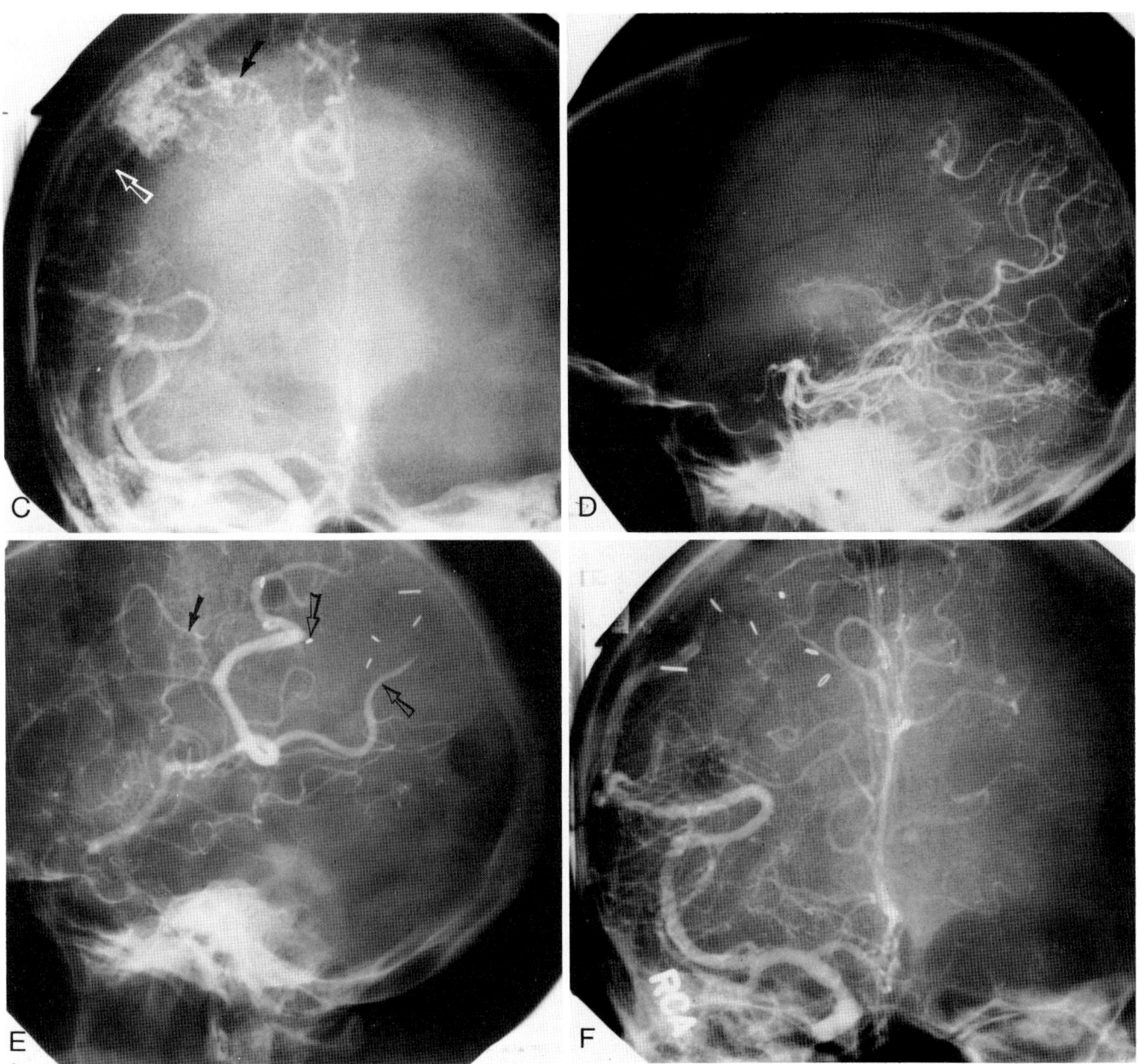

Figure 22.6 (*C* to *F*)

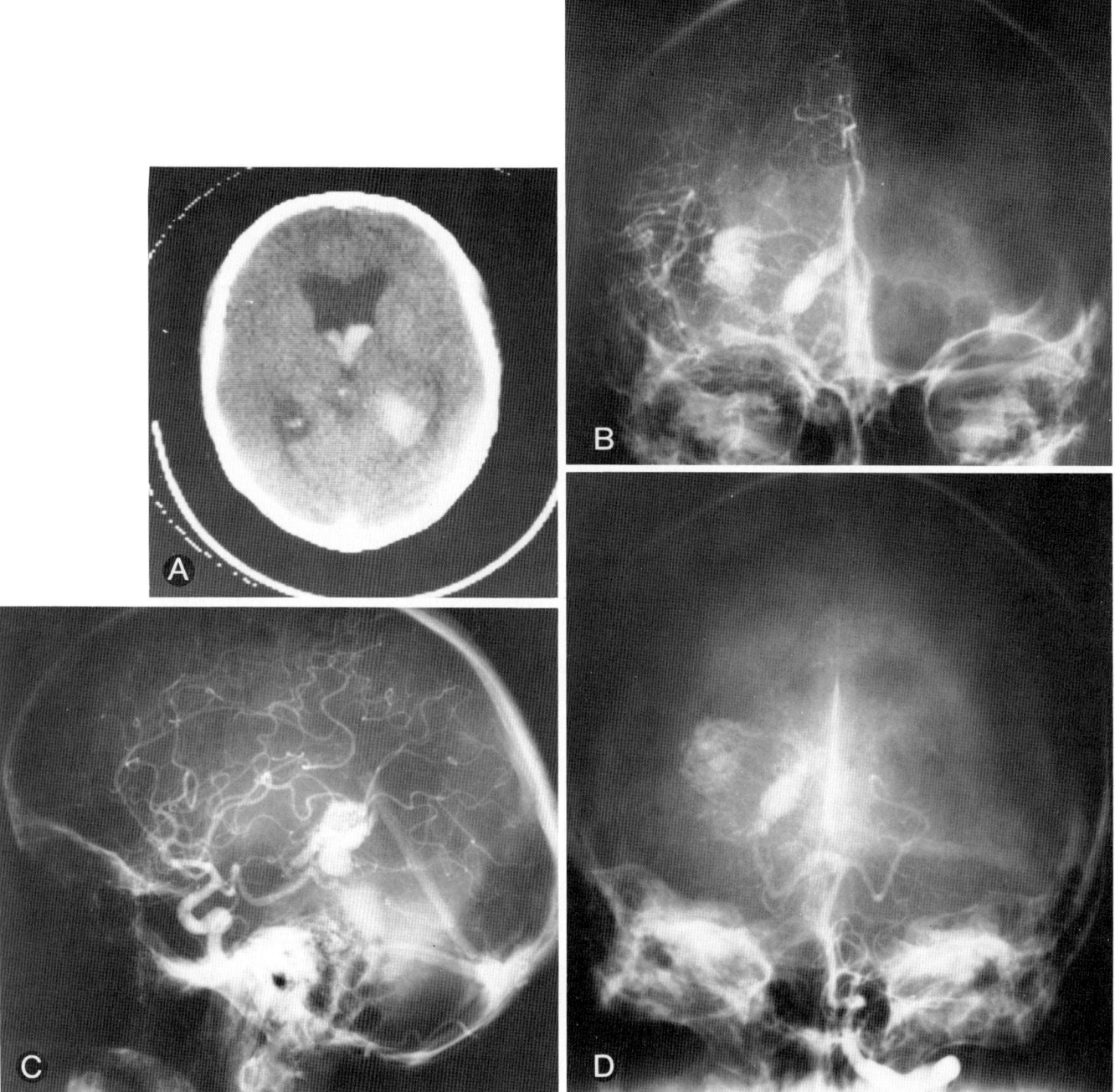

Figure 22.7 Medial temporal AVM approached through superior temporal gyrus and ventricle. *A*, CT scan shows a right posterior medial temporal lobe hematoma with a small amount of blood in the ventricles. *B* and *C*, right carotid angiogram outlines the AVM with primary blood supply from the enlarged right posterior cerebral artery but also middle cerebral artery supply. Venous filling is seen on the arterial phase. *D* and *E*, left vertebral angiogram. Note the washout in the right posterior cerebral artery due to flow from the carotid artery. *F* and *G*, postoperative left vertebral angiogram. The AVM was removed through a superior temporal gyrus approach.

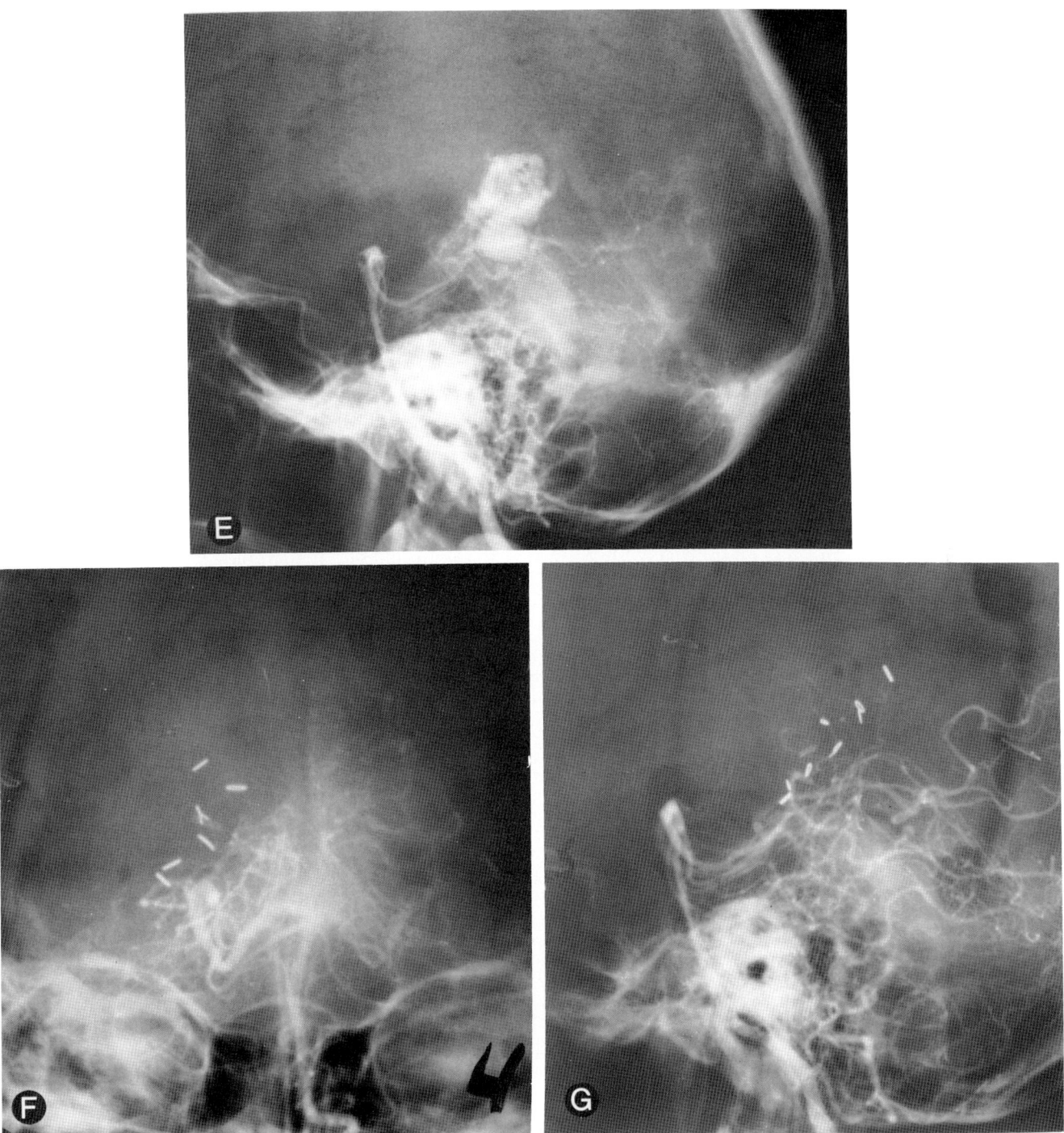

Figure 22.7 (E to G)

Arteriovenous malformations in the hippocampal area are often fed by branches of the posterior communicating and posterior cerebral arteries which must be preserved. A subtemporal approach can be used, but a transventricular approach through a superior temporal gyrus corticectomy, especially on the right side, and particularly in relation to the preexisting field deficit, can give a nice exposure of the medially placed lesion (Fig. 22.7). If the lesion is more posterior in the medial temporal-occipital region, a subtemporal approach is indicated and the cortex entered just lateral to the malformation (10). Heros has reviewed the literature relative to the surgical approach to medial temporal AVMs (15). He has used a transcortical incision through the inferior temporal lobe to reduce the risk of postoperative field defects and dysphasia when the dominant hemisphere is involved.

Cingulate AVMs may be exposed through a coronal incision with the bone flap crossing the midline, with a line of sight down the falx between the hemispheres (Fig. 22.8). Bilateral cerebral angiography and careful study of the venous drainage pattern will be needed to choose the appropriate side of approach. Ordinarily, one goes on the side of the lesion, but with an unfavorable venous drainage system, we have not hesitated to operate from the opposite side. It is important on the AP angiographic view to estimate the lateral extent of the lesion which may be quite difficult to reach through an interhemispheric approach. In one case, we found it necessary to make a separate superior frontal gyrus incision to excise a lateral extension of a cingulate gyrus lesion.

Callosal AVMs may also be approached along the falx through an interhemispheric exposure (45, 46). For lesions involving the anterior and middle portions of the corpus callosum, the patient is placed in the supine position with the head well elevated (Fig. 22.9). The bone flap is placed well across the midline. In planning surgery it is important to review the anatomy of the veins draining into the superior sagittal sinus on the angiogram. Ordinarily, one goes on the right, but with an adverse venous pattern, we have operated successfully from the left. Two self-retaining retractors are used, one against the falx and the other on the medial surface of the hemisphere. The anterior cerebral arteries must be preserved, and careful correlation of the anatomy seen at operation with the angiogram is helpful in locating the branches from the anterior cerebral arteries to the lesion. Excision of even large lesions of this region has not led to significant disconnection syndromes. Generally, a large draining vein into the third ventricle will be encountered at the conclusion of this dissection. AVMs involving the splenium of the corpus callosum are difficult to remove. Yasargil uses a sitting position and approaches the lesion along the falx in the parieto-occipital region (45).

In a few patients, lesions in the basal ganglia have been excised. According to Drake's experience and his review of the literature, AVMs lying in the anterior or posterior-superior thalamus and head of the caudate nucleus may be excised safely and without major sensory or motor deficit (10). Heros has reported three patients with AVMs of the medial temporal lobe with extension into the basal ganglia or the thalamus (15). These lesions were removed with low morbidity through a transcortical incision in the inferior portion of the temporal lobe.

AVMs may be predominately intraventricular with origin from the choroidal arteries and involvement of the choroid plexus (10). These lesions may involve the trigone of the lateral ventricle, the third or fourth ventricle.

When planning the approach to AVMs of the posterior fossa, the specific site of the lesion must be considered (10, 30, 40, 42). Most of these AVMs appear on the cerebellar surface and are exposed through a suboccipital craniectomy, usually in the sitting position. For some superomedial lesions, a subtemporal transtentorial or combined approach may be indicated (10) (see Chapter 18). Large AVMs of the cerebellar hemisphere may be removed successfully (Fig. 22.10). The vascular attachments to the tentorium must be carefully occluded as an early maneuver. For large hemisphere and vermis lesions, the fourth ventricle serves as an important landmark in the dissection.

Chou and Drake have reported surgical experiences in patients with AVMs involving the brain stem and cerebellopontine angle (4, 19). Their results are encouraging but the risks of surgery are high.

Results

In 27 patients in our series with surgical excision, 81% excellent or good function was attained postoperatively (Table 22.1) For good risk cases, excellent or good results were noted in 91% of cases. These results are comparable to those reported by others (5, 10, 14, 19, 28, 43). Following excision, the arterial vessels that were supplying the AVM progressively decreased in size.

In our series, there were three deaths, all due to hemorrhage, and two patients were in poor condition before operation. In one case of occipital AVM, severe hemorrhage was encountered from extensive tentorial feeding arteries which had not been recog-

Table 22.1
AVMs: Results of Surgical Excision

Preop status	Number	Results			
		Excellent	Good	Poor	Death
Good	23	15 (69%)	6 (26%)	1 (4%)	1 (4%)
Poor	4	—	1 (25%)	1 (25%)	2 (50%)
Total	27	15 (55%)	7 (26%)	2 (7%)	3 (11%)

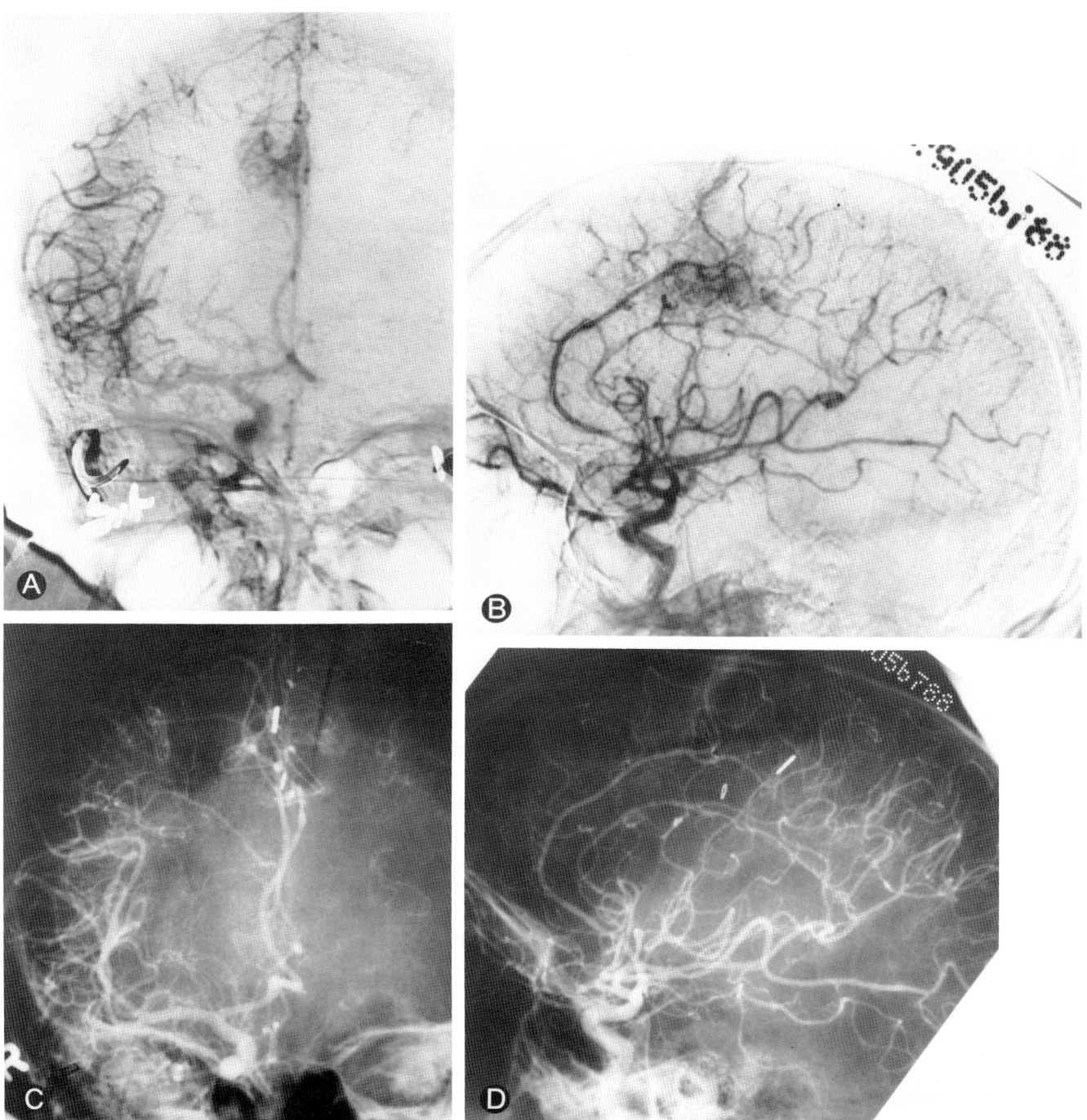

Figure 22.8 Cingulate AVM. *A* and *B*, right carotid angiogram (subtraction) shows an AVM with multiple small vessels involving the cingulate gyrus. The callosal marginal artery has a proximal origin. *C* and *D*, postoperative angiogram shows complete excision of the lesion.

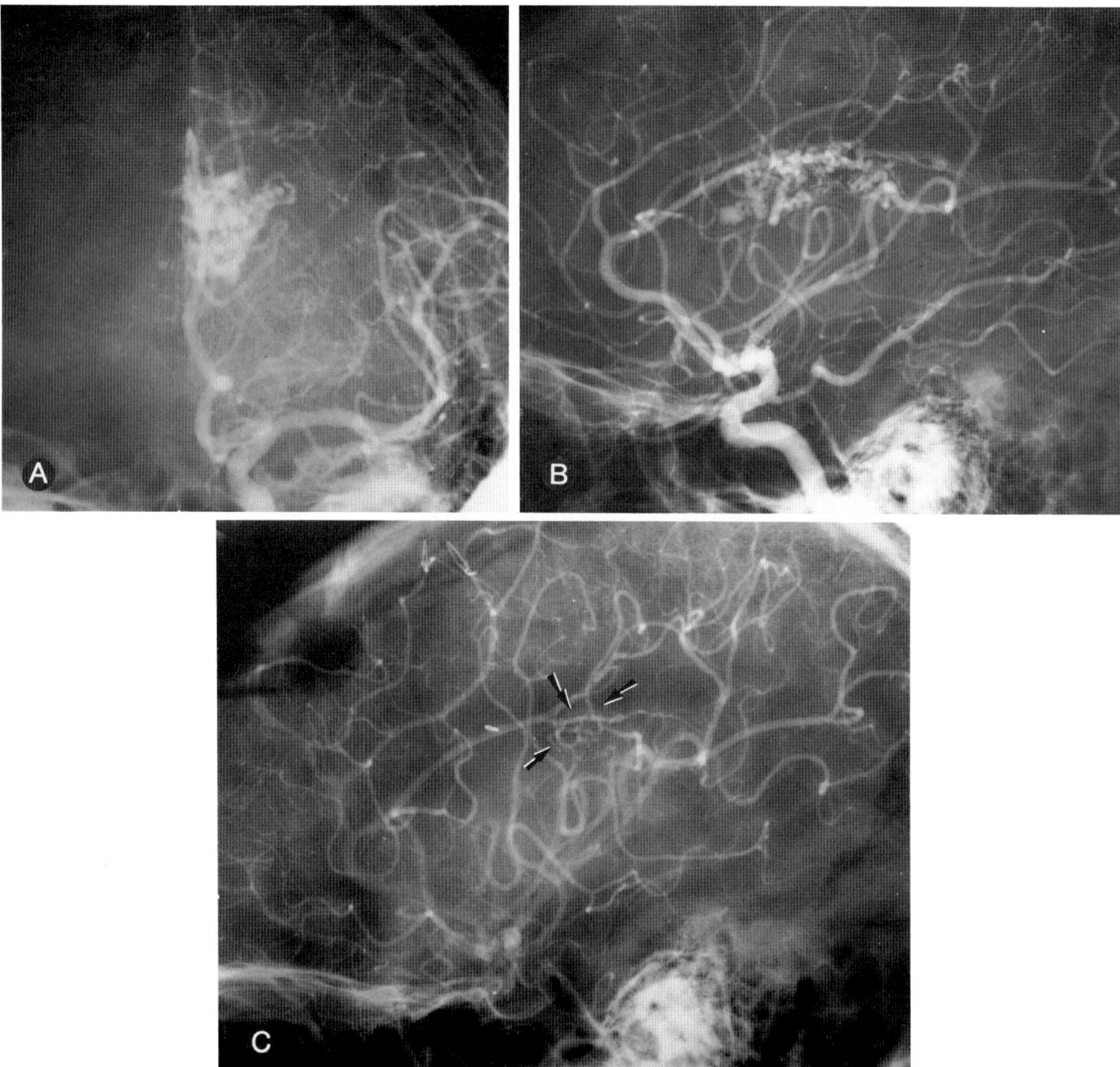

Figure 22.9 Callosal AVM. *A* and *B*, left carotid angiogram showing AVM involving the mid portion of the corpus callosum. *C*, postoperative angiogram shows small residual AVM (*arrows*). *D* and *E*, final angiogram shows complete removal of the AVM. Note occlusion of feeding branch from the pericallosal artery. Comment: This 17-year-old girl presented with SAH. The first postoperative angiogram showed residual AVM in the posterior portion of the lesion. Reoperation was done and a complete excision accomplished.

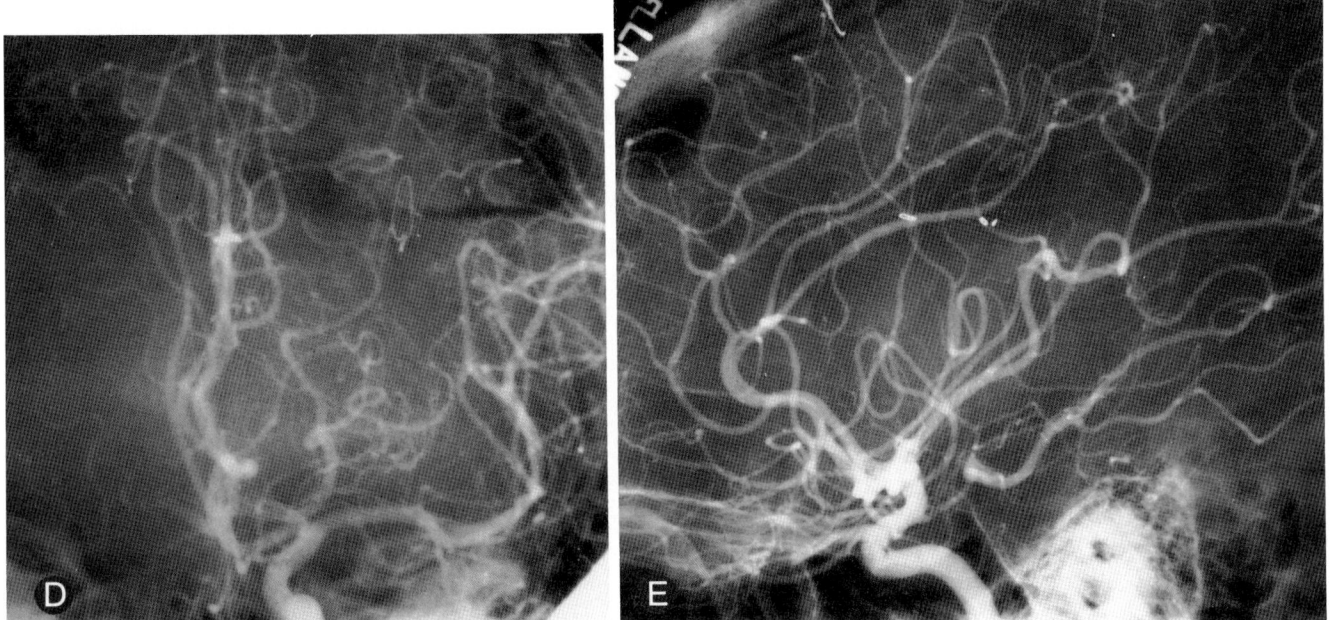

Figure 22.9 (*D* and *E*)

nized on angiography. In another case with a large Rolandic AVM, apparently successful excision was followed by uncontrollable edema and hemorrhage. Staged obliteration might have avoided this problem. The third death resulted from hemorrhage one day after complete excision of a large central AVM, which had been irradiated with proton beam; staged obliteration might also have helped in this patient. Lasting morbidity was recorded in four cases: hemiparesis in three, and mental change in one.

Total excision proved by angiography was achieved initially in all but three cases (88%). A reoperation was required in these three cases, two in the anterior corpus callosum. For the present, particularly for lesions in noncritical zones, and even for small lesions in eloquent zones except for the brainstem, excision remains the treatment of choice.

Parkinson has noted that patients suffering seizures before surgery were very likely to have seizures even after removal of the AVM (27). Our experience, in a few patients where the indication for excision of the AVM was difficulty in controlling the seizure disorder, demonstrated that while the patient was not made seizure-free, there was a marked reduction in the frequency and improvement in the ability to control the seizures with less medication.

PROTON BEAM THERAPY

While microsurgical resection is considered the treatment of choice for patients with AVM, some of these lesions are considered inoperable, and others have residual AVM post-excision. For these patients, proton beam therapy may be recommended. Dr. Raymond Kjellberg, who has developed the method at Massachusetts General Hospital has the most extensive experience with this form of treatment (17, 18).

The Bragg peak of proton irradiation delivers highly focused heavy particle energy to a deeply placed target. The proton beam is generated by a cyclotron (160 Mev) and administered via a stereotactic procedure performed under local anesthesia. Proton irradiation induces a thickening of AVM vascular channels which is thought to diminish the later risk of hemorrhage and death. The treatment itself has no immediate risk of morbidity.

Dr. Kjellberg has recently reviewed data on 258 patients with AVM treatment by proton beam. Four serious non-fatal non-hemorrhagic neurological complications were recorded in an early experience with 27 cases. Such complications have subsequently been avoided by lowering the proton dose for AVMs entwined in motor or visual pathways. The radiation reaction develops slowly over months with about 90% of the effect occurring in 2 years. The treatment confers no protection against hemorrhage in the first 12 months after proton irradiation, and three patients bled fatally during this unprotected interval.

The results of longer follow-up are impressive. In the 258 patients there have been cited no fatal rebleeds beyond 1 year. Four patients had non-fatal rebleeds; one patient who had four recurrent hemorrhages was subsequently retreated with the proton beam. None of these episodes of recurrent hemorrhage led to new neurological deficit.

Detailed evaluation of 75 patients followed more than 2 years is also encouraging. The frequency and disability associated with non-fatal rebleeding appear diminished after proton therapy. Seizure fre-

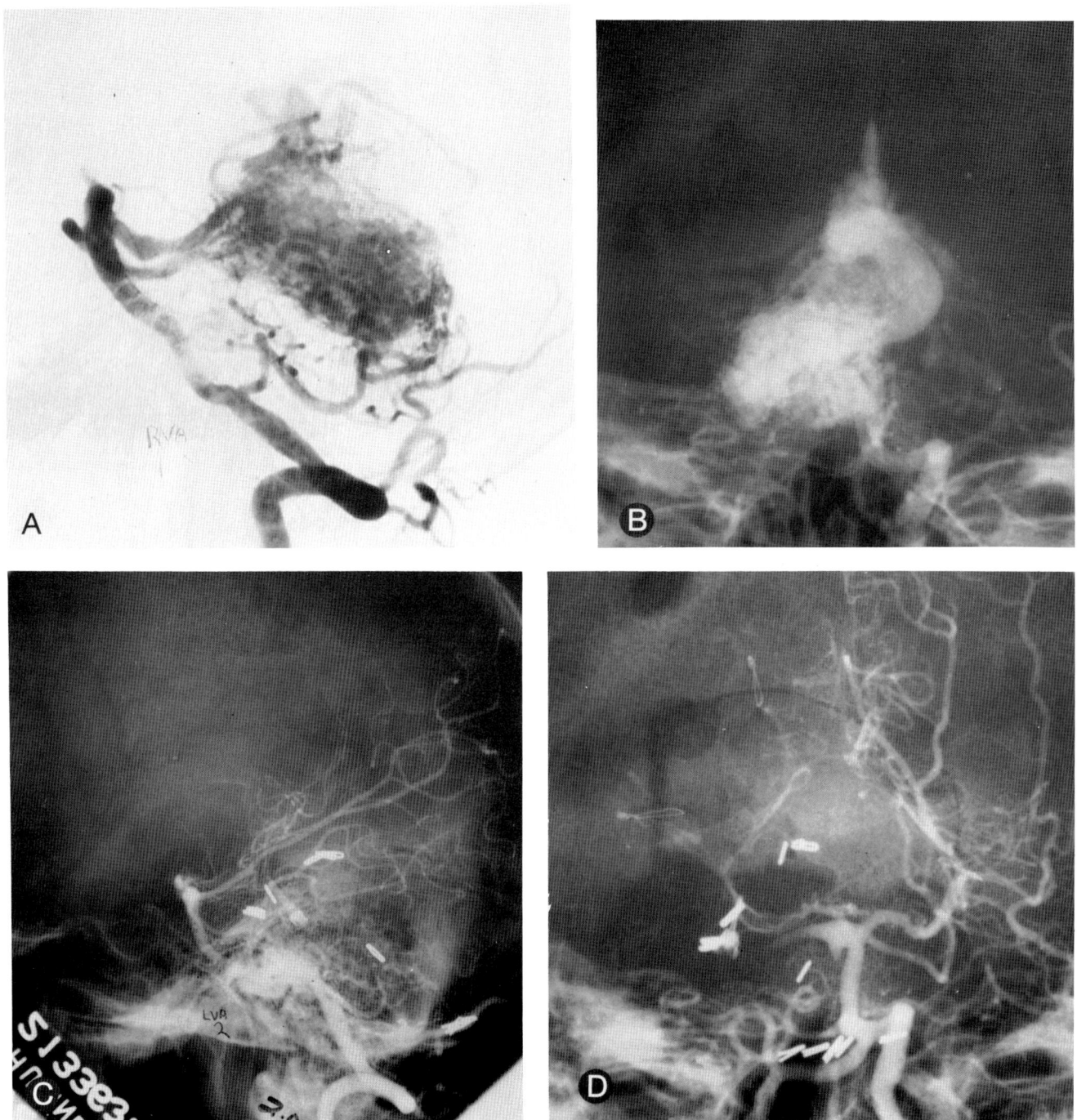

Figure 22.10 Cerebellar AVM. *A* and *B*, a large midline and right cerebellar hemisphere AVM is demonstrated. *C* and *D*, postoperative angiogram shows no evidence of the AVM. Comment: This patient had a history of seven SAHs which had left a significant neurological deficit, but he was still able to make decisions about his business. After operation he resumed his previous level of activity. The only new disability was an increase in difficulty with swallowing due to incoordination.

quency and pre-existing neurological deficits may improve or remain static. Angiography may show total, partial, or no obliteration of the AVM; and clinical improvement may or may not be correlated with the angiographic change (Figs. 22.11 and 22.12). Of AVMs studied 2–10 years after treatment, about a quarter showed total obliteration, and almost 80% showed some reduction in size.

It is likely that proton beam therapy will be established as the treatment of choice for unresectable lesions and possibly in the future for other lesions as well.

EMBOLIZATION

Artificial embolization of an intracranial arteriovenous malformation has been the subject of several reports (8, 12, 20, 21, 31, 32, 37). Initially, silastic spheres were injected into the internal carotid artery in the neck. Now, percutaneously placed catheters may be guided into the peripheral cerebral circulation for highly selective embolization of feeding arteries (8, 16). Debrun has developed a latex calibrated-leak balloon for intra-arterial navigation and embolization with bucrylate (8). This balloon can be used in vessels 1–4 mm in diameter without distending the vessel. In his series, two of 11 AVMs were completely obliterated. Embolization for staged occlusion of part of the AVM may help avoid the problems of cerebral hyperperfusion following resection (8, 31).

There are a number of possible complications that can occur with this embolization technique. The balloon and the catheter can become glued if the catheter is not withdrawn quickly enough. Fortunately, the occasional patient where this has occurred remained asymptomatic (8). The bucrylate may pass through the malformation and enter the venous system. Spontaneous hemorrhage may occur. If the venous drainage is occluded prematurely, hemorrhage and edema may follow. The bucrylate may be injected into or relex into normal cortical arteries. The immediate tissue reaction is variable and the long-term effects of the drug are unknown.

Intraoperative embolization of selected feeding arteries is used in large malformations where the AVM feeders cannot be reached safely from the transfemoral approach. In the series of 13 patients of Debrun et al., seven had partial intraoperative embolization with complete surgical resection in four and six had complete embolization with surgical resection in two, leaving only three patients with residual AVM (8). The same complications can be encountered as with percutaneous embolization and the injection must be monitored by fluoroscopy. In this series, three patients had permanent mild neurological deficits.

Embolization should usually be regarded as adjunctive in nature, since the total AVM can be obliterated in only a small number of patients. In some patients, injection of the adhesive makes excision more difficult, since a hard, polymerized mass is less easily retracted.

VEIN OF GALEN ANEURYSM

Primary aneurysms of the vein of Galen are due to multiple arterial vessels emptying directly into the vein of Galen. Secondary aneurysms occur when a separate arteriovenous malformation drains into the vein of Galen and causes it to enlarge.

The clinical syndromes caused by primary aneurysms of the vein of Galen have been presented in the review done by Amacher and Shillito (2). Four characteristic clinical groups were outlined and these are summarized in Table 22.2, together with a fifth group which we have added, comprising the thrombosed aneurysms.

In infancy, the malformation is associated with uncontrollable cardiac failure. Even with careful stepwise obliteration of the feeding arteries and intensive medical therapy, the prognosis in group 1 is poor with very few survivors being reported (1, 2, 23). When the symptoms develop after the first year, the cardiac failure will respond to surgical treatment of the malformation. In older children and adults, symptoms associated with hydrocephalus are more common. In Yasargil's series, four patients, all in the older age group, had subarachnoid hemorrhage (44). Thrombosed aneurysm of the vein of Galen usually presents with hydrocephalus (7, 34).

The diagnosis is suggested by the CT scan and confirmed by angiography. The arterial supply is usually bilateral and comes from the posterior cerebral arteries, as well as the anterior pericallosal, superior cerebellar, and thalamic perforating arteries, and occasionally from middle cerebral arteries (2, 44) (Fig. 22.13). A thrombosed aneurysm may show a blood fluid level within the aneurysm and marked

Table 22.2
Presenting Clinical Syndromes in Patients with Vein of Galen Aneurysms

Group[a]	Number of Patients	Age	Presenting Syndrome
1	11	Neonatal	Severe cardiac failure, cranial bruit
2	3	Neonatal or infancy	Mild heart failure (neonatal), then craniomegaly within 1–6 months; cranial bruit
3	22	1–12 months	Craniomegaly, cranial bruit
4	6	3.5–27 years	Headache, exercise syncope
5	9	6 months–45 years	Drowsy, irritable, hydrocephalus, spasticity

[a] Groups 1 to 4: modified from Ref. 2. Group 5: cases with thrombosed aneurysms from Refs. 7 and 34.

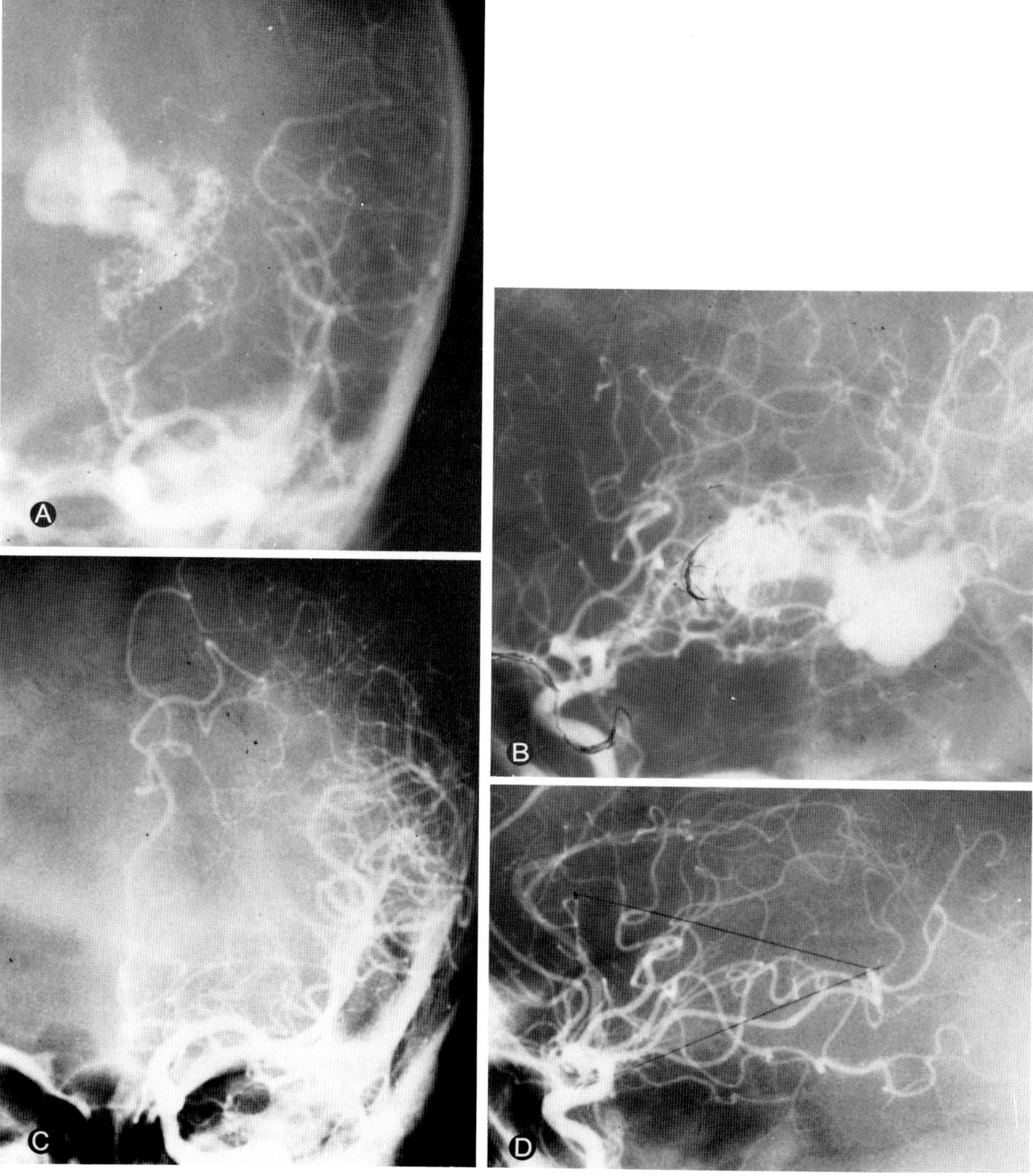

Figure 22.11 Treatment of AVM with proton beam. *A* and *B*, left carotid angiogram shows AVM involving the basal ganglia. *C* and *D*, repeat angiogram done 1 year after proton beam treatment showing obliteration of the AVM. Comment: This 39-year-old woman had two hemorrhages with a residual right hemiparesis. Proton beam treatment was given 4 months after the last hemorrhage. The patient remains well with a stable neurological deficit. (These pictures are reproduced through the courtesy of Dr. R. N. Kjellberg.)

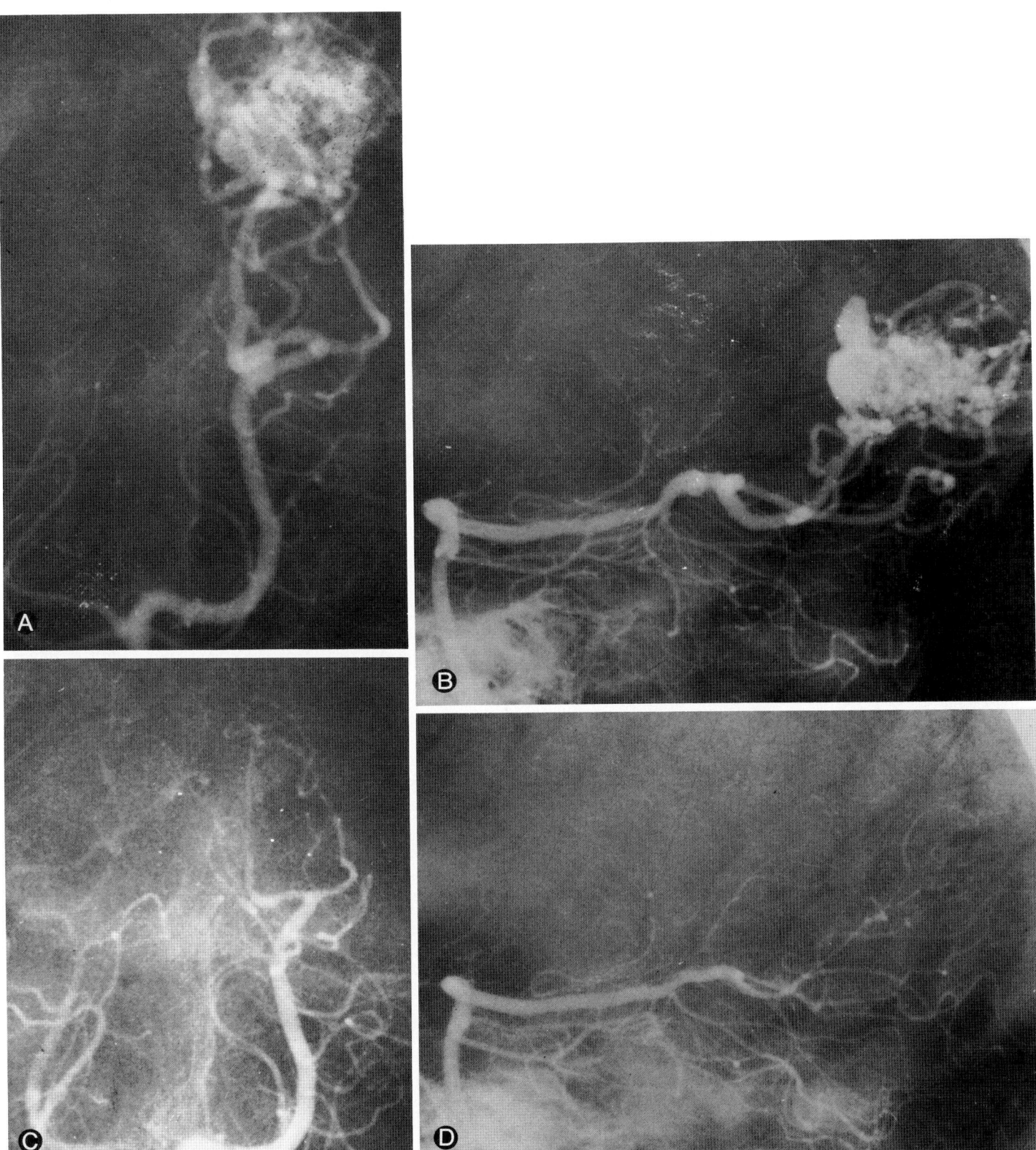

Figure 22.12 Treatment of AVM with proton beam. *A* and *B*, vertebral angiogram showing a left occipital AVM. *C* and *D*, repeat angiogram done 2 years after proton beam treatment. Only a small remnant of AVM remains. Comment: This 58-year-old woman was treated 1 month after a hemorrhage that was associated with a mild dyspasia. She is doing well. (These pictures are reproduced through the courtesy of Dr. R. N. Kjellberg.)

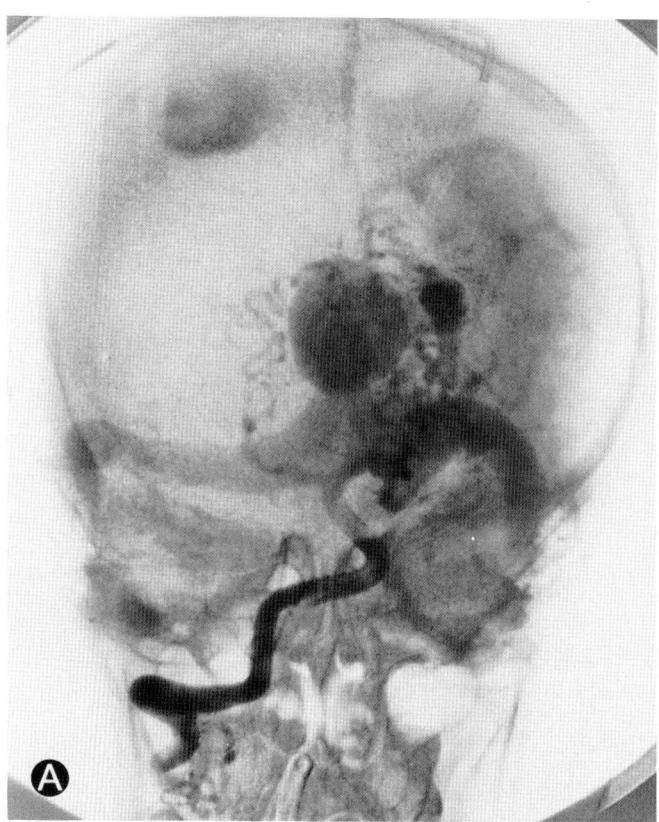
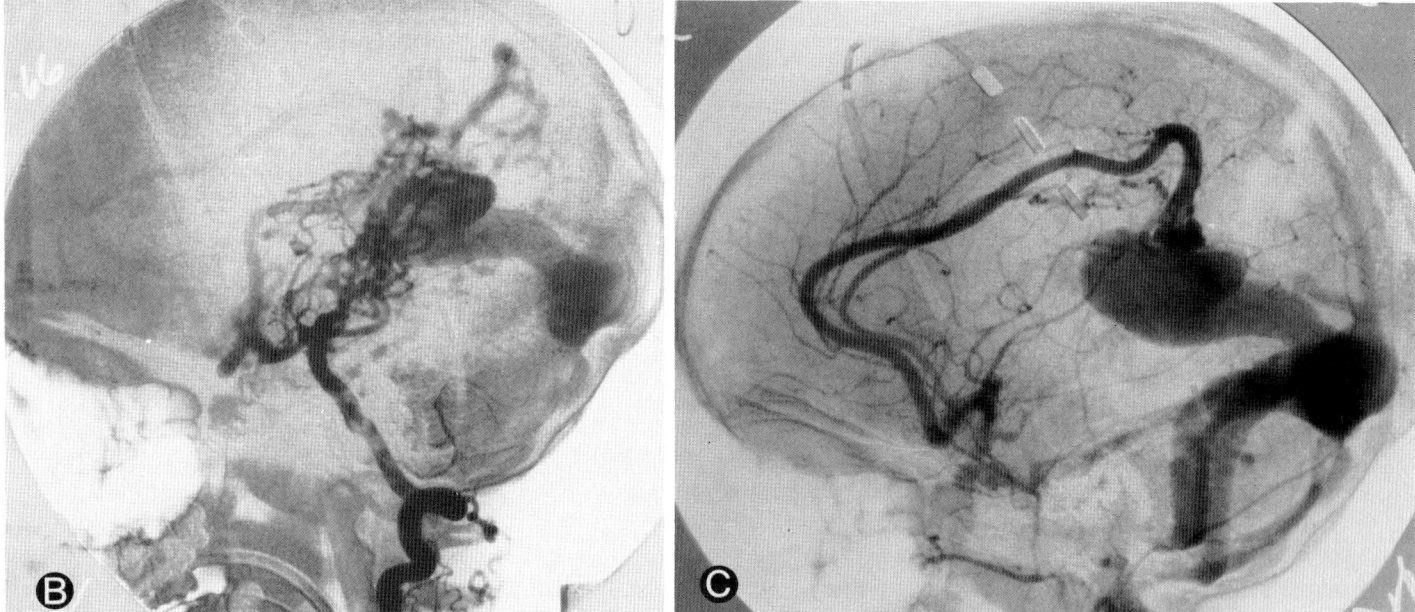

Figure 22.13 Vein of Galen malformation. *A* and *B*, AP and lateral vertebral angiogram shows arterial supply from both posterior cerebral arteries with filling of the vein of Galen aneurysm and transverse sinuses in the arterial phase of the study. Lateral vertebral angiogram better outlines the filling from the posterior branches of the left middle cerebral artery. *C*, branches from the pericallosal artery enter the top of the aneurysm. The ventricular portion of the shunt system is also seen.

enhancement of the periphery of the mass on the CT scan (34).

The lesion is exposed through a parietoccipital craniotomy and is approached along the falx. The technique has been described by Amacher and Shillito in five patients and subsequently by Yasargil in six patients (2, 44). Similar operative approach with good results has been used by others (3, 17, 23, 34). The sac of the aneurysm is identified in the region formed by the falx and tentorium posteriorly and under the splenium of the corpus callosum anteriorly. To expose the aneurysm, it may be necessary to split the splenium and divide the falx or tentorium.

Yasargil first occludes, the anterior pericallosal arteries, by going over the splenium, to the dome of the malformation (44). Then the right posterior cerebral artery is identified in the ambient cistern and followed to the malformation where feeders are divided. Next, the right superior cerebellar artery is identified behind the posterior cerebral artery in the ambient and quadrigeminal cisterns and is also followed to the malformation. After a flap is made in the falx, attention is turned to the left side of the aneurysm and the feeders from the left posterior cerebral and superior cerebellar arteries are occluded. In some cases, this will completely take care of the problem, but more often there will still be inflow through the large perforating posterior thalamic vessels from the peduncular segment of the posterior cerebral artery. The aneurysm is reflected inferiorly to expose these arteries as they enter at the anterior base. At times the aneurysm must be elevated to expose the posterior inferior surface to reach all the feeding arteries. The vein of Galen should now be blue. To further check on the completeness of the occlusion, the skull can be auscultated and a blood sample drawn from the vein of Galen for blood gas analysis. Because the sac is usually tough, it can be manipulated with relative safety. The sac is usually not excised.

Six et al. recommended that thrombosed aneurysms of the vein of Galen be decompressed but not removed, and this was also done by Dean. Both reports noted a much smoother postoperative course than when an attempt was made to excise the lesion (7, 34).

Postoperative complications include heart failure, subdural hematoma, hemiparesis, seizure, and hydrocephalus.

REFERENCES

1. Alvarez-Garijo JA, Mengual MV, Gomila DT, Martin AA: Giant arteriovenous fistula of the vein of Galen in early infancy treated successfully with surgery. J Neurosurg 53:703-706, 1980.
2. Amacher AL, Shillito J Jr: The syndromes and surgical treatment of aneurysms of the great vein of Galen. J Neurosurg 39:89-98, 1973.
3. Carson LV, Brooks BS, Gammal TE, Massey CE, Beveridge WD, Allen MB: Adult arteriovenous malformation of the vein of Galen: A case report with pre- and postoperative computed tomographic findings. Neurosurgery 7:495-498, 1980.
4. Chou SN, Erickson DL, Oritz-Surez HJ: Surgical treatment of vascular lesions in the brain stem. J Neurosurg 42:23-31, 1975.
5. Cophignon J, Thurel CL, Djindjian R, Rey A, Visot A, LeBesnerais Y, Houdart R: Cerebral arteriovenous malformations. Prog Neurol Surg 9:195-237, 1978.
6. Dahl RE, Kline DG: Intraparenchymal arteriovenous malformations with predominant external carotid artery contribution. J Neurosurg 41:681-687, 1974.
7. Dean DF: Management of clotted aneurysm of the vein of Galen. Neurosurgery 8:589-592, 1981.
8. Debrun G, Vinuela F, Fox A, Drake CG: Embolization of cerebral arteriovenous malformations with bucrylate. Experience in 46 cases. J Neurosurg (to be published).
9. Drake CG: Surgical removal of arteriovenous malformations from the brain stem and cerebellopontine angle. J Neurosurg 43:661-670, 1975.
10. Drake CG: Cerebral arteriovenous malformations: Considerations for and experience with surgical treatment in 166 cases. Clin Neurosurg 26:145-208, 1979.
11. Forster DMC, Steiner L, Hakanson S: Arteriovenous malformation of the brain. A long term clinical study. J Neurosurg 37:562-570, 1972.
12. French LA: Surgical treatment of arteriovenous malformations: a history. Clin Neurosurg 24:22-33, 1976.
13. Golden JB, Kramer RA: The angiographically occult cerebrovascular malformation. J Neurosurg 48:292-296, 1978.
14. Guidetti B, Delitala A: Intracranial arteriovenous malformations. Conservative and surgical treatment. J Neurosurg 53:149-152, 1980.
15. Heros RC: Arteriovenous malformations of the medial temporal lobe. Surgical approach and neuroradiological characterization. J Neurosurg (to be published).
16. Kerber C: Use of balloon catheters in the treatment of cranial arterial abnormalities. Stroke 11:210-216, 1980.
17. Kjellberg RN, Poletti CE, Robertson GH, and Adams RD: Bragg peak proton beam treatment of arteriovenous malformations of the brain, in Carrea R (ed): *Neurological Surgery (with Emphasis on Non-Invasive Methods of Diagnosis and Treatment)*. Proceedings of the Sixth International Congress of Neurological Surgery, Sao Paulo, June 19-26, 1977. Amsterdam, Excerpta Medica, 1978, pp 181-187.
18. Kjellberg R: Bragg peak proton beam therapy for arteriovenous malformations. Presented at Harvard neurosurgery postgraduate course, Boston, October, 1981.
19. Kunc Z: Surgery of arteriovenous malformations in the speech and motor sensory regions. J Neurosurg 40:293-303, 1974.
20. Kvam DA, Michelsen WJ, Quest DO: Intracerebral hemorrhage as a complication of artificial embolization. Neurosurgery 7:491-494, 1980.
21. Luessenhop AJ, Presper JH: Surgical embolization of cerebral arteriovenous malformations through internal carotid and vertebral arteries: long-term results. J Neurosurg 42:443-451, 1975.
22. Matsumura H, Makita Y, Someda K, Kondo A: Arteriovenous malformations in the posterior fossa. J Neurosurg 47:50-56, 1977.
23. Menezes AH, Graf CJ, Jacoby CG, Cornell SH: Management of vein of Galen aneurysms. Report of two cases. J Neurosurg 55:457-462, 1981.
24. Michelsen WJ: Natural history and pathophysiology of arteriovenous malformations. Clin Neurosurg 26:307-313, 1979.
25. Mullan S, Brown FD, Patronas NJ: Hyperemic and ischemic problems of surgical treatment of arteriovenous malformations. J Neurosurg 51:757-764, 1979.
26. Olivecrona H, Riives J: Arteriovenous aneurysms of the brain: their diagnosis and treatment. Arch Neurol Psychiat 59:567-602, 1948.
27. Parkinson D, Bachers G: Arteriovenous malformations. Summary of 100 consecutive supratentorial cases. J Neurosurg 53:285-299, 1980.

28. Pertuiset B, Galal A, Sichez JP, Effenterre RV, Goutorbe J, Dagreou F, Joly-Pottuz G: Exérèse totale par voie ventriculaire de deux malformations arterioveineuses pallidocaudus sous hypotension profonde. Rev Neurol 132:799-803, 1976.
29. Pool, JL: The treatment of arteriovenous malformations of the cerebral hemispheres. J Neurosurg 19:136-141, 1962.
30. Sahs AL, Perrett GE, Locksley HB, Niskioska H (eds): *Intracranial Aneurysms and Subarachnoid Hemorrhage*: A Cooperative Study. Philadelphia, JB Lippincott, 1969.
31. Samson D, Ditmore QM, Beyer CW Jr: Intravascular use of isobutyl 2-cyanoacrylate: Part 1 treatment of intracranial arteriovenous malformations. Neurosurgery 8:43-51, 1981.
32. Sano K, Jimbo M, Saito I, Baseiji N: Artificial embolization of inoperable angioma with polymerizing substance, in Pia HW, Gleave JRW, Gote E, Zierski J (eds): *Cerebral Angiomas: Advances in Diagnosis and Therapy*. Berlin, Springer-Verlag, 1975, pp 222-229.
33. Shuey HM Jr, Day AL, Quisling RG, Sypent, GW: Angiographically cryptic cerebrovascular malformations. Neurosurgery 5:476-479, 1979.
34. Six EG, Cowley AR, Kelly DL Jr, Laster DW: Thrombosed aneurysm of the vein of Galen. Neurosurgery 7:274-278, 1980.
35. Spetzler RF, Wilson CB: Enlargement of an arteriovenous malformation documented by angiography. J Neurosurg 43:767-769, 1975.
36. Spetzler RF, Wilson CB, Weinstein P, Mehdorn M, Townsend J, Telles D: Normal perfusion pressure breakthrough theory. Clin Neurosurg 25:651-672, 1978.
37. Stein BM, Wolpert SM: Surgical and embolic treatment of cerebral arteriovenous malformations. Surg Neurol 7:359-369, 1977.
38. Svien HJ, McRae JA: Arteriovenous anomalies of the brain; fate of patients not having definitive surgery. J Neurosurg 23:23-28, 1965.
39. Troupp H: *Natural History of Arteriovenous Malformations*. Presented at Symposium on Aneurysms, Arteriovenous Malformations and Carotid Cavernous Fistulae. Fiftieth Anniversary, University of Chicago, November, 1977.
40. Viale GL, Pau A, Viale ES: Surgical treatment of arteriovenous malformations of the posterior fossa. Surg Neurol 12:379-384, 1979.
41. Waltimo O: The relationship of size, density and localization of intracranial arteriovenous malformations to the type of initial symptom. J Neurol Sci 19:13-19, 1973.
42. Waltimo O: The change in size of intracranial arteriovenous malformations. J Neurol Sci 19:21-27, 1973.
43. Wilson CB, Hoi Sang U, Domingue J: Microsurgical treatment of intracranial vascular malformations. J Neurosurg 51:446-454, 1979.
44. Yasargil MG, Antic J, Laciga R, Jain K, Boone SC: Arteriovenous malformations of vein of Galen: Microsurgical treatment. Surg Neurol 6:195-200, 1976.
45. Yasargil MG, Jain KK, Antic J, Laciga R: Arteriovenous malformations of the splenium of the corpus callosum: microsurgical treatment. Surg Neurol 5:5-14, 1976.
46. Yasargil MG, Jain KK, Antic J, Laciga R, Kletter G: Arteriovenous malformations of the anterior and middle portions of the corpus callosum: Microsurgical treatment. Surg Neurol 5:67-80, 1976.

Chapter 23 DURAL ARTERIOVENOUS MALFORMATIONS

PATHOLOGY

Arteriovenous malformations (AVMs) involving the dura are caused by abnormal communications between branches of the external carotid, internal carotid, and vertebral arteries, and the venous sinuses within the dura, tentorium, or falx. Most dural AVMs involve the transverse and sigmoid sinuses (9). The next most common site is the cavernous sinus and these malformations are discussed in Chapter 24. A few cases of dural AVM involving the anterior fossa and the sphenoparietal sinus have been reported (3, 19).

Rarely is there a history of trauma (17). Some dural AVMs are probably developmental in origin (1, 17). It has been suggested that many are acquired lesions representing a form of arterial revascularization after thrombosis of the tranverse or sigmoid sinus with pathological examination showing multiple dysplastic-appearing vessels entering the sinus wall (9). Houser et al. reported two patients where angiography showed occlusion of the transverse or sigmoid sinus with no evidence of AVM, but within 4 years a dural AVM developed. We have seen one patient where, after partial obliteration of the sinus, multiple arterial communications developed from the dura and the occipital cortex to the sinus, and this was also observed in one patient by Houser et al. (9).

CLINICAL PRESENTATION

Dural AVMs of the transverse sinus can occur at any age and affect both sexes, but are more common in women who are more than 40 years of age. Pulsatile tinnitus is the most common presenting symptom, but other manifestations include headache, decreased vision, focal neurological deficits (transient or permanent), increased intracranial pressure, and, rarely, subarachnoid or intracerebral hemorrhage, normal pressure hydrocephalus syndrome, or seizure (8, 9, 11–13, 17).

On examination, a bruit is usually heard over the mastoid region. Papilledema may be associated with decreased visual acuity.

These lesions can be asymptomatic being an incidental finding at the time of angiography (1). Spontaneous thrombosis and disappearance of symptomatology have been reported (2, 5, 12, 14, 18).

RADIOGRAPHIC EVALUATION

Computerized tomography outlines ventricular size and may show abnormal decreased density in the white matter, patchy enhancement, and hemorrhage when this has occurred (16). The malformation itself is usually not seen but dilated veins may be outlined. In one case it was observed that after obliteration of the shunt, the decreased density in the white matter disappeared, suggesting that it was due to the edema from the raised venous sinus pressure (16).

Adequate angiography requires selective studies of the external and internal carotid and vertebral arteries (10, 12). Subtraction and special oblique views may be needed to characterize the fistulous communications. The center of the malformation is usually at the junction of the transverse and sigmoid sinuses (9) (Fig. 23.1). Kuhner et al. have classified the possible sources of blood supply into three groups (12). In the external group arteries from the scalp and neck reach the dura through perforations in the skull. This includes perforating branches from the occipital, superficial temporal, and posterior auricular arteries and muscular branches from the ascending cervical and vertebral arteries. In the medial group the meningeal branches from both the middle meningeal and vertebral arteries supply the malformation. The internal group includes the tentorial branches from the internal carotid artery and branches from the posterior and middle cerebral arteries.

Retrograde filling of the venous system may be striking. In some cases, thrombosis of a sinus may be seen (6). In the 14 patients reported by Houser et al., 10 had occlusion or narrowing of the transverse or sigmoid sinus (9).

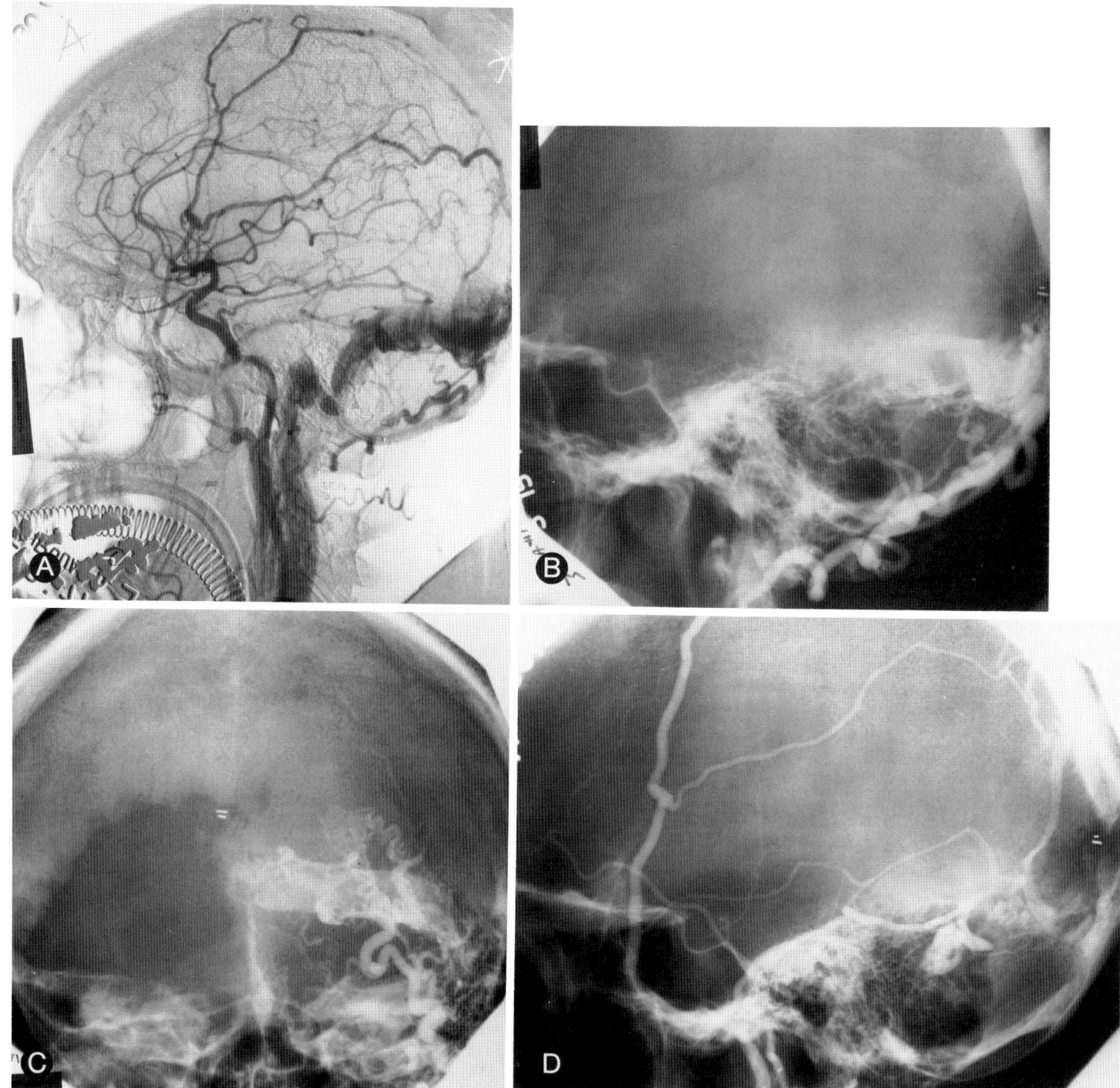

Figure 23.1 Dural arteriovenous malformation. This patient had a previous right dural AVM treated and now presented with a left-sided lesion. *A* to *D*, the transverse and sigmoid sinus are receiving direct communication from several branches of the hypertrophied occipital artery, the meningeal arteries, the tentorial artery, and the superficial temporal artery.

Dural Arteriovenous Malformations

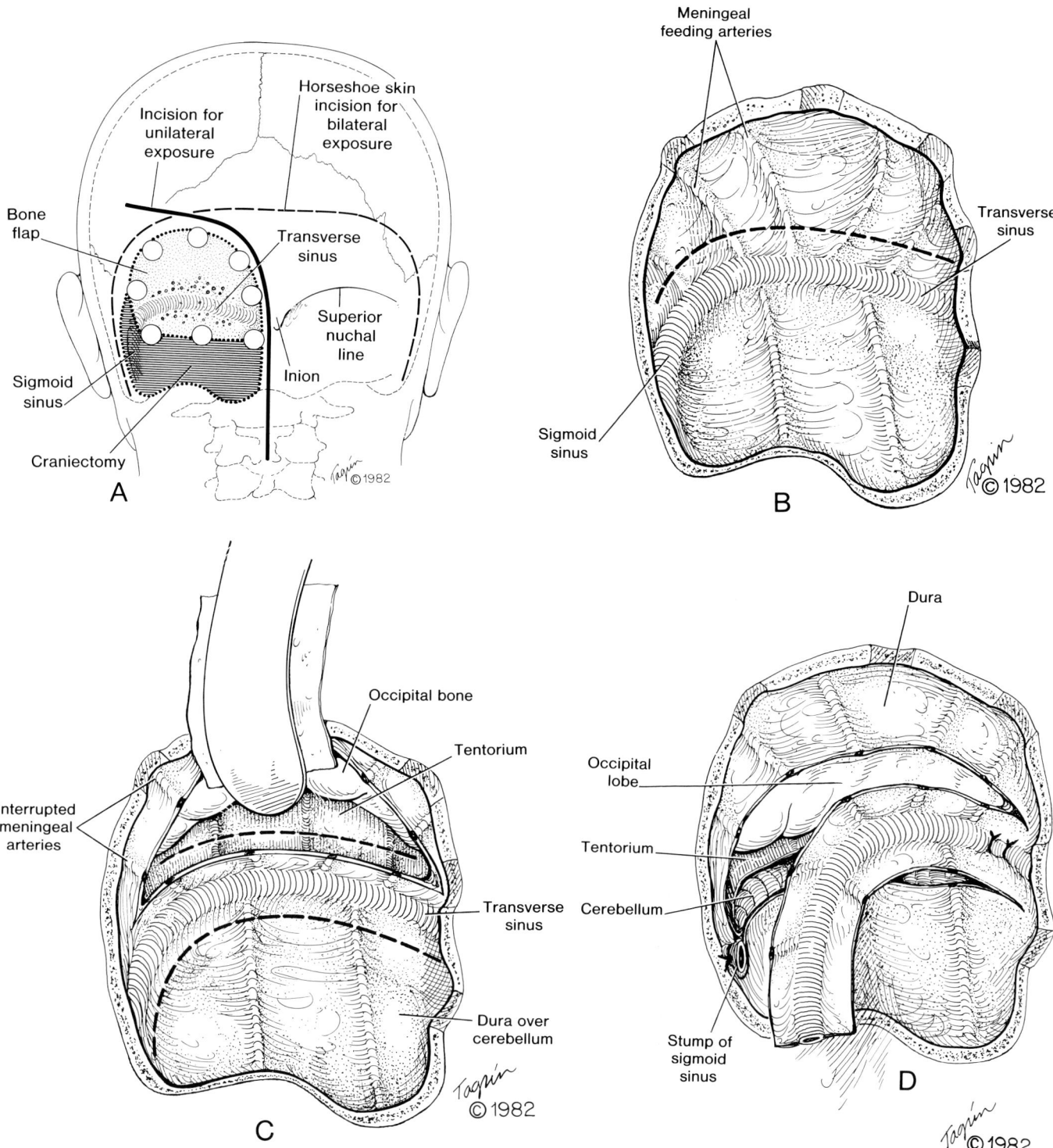

Figure 23.2 Surgical treatment of dural AVM of sigmoid and transverse sinuses. *A*, two types of skin incisions may be used. For wide exposure or bilateral lesions, a horseshoe incision is used. Alternatively, an incision may be made for a unilateral exposure. The bone often has a sieve-like appearance where arterial vessels have gone through the bone from the back of the scalp flap. The bone exposure is also outlined. *B*, numerous arterial branches may enter the sinus through the dura. The dura just above the transverse sinus is opened. *C*, the incision below the transverse sinus and in the tentorium is outlined. *D*, the transverse sinus has been ligated and is excised. If necessary, the sigmoid sinus is plugged with muscle.

TREATMENT

In most patients with progressive or disabling symptoms or in whom an intracranial hemorrhage has occurred, surgical treatment of the dural AVM is indicated. Several reports have concluded that surgical resection of the transverse and proximal sigmoid sinus is the preferred treatment and this has been our experience (9, 11, 17, 18). Hugosson and Bergstrom have described the exposure and dural incisions, and while they ligated the sinus, they did not resect it (10). In some patients, embolization may be an appropriate consideration (4, 5, 7). Occasionally, a shunt will be required for relief of hydrocephalus.

Surgical Technique

During the exposure, lasix and mannitol may be given. Depending on the extent of the lesion, either the prone position with a mastoid to mastoid horseshoe-shaped incision extending well above the muscle line or the lateral position with a unilateral exposure may be used (Fig. 23.2A). As the scalp flap is turned back individual perforating arteries entering the bone are coagulated and the bone waxed. In some patients, the bone may look like a sieve. The bone removal must extend above and below the transverse sinus. Usually a suboccipital craniectomy is done and a bone flap is turned over the sinus. In some cases, extensive dural bleeding requires the use of a craniectomy rather than a bone flap so bleeding can be controlled. The sigmoid sinus is uncovered using the high-speed air drill. The only area that cannot be exposed is the outer wall of the basal portion of the sigmoid sinus.

The dura is opened above, below and parallel to the sinus, occluding the feeding arteries as they are encountered (Fig. 23.2, B and C). The incision above the transverse sinus ends at the superior petrosal sinus. The incision in the cerebellar dura is carried along the transverse and sigmoid sinuses as close to the jugular foramen as possible (19). Great care must be taken to avoid injury to the congested brain since uncontrollable edema and bleeding may result even from minor injury to the hyperemic cortex. An incision is made in the tentorium anterior to the transverse sinus from just lateral to the torcular to the superior petrosal sinus.

The transverse sinus is then ligated lateral to the torcular and a second ligation, as far lateral as possible, is done and the sinus excised (Fig. 23.2D). If a portion of the sigmoid sinus cannot be removed and still has feeding arteries, the sinus is plugged with muscle or plastic. The dural defect is closed with a graft of pericranial tissue and the bone flap is replaced.

Embolization

In some patients, selective embolization of the feeding arteries has led to obliteration of the fistula (4, 7, 12, 15). Gelfoam, liquid silicone, silastic spheres, and silastic adhesive have been used. The disadvantages of this method are the possible further development of feeding arteries from other sources, the risk of emboli entering the venous circulation, neurological deficit, and scalp necrosis.

REFERENCES

1. Aminoff MJ, Kendall BE: Asymptomatic dural vascular anomalies. Br J Radiol 46:662–667, 1973.
2. Bitoh S, Sakaki S: Spontaneous cure of dural arteriovenous malformation in the posterior fossa. Surg Neurol 12:111–114, 1979.
3. Bitoh S, Arita N, Fujiwara M, Ozaki K, Nakao Y: Dural arteriovenous malformation near the left sphenoparietal sinus. Surg Neurol 13:345–349, 1980.
4. Djindjian R, Cophignon I, Rey A, Theron J, Merland JJ, Houdart R: Superselective arteriographic embolization by the femoral route in neuroradiology. Study of 50 cases. III. Embolization in craniocerebral pathology. Neuroradiology 6:143–152, 1973.
5. Endo S, Koshu K, and Suzuki J: Spontaneous regression of posterior fossa dural arteriovenous malformation. J Neurosurg 51:715–717, 1979.
6. Handa J, Yoneda S, Handa H: Venous sinus occlusion with a dural arteriovenous malformation of the posterior fossa. Surg Neurol 4:433–437, 1975.
7. Hilal SK, Michelsen JW: Therapeutic percutaneous embolization for extra-axial vascular lesions of the head, neck and spine. J Neurosurg 43:275–287, 1975.
8. Houser OW, Baker HL Jr, Rhoton AL Jr, Okazaki H: Intracranial dural arteriovenous malformations. Radiology 105:55–64, 1972.
9. Houser OW, Campbell JK, Campbell RJ, Sundt TM Jr: Arteriovenous malformation affecting the transverse dural venous sinus—an acquired lesion. Mayo Clin Proc 54:651–661, 1979.
10. Hugosson R, Bergstrom K: Surgical treatment of dural arteriovenous malformation in the region of the sigmoid sinus. J Neurol Neurosurg Psychiat 37:97–101, 1974.
11. Kosnik EJ, Hunt WE, Miller CA: Dural arteriovenous malformations. J Neurosurg 40:322–329, 1974.
12. Kühner A, Krastel A, Stoll W: Arteriovenous malformations of the transverse dural sinus. J Neurosurg 45:12–19, 1976.
13. Lamas E, Lobato RD, Esparza J, Escudero L: Dural posterior fossa AVM producing raised sagittal sinus pressure: case report. J Neurosurg 46:804–810, 1977.
14. Magidson MA, Weinberg PE: Spontaneous closure of a dural arteriovenous malformation. Surg Neurol 6:107–110, 1976.
15. Manaka S, Izawa M, Nawata H: Dural arteriovenous malformation treated by artificial embolization with liquid silicone. Surg Neurol 7:63–65, 1977.
16. Miyasaka K, Takei H, Nomura M, Sugimoto S, Aida T, Abe H, and Tsuru M: Computerized tomography findings in dural arteriovenous malformations. J Neurosurg 53:698–702, 1980.
17. Obrador S, Soto M, Silvela J: Clinical syndromes of arteriovenous malformations of the transverse-sigmoid sinus. J Neurol Neurosurg Psychiat 38:436–451, 1975.
18. Storrs DG, King RB: Management of extracranial congenital arteriovenous malformations of the head and neck. Report of five cases. J Neurosurg 38:584–590, 1973.
19. Waga S, Fujimoto K, Morikawa A, Morooka Y, Okada M: Dural arteriovenous malformation in the anterior fossa. Surg Neurol 8:356–358, 1977.

Chapter 24 CAROTID-CAVERNOUS FISTULA

Most fistulas between the carotid artery and cavernous sinus are due to trauma, but spontaneous communication can occur from a dural arterial malformation or rarely from rupture of an intracavernous aneurysm. The lesions due to trauma are frequently associated with a basal skull fracture. A fistula can also occur from attempting to pass a Fogarty catheter in an effort to remove a thrombus from the internal carotid artery and from surgical procedures near this area (7, 11).

POST-TRAUMATIC FISTULA

Clinical Presentation

Patients with carotid-cavernous fistula may present with exophthalmus, chemosis, extraocular palsies, visual failure, headache, ocular discomfort, or the hearing of a noise synchronous with the pulse. The bruit is the most common and often the most disturbing symptom but the changes in the eye may be severe. The exophthalmus is due to the retrograde flow of blood into the ophthalmic veins. Chemosis results from dilatation and arterialization of the small veins of the conjunctiva and sclera. Diplopia is usually secondary to cranial nerve palsy but can also be due to direct nerve injury at the time of trauma and mechanical restriction from the increased orbital mass (7). The major threat to vision is probably hypoxia (29). The lowered arterial pressure and elevated venous pressure reduce the ocular perfusion pressure. The hypoxic damage may be irreversible despite control of the fistula. On rare occasions, neurological symptoms relate to the steal of arterial blood from the brain or increased venous pressure in cortical veins (1, 3).

Bilateral fistulas are rare but may occur after trauma (5). A patient with a unilateral carotid-cavernous fistula may present with ipsilateral, contralateral, or bilateral signs (7). Occasionally, there may be no ocular signs. The extent of the involvement is determined by the pattern of venous drainage.

Angiography

The diagnosis is established by angiography. Characteristic angiographic findings include early dense opacification of the enlarged cavernous sinus, early filling of the ophthalmic or other veins draining the area, and reduced opacification of the intracranial arterial system. Although most post-traumatic fistulae appear to originate directly from one internal carotid artery, bilateral selective internal carotid injections should be done, as well as a vertebral study, to assess collateral circulation and to plan the operative procedure. Debrun was able to precisely locate the fistula on angiograms in all 54 cases he reported (9). In 51 of the patients, vertebral angiography with compression of the carotid artery in the neck on the side of the fistula showed retrograde filling of the internal carotid artery through the posterior communicating artery. Since the carotid artery below the fistula did not fill, it was possible to locate and measure the size of the opening in the internal carotid artery. In patients where the posterior communicating artery was too small, a double lumen balloon catheter was used. The balloon was inflated in the internal carotid artery just above the bifurcation, and contrast was injected through the other lumen. Most of the fistulae occurred in the horizontal or posterior ascending segment of the intracavernous internal carotid artery. The fistulae varied in size from 1 to 5 mm with an average of 3 mm. Rarely was more than one opening present in the internal carotid artery.

The venous drainage may be anterior through the superior ophthalmic vein, posterior through the inferior or superior petrosal sinus, superior through the Sylvian vein, and inferior into pterygoid plexus. There may be only one draining vein or any combination. Debrun et al. also noted that in post-traumatic fistula there was no contribution from external carotid branches, which is in striking contrast to the findings in spontaneous fistula (9).

Treatment

Indications for surgical treatment are preservation of vision, elimination of the bruit, and restoration of the orbit and its contents to normal while avoiding cerebral ischemia. Hemorrhage, either intracranial or into the sphenoid sinus, is very rare. Spontaneous remission is reported to occur in 5–10% of patients (7).

Prior to the development of catheter techniques, the preferred operative treatment for carotid-cavernous fistula was trapping of the fistula combined with muscle embolization (7, 14, 21). This involved a frontotemporal craniotomy for occlusion of the internal carotid artery proximal to the ophthalmic artery, or if this was not possible, occlusion of both the ophthalmic and intracranial internal carotid artery, and

Table 24.1
Results of Treatment in 54 Patients with Carotid-Cavernous Fistula using Detachable Balloon Catheters[a]

Total occlusion of the fistula	50 (93%)
Preservation of internal carotid flow	32 (59%)
Mortality (sepsis)[b]	1 (2%)
Complications	
Venous pouch or false aneurysm	
Small	19 (35%)
Large-requiring treatment	5 (10%)
Oculomotor palsy	
Transient	10 (19%)
Permanent	1 (2%)
Hemiparesis	
Transient[c]	2 (4%)
Permanent[d]	1 (2%)

[a] From Debrun et al. (9).
[b] Patient had increased eye symptoms after venous catheterization and then had a surgical procedure.
[c] In one patient this was associated with intraoperative injection of bucrylate.
[d] Occurred after surgical intracranial ligation of incompletely occluded fistula.

then muscle embolization in the internal carotid artery followed by ligation of that artery.

During the past few years, several techniques have been developed to obliterate the traumatic carotid-cavernous fistula, first by occluding the internal carotid artery by a balloon catheter (26) and more recently by occluding the fistulae with preservation of internal carotid flow (2, 4, 9, 12, 16, 17, 18, 22, 28, 30). These techniques have been summarized by Debrun et al. (9).

There are three types of treatment to consider in a patient with a carotid cavernous fistula: 1) intra-arterial detachable balloon catheter 2) intravenous detachable balloon catheter, and 3) surgical approach with various adjuncts. For the intraarterial detachable balloon the catheter is introduced into the internal carotid artery and enters the cavernous sinus through the hole in the wall of the artery. The balloon is inflated and detached to occlude the fistula leaving the artery patent. The use of a latex detachable balloon has been described by Serbinenko and Debrun et al. (8, 30) and of a calibrated-leak balloon and bucrylate by Kerber (17). The intravenous detachable balloon technique has been used to treat carotid-cavernous fistula that drain anteriorly through the superior ophthalmic vein or posteriorly through the inferior petrosal sinus (20, 22). The direct surgical approach to the cavernous sinus has been described by Parkinson (25). He has surgically occluded the fistula with the patient under cardiac arrest and deep hypothermia. Hosobuchi reported the use of electrothrombosis (16). Mullen described the use of thrombogenic needles or bronze wire to induce thrombosis (22). Drake has plugged the cavernous sinus with pieces of muscle (9). Samson et al. injected isobutyl-2-cyanoacrylate into the cavernous sinus at craniotomy with closure of the fistula (28).

Debrun et al. described the use of detachable balloon catheters in treating 54 patients with traumatic carotid cavernous fistula (9). All three approaches listed above were used. The results of this treatment are summarized in Table 24.1. In 45 patients, treatment was intra-arterial balloon catheterization; seven patients had this combined with either a venous or surgical approach, one patient was successfully treated by a venous approach alone, and one patient was treated by surgery after the venous approach failed.

In 50 of the 54 patients, total occlusion of the fistulae was accomplished with this balloon technique (Fig. 24.1). In some patients, more than one procedure was required to complete the occlusion. In two patients, the fistula recurred and was treated with a second balloon. In two patients with previous surgery, the cavernous sinus was punctured under direct vision and a balloon detached. There was often a minor stenosis from the balloon or a small false aneurysm which were asymptomatic findings. These tended to diminish on follow-up angiography. In three patients where both the fistula and the internal carotid artery were originally occluded by the balloon, the superior portion of the fistula was later found to be open and these patients had intracranial ligation of the supraclinoid portion of the internal carotid artery. This is a potentially serious complication because the patient can develop ischemic symptoms due to steal of blood through the fistula. In all patients, the goal was to preserve circulation in the internal carotid artery, but this was not possible in 22 cases. The reasons for this are listed in Table 24.2.

The complications from Debrun et al. are listed in Table 24.1 (9). There was one death due to sepsis in a patient who had both a venous catheterization and a surgical procedure. Venous pouch or false aneurysm occur when the balloon has deflated too quickly but the fistula usually remains occluded. Small pouches cause no symptoms but large pouches may cause intractable retro-orbital pain or oculomotor

Table 24.2
Reasons for Internal Carotid Occlusion when Attempting to Preserve Carotid Circulation in 22 Patients with Carotid-Cavernous Fistulas[a]

Failure to enter cavernous sinus	7
False aneurysm with symptoms	5
Cavernous sinus entered but fistula could not be occluded	4
Previous surgery	2
Balloon occluded artery below fistula	1
ICA thrombosis from procedure	2
ICA stenosis from balloon and traumatic dissection	1

[a] Modified from Debrun et al. (9).

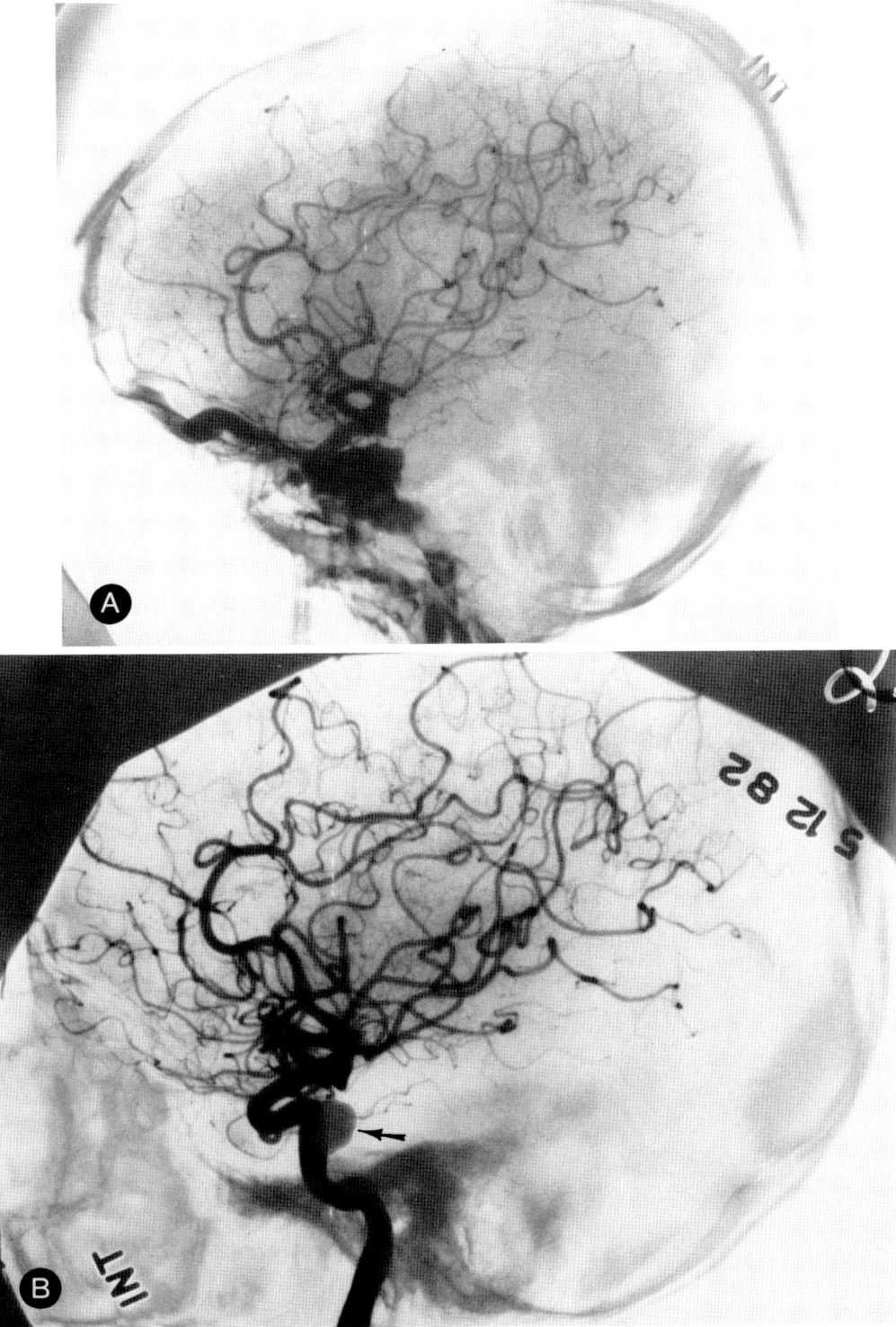

Figure 24.1 Post-traumatic carotid-cavernous fistula. *A*, lateral angiogram demonstrates a cartoid-cavernous fistula with anterior drainage into the superior ophthalmic vein. *B*, complete occlusion of the fistula after treatment with an intraarterial detachable balloon (*arrow*). The internal carotid circulation is preserved. (These pictures are reproduced through the courtesy of Dr. Gerard Debrun who treated the patient.)

palsy. If these symptoms develop, it is necessary to occlude the internal carotid artery and neck of the false aneurysm with a second detachable balloon. This had to be done in five of the 24 patients who developed a venous pouch or false aneurysm. With the use of silicone for injection, this complication should decrease. The incidence of hemiparesis is small, but an occasional patient may not tolerate the temporary balloon occlusion done prior to the permanent occlusion. In such patients, a bypass graft may be indicated (13, 31).

In the rare patient with bilateral carotid-cavernous fistula, the detachable balloon technique may also be used (9). Laws et al. (18) treated one such patient by combining balloon techniques with direct exposure of the fistula through a transphenoidal approach.

At the present time, the initial treatment to consider for a post-traumatic carotid-cavernous fistula is intra-arterial detachable balloon catheter techniques in an effort to preserve internal carotid circulation while occluding the fistula with a minimum risk. However, venous and surgical approaches must be kept in mind for particular problems. As new techniques develop, these must be considered. For example, there is not yet enough experience to know if the injection of a rapidly polymerizing plastic via a catheter or directly into the cavernous sinus at operation will give better results (9, 17, 28).

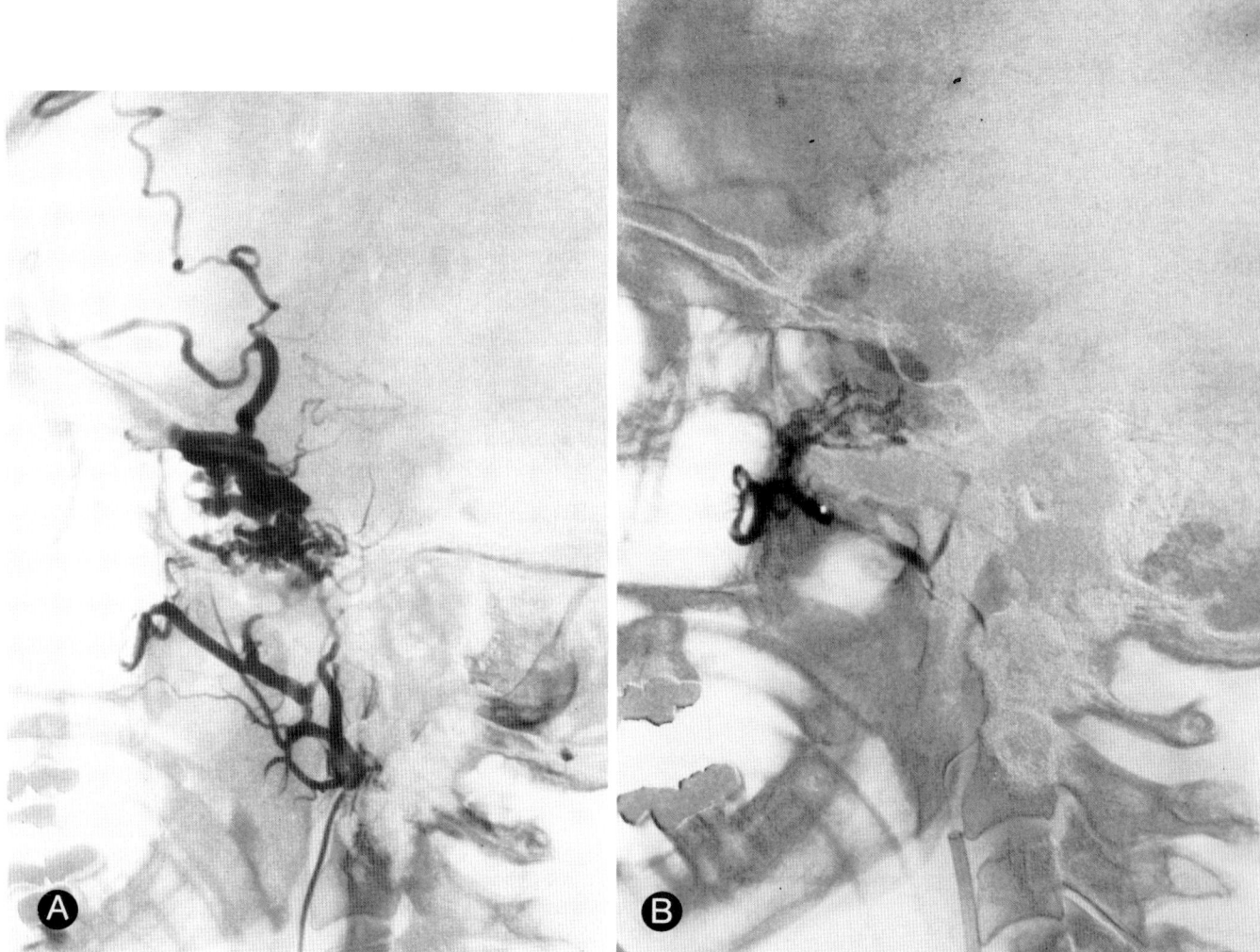

Figure 24.2 Spontaneous carotid-cavernous fistula. A, selective external carotid angiogram reveals a dural arteriovenous malformation with communication into the cavernous sinus. B, selective injection of internal maxillary artery outlines the multiple feeding arteries. C, selective internal carotid angiogram also fills the fistula from small internal carotid artery branches. D, common carotid angiogram after selective embolization of the internal maxillary artery. The external carotid supply is occluded and opacification from the internal carotid artery is much less. (These pictures are reproduced through the courtesy of Dr. Gerard Debrun who treated the patient.)

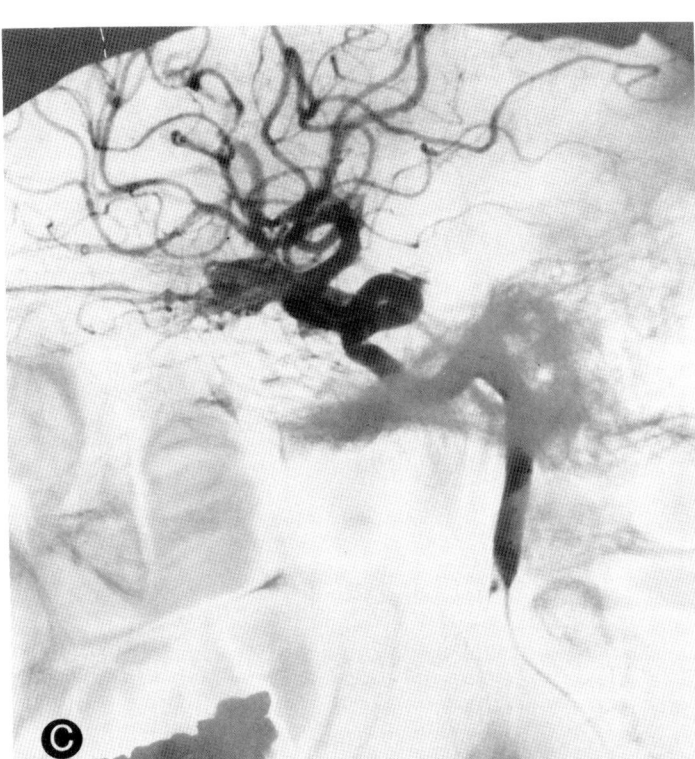
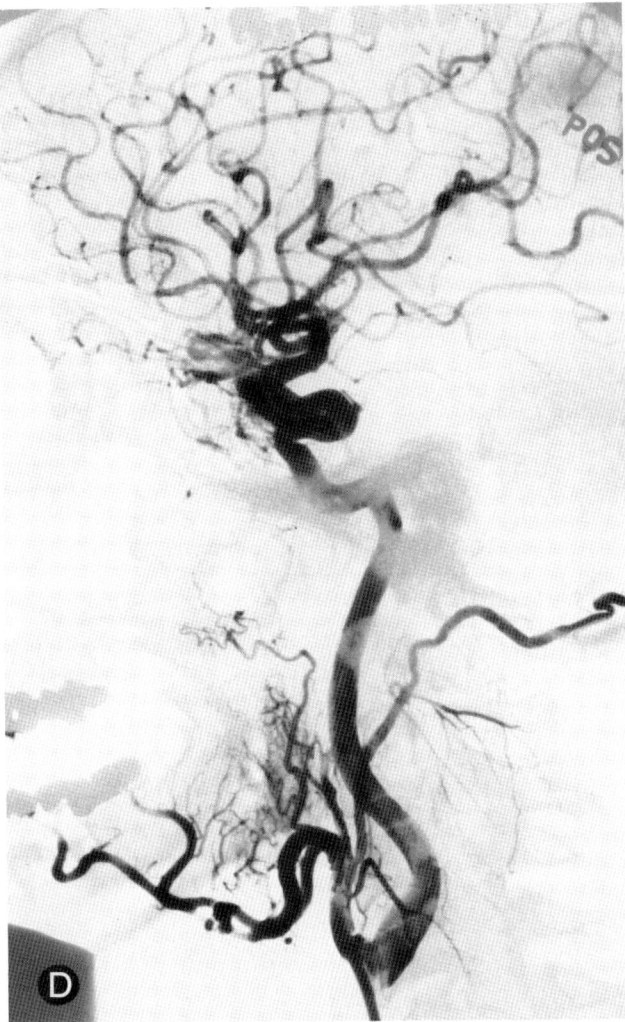

Figure 24.2 (*C* and *D*)

SPONTANEOUS FISTULA

The symptoms due to spontaneous carotid-cavernous fistula are often mild and may not develop abruptly. Mild unilateral headache, discomfort in the eye, or diplopia due to sixth nerve paresis may antedate the typical orbital signs by many months (7). Gradually, dilated conjunctival vessels and proptosis may develop. A bruit is noted by the patient in no more than one-half the reported cases.

Careful angiographic studies have shown that most of these spontaneous fistulae are secondary to a dural arteriovenous malformation see Chapter 23 (7, 10, 24, 32, 33). As such, they are low-flow and low-pressure fistulae. On rare occasion, rupture of an intracavernous aneurysm is the cause.

Most patients are middle aged, post-menopausal women (7, 32). However, onset may also occur during pregnancy (33). In the review of the literature by Pang et al., all patients were over 20 years of age except for one infant (24).

Complete selective internal and external carotid and vertebral angiography is essential. In 16 spontaneous carotid-cavernous fistulae, Debrun et al. found a contribution from the external carotid artery in all except one case of a ruptured cavernous aneurysm (9). External carotid branches that may supply the fistula include terminal meningeal branches of the internal maxillary ascending pharyngeal and pterygopalatine arteries (23, 24). The meningohypophyseal trunk is the usual feeding branch when the internal carotid artery also supplies the fistula.

Spontaneous resolution of the fistula may occur in patients with dural arteriovenous shunts. Newton and Hoyt reported that five of 11 such fistulae resolved completely (23). Spontaneous improvement was also noted in two patients where the onset was during pregnancy (33). In many patients, symptoms are mild and non-progressive and the patient may be followed (10, 32). If symptoms require surgical treatment, external carotid embolization is used (Fig. 24.2) (6, 15, 19, 24, 27). In the rare case of a spontaneous high-flow fistula due to a ruptured aneurysm, treatment is done by using a detachable balloon catheter as outlined for traumatic fistula.

REFERENCES

1. Ambler MW, Moon AC, Sturner WQ: Bilateral carotid-cavernous fistulae of mixed types with unusual radiological and neuropathological findings. Case report. J Neurosurg 48:117–124, 1978.
2. Bank WO, Kerber CW, Drayer BP, et al: Carotid-cavernous fistula: endarterial cyanoacrylate occlusion with preservation of carotid flow. J Neuroradiol 5:279–285, 1978.
3. Bartlow B, Penn RD: Carotid-cavernous sinus fistula presenting as a posterior fossa mass. Case report. J Neurosurg 42:585–588, 1975.
4. Benati A, Maschio A, Perini S, Beltramello A: Treatment of post-traumatic carotid-cavernous fistula using a detachable balloon catheter. J Neurosurg 53:784–786, 1980.
5. Conley FK, Hamilton RD, Hosobuchi Y: Successful surgical treatment of bilateral carotid-cavernous fistulas. Case report. J Neurosurg 43:357–361, 1975.
6. Costin JA, Weinstein MA, Berlin AJ, Hardy RW, Gutman FA: Dural arterio-venous malformations involving the cavernous sinus, a case report. Br J Ophthalmol 62:478–482, 1978.
7. Day AL, Rhoton Al Jr: Aneurysms and arteriovenous fistula of the intracavernous carotid artery and its branches, in Youmous JR (ed): *Neurological Surgery* 2nd Ed (to be published).
8. Debrun G, Lacour P, Caron JP, Hurth M, Comoy J, Keravel Y: Detachable balloon and calibrated-leak balloon techniques in the treatment of cerebral vascular lesions. J Neurosurg 49:635–649, 1978.
9. Debrun G, Lacour P, Vinuela F, Fox A, Drake CG, Caron JP. Treatment of 54 traumatic carotid-cavernous fistulas. J Neurosurg 55:678–692, 1981.
10. Edwards MS, Connolly ES: Cavernous sinus syndrome produced by communication between the external carotid artery and cavernous sinus. J Neurosurg 46:92–96, 1977.
11. Eggers F, Lukin R, Chambers AA, Tomsick TA, Sawaya K: Iatrogenic carotid-cavernous fistula following Fogarty catheter thromboendarterectomy. J Neurosurg 51:543–545, 1979.
12. Fierstien SB, DeFeo D, Nutkiewicz, A: Complete obliteration of a carotid cavernous fistula with sparing of the carotid blood flow using a detachable balloon catheter. Surg Neurol 9:277–280, 1978.
13. Guegan Y, Javalet A, Eon JY, Vallee B, Pecker J: Extra-intracranial anastomosis preliminary to treatment of carotid artery-cavernous sinus fistula. Surg Neurol 10:85–88, 1978.
14. Hamby WB: *Carotid-cavernous Fistulae*. Springfield, Illinois, Charles C. Thomas, 1966.
15. Hardy RW, Costin JA, Weinstein M, Berlin AJ Jr, Gutman FA: External carotid-cavernous fistula treated by transfemoral embolization. Surg Neurol 9:255–256, 1978.
16. Hosobuchi Y: Electrothrombosis of carotid-cavernous fistula. J Neurosurg 42:76–85, 1975.
17. Kerber C: Use of balloon catheters in the treatment of cranial arterial abnormalities. Stroke 11:210–216, 1980.
18. Laws ER Jr, Onofrio BM, Pearson BW, McDonald TJ, Dirrenberger, RA: Successful management of bilateral carotid-cavernous fistulae with a trans-sphenoidal approach. Neurosurgery 4:162–167, 1979.
19. Mahaley MS, Boone SC: External carotid-cavernous fistula treated by arterial embolization: Case report. J Neurosurg 40:110–114, 1974.
20. Manelfe C, Bernstein A: Treatment of carotid-cavernous fistulas by venous approach. J Neuroradiol 7:13–19, 1980.
21. Morley TP: Appraisal of various forms of management in 41 cases of carotid cavenous fistula, in Morley TP (ed): *Current Controversies in Neurosurgery*. Philadelphia, WB Saunders, 1976.
22. Mullan S: Experiences with surgical thrombosis of intracranial berry aneurysm and carotid-cavernous fistulas. J Neurosurg 41:657–670, 1974.
23. Newton TH, Hoyt WF: Dural arteriovenous shunts in the region of the cavernous sinus. Neuroradiology 1:71–81, 1980.
24. Pang D, Kerber C, Biglan AW, Ahn HS: External carotid-cavernous fistula in infancy: Case report and review of the literature. Neurosurgery 8:212–218, 1981.
25. Parkinson, D: Carotid cavernous fistula: Direct repair with preservation of the carotid artery. Technical note. J Neurosurg 38:99–106, 1973.
26. Prolo DJ, Burres KP, Hanbery JW: Balloon occlusion of carotid cavernous fistula: Introduction of a new catheter. Surg Neurol 7:209–214, 1977.
27. Pugatch RP, Wolpert SM: Transfemoral embolization of an external carotid-cavernous fistula: Case report. J Neurosurg 42:94–97, 1975.
28. Samson D, Ditmore QM, Beyer CW Jr: Intravascular use of isobutyl-2-cyanoacrylate: Part 2. Treatment of carotid-cavernous fistulas. Neurosurgery 8:52–55, 1981.
29. Sanders MD, Hoyt WF: Hypoxia ocular sequelae of carotid-cavernous fistulae. Study of the causes of visual failure before and after neurosurgical treatment in a series of 25 cases. Br J Ophthalmol 53:82–97, 1969.
30. Serbinenko FA: Balloon catheterization and occlusion of major cerebral vessels. J Neurosurg 41:125–145, 1974.
31. Shen, Al: Superficial temporal-middle cerebral artery anastomoses in the treatment of a carotid cavernous fistula. J Neurosurg 49:760–763, 1978.
32. Taniguchi RM, Goree JA, Odom GL: Spontaneous carotid-cavernous shunts presenting diagnostic problems. J Neurosurg 35:384–391, 1971.
33. Toya S, Shiobara R, Izumi J, Shinomiya Y, Shiga H, Kimura C: Spontaneous carotid-cavernous fistula during pregnancy or in the postpartum stage: Report of two cases. J Neurosurg 54:252–256, 1981.

Chapter 25 BRAIN HEMORRHAGE

Brain hemorrhage continues to be an important cause of death and neurological disability. Hemorrhage syndromes are sufficiently characterized to permit their clinical recognition in many patients. Computed tomography has revolutionized the management of brain hemorrhage by demonstrating these lesions with clarity and detail. The clinical and CT criteria for decisions regarding medical and surgical management continue to undergo change.

PATHOLOGY

Hypertensive brain hemorrhage tends to occur in specific sites: putamen, thalamus, cerebellum, and pons. Lobar hemorrhage may also be related to hypertension. Hemorrhage in any area of the brain, but especially lobar and cerebellar, may be due to a specific cause such as arteriovenous malformation, brain tumor, or coagulation disorders, and can occur in association with normal blood pressure and with no radiographic evidence of a specific etiologic factor.

In hypertensive hemorrhage, the most common sources of bleeding are the penetrating arteries from the Circle of Willis (the lenticulostriate and thalamoperforating arteries) and from similar branches (the paramedian) of the basilar artery (14). Though these vessels normally can withstand extremely high pressure without rupture, pathological changes lead to weakness. It has been suggested that microaneurysms were the cause of the hemorrhage, but careful histological studies indicate that fibrinoid necrosis is the cause of the weakness in the arterial wall (13, 49, 68). The final triggering mechanism for the rupture is not known, although it has been speculated that a sudden increase in blood pressure coincident with factors such as exertion or emotional stress may excede the tolerance of the vessel wall (70). This notion is supported by the finding that the setting for hemorrhage is usually during activity and infrequently during sleep (38).

Non-hypertensive brain hemorrhage may be associated with aneurysm or AVM, primary or metastatic brain tumor (26, 30, 41), infarction (23), anticoagulation (8, 28), endogenous coagulopathy, especially leukemia (28), and rare lesions such as amyloid angiopathy (31). In some hematomas, especially those in a lobar position, no source or cause for the hemorrhage may be found (48).

The hemorrhage produces both destruction and displacement of tissue. Pathologic studies demonstrate tracking of blood along tissue planes with displacement of tissue (14, 21). This latter effect is often more evident than is the destruction and provides the basis for hope that the ultimate outcome may be much better than indicated by the acute deficit. The hemorrhage is inferred to be of short duration in most cases, irrespective of size when the bleeding ceases. No correlation has been found between the hematoma size and blood pressure (9).

The mechanism of later clinical deterioration is less certain. Rebleeding is rare. In a study with chromium-labeled red cells injected at the time of admission for hypertensive hemorrhage, it was found that patients who died had virtually no evidence of labeling in the original hemorrhage although the Duret hemorrhages that reflected the post-admission fatal cerebral herniation were easily labeled (20). However, CT scan will occasionally document enlargement of the hematoma. Edema or ischemic necrosis around the lesion may extend and probably is the chief mechanism for subsequent worsening (10, 38). These changes relate to the development of hyperemia and disturbances of autoregulation and the blood brain barrier (22).

Reduction in the hematoma size is accomplished by reparative mechanisms over several months. The process is slow because macrophage activity must go on along the rim of the mass to reabsorb the hematoma. Within a year the hematoma site is converted to a slit-like cavity with orange-stained walls representing hemosiderin-laden macrophages surrounded by tissue which appears more or less normal (14).

DIAGNOSTIC STUDIES

CT Scan

Any patient suspected of having a brain hemorrhage should have an immediate CT scan. The scan gives a precise localization of the hemorrhage, outlines its size and configuration, shows the degree of hydrocephalus, indicates ventricular shift or compression, gives an indication of the degree of edema in adjacent brain tissue, and can be repeated as needed for evaluation of the subsequent clinical course (10, 18, 21, 35, 38, 52, 62).

Over several weeks, the high density seen on CT gradually becomes isodense, and then changes to a low density appearance. This change in the scan appearance is due to an alteration in photon absorption rather than actual resorption of the hematoma as shown by CT-autopsy correlation (32). From a few days to some months after hemorrhage, the CT scan with contrast administration will often show a ring-like enhancement around the hemorrhage which presumably represents the area of edema or local ischemic infarction (63, 69).

There is almost no indication for lumbar puncture in a patient suspected of having brain hemorrhage. It should not be used as a diagnostic study because large hemorrhages can lead to transtentorial herniation, and in small hemorrhages, the spinal fluid may be clear. CT scan provides the information needed.

Angiography

When the clinical syndrome and CT scan indicate a typical hypertensive brain hemorrhage, particularly in the putamen, thalamus, cerebellum, or pons, angiography is now rarely indicated. Prior to CT scanning, this was the most important diagnostic test (36). The direction of deviation of the lenticulostriate arteries has been used as a prognostic sign (33).

In cases where hypertension is not the likely cause and in lobar hemorrhages, angiography is needed to help decide whether there is a vascular malformation or tumor (18, 48). However, the procedure may fail to show either of these lesions, particularly in the acute phase. We recommend that if initial angiography is negative and no other cause for the hematoma is apparent, the study be repeated in 2-3 months when pressure from the hematoma has subsided. If no abnormality is seen at that time, we would continue to follow the patient with a CT scan at 4-6-month intervals to be certain that an underlying tumor is not being overlooked as a cause for the hemorrhage.

Coagulation Studies

Every patient with brain hemorrhage should have coagulation parameters checked. These should include prothrombin time (PT), partial prothromboplastin time (PPT), and platelet count. In patients known to be receiving aspirin, bleeding time should be measured.

SPECIAL CLINICAL PROBLEMS AND GUIDLINES FOR TREATMENT

Putaminal Hemorrhage

The most common site for hypertensive hemorrhages is the putamen. The hemorrhage may remain localized but can track into the white matter, into the frontal or temporal lobe, involve the internal capsule, or rupture into the ventricle. The larger the lesion, the greater the deficit and the worse the prognosis.

The clinical syndrome is well-described (15, 16, 21, 38). Patients are characteristically up and active when they become aware that something is wrong. Then a hemiparesis emerges smoothly and steadily which may progress to a hemiplegia, in some cases accompanied by a hemisensory loss, hemianopia, dysphasia if the dominant hemisphere is affected, unawareness of the deficit if the non-dominant hemisphere is involved, and conjugate deviation of the eyes to the side of the hemorrhage. The syndrome may stabilize at any point or continue to coma and death within a few hours. In 27 consecutive cases, a smooth onset characterized 62% while 30% developed symptoms so rapidly that observers felt the deficit was nearly maximal at onset (38). None of the patients experienced fluctuation of the deficit. Headache affected only 14% at onset and only 28% at any time, leaving nearly 72% free of headache even in the presence of substantial focal neurological deficit. Only 12% had a stiff neck. Vomiting occurred in nearly 40%. On examination, none showed papilledema or subhyaloid pre-retinal hemorrhages. Some form of motor deficit affected all cases, varying from mild to complete paralysis. Sensory disorder was not fully evaluated in some cases but approximately 65% of the patients tested showed some alteration in response to pin prick. A disorder in conjugate horizontal gaze deviation was found in 52% of patients. Thirty-seven per cent had no impairment in eye movement, while 11% showed other disorders in eye function usually related to mid-brain compression.

Most small and many moderate-sized hematomas in the putamen make a good recovery either spontaneously or with medical treatment (Fig. 25.1, A and B). With hematomas larger than 3 cm in diameter, the initial treatment is usually medical but if the patient is showing signs of increasing neurological deficit or decreasing state of consciousness in spite of medical therapy, surgical removal of the hematoma is considered (Fig. 25.1C).

In an evaluation of the CT scans in 24 patients with putaminal hemorrhage, three groups were defined (21). In the first group, patients comatose on admission were found to have massive hemorrhages and a poor prognosis. The second group were alert with substantial neurological deficit and moderate-sized hematomas. A few made acceptable recovery, but the majority were left with a significant deficit. The third group had only mild deficits, were found to have small hemorrhages on the CT scan, and generally made a good recovery. Whether surgery would have improved the outcome in the first two groups is not known.

Thalamic Hemorrhage

The classic features include, as initial deficit, a hemisensory loss, and if the internal capsule becomes involved, motor weakness occurs (3, 12, 13, 16, 61). Extension into the upper brain stem commonly leads to vertical gaze palsy, retraction nystagmus, skew deviation, loss of convergence, ptosis and miosis, anisocoria, or unreactive pupils. Dysphasia may occur. Headache is rare but compression of the cerebrospinal fluid pathways may cause hydrocephalus.

In 18 patients with hypertensive thalamic hemor-

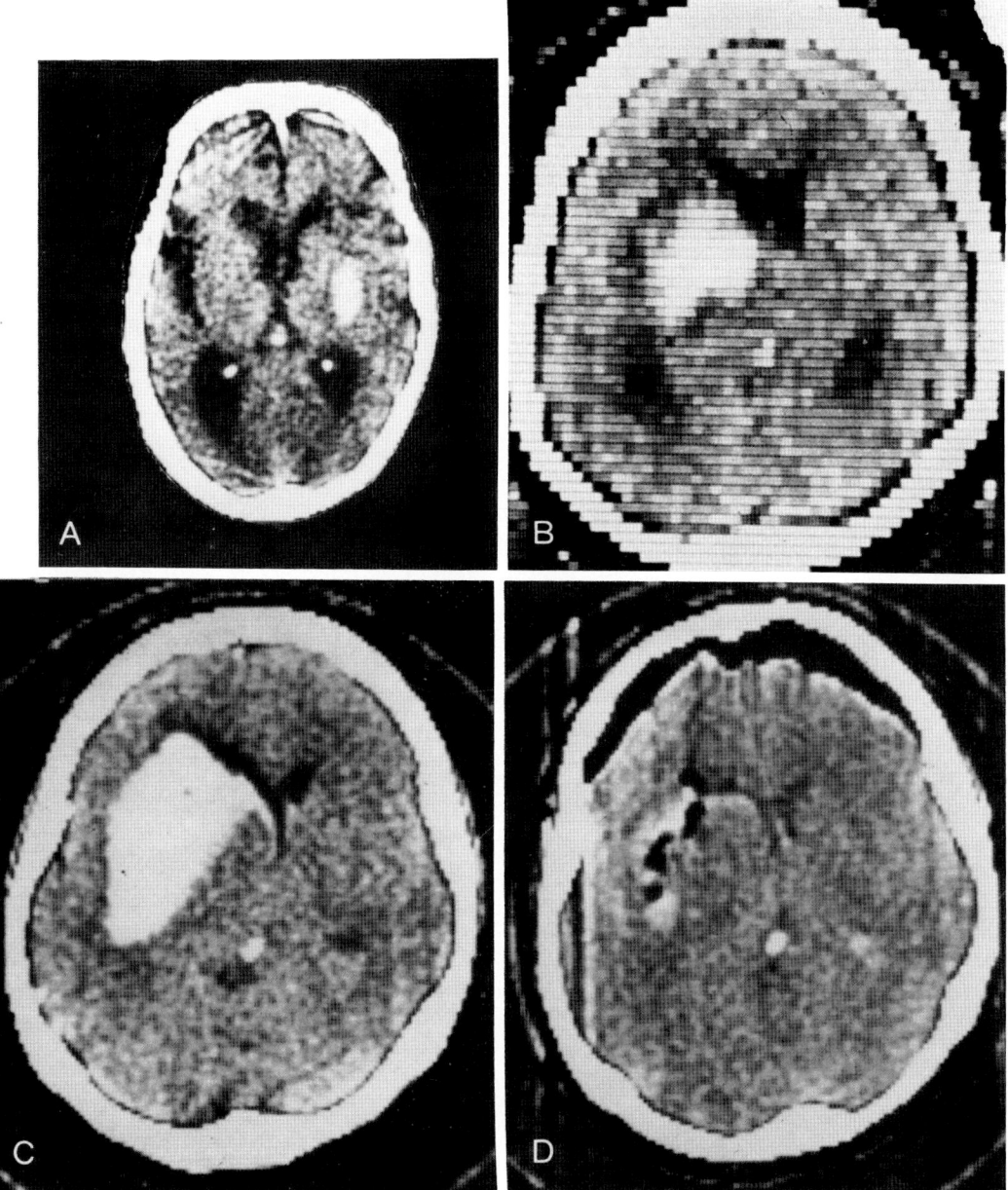

Figure 25.1 Hypertensive putaminal hemorrhage. *A,* small hematoma. Onset of mild deficit. Treated with steroids. Full recovery. *B,* Moderate hematoma. Onset of severe neurological deficit that worsened for 1 day then gradually improved. Speech cleared but residual hemiparesis persisted. *C,* large hematoma. Sudden onset of severe neurological deficit. Stable for 3 days on steroids. Then coma and evidence of increased intracranial pressure. Hematoma removed surgically. *D,* Scan done 3 hours postoperatively. There is air in the subdural space anteriorly. The hematoma has been removed but note that some hematoma remains on the walls of the cavity. This was left to minimize disturbance of the surrounding brain tissue. The patient recovered with residual hemiparesis. (From Ojemann RG, Mohr JP: Hypertensive brain hemorrhage, Ch. 17, in *Clinical Neurosurgery.* Baltimore, Williams & Wilkins, 1976, vol 23, pp 220–244, with permission.)

rhage, the diagnostic clinical features were limitations of vertical gaze, downward eye deviation, and small but reactive or sluggish pupils (61). All had a contralateral sensory-motor deficit. These findings were confirmed in another report of 23 patients (3). Headache was present in only 20–30% of these patients. The motor deficit was similar to that of putaminal hemorrhage. The sensory deficit was often of striking severity and widely distributed over the limbs, head, face, and trunk on the affected side.

In two reports of 41 patients with thalamic hemorrhage, it was found that all with a hematoma greater than 3.3 cm on the CT scan died (3, 61). Patients with smaller hematomas recovered but often with disability (Fig. 25.2).

Direct surgery on the hematoma should, therefore,

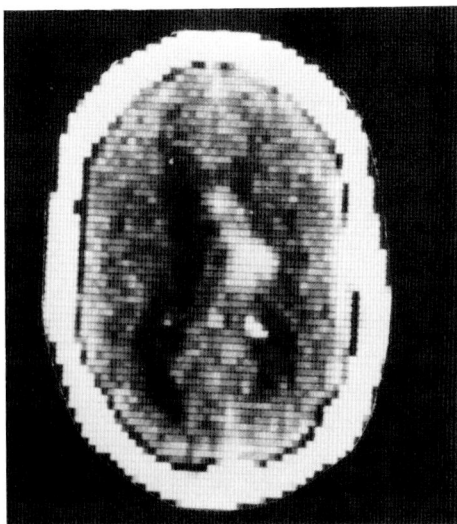

Figure 25.2 Hypertensive thalamic hemorrhage. Patient treated medically. Recovered to moderate neurological deficit.

be considered in patients with thalamic hematomas larger than 3 cm. The more common problem requiring surgery is the development of hydrocephalus which may require placement of a shunt (3, 60, 61).

Lobar Hemorrhage

Ropper and Davis have characterized the syndromes associated with lobar cerebral hemorrhages in 26 cases (48). Occipital hemorrhage (11 cases) caused severe pain around the ipsilateral eye and dense hemianopia (Fig. 25.3A). Left temporal hemorrhage (seven cases) began with mild pain in or just anterior to the ear, fluent dysphasia with poor auditory comprehension but relatively good repetition, and a partial hemianopic visual deficit (Fig. 25.3B). Frontal hemorrhage (four cases) caused a distinctive syndrome beginning with severe contralateral arm weakness, minimal leg and face weakness, and frontal headache. Parietal hemorrhage (three cases) begain with anterior temporal headache and hemisensory deficit, sometimes involving the trunk to the midline. A right temporal hemorrhage (one case) arrived in coma and no clinical syndrome could be assessed. The authors concluded that spontaneous lobar hemorrhage and branch artery embolization in the same region produced similar clinical syndromes. When there is hemorrhage, headache is the first prominent symptom with a rapid but not instantaneous onset over several minutes and, when combined with one of the typical syndromes, suggests lobar hemorrhage rather than another type of stroke.

The predisposing conditions which caused the hemorrhages were analyzed. Eight of the 26 patients were known to have had hypertension prior to hemorrhage, 14 had definite documentation of normal blood pressure, and in three the blood pressure was probably normal having been checked within a year before the illness, and in one a prior blood pressure was unknown. Two patients were on anticoagulants, two were found to have an AVM, and one had a metastatic tumor.

Most of the spontaneous or hypertensive lobar hematomas can be treated medically and will make a good recovery without surgical treatment (48). However, if the patient is showing signs of increasing neurological deficit in spite of medical therapy, then surgical removal of the hematoma is indicated.

Cerebellar Hemorrhage

Hemorrhage in the cerebellum causes a life-threatening syndrome which can be reversed by prompt surgical treatment. Classically, the onset of this hemorrhage is sudden, with nausea, vomiting, and inability to stand or walk (17). In a series of 56 patients with cerebellar hemorrhage, headache was present in 74%, dizziness in 55%, and loss of consciousness at onset in 14% (40). Examination showed appendicular ataxia in 78%, facial palsy in 60%, and ipsilateral gaze palsy in 54%. No distinctive clinical feature could be delineated in the acute state in noncomatose patients to predict those who would survive with minimal or mild disability and those who might progress to brain stem compression and coma.

The cerebellar hematoma represents a special situation regarding treatment. Deterioration due to brain stem compression is common, unpredictable, and often irreversible once set in motion. It is critically important to treat the patient before compression causes alteration in the state of consciousness and an unstable clinical situation. In our experience, 10 of 12 patients who were alert or drowsy preoperatively survived operation, while only four of 16 patients who were stuprous or comatose before surgery lived (40). The relationship of the level of consciousness to prognosis and the importance of not

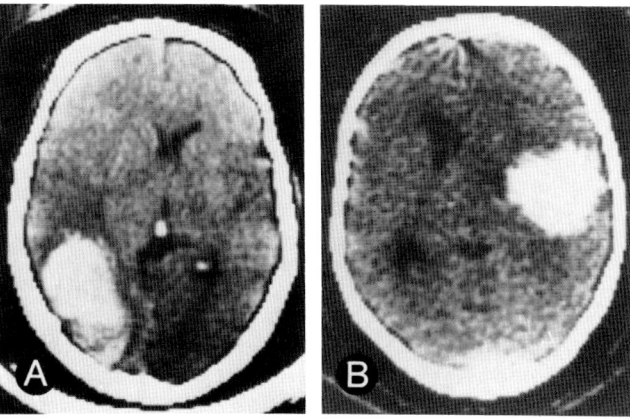

Figure 25.3 Lobar hemorrhage. A, occipital lobe hemorrhage. Patient on coumadin. Patient in coma at the time of hospital admission. Hematoma removed with good recovery. B, temporal lobe hemorrhage. Patient had mild neurological signs. Recovery with medical therapy.

delaying surgery in patients with acute cerebellar hematomas has been stressed in another review (6). Therefore, we generally recommend removal of hematomas that are greater than 3 cm in diameter on the CT scan (7, 8, 40, 51) (Fig. 25.4B). In one report of 10 patients with cerebellar hematoma, six had a progressive course with early brain stem compression and all had hematomas 3 cm or greater on CT scan (25).

Those patients with smaller lesions are monitored carefully in the intensive care unit. Many patients with small hematomas have a benign course (19) and CT scan evaluation confirms they may be treated medically with good results (25) (Fig. 25.4A).

Pontine Hemorrhage

This is one of the most dramatic and least treatable of all brain hemorrhages. A small hematoma often leads to immediate coma, rapid quadriplegia, decerebrate rigidity, pin-point pupils which may be barely reactive to light, and a variety of ocular motility disturbances. The uncommon smaller hemorrhage may cause the patient to be paralyzed but able to communicate by ocular movements ("Locked-in" state). Most patients do not survive the acute phase.

On rare occasions, successful removal of a pontine hematoma has been reported (4, 34). Sano and Ochiai reviewed 24 patients with pontine hematoma due to hypertension (50). Six with hematomas less than 1.0 cm in diameter as shown by CT survived but only one is working. All patients with hematomas larger than 1.0 cm died except for one. Four patients had suboccipital craniectomy for removal of the hematoma and several had ventricular drainage. It was concluded that direct operation was of doubtful value.

Intraventricular Hemorrhage

With the use of the CT scan, the degree of intraventricular hemorrhage associated with parenchymal brain hemorrhage can be easily defined. The spontaneous resolution of intraventricular hemorrhage was originally documented by pneumoencephalogram (37) and has been well demonstrated with the CT scan. A review of 54 patients with intraventricular hemorrhage on the CT scan revealed an association

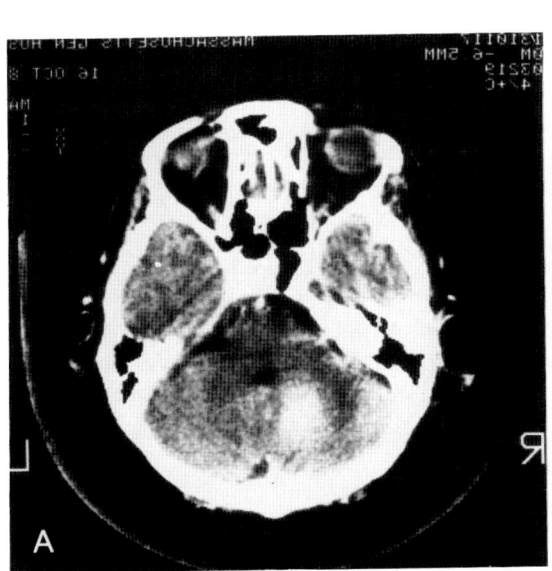
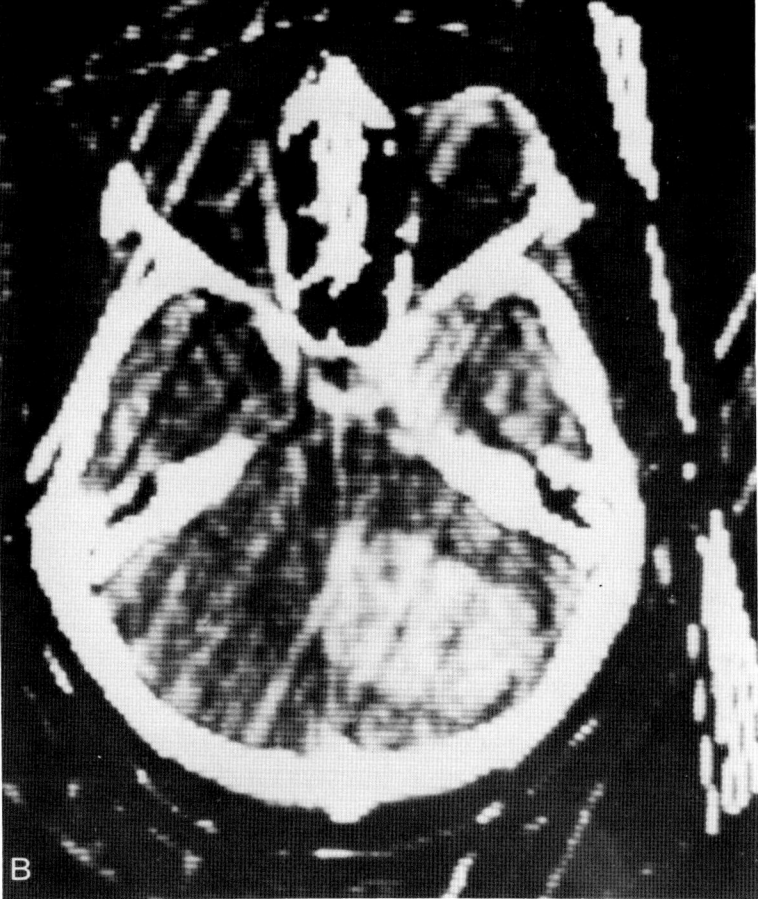

Figure 25.4 Cerebellar hemorrhage. A, hemorrhage less than 3 cm in diameter located in the medial aspect of the cerebellar hemisphere. Patient recovered on medical therapy. B, large hematoma causing brain stem compression. Emergency surgery was done to remove the hematoma. Patient recovered over several weeks. (From Mossy J, Reinmuth OM: *Cerebrovascular Disease.* New York, Raven Press, 1981, with permission.)

with a large number of disorders including hypertension, saccular and mycotic aneurysm, AVM, tumor, and coagulation disorders. Hypertensive hemorrhage in any of the common sites can rupture into the ventricle. In a report of 32 patients with hypertensive intracerebral hemorrhage, 62% had intraventricular rupture (63). Intraventricular hemorrhage also occurs from rupture of an aneurysm, and these hemorrhages are generally more extensive than those due to other causes.

The guidelines for surgical treatment are generally the same as those outlined for the parenchymal site of the hemorrhage. Ventricular drainage has usually not been helpful (24).

Hemorrhage Due to Amyloid Angiopathy

Amyloid angiopathy is an infrequent cause of spontaneous lobar brain hemorrhage (31). It usually occurs in patients over 60 years of age and may be associated with multiple hemorrhages (39, 58). When intracerebral hemorrhage is found in a normotensive elderly patient, this diagnosis must be considered (59). In such cases, it is important to biopsy the wall of the hematoma cavity if surgical treatment is indicated.

Hemorrhage Due to Coagulation Disorders

Anticoagulant and Antiplatelet Therapy

With the widespread use of anticoagulants for treatment of a variety of disorders, the number of patients with brain hemorrhage due to this cause has increased. The majority of patients who develop this complication are found to have either a prothrombin time longer than the therapeutic range or a local lesion such as infarction to account for bleeding (16). In contrast to most other bleeding disorders, an isolated intracerebral hemorrhage in a patient on anticoagulants may occur in the absence of bleeding in other areas of the body.

The initial evaluation and treatment is the same as described for spontaneous brain hemorrhage. Immediate transfusion of fresh frozen plasma reverses anticoagulation. To maintain hemostasis, parental administration of Vitamin K1 (phytonadione) preparation usually restores normal coagulation within 6 hours. With these measures, operation can usually be safely performed (Fig. 25.3A). Prothrombin time should be rechecked postoperatively to guard against rebound effects.

Occasionally, antiplatelet therapy may contribute to the development of brain hemorrhage. In such instances, platelet transfusions are needed to restore normal bleeding time, if intracranial surgery is needed.

Thrombocytopenia

The normal blood platelet count is 100,000 to 400,000 per mm^3. Thrombocytopenia is diagnosed when the platelet count is less than 80,000/mm^3 (1). This is a common cause of clotting deficiency. Intracerebral hemorrhage due to thrombocytopenia has been reported in idiopathic thrombocytopenic purpura and in a variety of disease states in which there is secondary thrombocytopenia. The latter includes conditions in which there is either failure of production of platelets due to suppression of bone marrow (drugs, septicemia and metastatic tumor) and myeloinfiltrative conditions (leukemia and multiple myeloma); or in which there is excessive destruction of platelets as in certain immune reactions. The initial symptoms of spontaneous intracranial bleeding in these patients is usually headache followed by deterioration in the level of consciousness. The onset is often insidious, coming on over several days. Usually the hemorrhage is intracerebral, but subdural hematoma can occur (1).

Surgery is hazardous if the platelet count is below 50,000 and is of concern when the count is 50,000–100,000. It is usually possible to achieve a hemostatic level by a combination of platelet transfusion and administration of corticosteroid drugs which have a number of effects not only in the hemostatic mechanisms but also in many instances on the underlying disease process. Guidelines for surgery on the hematoma are the same as previously stated. In a report on intracranial hemorrhage in children with idiopathic thrombocytopenia purpura, it was recommended that emergency splenectomy be done prior to neurosurgical intervention (64).

Hemophilia

Hemophilia is due to a deficiency in factor VIII, factor IX, or factor XI causing a prolonged partial thromboplastin time. The vast majority of patients are deficient in factor VIII, a small number in factor IX, and an occasional patient in factor XI. The problem has been summarized in several reports (53, 67).

Brain hemorrhage usually is associated with mild trauma but it can occur spontaneously. Any patient with hemophilia who complains of a persistent headache should have a CT scan. When hemorrhage is confirmed, appropriate replacement treatment should be started immediately. To prevent further spontaneous, intra-operative or postoperative hemorrhage, it is necessary to maintain a minimum level of at least 20% of the deficient factor with transfusions of the appropriate concentrate. If an operation is done, replacement needs to be given until the incision is healed (39). The indications for operation are the same as those previously outlined.

MEDICAL TREATMENT

When a diagnosis of brain hemorrhage has been established by CT scan, measures are taken to normalize blood pressure, prevent hemorrhage, reduce mass affect, control edema, and prevent seizures. Since most hemorrhages appear to have stopped before the patient arrives in the hospital, it has been difficult to assess efforts to stop hemorrhage in the occasional case of continued bleeding. Recurrence of hemorrhage is rare, except when the etiology is an aneurysm. Epsilon-aminocaproic acid has not been recommended.

Hypertension is controlled with drug therapy. If the blood pressure is exceedingly high, intravenous nitroprusside is utilized. We prefer hydralazine for longer-term control. This drug does not cause alteration in consciousness, which may occasionally occur with some of the other antihypertensive medications (e.g., α- methyldopa).

Control of intracranial pressure (ICP) requires several considerations. When indicated, the patient is intubated to insure adequate ventilation and the maintenance of a normal or reduced pCO2. Steroids may be helpful. We have noted temporary worsening after premature taper of steroid therapy with improvement on restoring high dosage. However, the benefit of this therapy in a large series of cases has not been established. One controlled study showed no benefit, but the majority of patients were in coma or deep stupor (57).

The role of continuous monitoring of ICP in the management of patients with large hematomas has been reported (11). In 12 patients, all with hematoma greater than 4.0 cm on the CT scan, the use of osmotic diuretics was governed by continuous monitoring of ICP. In that study, treatment with urea or mannitol was given whenever the ICP exceeded 40 mm Hg or cerebral perfusion pressure was less than 50 mm Hg. The mean arterial pressure was kept above 80 mm with either colloid or IV dopamine. Four patients returned to full activity, six were partially disabled, one totally disabled, and one other partially disabled patient died from a myocardial infarction. Whether surgery could have improved the outcome is unknown.

Careful management of fluid and electrolytes is required in all patients. One must watch for inappropriate antidiuretic hormone secretion which is not uncommon in these cases. In lobar lesions, the patient is given diphenylhydantoin.

SURGICAL TREATMENT

Indications

The indications for surgical therapy for brain hemorrhage continue to be modified. Although clear-cut indications are not yet available for all patients, clinical and CT guidelines for therapy are emerging (8, 21, 44, 47, 53). The smaller hematomas will generally respond to medical therapy as will most of the moderately sized hematomas (8, 38, 47, 65). When the hematoma is larger than 3.0 cm in diameter, surgical therapy is considered. If the patient is showing signs of increasing neurological deficit or decreasing state of consciousness in spite of medical therapy, then surgical removal of the hematoma is usually done.

The best guide to prognosis has been the state of consciousness (5, 29, 44).

Several reports have attempted to determine the indications for timing of operation in patients with hypertensive hemorrhage. Benefit of delayed operation has been assessed by some (5, 42, 46, 56) and of immediate operation by others (27, 54). Surgery can be life saving in the deteriorating patient (2, 8, 27, 45, 56, 65). It has not been established whether morbidity can be lessened by removal of a hematoma in a patient with a stable, moderate, or severe neurological deficit immediately or several days or weeks after onset. Reports of single cases and small series suggest that surgery may diminish late morbidity (8, 42, 43, 45, 46, 56, 65, 66). The special problem of cerebellar hemorrhage has been discussed.

When a hematoma in any location is associated with a history and finding of severely increased intracranial pressure and brain stem compression, emergency surgery is considered depending on the findings on CT scan and physical examination. Mannitol (100 gm in 500 ml) is given intravenously over 15–20 minutes while the CT scan is being done. Surgery is generally not undertaken if there is massive hemorrhage with loss of pupillary reaction and brain stem function and no response to the medical therapy.

Preoperative Preparation

If the patient has been treated medically for several days, care is taken to be sure that there is adequate hydration and the electrolytes are normal. Prior to induction of anesthesia, a radial artery catheter is placed for continuous monitoring of intraarterial blood pressure and intermittent blood gas determinations. Care is taken to avoid hypertension during induction of anesthesia. A Foley catheter is placed. After induction of anesthesia, 10–20 mg of furosemide is given and 50–100 gm of mannitol is infused while the craniotomy is being performed.

Operative Technique

In putaminal and lobar hemorrhages, the patient is placed in a semi-lateral position with the head turned to the appropriate side and held with a three-point skeletal fixation head rest. A wide exposure is made and a free bone flap elevated.

We operate cerebellar hemorrhages in the prone position with the head moderately flexed and held with the skeletal fixation headrest. This avoids the risk of hypotension. An occipital burr hole permits ventricle puncture. A midline incision allows a wide suboccipital craniectomy and removal of the posterior rim of the foramen magnum.

With the precise localization from the CT scan, a direct approach to the hemorrhage is usually possible. It is not possible to adequately evacuate an acute hematoma through a ventricular needle or catheter. Direct exposure of the hematoma is required for

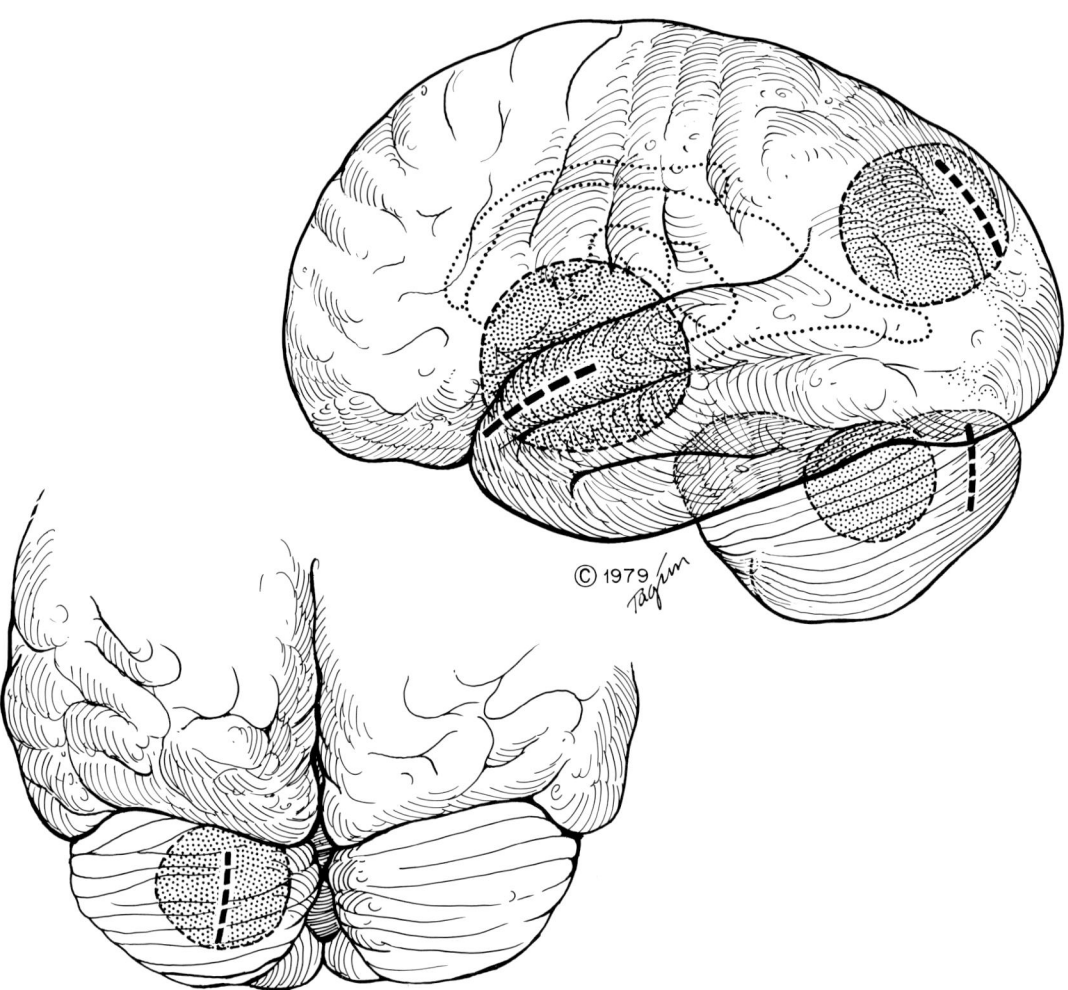

Figure 25.5 Common sites for brain hemorrhage requiring surgical treatment. Putamen, lobar (parietal-occipital), and cerebellum. The location of the cortical incisions are outlined for the easiest access with the least trauma to normal brain tissue. (From Mossy J, Reinmuth OM: *Cerebrovascular Disease.* New York, Raven Press, 1981, with permission.)

satisfactory removal. A cortical incision is performed in the appropriate area (Fig. 25.5). For temporal or putaminal lesions, an anterior superior temporal gyrus approach is used. A trans-Sylvian approach has been described (55). For parietal-occipital lesions, a superior posterior parietal lobule incision is chosen. For a frontal lesion, we prefer a superior frontal gyrus incision anterior to the motor strip. For cerebellar lesions, a paramedian approach is made depending on the lesion's location. The cortisectomy is made 2–3 cm long with the aid of bipolar cautery and microscissors (Fig. 25.6A, p. 306). Loupes and headlights permit satisfactory visualization. On occasion, the operating microscope is useful if an unexpected AVM is found or in controlling hemorrhage from a deep vessel.

Evacuation of the hemorrhage is achieved with gentle suction and irrigation (Fig. 25.6B, p. 307). Sometimes a tumor forceps can deliver a large clot. Most of the hematoma is removed to achieve decompression but the last adherent bits of clot may be left behind (Fig. 25.1D). This is done to avoid injury and bleeding from the walls of the cavity. Great care is taken to keep instruments, particularly the sucker, away from the adjacent edematous brain tissue. This is aided by the use of self-retaining retractors. Any abnormal appearing brain tissue should be biopsied.

Hemostasis is achieved using bipolar cautery (Fig. 25.6C, p. 307). Occasionally a clip is needed. Surgicel is used to line the hematoma cavity. Hemostasis must be meticulous to avoid recurrence. We raise the blood pressure for 5–10 minutes to 150 mm Hg in order to check hemostasis. Great care must be taken to avoid hypertension. Closure is performed in the usual fashion without a drain. In some cases of cerebellar hemorrhage, a ventricular catheter may be left in for a few days.

Postoperative Care

Postoperative care must be meticulous in order to avoid recurrence. Blood pressure must be controlled as the anesthesia wears off. The radial artery catheter permits careful monitoring of pressure. An intravenous medication (either sodium nitroprusside or trimethapan camsylate) is ready at all times. Continuous monitoring of blood pressure must be done particularly during the transfer of the patient from operating table to bed and to the recovery room area. Steroid medication is continued to control brain swelling. In supratentorial lesions, diphenylhydantoin is started. Electrolytes are checked regularly. If the patient's state of consciousness is reduced, intubation may be continued. The place of continuous intracranial pressure monitoring in postoperative management has not been established.

Any evidence of worsening should lead to a CT scan for evaluation. Postoperative complications include recurrence of bleeding, hydrocephalus, and infection.

REFERENCES

1. Almaani WS, Awid AS: Spontaneous intracranial bleeding in hemorrhagic diathesis. Surg Neurol (to be published).
2. Arana-Iniquez R, Wilson E, Bastarrica E, Medici M: Cerebral hematomas. Surg Neurol 6:45–52, 1976.
3. Barraquer-Bordas L, Illa A, Escartin J, Ruscalleda J, Marti-Vilalta JL: Thalamic hemorrhage. A study of 23 patients with diagnosis by computed tomography. Stroke 12:524–527, 1981.
4. Becker DH, Silverberg GD: Successful evacuation of an acute pontine hematoma. Surg. Neurol 10:263–265, 1978.
5. Benes V, Koukolik F, Obrovska D: Two types of spontaneous intracerebral hemorrhage due to hypertension. J Neurosurg 37:509–513, 1972.
6. Brennan RW, Bergland RM. Acute cerebellar hemorrhage. Analysis of clinical findings and outcome in 12 cases. Neurology 27:527–532, 1977.
7. Crowell RM, Ojemann RG: Cerebellar Hemorrhage, in Buchheit WA, Truex RC Jr (eds): Surgery of the Posterior Fossa. New York, Raven, 1979, pp 135–142.
8. Crowell RM, Ojemann RG: Surgery for Brain Hemorrhage, in Mossy J, Reinmuth OM (eds): Cerebrovascular Disease. New York, Raven, 1981, pp 233–254.
9. Dinsdale HB: Spontaneous hemorrhage in the posterior fossa. Arch Neurol 10:200–217, 1964.
10. Dolinskas CA, Bilaniuk LT, Zimmerman RA, Kuhl DE, Alavi A: Computed tomography of intracerebral hematomas. II. Radionuclide and transmission CT studies of the perihematoma region. Am J Roentgenol 129:689–692, 1977.
11. Duff TA, Ayeni S, Levin AB, Javid M: Nonsurgical management of spontaneous intracerebral hematoma. Neurosurgery 9:387–393, 1981.
12. Fazio C, Sacco G, Bugiani O: The thalamic hemorrhage. An anatomo-clinical study, Eur Neurol 9:30–43, 1974.
13. Fisher CM: The pathologic and clinical aspects of thalamic hemorrhage. Trans Am Neurol Assoc 84:56–59, 1959.
14. Fisher CM: The Pathology and Pathogenesis of Intracerebral Hemorrhage, in Field WS (ed): Pathogenesis and Treatment of Cerebrovascular Disease. Springfield, Illinois, Charles C Thomas, 1961, pp 295–317.
15. Fisher CM: Clinical Syndromes in Cerebral Hemorrhage, in Fields WS (ed): Pathogenesis and Treatment of Cerebrovascular Disease. Springfield, Illinois, Charles C Thomas, 1961, pp 318–338.
16. Fisher CM, Mohr JP, Adams RD: Cerebrovascular Diseases, in Wintrobe MM, Thorn GW, Adams RD, Braunwald E, Isselbacher KJ, Petersdorf RG (ed): Harrison's Principles of Internal Medicine. New York, McGraw-Hill, 1974, pp 1743–1780.
17. Fisher CM, Picard EH, Polak A, Dalal P, Ojemann RG: Acute hypertensive cerebellar hemorrhage: diagnosis and surgical treatment. J Nerv Ment Dis 140:38–57, 1965.
18. Hayward RD, O'Reilly GVA: Computerized tomography and intracerebral hemorrhage. Am Heart J 93:126–127, 1977.
19. Heiman TD, Satya-Murti S: Benign cerebellar hemorrhages. Ann Neurol 3:366–368, 1978.
20. Herbstein DS, Schaumburg HH: Hypertensive intracerebral hematoma. An investigation of the initial hemorrhage and rebleeding using chromium Cr51-labeled erythrocytes. Arch Neurol 30:412–414, 1974.
21. Hier DB, Davis KR, Richardson EP Jr, Mohr JP: Hypertensive putaminal hemorrhage. Ann Neurol 1:152–159, 1977.
22. Kawakami H, Kutsuzawa T, Uemura K, Sakurai Y, Nakamura T: Regional cerebral blood flow in patients with hypertensive intracerebral hemorrhage. Stroke 5:207–212, 1974.
23. Lieberman A, Hass WK, Pinto R, Isom WO, Kupersmith M, Bear G, Chase R: Intracranial hemorrhage and infarction in antiocoagulated patients with prosthetic heart valves. Stroke 9:18–24, 1978.
24. Little JR, Blomquist GA Jr, Ethier R: Intraventricular hemorrhage in adults. Surg Neurol 8:143–149, 1977.

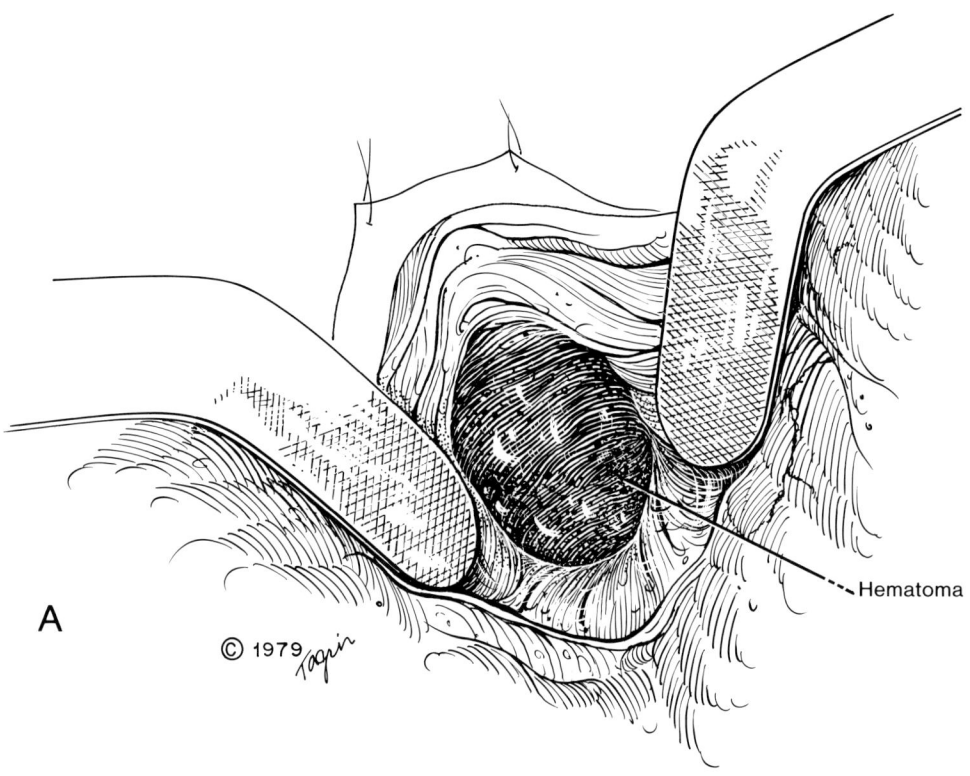

Figure 25.6 Surgical technique for removal of brain hemorrhage. *A,* exposure of the hematoma after the cortical incision has been made. Self-retaining brain retractors provide gentle steady exposure with minimum trauma. *B,* removal of hematoma. Careful suction and irrigation removes the clot with minimal injury to the cavity walls. It is not necessary to remove every last fragment of hematoma from the wall. *C,* hemostasis is achieved with bipolar coagulation and Surgicel. Abnormal tissue is biopsied (*arrow*). (From Mossy J, Reinmuth OM: *Cerebrovascular Disease.* New York, Raven Press, 1981, with permission.)

Brain Hemorrhage

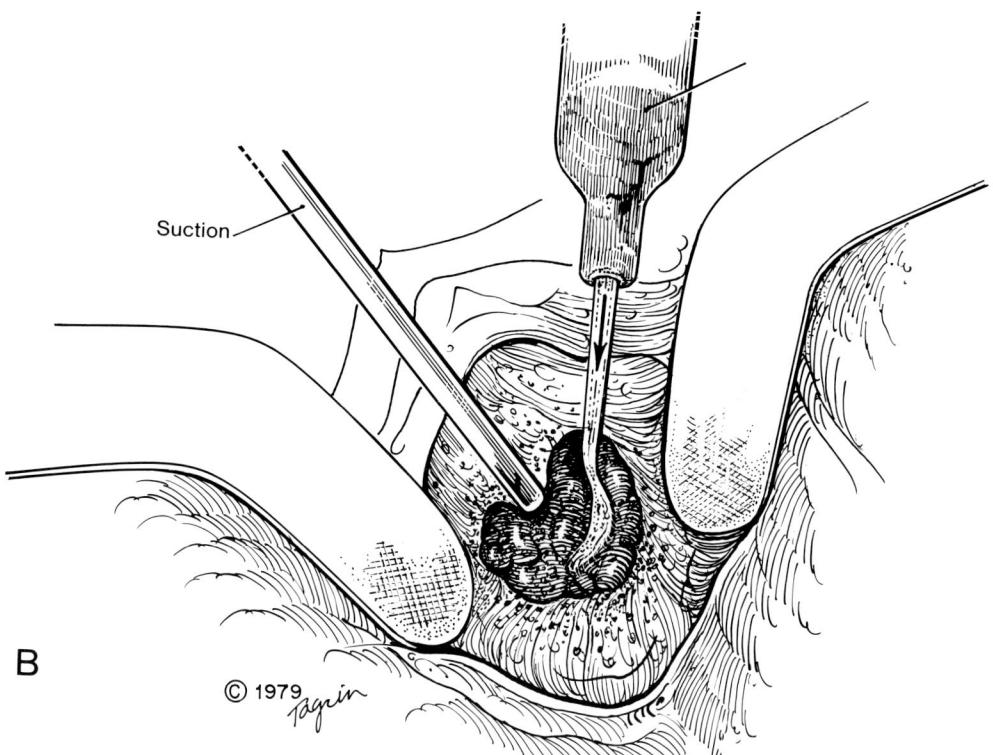

Figure 25.6 (*B*)

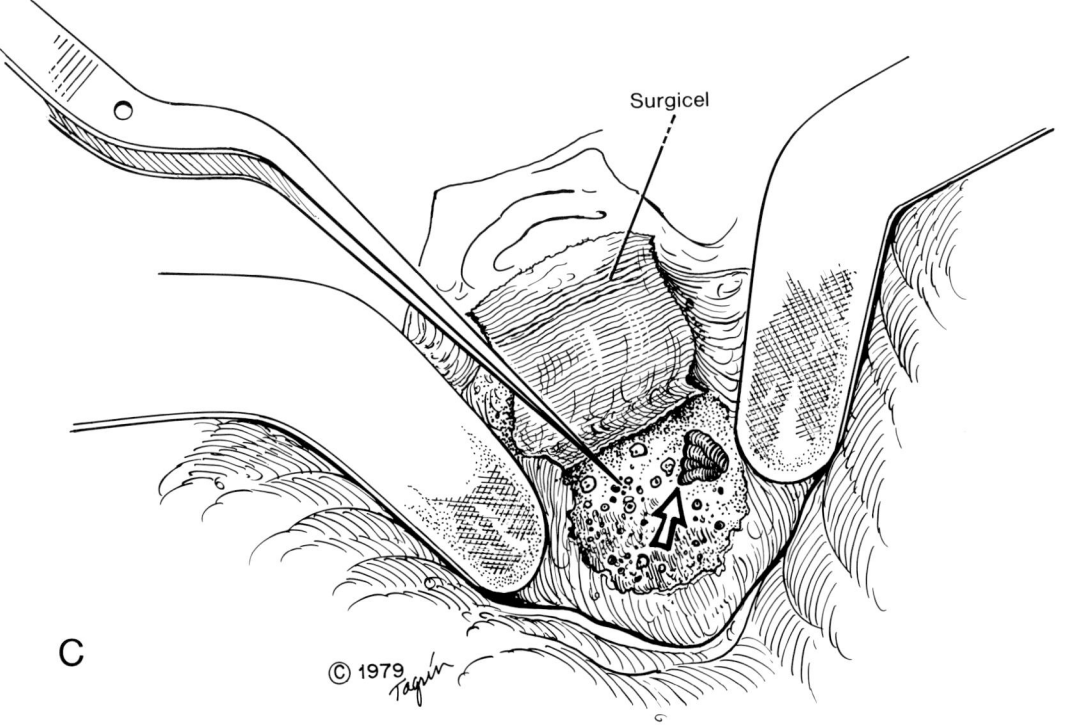

Figure 25.6 (*C*)

25. Little JR, Tubman DE, Ethier R: Cerebellar hemorrhage in adults. Diagnosis by computerized tomography. J Neurosurg 48:575-579, 1978.
26. Little JR, Dial B, Belanger G, Carpenter S: Brain hemorrhage from intracranial tumor. Stroke 10:283-288, 1979.
27. Luessenhop AJ, Shevlin WA, Ferrero AA, Ferrero AA, McCullough DC, Barone AM: Surgical management of primary intracerebral hemorrhage. J Neurosurg 27:419-427, 1967.
28. McCormick WF, Rosenfield DB: Massive brain hemorrhage: A review of 144 cases and an examination of their causes. Stroke 4:946-954, 1973.
29. McKissock W, Richardson A, Taylor J: Primary intracerebral hemorrhage: A controlled trial of surgical and conservative treatment in 180 unselected cases. Lancet 2:221-226, 1961.
30. Mandybur TI: Intracranial hemorrhage caused by metastatic tumors. Neurology 27:650-655, 1977.
31. Mandybur TI, Bates SRD: Fatal massive intracerebral hemorrhage complicating cerebral amyloid angiopathy. Arch Neurol 35:246-248, 1978.
32. Messina AV, Chernik NL. Computed tomography: The "resolving" intracerebral hemorrhage. Radiology 118:609-613, 1976.
33. Mizukami M, Araki G, Mihara H: Angiographic sign of good prognosis for hemiplegia in hypertensive intracerebral hemorrhage. Neurology 24:120-126, 1974.
34. Murphy MG: Successful evacuation of acute pontine hematoma. J Neurosurg 37:224-225, 1972.
35. New PFJ, Scott WR, Schnur JA, Davis KR, Taveras JM: Computerized axial tomography with the EMI scanner. Radiology 110:109-123, 1974.
36. Ojemann RG: Intracerebral and intracerebellar hemorrhage, in Youmans JR (ed): *Neurologica! Surgery*. Philadelphia, WB Saunders, 1973, vol 2, pp 844-851.
37. Ojemann RG, New PFJ: Spontaneous resolution of an intraventricular hematoma. J Neurosurg 20:899-902, 1963.
38. Ojemann RG, Mohr JP: Hypertensive brain hemorrhage. Clin Neurosurg 23:220-244, 1975.
39. Okazak H, Reagan TJ, Campbell RJ: Cliniopathologic studies of primary cerebral amyloid angiopathy. Mayo Clin Proc 54:22-31, 1979.
40. Ott KH, Kase CS, Ojemann RG, Mohr JP: Cerebellar hemorrhage: Diagnosis and treatment. A review of 56 cases. Arch Neurol 31:160-167, 1974.
41. Padt JP, DeReuck J, vander Eecken H: Intracerebral hemorrhage as initial symptom of a brain tumor. Acta Neurol Belg 73:241-251, 1973.
42. Paillas JE, Alliez B: Surgical treatment of spontaneous intracerebral hemorrhage. Immediate and long-term results in 250 cases. J Neurosurg 39:145-151, 1973.
43. Pia HW: The surgical treatment of intracerebral and intraventricular hematomas. Acta Neurochir 27:149-164, 1972.
44. Pia HW, Langmaid C, Zierski J (eds): *Spontaneous Intracerebral Hematomas*. New York, Springer-Verlag, 1980.
45. Ransohoff J, Derby B, Kricheff I: Spontaneous intracerebral hemorrhage. Clin Neurosurg 18:247-266, 1971.
46. Richardson A: Surgical Therapy of Spontaneous Intracerebral Haemorrhage, in Krayenbull H, Maspes PE, Sweet WH (eds): *Progress in Neurological Surgery*. Basel, Karger, 1969, vol 3, pp 397-418.
47. Richardson A: Spontaneous intracerebral and cerebellar hemorrhage, in Russell RW (ed): *Cerebral Arterial Disease*. New York, Churchill Livingstone, 1976, pp 210-230
48. Ropper AH, Davis KR: Lobar cerebral hemorrhages: Acute clinical syndromes in 26 cases. Ann Neurol 8:141-147, 1980.
49. Russell DS, Falconer MA, Beck DJK, McMenemey WH: The pathology of spontaneous intracranial hemorrhage. Proc R Soc Med 47:689-704, 1954.
50. Sano K, Ochiai C: Brain Stem Hematomas: Clinical Aspects with Reference to Indications for Treatment, in Pia HW, Langmaid C, Zierski J (eds): *Spontaneous Intracerebral Hematomas*. New York, Springer-Verlag, 1980, pp 366-371.
51. Sano K, Yoshida S: Cerebellar Hematomas, in Pia HW, Langmaid C, Zierski J (eds): *Spontaneous Intracerebral Hematomas*. New York, Springer-Verlag, 1980, pp 348-356.
52. Scott WR, New PFJ, Davis KR, Schnur JA: Computerized axial tomography of intracerebral and intraventricular hemorrhage. Radiology 112:73-80, 1974.
53. Seeler RA, Imana RB: Intracranial hemorrhage in patients with Hemophilia. J Neurosurg 39:181-185, 1973.
54. Suzuki J, Sato T: Grading and Timing of Operation in Putaminal ICH, in Pia HW, Langmaid C, Zierski J (eds): *Spontaneous Intracerebral Hematomas*. New York, Springer-Verlag, 1980, pp 274-279.
55. Suzuki J, Takaku A: Trans-Sylvian Approach to Putaminal Haematomas, in Pia HW, Langmaid C, Zierski J (eds): *Spontaneous Intracerebral Hematomas*. New York, Springer-Verlag, 1980, pp 384-386.
56. Tedeschi G, Bernini FP, Cerillo A: Indications for surgical treatment of intracerebral hemorrhage. J Neurosurg 43:590-595, 1975.
57. Tellez H, Bauer RB: Dexamethasone as treatment in cerebrovascular disease. 1. A controlled study in intracerebral hemorrhage. Stroke 4:541-546, 1973.
58. Tucker WS, Bilbao JM, Klodawsky H: Cerebral amyloid angiopathy and multiple intracerebral hematomas. Neurosurgery 7:611-614, 1980.
59. Vinters HV, Gilbert JJ: Amyloid angiopathy: Its incidence and Complications in the Aging Brain. Stroke 12:118, 1981.
60. Waga S, Okada M, Yamamoto Y: Reversibility of parinaud syndrome in thalamic hemorrhage. Neurology 29:407-409, 1979.
61. Walshe TM, Davis KD, Fisher CM: Thalamic hemorrhage: A computed tomographic-clinical correlation. Neurology 27:217-222, 1977.
62. Weisberg LA: Computerized tomography in intracranial hemorrhage. Arch Neurol 36: 422-426, 1979.
63. Wiggins WS, Moody DM, Toole JF, Laster DW, Ball MR: Clinical and computerized tomographic study of hypertensive intracerebral hemorrhage. Arch Neurol 35:832-833, 1978.
64. Woerner FJ, Abildgaard CF, French BN: Intracranial hemorrhage in children with idiopathic thrombocytopenia pupura. Pediatrics 67:453-460, 1981.
65. Yarnell P, Earnest MP: Primary non-traumatic intracranial hemorrhage. A municipal emergency hospital viewpoint. Stroke 7:608-610, 1976.
66. Yashon D, Kosnik EJ: Chronic intracerebral hematoma. Neurosurgery 2:103-106, 1978.
67. Yoshida M, Hayashi T, Kuramoto S, Hiyoshi Y, Yokoyama T: Traumatic intracranial hematomas in hemophiliac children. Surg Neurol 12:115-118, 1979.
68. Zimmerman HM: Cerebral apoplexy: mechanism and differential diagnosis. N Y St J Med 49:2153-2157, 1949.
69. Zimmerman RD, Leeds NE, Naidich TP: Ring blush associated with intracerebral hematoma. Radiology 122:707-711, 1977.
70. Zülch KJ: Pathological aspects of cerebral accidents in arterial hypertension. Acta Neurol Belg 71:196-221, 1971.

Index

Abscess, brain
  postoperative after treatment of middle cerebral aneurysm, 154
  with bacterial aneurysm, 260–262
Amaurosis fugax (*see* transient ischemic attacks, monocular blindness), 1
Anesthetic management
  aneurysm surgery, 141–143
  carotid endarterectomy, 30
Aneurysm
  and AVM, 129
  and carotid stenosis, 22, 23
  angiography, 136
  anterior communicating
    angiography, 143, 182, 190
    evaluation, 183
      angiography, 184, 185
      giant, 249, 251
    presentation, 183
    surgical treatment, 142
      initial exposure, 183
      microsurgical dissection, 189–191
      obliteration of the aneurysm, 191–194
      position, 183
      results, 194, 195
      timing, 181
  asymptomatic, 237–239
    management, 237
    natural history, 237
    surgical treatment
      indications, 237
      results, 237
  bacterial intracranial
    bacteriology, 255, 256
    clinical manifestations, 255, 256
    diagnostic studies, 256–258
      angiography, 256–258, 260, 261
      CT scan, 256, 260
    etiology
      cavernous sinus thrombophlebitis, 262
      endocarditis, 255
      meningitis, 262
    management, 258, 259, 262
    multiple, 259
    surgical treatment
      indications, 258–259
      results, 258–259
  basilar bifurcation
    evaluation, 210
      angiography, 210, 216, 217, 220, 221
    giant, 253, 254
    operative technique, 210–222
      anterior pointing lesion, 218, 219
      dural opening, 211
      incision and craniotomy, 210
      low-lying bifurcation, 220, 222
      microsurgical dissection, 211–214
      obliteration, 214–217
      posterior pointing lesion, 215, 218
      pterional approach, 219, 222
    presentation, 210
    surgical treatment
      complications, 222
      results, 222
  basilar trunk-anterior inferior cerebellar
    evaluation
      angiography, 224
      operative technique, 223, 225
    presentation, 223
    surgical treatment
      results, 226
  basilar trunk-anterior inferior cerebellar artery
    operative technique
      approach, 225
    presentation, 223
  basilar trunk-superior cerebellar
    operative technique, 223
    presentation, 223
    surgical treatment
      results, 223
  carotid-ophthalmic
    CT scan, 134
    giant, 244, 246, 247
    operative technique
      approach, 171–174
      clipping, 179–180
      clipping contralateral aneurysm, 180–181
      dissection of aneurysm, 178–179
      removal of clinoid process, 173–178
    presentation, 171
    surgical treatment
      carotid occlusion, 181
      postoperative complications, 181–182
      results, 181
    unruptured symptomatic, 237
  clinical presentation, 132–135
  clips, 149–150
  distal anterior cerebral
    evaluation, 196
      angiography, 200
    operative technique, 196–197
      initial exposure, 196
      microsurgical dissection, 196–197
      obliteration, 197
      preparation and positioning, 196
    presentation, 196
    surgical treatment
      results, 197
  etiology, 129
  false, after carotid endarterectomy, 59
  familial, 129
  fibromuscular dysplasia, association with, 107, 108
  fungal, 262
  giant
    anterior communicating, 249, 251
    basilar bifurcation, 253, 254
    clinical presentation, 240
    incidence, 240
    internal carotid, 246, 247, 249, 250
      surgical results, 246, 247
    intracavernous, 247, 248
    middle cerebral, 252
    pathology, 240
    surgical management, 240–244
      bypass graft, 240
      detachable balloon technique, 244, 245
      extracranial occlusion of carotid artery, 244
      intracranial arterial occlusion, 244
      intracranial operation, 240–241
  internal carotid
    evaluation, 157
      angiography, 158
    giant, 244, 246, 247, 249, 250
      treatment using bypass graft, 71
    operative technique
      at origin anterior choroidal artery, 166–167
      at origin of posterior communicating artery, 144, 145, 154, 162–165
      incision and scalp flap, 157–159
      initial exposure, 160–162
      microsurgical dissection, 162
      position, 157
    presentation, 157
    surgical treatment
      results, 166
    timing of operation, 157
    unruptured symptomatic, 237, 238
  internal carotid bifurcation
    operative technique
      at internal carotid bifurcation, 166–170
    surgical treatment, 169
      results, 168, 170
  intracavernous, 247, 248
  middle cerebral
    asymptomatic, 239
    evaluation, 201
    giant, 252
    operative technique
      subfrontal-sylvian fissure approach, 207, 208
      superior temporal gyrus approach
        initial exposure, 204, 205
        microsurgical dissection, 206, 207
    presentation, 201
    surgical approaches, 201–208
      complications, 208–209
      results, 208, 209
      subfrontal, 201, 207–208
      superior temporal gyrus, 201–207
  multiple, 129, 172, 173
    bacterial, 259
    evaluation, 233
      angiography, 233, 234–236
      CT scan, 233
    incidence, 233
    management, 233
    operative technique, 233–236
  operative technique
    bipolar coagulation, 151
    clips, 149, 150

Aneurysm—continued
  operative technique
    closure, 153
    cranial approaches, 146–148
    instrumentation, 145
    intraoperative rupture, 151–153
    ligature, 151, 152
    microsurgical dissection, 149
    obliteration of the aneurysm, 150–153
    operating room layout, 145, 146
    positioning, 145, 146, 147
    retraction, 147, 149
    tissue adhesive, 153
  pathology, 129
  pathophysiology, 129–132
  premonitory symptoms, 132
  prevalence, 128, 129
  surgical management, 141–156
    anesthesia
      controlled hypotension, 142–143
      induction, 142
      premedication, 141
      preparation, 141–142
      reduction of brain tension, 142
    occlusion of feeding artery, 155, 156
    postoperative complications, 153
      slipped clip, 154, 156, 231
      vasospasm, 153
    postoperative management, 153–156
  relation to age, 128
  relation to size, 128
  timing, 141, 143, 181
  unruptured symptomatic
    management, 237
    symptoms, 237
  vein of Galen, 281, 284, 285
    clinical syndromes, 281
    evaluation
      angiography, 281, 284
      CT scan, 281
    operative technique, 281, 285
  vertebral-posterior inferior cerebellar artery
    angiography, 155
    evaluation, 226
    operative technique, 226–231
    presentation, 226
    surgical treatment, 155
    results, 231–232
Angiography
  acute stroke, 25
  aneurysms, 136
    after use of tissue adhesive, 151, 153
    anterior communicating, 137, 143, 184, 185, 192, 193
      giant, 251
    basilar bifurcation, 210, 216, 217, 220, 221, 253
    basilar trunk-anterior inferior cerebellar artery, 224
    brain hemorrhage, 296
    carotid-ophthalmic, 172
    giant, 246
    distal anterior cerebral, 200
    internal carotid, 157
      unruptured symptomatic, 238
    internal carotid bifurcation, 168
    internal carotid, giant, 250
      treatment with balloon catheter, 245
    internal carotid-posterior communicating, 144, 145, 158

surgical treatment, 154
intracavernous, 247, 248, 249
intracranial aneurysm with carotid stenosis, 24
middle cerebral, 201, 202, 203
  asymptomatic, 239
  giant, 252
  multiple, 234–236
    identification of ruptured lesions, 233
  vertebral-posterior inferior cerebellar artery, 155
  postoperative studies, 153
  vein of Galen, 281, 284
arteriovenous malformation, brain, 265, 266
  callosal, 278, 279
  cerebellar, 280
  cingulate, 277
  convexity, angular gyrus, 270–271
  convexity, motor-sensory area, 272–273
  medial temporal, 274, 275
  on delayed study, 267, 268
  proton beam therapy results, 282, 283
arteriovenous malformation, dural, 287, 288
asymptomatic carotid bruit, 67
bacterial aneurysm, 256, 258, 260, 261
carotid atherosclerosis
  carotid "slim" sign, 3
  carotid stenosis, bilateral with TIAs, 18
  carotid stenosis with intracranial aneurysm, 24
  collateral circulation, 8
  common carotid artery, 25
  importance of delayed films, 8
  internal carotid occlusion, 16
    characteristics, 3, 7
  intracranial "pseudostenosis," 9
  measurement of degree of stenosis, 2
  need for multiple views with stenosis and ulceration, 4, 5
  occlusion, collateral circulation, 20
  occlusion, proximal stump, 21
  significance of degree of stenosis, 3
  stenosis and vertebral basilar TIAs, 22
  stenosis, bilateral with TIAs, 17
  stenosis, origin internal carotid artery types, 6
  stenosis, tandem lesions, 19
  stenosis with associated thrombus, 14
  stenosis with delayed flow, 13
  ulceration, 10, 15
carotid cavernous fistula
  postraumatic, 293
dissection, spontaneous, 112, 114, 115, 116, 117
fibromuscular dysplasia, 107, 108, 109
middle cerebral artery occlusion, 124
subarachnoid hemorrhage, 136, 137
vasospasm, 133, 136
vertebral
  importance with internal carotid aneurysm, 158
vertebrobasilar atherosclerosis
  basilar artery stenosis, 93
  subclavian steal, 96
  vertebral artery stenosis, 94
Angioplasty, transluminal
  dissection, spontaneous, 118

fibromuscular dysplasia, 109
subclavian and innominate artery stenosis, 100
vertebral artery stenosis, 99
Amyloid angiopathy, 297
  brain hemorrhage, 302
Anterior clinoid process
  removal in aneurysm surgery 166, 173–178
Anterior communicating aneurysm
  angiography, 137, 142, 184, 185
  evaluation, 183
  giant, 249, 251
  presentation, 183
  surgical treatment
    initial exposure, 183
    microsurgical dissection, 189–191
    obliteration of the aneurysm, 191–194
    results, 194, 195
Anticoagulation
  as cause of brain hemorrhage
    treatment, 302
  following carotid endarterectomy, 53
  use in internal carotid occlusion, 22
Antiplatelet therapy
  use in asymptomatic bruit, 67
Arteriovenous malformation, brain
  angiography, 265, 266
    callosal, 278, 279
    cerebellar, 280
    cingulate, 277
    convexity, angular gyrus, 270–271
    convexity, motor-sensory area, 272–273
    medial temporal, 274, 275
  aneurysm, association, 264
  clinical presentation, 264–265
  CT scan, 265, 266, 267
    medial temporal, 274
  embolization, 281
    complications, 281
    indications, 281
  evaluation, 265, 266
  incidence, 264
  pathology, 264
  proton beam therapy, 279, 281–283
    results, 279, 281–283
      angiography, 282, 283
    technique, 279
  recurrent hemorrhage, risk, 264
  surgical excision, 266–279
    operative technique, 269, 276
      basal ganglia, 276
      brainstem, 276
      callosal, 276
      cingulate, 276
      convexity lesion, 269
      intraventricular, 276
      lesion of falx and tentorium, 269
      medial temporal-occipital region, 276
      posterior fossa, 276
    results, 276, 279
    timing, 266, 269
    two-stage operation, 269
  thrombosed, 266
    CT scan, 266, 268
Arteriovenous malformation, dural
  angiography, 287, 288
  clinical presentation, 287
  embolization, 290
  etiology, 287

Index

evaluation, 287
pathology, 287
surgical technique, 289, 290
Artery
  ascending pharyngeal
    dissection in carotid endarterectomy, 35
  anterior cerebral
    exposure for anterior communicating aneurysm, 183–187
    occlusion, 168, 244
    variations, 183–188
  anterior choroidal
    internal carotid aneurysm, 164, 167
    occlusion, 166
  anterior inferior cerebellar
    aneurysm, 223, 225
  basilar
    bypass procedures for occlusive disease, 103
  callosal-marginal
    distal anterior cerebral aneurysm, 197
  common carotid
    dissection in carotid endarterectomy, 33
    in carotid-subclavian graft, 100
    stenosis and occlusion, carotid endarterectomy, 52
    stenosis and occlusion with TIAs, 23
  external carotid
    stenosis, 16, 21
    stenosis and asymptomatic bruit, 66
    stenosis, endarterectomy, 51, 52
  hypoglossal, 22
  innominate
    atherosclerosis, 95
    endarterectomy, 99, 100
    stenosis and asymptomatic bruit, 66
  internal carotid, extracranial
    carotid occlusive disease and intracranial aneurysm, 22, 23
    dissection, 111–121
    fibromuscular dysplasia, 107–110
    occlusion
      angiography, collateral circulation, 9
      associated with acute stroke, 25, 26
    occlusion, with TIAs, 16, 21, 22
    stenosis and ulceration
      angiography, 7
      significance, 3, 4
    stenosis and asymptomatic bruit, 66
      associated with acute stroke, 25, 26
      bilateral with TIAs, 16
      tandem with TIAs, 16
      TIAs with ipsilateral stenosis and contralateral occlusion, 16
      types, 6
      unilateral with TIAs, 13
      stump, as source of emboli, 52
    ulceration
      angiography, 10
      asymptomatic, 67
  lenticulostriate, 162
    in hypertensive brain hemorrhage, 297
    internal carotid aneurysm, 168
  middle cerebral
    embolic occlusion, 122–125
    use in bypass graft, 71–92
    with bacterial aneurysm, 256–258
  middle meningeal
    use in bypass graft, 90
  occipital
    anastomosis to MCA, 90
    in occipital-PICA bypass, 103
    use in bypass graft, 72
  perforating
    from anterior cerebral, 183–185
    from posterior cerebral, 213, 217
  pericallosal
    distal anterior cerebral aneurysm, 196, 197
  posterior cerebral
    in exposure of basilar bifurcation aneurysm, 211–232
    use in bypass procedure, 103
  posterior communicating
    and internal carotid aneurysm, 144–145
    in approach to basilar bifurcation aneurysm, 218–221
  posterior inferior cerebellar
    aneurysm, 226
    in occipital-PICA bypass, 103
  recurrent of Heubner
    anterior communicating aneurysm, 184
    internal carotid aneurysm, 162
    internal carotid bifurcation aneurysm, 168
  subclavian
    asymptomatic bruit, 66
    atherosclerosis, 95
    dissection in supraclavicular exposure, 95, 97, 98
    endarterectomy, 99, 100
    in carotid-subclavian graft, 100
  subclavian steal, 95
  superficial temporal
    use in bypass graft, 71–92
  superior cerebellar
    aneurysm, 223
    in exposure of basilar bifurcation aneurysm, 212–215
    use in bypass procedure, 103
  superior thyroid
    dissection in carotid endarterectomy, 35
  sterno-cleidomastoid
    dissection in carotid endarterectomy, 33
  trigeminal, 22
  vertebral
    atherosclerotic occlusive disease, 93–105
    dissection in supraclavicular exposure, 95, 97, 98
    removal of foreign bodies, 103, 105
    spontaneous, dissection, 118, 119
Asymptomatic carotid bruit (see bruit, asymptomatic carotid), 66–70
Asymptomatic carotid stenosis
  treatment, 66–70
Asymptomatic internal carotid
  ulcer, 67
Atherosclerosis
  with intracranial aneurysms, 240, 241

Bacterial intracranial aneurysms
  clinical manifestations, 255, 256
  bacteriology, 255, 256
  diagnostic studies, 256–258
  angiography, 256–258, 260, 261
  CT scan, 256, 260
  etiology
    cavernous sinus thrombophlebitis, 262
    endocarditis, 255
    meningitis, 262
  multiple
    angiography, 259
    management, 259
  surgical treatment
    indications, 258–259
    results, 258–259
Balloon catheter occlusion
  carotid-cavernous fistula, 292–294, 296
  carotid-ophthalmic aneurysm, 181, 182
  giant aneurysm, 244
Basilar bifurcation aneurysm
  evaluation, 210
    angiography, 210, 216, 217, 220, 221
  giant, 253, 254
  operative technique, 210–222
    anterior pointing lesion, 218, 219
    dural opening, 211
    incision and craniotomy, 210
    low-lying bifurcation, 220, 222
    microsurgical dissection, 211–214
    obliteration, 214–217
    posterior pointing lesions, 215, 218
    pterional approach, 219, 222
  presentation, 210
  surgical treatment
    complications, 222
    results, 222
Basilar trunk-anterior inferior cerebellar artery aneurysm
  evaluation
    angiography, 224
  operative technique
    approach, 225
  presentation, 223
  surgical treatment
    results, 226
Basilar trunk-inferior cerebellar artery aneurysm
  operative technique, 223, 225
Basilar trunk-superior cerebellar aneurysm
  operative technique, 223
  presentation, 223
  surgical treatment
    results, 223
Bipolar coagulation
  use in aneurysm surgery, 150, 179
Blood flow measurement
  electromagnetic flow meter
    in vertebral artery transposition, 100
Brain abscess
  after aneurysm surgery, 154
  with bacterial aneurysm, 260–262
Brain hemorrhage, 297–308
  amyloid angiopathy, 302
  aneurysm, 129, 130, 132, 201, 203
  arteriovenous malformation, 264
  cerebellar
    clinical syndrome, 300–301
    CT scan, 301
    indications for medical and surgical treatment, 300–301
    natural history, 300–301
    surgical treatment, 305
  coagulation disorders, 302
    anticoagulation therapy treatment, 302

Brain hemorrhage—continued
　coagulation disorders—continued
　　thrombocytompenia, 302
　CT scan, 298
　　aneurysm, 201, 203
　　arteriovenous malformation, 265, 266, 267, 270
　diagnostic studies
　　angiography, 298
　　coagulation, 298
　　CT scan, 298
　etiology, 297
　hypertensive
　　location, 297
　　natural history, 297
　　pathology, 297
　intraventricular
　　CT scan, 301-302
　　etiology, 301-302
　lobar
　　clinical syndromes, 300
　　CT scan, 300
　　etiology, 300
　　treatment, 300
　medical treatment, 302-303
　non-hypertensive causes, 297
　pathology, 297
　pontine
　　natural history, 301
　　surgical treatment, 301
　putaminal
　　clinical syndrome, 298
　　CT scan, 298, 299
　　indications for surgery, 298, 299
　　natural history, 298
　　surgical treatment, 303-305
　surgical treatment, 303-307
　　incisions, 304
　　indications, 303
　　operative technique, 303-307
　　postoperative care, 305
　　preoperative preparations, 303
　thalamic
　　clinical syndrome, 298-300
　　CT scan, 300
　　indications for surgery, 299-300
　　natural history, 299-300
Brain tumor
　and brain hemorrhage, 297
Bruit
　a symptomatic, 66-70
　　results of surgical treatment, 13
　carotid cavernous fistula
　　spontaneous, 294-295
　carotid stenosis
　　characteristics, 1
　evaluation
　　phonoangiography, 12
　fibromuscular dysplasia, 107
　with carotid cavernous fistula, 291
　with dural arteriovenous malformation, 287
Bruit, asymptomatic carotid
　angiography, 67
　characteristics, 67
　characteristics of atheromatous plaque causing, 66
　clinical evaluation, 67
　etiology, 66
　indications for treatment, 67
　natural history, 66, 67
　non-invasive tests, 66, 67

risk of stroke, 67
risk of stroke during major surgery, 69, 70
treatment
　carotid endarterectomy, 67
　risks, 69
　indications, 69
　medical therapy, 67
Bypass procedures
　carotid-subclavian, 100
　external carotid to posterior cerebral with vein graft, 103
　for basilar artery occlusive disease, 103
　for fibromuscular dysplasia, 109
　meningeal-MCA, 90
　occipital artery-MCA, 90
　occipital-PICA
　　operative technique, 103, 104
　　results, 103
　omental graft, 90
　STA to superior cerebellar, 103
　superficial temporal artery-middle cerebral artery (see STA-MCA bypass), 71-92

Carotid cavernous fistula
　etiology, 291
　posttraumatic, 291
　　angiography, 291, 293
　　bilateral, 291
　　clinical presentation, 291
　　treatment, 291-294
　　　balloon catheter, 292-294
　　　　complications, 292
　　　preservation of carotid circulation, 292-294
　　　results, 292
　　　indications for surgery and embolization, 291, 292
　spontaneous
　　angiography, 295-296
　　clinical presentation, 295-296
　　etiology, 295
　　natural history, 295
　　treatment, 295-296
Carotid endarterectomy
　abnormal anatomy
　　internal carotid artery loop, 50
　anesthetic management, 30
　brain protection, 30
　contraindications for surgery, 29
　indications
　　acute stroke, 23, 25, 26
　　carotid stenosis with intracranial aneurysm, 22, 23
　　common carotid stenosis or occlusion, 23
　　established stroke, 23
　　external carotid stenosis, 16, 21
　　fibromuscular dysplasia, 109
　　internal carotid occlusion, 16, 21, 22
　　TIAs with bilateral carotid stenosis, 16
　　TIAs with ipsilateral internal carotid stenosis and contralateral internal carotid occlusion, 16
　　TIAs with tandem stenosis, 16
　　TIAs with unilateral carotid stenosis, 13, 14, 16
　　TIAs with unilateral carotid ulceration, 13, 15, 16
　　TIAs with unilateral stenosis, 22

asymptomatic bruit, 67
asymptomatic carotid ulcer, 67
intraoperative hypertension, 30
medical risk factors, 29
　cardiopulmonary, 29
monitoring, 30
　electroencephlogram, 31
　pulmonary artery catheter, 29
operating room setup, 32
operative technique, 31
　abnormal arterial anatomy, 48, 50
　arteriotomy, 35, 38
　arteriotomy, closure, 40, 42
　arteriotomy, management of bleeding from suture line, 40
　carotid sinus, blocking of, 33, 35
　common carotid artery stenosis and occlusion, 52, 53, 55
　dissection of ascending pharngeal artery, 35
　dissection of common carotid artery, 33, 34
　dissection of descendans hypoglossi nerve, 35
　dissection of hypoglossal nerve, 33
　dissection of internal carotid artery, 35
　dissection of internal jugular vein, 34, 35
　dissection of plaque, 37, 38, 39, 40, 41
　dissection of sternocleidomastoid muscle, 33
　dissection of superior thyroid artery, 35
　dissection of vagus nerve, 33, 35
　exposure, stenosis
　　C2 level, 46, 48
　external carotid stenosis, 51, 52
　incision, 32
　internal carotid artery
　　occlusion, 48, 51, 53
　　stump, 52, 54, 55
　intimal flap, management of
　　in external carotid artery, 43
　　in internal carotid artery, 40, 41
　patch graft, 44, 46, 47
　shunt, 31, 43, 45
　use of heparin, 35
　use of hypertension, 35
　vascular clamps and clips, 35, 37
pathology of carotid endarterectomy specimen, 59-61
　hemorrhage into plaque, 60
　mural thrombus, 60
postoperative complications
　angiography, 56
　cardiopulmonary, 29, 59
　cerebral emboli, 58
　cerebral ischemia, 56
　cranial nerve injury
　　facial nerve (mandibular branch), 57
　　hypoglossal nerve, 59
　　superior laryngeal nerve, 57
　　vagus nerve, 57
　false aneurysm, 59
　headache, 56
　intracerebral hemorrhage, 56, 59
　seizures, 56
　wound hematoma, 59
　wound infection, 59
postoperative management

Index

angiography, 53, 56, 57
anticoagulation, 43
medical therapy, 53
treatment of hypertension, 53, 69
treatment of hypotension, 53
preoperative evaluation, 29
cardiac function, 29
recurrent stenosis, 56
angiographic appearance, 62, 63
incidence and pathology, 60
technical points, 60, 63
results
assymptomatic carotid stenosis, 14
stroke, acute, 26
stroke, established, 14, 23
TIAs with carotid stenosis, 14
unilateral stenosis and contralateral occlusion, 16
with myocardial revascularization, 29
Carotid ligation
detachable balloon method, 244
internal vs. common, 241
pressure recording, 241, 243
risk of ischemia, 241
technique, 241-244
Carotid-ophthalmic aneurysm
evaluation, 171
operative technique
approach, 171-174
clipping, 179-180
clipping contralateral aneurysm, 180-181
dissection of aneurysm, 178-179
removal of anterior clinoid process, 173-178
presentation, 171
surgical treatment
carotid occlusion, 181
craniotomy, 171-181
postoperative complications, 181-182
results, 181
unruptured symptomatic, 237
Carotid-subclavian artery graft
operative technique, 102
Catheter, balloon
treatment of aneurysms, 181, 182, 244
treatment of carotid cavernous fistula, 291-294
Central venous pressure
management of postoperative hypotension, 63
Cerebellar hemorrhage
clinical syndrome, 300-301
CT scan, 301
indications for medical and surgical treatment, 301-302
natural history, 300-301
surgical treatment, 305
Cerebellar infarction, 126-127
clinical presentation, 126-127
CT scan, 126, 127
diagnosis, 126-127
etiology, 126
surgical treatment, 126
treatment, 127
Cerebral blood flow
STA-MCA bypass, preoperative evaluation, 71
Coagulation disorders
anticoagulant therapy, 302
brain hemorrhage, 297
hemophilia, 302

Thrombocytopenia, 302
Coumadin
use in spontaneous dissection, 115
Crutchfield clamp, 241-242
CT scan
aneurysm
anterior communicating, giant, 251
giant internal carotid-ophthalmic, 134
middle cerebral, 201, 203
multiple
identification of ruptured lesion, 233
mural thrombus, 134, 210, 250, 251, 253
postoperative brain abscess, 154
arteriovenous malformation, brain, 265-267
medial temporal, 274
thrombosed, 266, 268
arteriovenous malformation, dural, 287
bacterial aneurysm, 256, 260
brain hemorrhage, 297-298
carotid occlusive disease, 10
cerebellar hemorrhage, 301
cerebellar infarction, 127
cerebral infarction
appearance, 11, 12
after surgical treatment of aneurysm, 169
middle cerebral artery occlusion, 124
vasospasm, 134
intraventricular hemorrhage, 301-302
lobar hemorrhage, 300
putaminal hemorrhage, 299
subarachnoid hemorrhage, 135, 184
infarction, 133, 137
vasospasm, 128
thalamic hemorrhage, 300

Dissection, spontaneous
internal carotid artery
angiography
characteristics, 111
pouch, 114, 115, 116
string sign, 112, 114, 117
asymptomatic bruit, 66
clinical manifestations, 111-113
embolism, 111
natural history, 113
pathogenesis, 111
relationship to fibromuscular dysplasia, 111
treatment, 115, 118
indications for surgery, 115
intracranial arteries
angiography, 118
clinical manifestations, 118
pathogenesis, 118
treatment, 118
Dissection, traumatic
internal carotid artery
clinical manifestations, 119, 120
diagnosis, 119, 120
pathogenesis, 118, 119
treatment, 119, 120
Distal anterior cerebral aneurysm, 196, 197
angiography, 200
evaluation, 196, 197
operative technique, 196, 197, 199
initial exposure, 196
microsurgical dissection, 196-197
obliteration of the aneurysm, 197

preparation and positioning, 196
presentation, 196, 197
surgical treatment
results, 197
Digital subtraction angiography
aneurysms, 136, 237
carotid occlusive disease, 7, 10, 11
Doppler imaging, 12, 13
Dural arteriovenous malformations, 287-290
Electrocardiogram after SAH, 131
Electroencephalogram
in carotid endarterectomy, 31
postoperative evaluation, 56
in carotid-subclavian artery graft, 100
in vertebral artery transposition, 100
Endarterectomy, carotid (see carotid endarterectomy), 29-65
anesthetic management, 29-30
brain protection, 30-31
monitoring, 30-31
operative technique, 31-43
common carotid artery stenosis and occlusion, 52-53
complete internal carotid artery occlusion, 48, 51
external carotid stenosis, 51-52
stenosis and ulceration, internal carotid artery, 31-43
patch, insertion of, 44-46
pathology, 59-61
postoperative complications, 56-59
postoperative management, 53, 56
preoperative management, 29
recurrent stenosis, 60-64
shunt, use of, 43-45
Embolectomy
middle cerebral artery, 123-125
indications for operation, 125
operative technique, 123, 125
results, 125
Embolism, 122-125
as cause of cerebellar infarction, 126
carotid artery, 123
diagnosis, 123
treatment, 123
clinical manifestations, 122
diagnosis, 122, 123
etiology, 122
in association with carotid occlusion, 16
middle cerebral artery, 123-125
Embolization
dural AVM, 290
intracranial AVM, 281
Endarterectomy, carotid, 26-65
Endarterectomy, subclavian and innominate, 99-100
Endarterectomy, vertebral, 98-99
Endocarditis
incidence of neurological problems, 255
Epsilon amino caproic acid in SAH, 136

Fibromuscular dysplasia
age and sex distribution, 108
angiography, 107, 108, 109
asymptomatic bruit, 66
clinical presentation, 107
natural history, 107
pathogenesis, 107
treatment
operative technique, 108
results, 108, 109

Foreign body
  removal from vertebral artery, 103, 105
Fungal intracranial aneurysms, 262

Giant aneurysm
  anterior communicating, 249, 251
  basilar bifurcation, 253, 254
  incidence, 240
  internal carotid, 249, 250
    surgical results, 246, 247
  intracavernous, 247, 248
  middle cerebral, 252
  pathology, 240
  surgical management, 240–244
    detachable balloon technique, 244, 245
    extracranial occlusion of carotid artery
      technique, 241
    intracranial arterial occlusion, 244
    intracranial operation, 240, 241

Headache
  aneurysm
    vertebral-posterior inferior cerebellar artery, 226
    unruptured, 237
  dissection, intracranial, 118
  dissection, spontaneous, 111, 112
  following carotid endarterectomy, 56
  with arteriovenous malformation, brain, 265
  with cerebellar hemorrhage, 300
  with lobar hemorrhage, 300
  with putaminal hemorrhage, 298
  with subarachnoid hemorrhage, 132–135
  with thalamic hemorrhage, 299
Hemophilia
  as cause of brain hemorrhage, 302
Hemorrhage, brain, 297–308
  amyloid angiopathy, 302
  arteriovenous malformation, 265, 266, 267, 270
  cerebellar
    clinical syndrome, 300–301
    CT scan, 301
    indications for medical and surgical treatment, 300–301
    natural history, 300–301
    surgical treatment, 305
  coagulation disorders, 302
    anticoagulation therapy treatment, 302
    thrombocytopenia, 302
  diagnostic studies
    angiography, 298
    coagulation, 298
    CT scan, 298
  etiology
    aneurysm, 129, 130, 132
  hypertensive
    location, 297
    natural history, 297
    pathology, 297
  intraventricular
    CT scan, 301–302
    etiology, 301–302
  lobar
    clinical syndromes, 300
    CT scan, 300
    etiology, 300
    management, 300
    surgical treatment, 303–305

  medical treatment, 302–303
  non-hypertensive
    causes, 297
    pathology, 297
  pontine
    clinical syndrome, 301
    natural history, 301
    surgical treatment, 301
  putaminal
    clinical syndrome, 298
    CT scan, 298, 299
    indications for surgical treatment, 298, 299
    natural history, 298
  surgical treatment, 303–307
    incisions, 304
    indications, 303
    operative technique, 303–307
    postoperative care, 305
    preoperative preparations, 303
  thalamic
    clinical syndrome, 298–300
    CT scan, 300
    indications for surgery, 299–300
    natural history, 299–300
Heparin
  use following embolism, 123
  use in carotid endarterectomy, 35, 40, 53
  use in spontaneous dissection, 115
  use in STA-MCA bypass, 72
  use in traumatic dissection, 120
  use prior to STA-MCA bypass, 72
Hydrocephalus
  after subarachnoid hemorrhage, 129, 133
  in thalamic hemorrhage, 300
  with cerebellar infarction, 127
Hypertension
  brain hemorrhage
    pathology, 297
  in carotid endarterectomy, 30
  treatment following carotid endarterectomy, 53
  treatment in brain hemorrhage, 303
Hypotension
  for aneurysm surgery, 142–143
    anterior communicating, 190
    middle cerebral, 206
  giant, 241
  treatment following carotid endarterectomy, 53
  treatment for SAH, 136, 138
Hypothalamus
  disturbance with SAH, 131, 183

Infarction
  associated with brain hemorrhage, 297
  cerebellar, 126–127
    clinical presentation, 126–127
    CT scan, 126, 127
    diagnosis, 126–127
    etiology, 126
    treatment, 127
  cerebral, 89, 126
    surgical treatment, 126
    treatment with craniectomy, 26
    vasospasm-CT scan, 133
    with vasospasm, 131
  CT scan appearance, 10
  emboli
    bacterial from endocarditis, 255
    pathology, 126
  vertebrobasilar, 93

Innominate artery endarterectomy, 99, 100
Internal carotid aneurysm
  evaluation, 157
    angiography, 158
  giant, 249, 250
    surgical management, 244, 246, 247
  operative technique
    at internal carotid bifurcation, 166–170
    at origin anterior choroidal artery, 166, 167
    at origin posterior communicating artery, 162–165
    incision and scalp flap, 157–159
    initial exposure, 160–162
    microsurgical dissection, 162
    position, 157
  presentation, 157
  surgical treatment
    planning, 157
    results, 166
  timing of operation, 157
  unruptured, symptomatic, 237, 238
Internal carotid bifurcation aneurysm
  surgical treatment, 169
  results, 168, 170
Intracavernous aneurysm, 247, 248
Intracerebral hemorrhage
  see brain, hemorrhage, 297–308
  after carotid endarterectomy, 56, 59
Intraventricular hemorrhage
  etiology, 301–302
  with aneurysms
    middle cerebral, 201, 203, 204
Intracranial pressure
  control in aneurysm surgery, 142
  management after brain hemorrhage
    monitoring, 303
    treatment, 303
  management after subarachnoid hemorrhage, 129, 138
Intraventricular hemorrhage
  CT scan, 301–302

Lacunar stroke, 10
Lobar hemorrhage
  clinical syndrome, 300
  CT scan, 300
  etiology, 300
  surgical treatment, 303–305
  treatment, 300
Lumbar puncture
  in subarachnoid hemorrhage, 136

Microscope
  use in aneurysm surgery, 145, 162
  use in STA-MCA bypass, 72
Middle cerebral aneurysm
  asymptomatic, 239
  evaluation, 201
  operative technique
    subfrontal-sylvian fissure approach, 207, 208
    superior temporal gyrus approach
      initial exposure, 204, 205
      microsurgical dissection, 206, 207
      position, 204
  presentation, 201
  surgical approaches, 201–208
  results, 208, 209
Middle cerebral artery stenosis

Stroke—continued
  in association with carotid stenosis, 53, 56
Monitoring
  in aneurysm surgery, 141–143
  in carotid endarterectomy, 30
Nerve
  descendens hypoglossi
    dissection in carotid endarterectomy, 33
  facial nerve (mandibular branch)
    dissection in carotid endarterectomy, 31
    injury in carotid endarterectomy, 57, 143–156
  fourth cranial
    in exposure of basilar bifurcation aneurysm, 211–212
  great auricular
    dissection in carotid endarterectomy, 31
  hypoglossal
    dissection in carotid endarterectomy, 33
    injury in carotid endarterectomy, 59
  phrenic
    dissection in supraclavicular exposure, 95, 97
    dissection in vertebral artery transposition, 100
  recurrent laryngeal
    dissection in carotid endarterectomy, 31
  sixth cranial
    basilar trunk-anterior inferior cerebellar artery aneurysm, 223
    vertebral-posterior inferior cerebellar artery aneurysm, 222
  superior laryngeal
    dissection in carotid endarterectomy, 33
    injury in carotid endarterectomy, 59
  third cranial
    basilar trunk-superior cerebellar aneurysm, 223
    exposure of basilar bifurcation aneurysm, 211–222
    with basilar bifurcation aneurysm, 210
    with internal carotid aneurysm, 157
  vagus
    dissection in carotid endarterectomy, 33
    injury in carotid endarterectomy, 57
Nitroglycerine
  in carotid endarterectomy, 30
Non-invasive carotid studies, 7–9
  use in asymptomatic carotid bruit, 68, 69

Oculoplethysmography, 12
Operating room layout
  carotid endarterectomy, 32
  aneurysm surgery, 144–146
Operative procedures
  bypass for basilar artery occlusive disease, 103
  carotid endarterectomy
    anesthetic management, 29, 30
    brain protection, 30, 31
    monitoring, 30, 31
    operative technique, 31–53
    postoperative complications, 56–59
    postoperative management, 53–56
    preoperative evaluation, 29
  carotid-subclavian artery graft, 100
  carotid-subclavian graft, 102
  cervical exposure of subclavian and vertebral arteries, 95, 97, 98
  craniectomy for cerebral infarction, 126
  embolectomy, middle cerebral artery, 123–125
  for aneurysms, 143–156
    anterior communicating, 183–195
    asymptomatic, 237
    basilar bifurcation, 210–222
    basilar trunk-anterior inferior cerebellar artery, 223, 225
    basilar trunk-superior cerebellar artery, 223
    carotid-ophthalmic, 170–182
    distal anterior cerebral, 196, 197
    general aspects, 143–156
    internal carotid, 157–169
    middle cerebral, 204–208
    multiple, 233–236
    unruptured symptomatic, 237
    vein of Galen, 281, 285
    vertebral-posterior inferior cerebellar artery, 226–231
  for arteriovenous malformation, dural, 289–290
  for carotid cavernous fistula, 291–295
  for cerebellar infarction, 127
  for dissection, 112, 117, 118
  for fibromuscular dysplasia, 108
  middle cerebral artery embolectomy
  occipital artery-middle cerebral artery anastomosis, 90
  occipital-PICA bypass, 103, 104
  STA-MCA bypass
    anesthesia, 72
    indications, 71
    operative technique, 72
    postoperative complications, 85
    postoperative management, 85
    preoperative evaluation, 71
  subclavian and innominate endarterectomy, 99, 100
  subclavian endarterectomy, 95
  vertebral artery endarterectomy, 98, 99
  vertebral artery transposition, 95, 100, 101
Ophthalmodynamometry, 12

Pathology
  aneurysms and SAH, 129–130
  carotid endarterectomy specimens, 60
Phenylephrine hydrochloride
  in carotid endarterectomy, 30
Phonoangiography, 12
  asymptomatic bruit, 68
  in postoperative evaluation, carotid endarterectomy, 56
Pontine hemorrhage
  clinical syndrome, 301
  natural history, 301
  surgical treatment, 301
Propranolol
  use in aneurysm surgery, 141–142
Putaminal hemorrhage
  clinical syndrome, 298
  CT scan, 298, 299
  indications for surgical treatment, 298, 299
  natural history, 298
  surgical treatment, 303–305
Seizure
  following carotid endarterectomy, 56
  with arteriovenous malformation, brain, 264
    and surgical treatment, 270–271
  with subarachnoid hemorrhage, 131, 132
  with unruptured aneurysm, 237, 238
STA-MCA bypass
  alternative procedures
    long-graft from cervical arteries to MCA, 90
    occipital-MCA anastomosis, 90
  anesthesia, 72
  for treatment of giant aneurysm, 241
  indications
    amaurosis fugax, 72
    carotid atherosclerosis, inaccessible stenosis, 16
    dementia, 71
    dissection, spontaneous, 118
    giant aneurysm, 71, 240
    stroke, acute, 72
    moyamoya syndrome, 71
    stroke, established, 71
    transient ischemic attacks, 71
    vertebral artery stenosis, 94
  operative technique
    anastomosis, 84, 85
    closure, 85, 86
    instruments, 72
    middle cerebral artery, exposure, 81
    middle cerebral artery, preparation, 81, 82, 83
    positioning, 72
    scalp incision, 72, 73, 74
    selection of arteries, 72
    STA preparation, 73, 75, 76, 77, 78
    catheter for irrigation and pressure measurement, 79
    tip, 80
  use of vein graft, 72
  postoperative complications, 85, 87
    delayed stroke, 87
    internal carotid occlusion, 88
    intraoperative thrombosis, 87
  postoperative management, 85, 87
    angiography, 88
  preoperative evaluation, 71, 72
    angiography, 72
    use of antiplatelet therapy, 72
  results, 71, 87, 88
    angiogram, 87
Stenosis, asymptomatic carotid
  pathology of endarterectomy specimens, 60
Stroke
  acute
    angiography, 3
    carotid occlusive disease, 25, 26
      correlation of surgical findings and outcome, 26
      evaluation, 25
      indications for surgical treatment, 23, 25, 26
      progressive or fluctuating deficit, 25, 26
    diagnostic studies, 2
    dissection, spontaneous, 115
    fibromuscular dysplasia, 107
    use of STA-MCA bypass, 71
  established
    carotid occlusive disease

Stroke—continued
  established—continued
    indications for surgical treatment, 23
    results of surgical treatment, 13
  diagnostic studies, 2
    CT scan, 10, 11, 12
    evaluation, 23
    progressive deficit due to chronic ischemia, 23
  following carotid endarterectomy, 56
  lacunar, 10
  relationship to TIAs, 2
Subarachnoid hemorrhage
  angiography, 136
    normal initial study, 138
  arteriovenous malformation, 64
  cardiac abnormalities, 131, 132
  classification, 133, 134
  complications, 132
  CT scan, 135
  dissection, spontaneous, 118
  etiology, 129
    bacterial aneurysm, 255
    giant aneurysms, 240
  hydrocephalus, 133
  hypothalamic disturbance, 131
  incidence, 128-129
  lumbar puncture, 136
  medical evaluation, 135-136
  medical management, 135, 138
    prevention of recurrent hemorrhage, 136, 138
  multiple aneurysms, 233
  neurological complications, 131
  pathophysiology, 129-132
  pregnancy, 129
  recurrent hemorrhage, 134-135
  risk in asymptomatic aneurysm, 237
  vasospasm, 128, 144, 145
    treatment, 138
Subclavian endarterectomy, 99, 100
Subclavian steal, 95
  angiography, 95, 96
  etiology, 95
  symptoms, 95
  treatment, 95

Thalamic hemorrhage
  clinical syndrome, 298-300
  CT scan, 300
  indications for surgery, 299-300
  natural history, 299-300
Thoracic duct
  dissection in supraclavicular exposure, 98

dissection in vertebral artery transposition, 100
Transient ischemic attacks
  angiography, 5, 6, 7
    clinical correlation, 8, 10
  anticoagulation therapy, 67
  antiplatelet therapy, 67
  clinical correlation, 3
  diagnostic studies
    angiography, 3
    angiography, digital subtraction, 7
    guidelines, 2
    non-invasive studies, carotid circulation, 12
  differential diagnosis, 2
  etiology
    carotid atherosclerosis, 1
    common carotid stenosis, 25
    dissection, spontaneous, 111
    fibromuscular dysplasia, 107
    intracranial aneurysm, 24, 233, 237
    internal carotid occlusion, 16
  following carotid endarterectomy, 56
  hemispheral, 2
    characteristics, 1
  indications for surgical treatment, 13-23
    bilateral internal carotid stenosis, 16
    carotid stenosis with intracranial aneurysm, 22, 23
    carotid stenosis with posterior circulation TIAs, 22
    common carotid stenosis or occlusion, 23
    external carotid stenosis, 16, 21
    ipsilateral carotid stenosis and contralateral carotid occlusion, 16
    ipsilateral internal carotid occlusion, 16, 21, 22
    tandem stenosis, 16
    unilateral internal carotid artery stenosis, 13, 14, 16
    unilateral internal carotid artery ulceration, 13, 15, 16
  monocular blindness, 2
    characteristics, 1
  pathophysiology, 1
  results of surgical treatment, 13, 16
  vertebrobasilar, 93
    characteristics, 22
Transluminal angioplasty
  dissection, spontaneous, 118
  fibromuscular dysplasia, 109
  subclavian and innominate artery stenosis, 100
  vertebral artery stenosis, 99

Ulcer
  internal carotid
    angiography, 10
    asymptomatic bruit, 67
    treatment, indications, 9

Vasospasm, 128, 131, 133
  angiography, 136
  classification, 136
  clinical manifestations, 134-135
  CT scan, 135
  etiology, 131
  postoperative, 154
  subarachnoid hemorrhage, 144, 145
  treatment, 138
Vein
  internal jugular
    dissection in carotid endarterectomy, 33
Vein graft
  common carotid artery to middle cerebral artery, 90, 91
  extracranial-intracranial graft, 90
Vein of Galen aneurysm, 281, 284, 285
  clinical syndromes, 281
  evaluation
    angiography, 281, 284
    CT scan, 281
  operative technique, 281, 285
Vertebral artery endarterectomy
  intradural, 99
  operative technique, 98, 99
  results, 98
Vertebral artery transposition, 100
  operative technique, 101
Vertebral-posterior inferior cerebellar artery aneurysm
  angiography, 155, 226
  operative technique, 226-231
  presentation, 226
  surgical treatment
    results, 231-232
Vertebrobasilar ischemia, 93-95
  etiology, 93
  subclavian steal, 95
  symptoms, 93
  treatment, 93
  with neck motion and manipulation
    angiography, 95
    etiology, 95
    treatment, 95
Visual impairment
  carotid cavernous fistula, 291
  carotid ophthalmic aneurysm 171, 182